METAL IONS IN
BIOLOGICAL SYSTEMS

METAL IONS IN BIOLOGICAL SYSTEMS

Edited by

Astrid Sigel
and Helmut Sigel

Institute of Inorganic Chemistry
University of Basel
CH-4056 Basel, Switzerland

VOLUME 37

Manganese and Its Role in Biological Processes

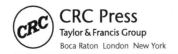

CRC Press
Taylor & Francis Group
Boca Raton London New York

CRC Press is an imprint of the
Taylor & Francis Group, an **informa** business

CRC Press
Taylor & Francis Group
6000 Broken Sound Parkway NW, Suite 300
Boca Raton, FL 33487-2742

First issued in paperback 2019

ISBN-13: 978-0-8247-0288-5 (hbk)
ISBN-13: 978-0-367-39893-4 (pbk)

**Visit the Taylor & Francis Web site at
http://www.taylorandfrancis.com**

**and the CRC Press Web site at
http://www.crcpress.com**

Library of Congress Cataloging-in-Publication Data

Manganese and its role in biological processes/edited by Astrid Sigel and Helmut Sigel.
    p. cm. — (Metal ions in biological systems; v. 37)
    Includes bibliographical references and index.
    ISBN 0-8247-0288-3
    1. Manganese—Physiological effect. 2. Manganese—Metabolism. 3. Manganese enzymes. I. Sigel, Astrid. II. Sigel, Helmut. III. Series.

QP532.M47 vol. 37
[QP535.M6]
572'.51 s—dc21
[572'.52541]

                          99-058164

The figure on the dustcover corresponds to Figure 6 of Chapter 17
by M. H. Gold et al.; reprinted with permission from *Biochemistry 38*
(1999) 11487. Copyright 1999 American Chemical Society.

Preface to the Series

Recently, the importance of metal ions to the vital functions of living organisms, hence their health and well-being, has become increasingly apparent. As a result, the long-neglected field of "bioinorganic chemistry" is now developing at a rapid pace. The research centers on the synthesis, stability, formation, structure, and reactivity of biological metal ion-containing compounds of low and high molecular weight. The metabolism and transport of metal ions and their complexes is being studied, and new models for complicated natural structures and processes are being devised and tested. The focal point of our attention is the connection between the chemistry of metal ions and their role for life.

No doubt, we are only at the brink of this process. Thus, it is with the intention of linking coordination chemistry and biochemistry in their widest sense that the *Metal Ions in Biological Systems* series reflects the growing field of "bioinorganic chemistry". We hope, also, that this series will help to break down the barriers between the historically separate spheres of chemistry, biochemistry, biology, medicine, and physics, with the expectation that a good deal of future outstanding discoveries will be made in the interdisciplinary areas of science.

Should this series prove a stimulus for new activities in this fascinating "field", it would well serve its purpose and would be a satisfactory result for the efforts spent by the authors.

Fall 1973

Helmut Sigel
Institute of Inorganic Chemistry
University of Basel
CH-4056 Basel, Switzerland

Preface to Volume 37

Manganese, element 25 in the Periodic Table, is the third most abundant transition metal in the Earth's crust after iron and titanium. Its geochemical distribution in the hydrosphere, lithosphere, and atmosphere (dust particles) involves oxidation states II, III, and IV. Manganese is an essential element for many living systems, including mammals, with more than 20 identified functions in enzymes and proteins, yet in excess it is toxic.

These more general aspects, including uptake and transport of manganese by microorganisms and plants as well as its interrelations with other metal ions in health and disease, are discussed in the first five chapters. The next two contributions summarize how Mn^{2+} may be employed to elucidate the role of other divalent metal ions in ribozymes and proteins; the same aspect regarding restriction endonucleases is dealt with in Chapter 11. Chapter 8 presents an overview of enzymes and proteins containing manganese, which is then followed by contributions devoted to the role of the element in, for example, concanavalin A and other lectins (which are important for carbohydrate recognition in plants), phosphatases, xylose isomerase (one of the most widely used industrial enzymes), and arginase which catalyzes the hydrolysis of L-arginine to L-ornithine and urea.

The use of model complexes to elucidate the structure and function of manganese redox enzymes is summarized in Chapter 14, which is followed by four contributions covering catechol extradiol dioxygenases, manganese catalases, and peroxidases as well as superoxide dismutases. In the terminating Chapters 19 and 20, photosynthetic water oxidation is highlighted, a very important reaction which is the source of nearly all oxygen in the atmosphere and thus, indirectly, of nearly all biomass on Earth. Duplication of the catalytic ability of this splendidly effective catalyst in industrial settings would have significant economic benefits; in order to achieve this, a solid understanding of the mechanism of the biological catalyst is required.

It is the hope of the authors and the editors that this book will facilitate further research on the fascinating role of manganese in biological systems.

Astrid Sigel
Helmut Sigel

Contents

Contributors

Numbers in parentheses indicate the pages on which the authors' contributions begin.

David E. Ash   Department of Biochemistry, Temple University School of Medicine, Philadelphia, PA 19140, USA (407)

Gerald T. Babcock   Department of Chemistry, Michigan State University, 320 Chemistry Building, East Lansing, MI 48824-1322, USA (Fax: +1-517-353-1793; <babcock@cem.msu.edu>) (613)

Geoffrey S. Baldwin   Department of Biochemistry, School of Medical Sciences, University of Bristol, University Walk, Bristol, BS8 1TD, UK (Fax: +44-117-928-8274; <g.baldwin@bristol.ac.uk>) (345)

Ralf Bogumil   Fakultät für Biologie, Universität Konstanz, Fach X 910-Sonnenbühl, D-78457 Konstanz, Germany (365)

Alex W. K. Chan   Imperial College Reactor Centre, University of London, Silwood Park, Ascot, Berkshire, SL5 7PY, UK (123)

David W. Christianson   Roy and Diana Vagelos Laboratories, Department of Chemistry, University of Pennsylvania, Philadelphia, PA 19104-6323, USA (Fax: +1-215-573-2201; <chris@xtal.chem.upenn.edu> or <chris@rock.chem.upenn.edu>) (407)

Michael S. Clegg   Department of Nutrition, University of California at Davis, One Shields Avenue, Davis, CA 95616, USA (89)

J. David Cox   Roy and Diana Vagelos Laboratories, Department of Chemistry, University of Pennsylvania, Philadelphia, PA 19104-6323, USA (407)

James D. Crowley School of Chemical and Physical Sciences, Victoria University of Wellington, P.O. Box 600, Wellington, New Zealand (209)

Valeria Cizewski Culotta Department of Environmental Health Sciences, Johns Hopkins University, School of Hygiene and Public Health, Room 7032, 615 N. Wolfe Street, Baltimore, MD 21205, USA (<vculotta@jhsph.edu>) (35)

Richard J. Debus Department of Biochemistry, University of California, Riverside, CA 92521-0129, USA(<richard.debus@ucr.edu>) (657)

Jodi L. Ensunsa Department of Nutrition, University of California at Davis, One Shields Avenue, Davis, CA 95616, USA (<jlensunsa @ucdavis.edu>) (89)

Andrew L. Feig Department of Chemistry and Biochemistry, University of Colorado, Campus Box 215, Boulder, CO 80309, USA. Present Affiliation: Department of Chemistry, Indiana University, 800 E. Kirkwood Avenue, Bloomington, IN 47405, USA (<afeig@indiana.edu>) (157)

Michael H. Gold Department of Biochemistry and Molecular Biology, Oregon Graduate Institute of Science and Technology, 20000 NW Walker Road, Beaverton, OR 97006-8921, USA (<mgold@bmb.ogi. edu>) (559)

Niall A. Gormley Department of Biochemistry, School of Medical Sciences, University of Bristol, University Walk, Bristol, BS8 1TD, UK (345)

Jarjis Habash Section of Structural Chemistry, Department of Chemistry, University of Manchester, Manchester M13 9PL, UK (279)

Stephen E. Halford Department of Biochemistry, School of Medical Sciences, University of Bristol, University Walk, Bristol, BS8 1TD, UK (Fax: +44-117-928-8274; <s.halford@bristol.ac.uk) (345)

John R. Helliwell Section of Structural Chemistry, Department of Chemistry, University of Manchester, Manchester M13 9PL, UK (Fax: +44-161-275-4734; <john.helliwell@man.ac.uk>) (279)

Curtis W. Hoganson Department of Chemistry, Michigan State University, Chemistry Building, East Lansing, MI 48824-1322, USA (<hoganson@dplus.net>) (613)

Wen-Yuan Hsieh Department of Chemistry, University of Michigan, Ann Arbor, MI 48109-1055, USA (<hsiehw@umich.edu>) (429)

Nicola S. Hunter Section of Structural Chemistry, Department of Chemistry, University of Manchester, Manchester M13 9PL, UK (279)

Jürgen Hüttermann Fachrichtung Biophysik und Physikalische Grundlagen der Medizin, Universität des Saarlandes, Klinikum, Bau 76, D-66421 Homburg (Saar), Germany (Fax: +49-6841-166227; <bpjhue @krzsun.med-rz.uni-sb.de>) (365)

Jungwon Hwang Department of Chemistry, University of Michigan, 930 North University Avenue, Ann Arbor, MI 49109, USA (<jugwonh @umich.edu>) (527)

A. Joseph Kalb(Gilboa) Department of Structural Biology, The Weizmann Institute, Rehovot, Israel (<bfgilboa@wis.weizmann.ac.il>) (279)

Reinhard Kappl Fachrichtung Biophysik und Physikalische Grundlagen der Medizin, Universität des Saarlandes, Klinikum, Bau 76, D-66421 Homburg (Saar), Germany (365)

Carl L. Keen Department of Nutrition, University of California at Davis, One Shields Avenue, Davis, CA 95616, USA (<clkeen@ucdavis. edu>) (89)

James C. K. Lai Department of Pharmaceutical Sciences, College of Pharmacy, Idaho State University, Pocatello, ID 83209-8334, USA (Fax: +1-208-236-4482; <lai@otc.isu.edu>) (123)

Louis Lim Institute of Neurology, University of London, Queen Square, London, WCIN 2NS, UK (123)

Margaret J. Minski Imperial College Reactor Centre, University of London, Silwood Park, Ascot, Berkshire, SL5 7PY, UK (123)

James J. Morgan Environmental Engineering Science, California Institute of Technology, W.M. Keck Laboratories 138-78, Pasadena, CA 91125, USA (Fax: +1-818-395-3170; <jjjbm@cco.caltech.edu>) (1)

Vincent L. Pecoraro Department of Chemistry, University of Michigan, Ann Arbor, MI 48109-1055, USA (<vlp@chem.lsa.umich.edu>) (429)

CONTRIBUTORS

James E. Penner-Hahn Department of Chemistry, University of Michigan, 930 North University Avenue, Ann Arbor, MI 49109-1055, USA (Fax: +1-734-647-4865; <jeph@umich.edu>) and Section de Bio-énergétique, CNRS URA 2096, DBCM CEA Saclay, F-91191 Gif-sur-Yvette Cedex, France (527)

Russell R. Poyner Institute of Enzyme Research and Department of Biochemistry, University of Wisconsin, 1710 University Avenue, Madison, WI 53705, USA (183)

Helen J. Price Section of Structural Chemistry, Department of Chemistry, University of Manchester, Manchester M13 9PL, UK (279)

Lawrence Que, Jr. Department of Chemistry and Center for Metals in Biocatalysis, University of Minnesota, 207 Pleasant Street SE, Minneapolis, MN 55455, USA (Fax: +1-612-624-7029; <que@chemsun. chem.umn.edu>) (505)

James Raftery Section of Structural Chemistry, Department of Chemistry, University of Manchester, Manchester M13 9PL, UK (279)

George H. Reed Institute of Enzyme Research and Department of Biochemistry, University of Wisconsin, 1710 University Avenue, Madison, WI 53705, USA (<reed@enzyme.wisc.edu>) (183)

Zdenko Rengel Soil Science and Plant Nutrition, Faculty of Agriculture, University of Western Australia, Nedlands, WA 6907, Australia (Fax: +61-8-9380-1050; <zrengel@agric.uwa.edu.au) (57)

Mark F. Reynolds Department of Chemistry and Center for Metals in Biocatalysis, University of Minnesota, 207 Pleasant Street SE, Minneapolis, MN 55455, USA (505)

Frank Rusnak Department of Biochemistry and Molecular Biology, Section of Hematology Research, Mayo Clinic and Foundation, 200 First Street S.W., Rochester, MN 55905, USA (Fax: +1-507-284-8286; <rusnak@mayo.edu>) (305)

Maarten D. Sollewijn Gelpke Department of Biochemistry and Molecular Biology, Oregon Graduate Institute of Science and Technology, 20000 NW Walker Road, Beaverton, OR 97006-8921, USA (559)

Deborah A. Traynor School of Chemical and Physical Sciences, Victoria University of Wellington, P.O. Box 600, Wellington, New Zealand (209)

David C. Weatherburn School of Chemical and Physical Sciences, Victoria University of Wellington, P.O. Box 600, Wellington, New Zealand (Fax: +64-4-495-5241; <david.weatherburn@vuw.ac.nz>) (209)

James W. Whittaker Department of Biochemistry and Molecular Biology, Oregon Graduate Institute of Science and Technology, 20000 NW Walker Road, Beaverton, OR 97006-8921, USA (<jim@bmb.ogi.edu>) (587)

Derek W. Yoder Department of Chemistry, University of Michigan, 930 North University Avenue, Ann Arbor, MI 49109-1055, USA (<derekwy@umich.edu>) (527)

Heather L. Youngs Department of Biochemistry and Molecular Biology, Oregon Graduate Institute of Science and Technology, 20000 NW Walker Road, Beaverton, OR 97006-8921, USA (559)

Contents of Previous Volumes

---

*Out of print.

---

*Out of print.

---

*Out of print.

Comments and suggestions with regard to contents, topics, and the like for future volumes of the series are welcome.

The following Marcel Dekker, Inc. books are also of interest for any reader dealing with metals or other inorganic compounds:

Handbook on Toxicity of Inorganic Compounds
edited by Hans G. Seiler and Helmut Sigel, with Astrid Sigel
In 74 chapters, written by 84 international authorities, this book covers the physiology, toxicity, and levels of tolerance, including prescriptions for

detoxification, for all elements of the Periodic Table (up to atomic number 103). The book also contains short summary sections for each element, dealing with the distribution of the elements, their chemistry, technological uses, and ecotoxicity as well as their analytical chemistry.

Handbook on Metals in Clinical and Analytical Chemistry
edited by Hans G. Seiler, Astrid Sigel, and Helmut Sigel
This book is written by 80 international authorities and covers over 3500 references. The first part (15 chapters) focuses on sample treatment, quality control, etc., and on the detailed description of the analytical procedures relevant for clinical chemistry. The second part (43 chapters) is devoted to a total of 61 metals and metalloids; all these contributions are identically organized covering the clinical relevance and analytical determination of each element as well as, in short summary sections, its chemistry, distribution, and technical uses.

1

Manganese in Natural Waters and Earth's Crust: Its Availability to Organisms

James J. Morgan

Environmental Engineering Science, California
Institute of Technology, Pasadena, CA 91125, USA

1.   INTRODUCTION

1.1.   Overview

Manganese, element 25 (atomic weight 54.93805), is the third most abundant transition metal in Earth's crust ($\sim$0.019 mol kg^{-1}), considerably less abundant than iron ($\sim$1.1 mol kg^{-1}), and the eighth most abundant crustal metal overall [1–3]. The manganese abundance of the ocean crust is about 60% greater than that of the continental crust. (In the solar system, the relative abundance of Fe and Mn is about 10^2 [2].) Manganese is an essential element in living systems, with some 20 identified functions in enzymes and proteins [3]. Major biological roles of manganese are in making O_2 (photosystem II) and in disposing of superoxide radicals (superoxide dismutase) [3]. The geochemical distribution of manganese in the hydrosphere, lithosphere, and atmosphere (dust particles) involves oxidation states Mn(II), Mn(III), and Mn(IV) [4], which show a wide range of strengths as Lewis acids, and whose coordination chemistries reflect a strong preference for oxygen donor ligands [3,5,6]. The biota exert a strong influence on the geochemistry of manganese through bacterial oxidation and reduction [7–9], and through Mn incorporation in new biomass production. Because of the high reduction potentials of the IV and III oxidation states of manganese in aquatic systems, manganese cycles are linked to a significant degree with the geochemical cycles of carbon, oxygen, iron, sulfur, arsenic, and other redox elements [4,7]. Linkage between the oxygen and manganese cycle is exemplified by the redox reaction

$$O_2 + 4Mn^{2+} + 6H_2O \longrightarrow 4MnOOH(s) + 8H^+ \tag{1}$$

(and similarly for the further oxidation of Mn(III) to MnO_2). Linkage between the carbon and manganese cycle may be symbolized by the redox reaction:

$$H_2CO(aq) + 2MnO_2(s) + 4H^+ \longrightarrow 2Mn^{2+} + CO_2(aq) + 3H_2O \tag{2}$$

in which H_2CO is formaldehyde, the carbohydrate building block. Both reactions (1) and (2) are energetically favorable under the conditions in most natural waters and sediments; both are microbially mediated.

For natural systems, some of the more important aqueous species and mineral phases of manganese can be summarized in a "manganese triangle":

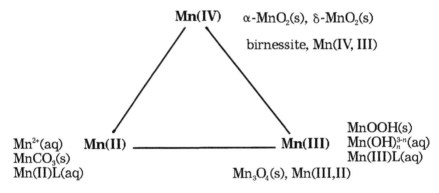

where L stands for a ligand forming aqueous Mn complexes (e.g., OH^-, Cl^-, SO_4^{2-}, citrate, humic acid, etc.). The observed distributions and speciation of manganese in aqueous and crustal environments can be reasonably well understood on the basis of thermodynamic and kinetic connections among the three oxidation states of manganese. The kinetics of manganese transformation concern chemical, biochemical, and photochemical reactions.

1.2. Concentrations and Fluxes

It will be helpful at the outset to have a synoptic view of the overall distribution of manganese on a global basis. Figure 1 indicates important concentrations of manganese in different environments and fluxes between different environments. Major *sources* of manganese to the world oceans are wind-blown dust (aeolian), rivers, diffusion out of sediments, and hydrothermal vents. In addition to the fluxes indicated, vertical advection and mixing play an important role in shaping the profiles of dissolved and particulate manganese in the world oceans. The oceans are stratified, with large temperature differences (~20 C°) between top and the deepest open-ocean waters. The ocean mixed surface layer has a thickness that changes seasonally, with depths ranging from perhaps 25 to 300 m.

Chemical consequences of this stratification will be discussed below. Fjords are also stratified, with freshwater over salty waters and may be periodically mixed by marine incursions [8,10]. Metal-rich manganese-iron mineral concretions known as nodules are widely distributed over sea floors [11,12]. The concentrations of manganese (and several other elements) *within* the hydrothermal fluids emerging from ridge spreading areas have been found to be very high, ranging up to some 25 mM in the end-member hot waters with estimated temperatures of near 350°C [13–16]. Table 1 offers some approximate values of manganese concentrations and fluxes.

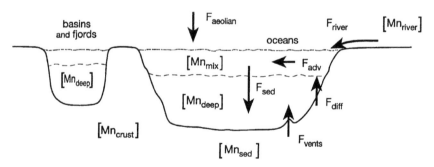

FIG. 1.   A descriptive view of some important manganese concentrations [Mn_i] and global fluxes, F_{Mn}. (Approximate values for concentrations and fluxes are given in Table 1.)

TABLE 1

Approximate Ranges of Manganese Concentrations and Global Fluxes (F)

$[Mn_i]$, mol kg^{-1}		Ref.	F_{Mn}, mol y^{-1}		Ref.
Crust	0.015–0.028	17			
River		18	River		18,19
Dissolved	2×10^{-7}		Dissolved	5×10^{9}–2×10^{10}	
Particles	8×10^{-6}		Particles	2×10^{11}–4×10^{11}	
Ocean		19	Aeolian	2×10^{9}	19
Mixed	5×10^{-10}–3×10^{-9}		Vents	5×10^{10}–2×10^{11}	15,16
Deep	8×10^{-11}–5×10^{-10}				
Pelagic sediments		20	Sedimentation		22
Solids	0.1		Pelagic	5×10^{10}	
Pore waters	10^{-8}–10^{-4}		Margins	1.5×10^{11}–3.5×10^{11}	18
Nodules	0.5–6				
Deep basins	3×10^{-6}–1×10^{-5}	21			
Fjords	5×10^{-6}–2×10^{-5}	10			

A global distribution picture for manganese may be summarized thus. Continental crust is weathered, releasing its manganese to soils and freshwaters. The soils lose Mn-containing dust (with still greater Fe, Al, Ca, and Si) to the winds, which deposit dissolvable Mn particles in the ocean mixed layer. Rivers bring both dissolved and particulate Mn to the marginal zones of the oceans at *total* concentrations on the order of 8 μM. Hydrothermal vents, e.g., on the East Pacific Rise, discharge hot waters of high Mn content, which react with colder seawater to produce both nearby and far-field deposits rich in Mn. Dissolved concentrations of Mn in the surface waters of the world oceans are typically 0.5–3 nmol kg^{-1} (hereinafter nM, for brevity). Deep ocean waters have dissolved manganese concentrations in the range 0.08–0.5 nM [19]. The present day partitioning of manganese between seawater and crust, $[Mn]_{sea}/[Mn]_{crust}$, is on the order of 10^{-8} (compare $[Fe]_{sea}/[Fe]_{crust} \sim 10^{-9}$) [23]. Concentrations of dissolved Mn in present day oceans are thought to be much lower than those of ancient oceans of the Precambrian era, estimated to have reached concentrations as high as 20 μM [24] to more than millimolar [25], possibly under the control of $MnCO_3(s)$ equilibrium. The development of an O_2 atmosphere as a result of photosynthesizing organisms some 2.7×10^9 years ago [3] has lowered the dissolved Mn in the oceans by many orders of magnitude. Deep basins and fjords show high concentrations of dissolved Mn in deeper, anoxic waters, and characteristically low dissolved Mn in oxygenated waters in the surface region. For example, the anoxic waters of the Black Sea below about 150 m have dissolved Mn levels approaching 10 μM [26].

2. CHEMICAL PROPERTIES

2.1. Oxidation States, Electronic Structures, and Coordination

Manganese, with an electronegativity of 1.55, has a preference for bonding of predominately ionic character to oxide, hydroxide, and carbonate ligands. The Pauling electronegativity difference, Δ_χ, between O and Mn is 1.9 [6]. Whitfield and Turner [27] correlated the seawater/crust partitioning of elements with $(\Delta_\chi)^2$ and grouped manganese with those lithophile elements that partition into seawater to a very small extent.

TABLE 2

Some Physical-Chemical Properties of Manganese Ions

Ion	a (pm)[a]	Electron configuration[b]		k_{-w} (s^{-1})[c]	$\log K_{OH^-}$	$\log K_{CIT^{3-}}$
Mn^{2+}	91	d^5	$t_{2g}^3 e_g^2$	10^7	3.4	5.0
Mn^{3+}	70	d^4	$t_{2g}^3 e_g^1$	10^5	14.4	~15
Mn^{4+}	52	d^3	t_{2g}^3	10^{-2}	>15	—

[a]Ionic radius a in picometers.
[b]High-spin complexes.
[c]Water exchange rate.
CIT, citrate.

Some relevant properties of manganese in the II, III, and IV oxidation states are summarized in Table 2. The Lewis acid strength of manganese ions increases greatly with oxidation state, and the exchange rate of water (related to rates of ligand binding) of the ion coordination sphere decreases dramatically. The ionic radius of Mn^{2+}, 91 pm, lies between that of Ca^{2+} (106 pm) and Mg^{2+} (78 pm), and is considerably larger than that of Cu^{2+} (72 pm). The electronic configuration of Mn^{2+} has five unpaired electrons in almost all of its complexes, providing no ligand field stabilization energy (LFSE) and resulting in complexes of usually lower stability compared to those of the other bivalent 3d transition metal ions. For example, the stability constant of the Mn(II)(citrate)$_{aq}^-$ complex is $10^{5.5}$, while that for Cu(II)(citrate)$_{aq}^-$ is $10^{7.2}$ [4]. The preference of an O/N ligand such as glycine for Cu with respect to Mn is still greater: $10^{8.4}$ vs. $10^{4.0}$. Mn(III) ion, with greater charge, smaller ionic radius, and an LFSE of $0.6\Delta_0$ (the ligand field splitting energy) in high-spin complexes [5,6], forms much more stable aqueous complexes with O-donor (and also N-donor) ligands. The coordination is usually octahedral or distorted tetragonal in the compounds of the manganese II, III, and IV ions [3,6]. The coordination environments of the II, III, and IV states establish the energetics of electron transfer. For example, in excess of citrate ligand, the reduction potential of the Mn(III)/Mn(II) couple is lowered by ~0.5 V.

2.2. Redox Energetics

$Mn^{2+}(aq)$ is a weak reductant. $Mn^{3+}(aq)$ is a strong oxidant, as is $MnO_2(s)$. At 25°C,

$$Mn^{3+} + e^- = Mn^{2+} \qquad E_H^\circ = 1.5 \text{ V},$$

$$\text{or } pE^\circ = E_H^\circ/0.0592 = 25.3 \tag{3}$$

(We use the variable $pE = -\log\{e^-\}$ for redox energetics; it scales as pH and log K for reactions (4).) For the reduction of $MnO_2(s)$,

$$MnO_2(s) + 2e^- + 4H^+ = Mn^{2+} + 2H_2O \qquad pE^\circ = 21.8 \tag{4}$$

The Mn(III) phase manganite also is a strong oxidant:

$$MnOOH(s) + e^- + 3H^+ = Mn^{2+} + 2H_2O \qquad pE^\circ = 25.0 \tag{5}$$

The mineral hausmannite, $Mn_3O_4(s)$, has a domain of stability at higher pH and lower pE. The reduction reaction is

$$Mn_3O_4(s) + 2e^- + 8H^+ = 3Mn^{2+} + 4H_2O \qquad pE^\circ = 19.9 \tag{6}$$

The Mn(III) state is subject to disproportionation (simultaneous oxidation and reduction) to form Mn(II) and Mn(IV) compounds. For example,

$$Mn_3O_4(s) + 2H^+ = 2\gamma\text{-}MnOOH(s) + Mn^{2+}$$

$$\Delta G^\circ = -102 \text{ kJ mol}^{-1} \tag{7}$$

For μM Mn^{2+} concentrations, reaction (7) is spontaneous at pH < 11.

A pE–pH stability diagram for manganese is presented in Fig. 2. Two concentration levels for $Mn^{2+}(aq)$ are illustrated, i.e., 1 nM for ocean surface waters and 1 μM for river waters. The O_2–H_2O pE vs. pH line for air-saturated conditions indicates that MnO_2 can be formed at pH > 6 for μM aqueous Mn. In the pH region of open-ocean waters, $MnOOH(s)$ could form, but the "window" for $Mn_3O_4(s)$ is open only at higher Mn^{2+} activity. Although not shown here, $MnCO_3(s)$ has a domain of stability for a total dissolved inorganic carbon concentration C_T, of 1 mM for pH between ~9.3 and 10 and pE <2, if $[Mn^{2+}]$ is 1 μM. Thus, $MnCO_3(s)$ may form in the circumneutral pH region only at higher Mn^{2+} activities (say, >10 μM), such as can be found in sedimentary pore waters, e.g., reaction (2), or are thought to have existed in Precambrian oceans. Under conditions of low O_2 partial pressure (*anoxic* environ-

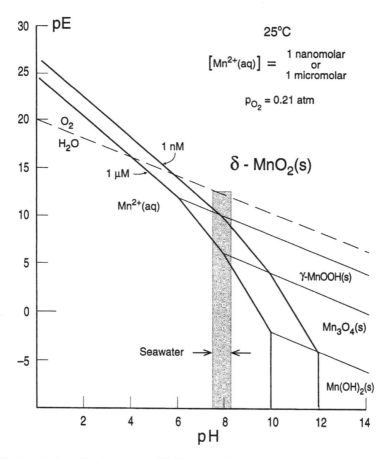

FIG. 2. A simplified pE vs. pH diagram for some major manganese solid phases and their equilibrium boundaries with aqueous manganese(II) at two environmentally relevant locations. The position of the atmospheric O_2–H_2O reduction energy vs. pH is also shown. (pE is the nondimensional reduction potential. See text for details.)

ments) and in the pH range from ~6 to 8, Mn(II) species (i.e., the aqueous ion and its complexes) have high stability. Where conditions are *oxic*, e.g., throughout most of the open oceans, in the surface mixed layers of basins and fjords, in the surface waters of lakes, and at the air/ crust or air/soil boundaries, MnOOH and MnO_2 are stable at the ex-

pense of Mn(II). However, interpreting the actual aquatic and geochemical distributions of manganese usually calls for insights about
rates of redox and coordination reactions under natural conditions.
Speciation is a prerequisite for understanding manganese kinetics.

2.3. Speciation

To paraphrase an observation reported by Pecoraro in 1992 [28] regarding earlier manganese chemistry, Mn(II) was boring, Mn(III) was
tricky, and Mn(IV) existed as the dioxide. The context was biochemistry, but similar preconceptions have existed concerning manganese in
the *milieu externe*.

2.3.1. Mn(IV)

First, as to Mn(IV), its complexity in nature is reflected in the many
varieties of "the dioxide" and their distinctive structures and surface
properties, and the presence in them of Mn^{3+} and other metal ions as
in, e.g., birnessite. Total manganese contents and average oxidation
states of marine sediments and ferromanganese nodules from the floor
of the Pacific Ocean have been reported [29]. For nodules, it was found
that the Mn was entirely in the IV oxidation state (less than 1% Mn(II)),
and that Mn/Fe ratios ranged from about 6 to 70. In sedimentary cores
to depths as great as ~50 cm, the oxidation state of the Mn in the solids
ranged from close to IV under oxic conditions to III or lower in sediments that undergo reduction by the depositing organic carbon (biomass from surface ocean water productivity). Ferromanganese nodules
of the Pacific contain as much as 30–40% Mn; average Mn contents of
nodules in the major oceans are about 15–20% [11,20]. Marine nodules
are often rich in transition metals such as Ni, Cu, and Co [11,12].
    Some of the manganese dioxide minerals found in natural deposits
include birnessite, todorokite, vernadite, pyrolusite, and hollandite. We
cannot discuss this particular and important aspect of environmental
manganese chemistry here. Accounts of advances related to Mn(IV, III)
oxide chemistry should be consulted [12,30–32].

2.3.2. Mn(III)

Research on Mn(III) chemistry in the environment has centered on MnOOH and Mn_3O_4 solid phases [10,33,34]. Combined kinetic and equilibrium models have postulated the processes: (1) $Mn(OH)_2(s)$ oxygenation to form $Mn_3O_4(s)$ and/or MnOOH(s), followed (2) by possible disproportionations to yield MnO_2 and Mn(II). Oxygenation of Mn(II) (probably initially $Mn(OH)_2(s)$) yielded Mn_3O_4 (hausmannite), followed by β-MnOOH (feitknechtite) and then γ-MnOOH (manganite), identified as an Mn(III) solid phase [33]. Kessick and Morgan [35] observed formation of an MnOOH solid during laboratory oxygenation of an initially homogeneous solution at pH 8.9; prolonged oxygenation then yielded solid particles containing an increasing proportion of Mn(IV) relative to Mn(III). A partial thermodynamic model (using observed dissolved O_2 profiles) of $[Mn^{2+}]$ vs. ocean depth to ~5000 m was proposed by Gramm-Osipov [36], who claimed $[Mn^{2+}]$ solubility control by $Mn_3O_4(s)$ (surface ocean) or MnOOH(s) (deep ocean).

Suggestions have been put forward that *dissolved* Mn(III) species might play a role in manganese cycles in water [37,38]. Mn(III) would be kinetically stable only in the presence of suitably strong ligands. Candidate paths could include (1) dissolution of MnOOH, (2) reduction of MnO_2, (3) oxidation of Mn(II) complexes. Among Mn(III) complexes that have been examined in laboratory studies are those of pyrophosphate, citrate, ethylenediaminetetraacetate [38], and tartrate [39]. Manganese peroxidase enzyme (from a white-rot basidomycete oxidizes Mn(II)tartrate to Mn(III)tartrate, which is in turn able to oxidize aromatic pollutants [39]. Complexes of Mn(III) with pyrophosphate, citrate, and ethylenediaminetetraacetate, while generally *thermodynamically* unstable with respect to disproportionation, can have appreciable *kinetic* stability in circumneutral solutions [38].

2.3.3. Mn(II)

It can be anticipated on the basis of the chemical properties of Mn(II) (Table 2) that $Mn^{2+}(aq)$, the hydrated cation, should be an important species in most natural waters. The O-donor ligands are OH^-, SO_4^{2-},

CO_3^{2-}, PO_4^{3-}, phenolate, and carboxylate groups. As a "hard"-type Lewis base, Mn^{2+} will not form strong complexes with Cl^- ion. However, chloride is the most abundant anion in seawater (~0.55 M), and total sulfate (much of it complexed by major cations) is present in seawater at ~28 mM, so that equilibrium models have proved essential for quantitative assessment of natural water speciation. Turner et al. [40] predicted the following speciation for Mn(II) for average seawater (pH 8.2, 25°C, 1 atm): Mn^{2+}, 58%; $MnCl_n^{2-n}$, 37%; $MnSO_4$, 4%; $MnCO_3^0$, 1%. They also made approximate calculations for aqueous "Mn-humate" complexing in seawater and estimated only 0.01% Mn in organic-bound form (contrasted with a 47% estimate for aqueous "Cu-humate"). For a model freshwater (pH 6), they computed 98% Mn^{2+} and 2% $MnSO_4$. Freshwater speciation at pH 9 shifted appreciably: 62% Mn^{2+}, 35% $MnCO_3^0$, and 1% each of $MnOH^+$ and $MnSO_4$.

Experimental confirmation of the general results predicted for Mn(II) in seawater came from electron spin resonance (ESR) measurements by Carpenter [41]. The ESR method yielded these results: Mn^{2+}, 72%; $MnCl_n^{2-n}$, 15%; and $MnSO_4$, 10%. Influences of temperature and pH on metal speciation in seawater were subsequently computed by Byrne et al. [42]. For pH 8.2, the computed 25°C speciation of Mn(II) was: Mn^{2+}, 72%; $MnCl_n^{2-n}$, 21%; $MnSO_4$, 5%; and $MnCO_3^0$, 2%. Shifting the temperature to 5°C resulted in only a minor increase in free Mn(II) from 72% to 74%. Lowering the pH to 7.6 produced only a 1% increase in free manganese. A firm conclusion from Mn(II) speciation research is that the free (hydrated) metal ion, $Mn^{2+}(aq)$, predominates in natural waters under nearly all conditions (apart, possibly, from unique estuarine environments or higher salinity seas rich in complexing ligands). It is clear that the high proportion of Mn(II) in the free form indicates high biological availability in most natural waters. The speciation of Mn(II) in seawater is akin to those of Ni(II), Fe(II), and Zn(II), but is quite different from the inorganic speciations of Cu(II) (~5% free ion), Cu(I) (0.001% free ion), and Cd(II) (3% free ion).

A speciation model for trace metals, including Mn(II), vs. water depth in the center of the Black Sea was generated by Landing and Lewis [26]. The measured $[Mn(II)]_T$ vs. depth was combined with the observed distributions of the pH, major cations and anions (salinity), and the ligands carbonate, sulfate, chloride, and sulfide to compute equilibrium speciation using selected thermodynamic data. The result

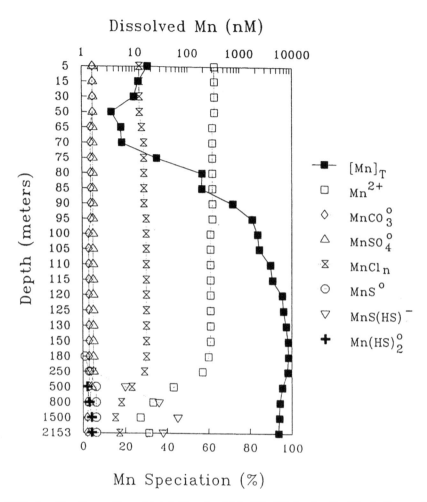

FIG. 3. Depth profiles of total dissolved Mn(II), $[Mn]_T$, in the Black Sea and computed annual speciation [26].

is shown in Fig. 3. To depths of 250 m the computed speciation is ~60% Mn^{2+} and ~30% chloro species. As the transition from oxic to sulfide-rich waters develops ($[S(-II)]_T$ increases to ~10 μM at 125 m depth and to over 100 μM at 250 m), increasing Mn(II) sulfide aqueous species are predicted. These authors also conjectured that total Mn(II) solubility in very deep waters (greater than 500 m) might be controlled by the phase $MnS_2(s)$ (haurite).

3. RATES OF MANGANESE REACTIONS IN WATER

3.1. Overview

Oceanic *residence time* for Mn, i.e., *the mass of Mn in the oceans divided by the total removal rate of Mn in a steady-state ocean*, was earlier thought to be long, perhaps ~10^3 years or more [43]. Turnover time scales for manganese in lakes and rivers were recognized to be highly variable and related to chemical stratification, e.g., for O_2, pH, carbon, and sulfur, and to suspended particles. Contemporary understanding of manganese oxidation and reduction processes in nature recognizes a wide diversity of reaction modes, including homogeneous and hetero-geneous chemical, biological, and photochemical processes that produce oxidation, reduction, and scavenging (sorption, precipitation) pro-cesses, imparting distinctive manganese profiles over the depths of the oceans. The ocean environment is increasingly understood to be diverse, as are freshwaters. The earlier notion of an *overall ocean resi-dence time* for biologically influenced elements is not as informative as recognition of relevant residence times of manganese in surface waters, coastal margins, hydrothermal vent areas, and abyssal deep water. It is not surprising to know that time scales of manganese oxidation in nature can range from days to centuries or more.

3.2. Laboratory Studies of Manganese Oxidation Kinetics

Oxygenation rates of Mn(II) in water were first investigated in labora-tory experiments at low ionic strength and pH greater than 9 some 35 years ago [44–46]. The autocatalytic character of the oxidation process was established by Morgan and Stumm [45,46] under abiotic condi-tions. A two-term rate law described the *homogeneous* and *hetero-geneous* paths of the process:

$$-\frac{d[\text{Mn(II)}]}{dt} = k[\text{Mn(II)} + k_s[\text{MnO}_x][\text{Mn(II)}] \tag{8}$$

in which the observed first-order rate constant, k, depends on $[O_2]$, pH, temperature, and speciation of Mn(II) in solution. The second-order rate constant, k_s, depends on the same parameters and the nature of the MnO_x (e.g., MnO_2 or MnOOH) surface formed in the reaction. A provocative question was raised 15 years ago concerning the homogeneous path: is Mn(II) oxidized in the absence of precipitate or surfaces [47]? A satisfactory answer called for experiments at lower pH and lower Mn(II) concentrations.

Subsequent experiment of Davies and Morgan [48] extended the pH domain of k for the homogeneous oxidation to lower values, confirming a strong pH influence on the rate. Very recently, rates of Mn(II) oxygenation have been studied by Von Langen et al. [49] in filtered coastal seawater with pH adjusted to different values and with Mn(II) initial concentrations of ~20 nM. They interpreted their kinetic data as describing *homogeneous* oxidation, and compared their observations with those of Morgan and Stumm [45] and Davies and Morgan [48]. Figure 4 shows homogeneous first-order rate constants for three groups of experiments [45,48,49]. These results are consistent with the expression for k:

$$k = k_1[O_2][OH^-]^2 \tag{9}$$

where k_1 is in the range from 1×10^{12} M^{-3} day^{-1} to 2×10^{12} M^{-3} day^{-1} at 25°C. Manganese *is* oxidized in the absence of precipitate or surfaces, but slowly.

3.3. Slowness of Homogeneous Mn(II) Oxidation by O_2

Homogeneous oxidation of Mn(II) by O_2 is 10 million times slower than that of Fe(II) at pH 8 and 25°C. This observation might be expected, in part, on the basis of the large difference in standard reduction potentials for Fe^{3+} and Mn^{3+}, 0.7 V, i.e., the manganous ion is energetically quite stable. As already mentioned, oxygenation of Mn(II) in slightly alkaline solution gives initially an Mn(III)-containing oxohydroxide

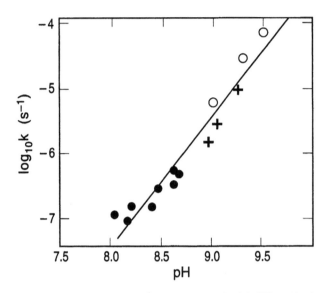

FIG. 4. Homogeneous first-order rate constants for Mn(II) oxidation at different pH values, normalized to unit O_2 partial pressure and 25°C. + [48], • [49], and ○ [45].

product. Suppose that the rate-determining reaction for manganese oxidation is,

$$Mn(OH)_2(aq) + O_2(aq) \longrightarrow Mn(OH)_2^+ + O_2^{-\bullet} \qquad (10)$$

The *predicted* rate expression would then be

$$-\frac{d\,[Mn(OH)_2]}{dt} = k_2[O_2]\beta_2[OH^-]^2[Mn^{2+}]$$

$$\cong k_2[O_2]\beta_2[OH^-]^2[Mn(II)] \qquad (11)$$

β_2 is the cumulative formation constant for the complex $Mn(OH)_2(aq)$. From the data in Fig. 4, and with $\beta_2 \cong 10^6$ M^{-2}, we estimate a *bimolecular* rate constant for the proposed slow step: $k_2 \cong 50 \pm 10$ M^{-1} s^{-1}. The (unfavorable) standard free energy, ΔG°, for reaction (10) is about +35 kJ mol^{-1}. (For comparison with Fe(II) oxidation $k_2 \sim 10^7$ and $\Delta G^\circ \sim +15$ kJ mol^{-1}.) It is not yet clear as to whether the predominant path for Mn(II) oxygenation is outersphere or innersphere.

3.4. Catalysis of Mn(II) Oxygenation by Oxide Surfaces

The rate term $k_s[MnO_x][Mn(II)]$ describing catalysis of Mn(II) oxidation by manganese oxide reaction products was also examined by Morgan and Stumm [45] and by Brewer [50]. It was found that the observed rate constant k_s depended on temperature, pH, and O_2 concentration. Observations of Mn(II) and MnO_x vs. time were described by

$$k_s = k_{Mn}[OH^-]^2[O_2] \tag{12}$$

with $k_{Mn} \sim 5 \times 10^{18}$ M^{-4} day^{-1}.

The behavior of the manganese oxide reaction product raised the question of whether other oxohydroxide solid surfaces might play a similar catalytic role. Catalysis by iron oxide would provide a kinetic link with manganese redox cycles. Sung and Morgan [51] showed that the surface of the iron oxide γ-FeOOH (lepidocrocite) greatly accelerated the oxygenation of Mn(II) over the homogeneous rate at the same pH and temperature. The oxidized manganese progressively coated the iron oxide surface, and after full coverage with MnO_x deposit was attained, the ensuing kinetics were then described by the expression $k_s[MnO_x][Mn(II)]$. Mn(II) oxidation catalysis was further investigated by Davies and Morgan [48] who compared γ-FeOOH, α-FeOOH, SiO_2, and Al_2O_3 surfaces. A rate law of the form

$$-\frac{d[Mn(II)]}{dt} = k^*\{(\equiv SO)_2Mn^{II}\}A \times [O_2] \tag{13}$$

was found, in which $\{(\equiv SO)_2Mn^{II}\}$ is the mole concentration Mn(II) *bound* to a surface site, $\equiv SOH$, and the surface-bound fraction depends on surface site density and structure as well as on pH and [Mn(II)] speciation in solution. A is the mass concentration of oxide particles. At low surface coverage, the observed kinetics are first order in [Mn(II)], and at high surface coverage (near saturation) the kinetics become zero order, i.e., independent of [Mn(II)]. Davies [52] illustrated the range of time scales for Mn(II) oxidation catalyzed by γ-FeOOH. For example, at pH 8, [Mn(II)] = 0.2 μM, and [γ-FeOOH] = 10 μM; the time for 50% oxidation of Mn(II) is about a month.

The rate of a surface-catalyzed reaction is subject to influence by metals and ligands in natural waters. Metal ions can inhibit catalysis by competing for adsorption sites on the surface, e.g., Ca^{2+}, Mg^{2+}, and other cations. Ligands can retard oxidation by lowering the free Mn(II) ions in solution, thereby decreasing adsorption to reactive sites [53].

The rate of catalyzed oxidation, r_s, for a surface-dependent process takes the general form:

$$r_s = -\frac{d\,[Mn(II)]}{dt} = \frac{r_{s,max}[Mn(II)]}{K_s + [Mn(II)]} \tag{14}$$

in which K_s is a function of the kinetic constants for adsorption, e.g., an equilibrium constant in the simplest case. The maximum rate, $r_{s,max}$, depends on the density of surface groups and their structure and reactivity. Accelerations of Mn(II) oxygenation by MnO_2, FeOOH, and SiO_2 [48] and by bacterial spores [54] can be described by a saturation expression such as (14), because they all entail surface site binding of Mn(II).

3.5. Bacterial Mediation of Mn(II) Oxidation

Detailed observations in a wide variety of natural water environments, e.g., the oxic/anoxic transition in fjords [8,10] and marine basins [55], estuaries [56,57], coastal waters [58,59], Sargasso Sea surface waters [59,60], and in the vicinity of hydrothermal vents [61,62], reveal rapid oxygenation of Mn(II) by marine bacteria in comparison to homogeneous or heterogeneous rates. The mechanisms of microbial Mn(II) oxidation have not yet been established; a thorough review of current knowledge was recently provided [9].

Oxidative removal times and absolute removal rates of Mn(II) in incubated environmental water samples (both in situ and shipboard) have been quantified by use of a [54]Mn(II) radiotracer. Metabolic poisons were used to distinguish nonoxidative sorption from bacterially mediated Mn(II) oxidation by O_2 [55,63]. The quantitative framework for interpreting rates of bacterially mediated Mn(II) oxidation is a "Michaelis-Menten" saturation function, in analogy with enzyme kinetics [55]:

$$V_0 = \frac{V_{0,max}[Mn(II)]}{K_m + [Mn(II)]} \tag{15}$$

in which the 0 subscript signifies initial rate, $V_{0,max}$ is the maximum rate, and K_m is a "Michaelis constant", which equals the Mn(II) concentration giving one-half maximum rate.

Tebo and Emerson [55] reported $V_{0,max}$ values ranging from ~4 to 12 nM h^{-1} for Sannich Inlet waters just above the oxic/anoxic boundary (85–115 m depths). K_m values ranged from 0.4 to 0.9 μM. In the environment studied, [Mn(II)] was greater than K_m, and kinetics were less than first order, approaching zero order. Microbial oxidation in the Newport River Estuary [57] was characterized by $V_{0,max}$ of 12 nM h^{-1} and K_m of 0.19 μM. Sunda and Huntsman [57] remarked that the implied conditional binding constant for Mn^{2+} to a surface site should be more than 7×10^6 M^{-1}. Moffett and Ho [59] reported $V_{0,max}$ ~55 nM h^{-1} and K_m ~0.8 μM for Mn(II) oxidation in bay water on the Massachusetts coast.

Examples of [Mn(II)] oxidation rates in natural waters attributed to bacteria are presented in Table 3. The highest rates appear to be observed in zones of lower O_2 concentrations. In surface waters of high light intensity, photoinhibition of bacterial oxidation has been proposed [58,60]. At 500 m depth in the Sargasso Sea, the measured rate of 0.0004 nM h^{-1} corresponds to a residence time with respect to oxidation of approximately 100 days. The highest rates attributed to bacterial oxidation of Mn(II) are in the nearshore waters of the Black Sea [63].

TABLE 3

Mn(II) Oxidations Attributed to Bacteria

Water	[Mn(II)], μM	V, nM h^{-1}	Condition	Ref.
Black Sea, central	2	6	100 m	55
Black Sea, nearshore	4	67	160 m	55
Newport Estuary	0.2	3.5	pH 8.2, salty	57
Sargasso Sea	0.004	0.0004	25 m	60
	0.002	0.0037	120 m	
	0.001	0.0004	500 m	
Galapagos Vent	0.20	0.06	2000 m	62
Juan de Fuca Ridge	0.07	0.002	2100 m	61

3.6. Rates of Reduction and Dissolution of Mn(III,IV) Oxides

Reductions of MnO_2 by organic compounds and a variety of inorganic reductants, e.g., sulfide, Fe(II), arsenite, Cr(III), etc., are energetically favorable under most natural water conditions. For example, reaction (2), $H_2CO(aq) + 2MnO_2(s) + 4H^+ \rightarrow 2Mn^{2+} + CO_2(aq) + 3H_2O$, has a reaction free energy, ΔG of about -420 kJ mol^{-1}, or a potential driving force of ~1 Volt, or $\Delta\ pE$ ~ 17, at pH 7.0, $[H_2CO] = 10\ \mu M$ and $[Mn^{2+}] = 1$ μM. What are the rates of some of different kinds of redox reactions that lead to dissolution of manganese oxides and an increase of dissolved Mn in natural waters? The rate processes may be chemical, photochemical, or microbial. Only a brief indication of answers to this question can be provided here.

3.6.1. Chemical Reduction

Chemical reduction rates of an Mn(III,IV) oxide by some two-dozen simple, low molecular weight (LMW) compounds (e.g., hydroquinone, oxalate) in the neutral pH region were reported by Stone and Morgan [64]. Rates of reduction with these simple organic compounds ranged over two orders of magnitude (5×10^{-3}–20 M^{-1} s^{-1}). Reduction of MnO_2 by humic substances (fulvic acid) yielded a variety of LMW compounds, including pyruvate, acetone, and formaldehyde [65]. Rates of LMW product formation were fit by a saturation function [similar in form to Eq. (14)] with an $r_{s,max}$ value of ~36 nM h^{-1} for pyruvate production. Sunda and Kieber [65] suggest that the reduction of MnO_x by biologically refractory humic substances could provide an important source of microbial substrates in natural waters.

3.6.2. Photoreductive Dissolution

Photoreductive dissolution of MnO_x particles in eastern Caribbean surface waters was measured by Waite and Szymczak [66]. Rates of production of dissolved Mn (less than 0.22-μm-pore membrane filters) from 10 sampling locations were found to range from ~20 to 1300 pM h^{-1} at 365 nm wavelength irradiation. The rate of dissolved Mn(II) production by photodissolution was proportional to absorbance of 365-nm light. The authors proposed a rapid surface equilibrium reaction:

$$\equiv Mn(IV)OH + HA = \equiv Mn(IV)A + H_2O \tag{16}$$

where $\equiv Mn(IV)OH$ represents an oxide surface site, HA organic compounds in the surface water, and $\equiv Mn(IV)A$ a surface precursor complex. A steady-state treatment for the (chromophore) precursor yields, as an approximation,

$$d[Mn(II)]_{aq}/dt \approx k_2 \, [\equiv Mn]_T [HA]_T \tag{17}$$

where k_2 is proportional to light absorbance and the binding constants and $[...]_T$ means the total concentration.

3.6.3. Bacterial Reduction

The MnO_2 solid [7] and the Mn(III)pyrophosphate solution complexes [37] have each been found to serve as terminal electron acceptors for bacterial respiration, releasing Mn(II) to solution. The bacterium *Alteromonas putrefaciens* MR-1 (isolated from anoxic Lake Oneida sediment) requires physical contact with MnO_2 for growth. With lake water medium containing acetate or succinate as carbon source, rates of reduction of MnO_2 were observed to be $\sim 1 \times 10^{-9}$ μmol cell^{-1} h^{-1}. With a bacteria concentration of 1.87×10^9 cell L^{-1}, the reduction rate was ~2 μM h^{-1}.

Manganese-reducing bacteria (genus *Shewanella*) were isolated from the suboxic waters (less than 5 μM O_2) of the Black Sea in the Mn(IV) reducing zone at 80–90 m depth [67]. This zone is absent of sulfide, so that direct reduction by HS$^-$ does not take place. *Shewanella* cell densities were on the order of 1–5×10^8 L^{-1} in this zone. Mn(IV) reduction rates were estimated to be in the range 0.15–0.5 μM h^{-1}.

4. MANGANESE PROFILES IN THE OCEANS

4.1. General Observations

During the past two decades knowledge of trace element concentrations actually present in the ocean waters has grown enormously, and in parallel there have been major advances in the understanding of chemical and biological processes that bring about observed spatial and temporal variations. A concise overview of all trace element profiles in the Pacific has recently been presented by Nozaki [68]. Manganese in the oceans has a profile of dissolved concentration vs. depth with high values in surface waters and lower concentration at great depth. Manganese belongs to that group of trace elements called "scavenged", i.e., taken from the water onto and into particles with depth.

4.2. Atlantic

Profiles of dissolved and particulate forms of manganese in the southwestern Sargasso Sea measured by Sunda and Huntsman are shown in Fig. 5 [60]. Figure 5A shows dissolved (passing through 0.4-μm-pore filters) Mn, which is in the II oxidation state. Figure 5B gives information on two forms of particulate Mn in the water column: a small fraction of mineral particles resistant to reduction by ascorbic acid, and the major fraction, readily reduced and dissolved by ascorbic acid and understood to comprise oxide particles of Mn(IV) and Mn(III). The authors interpret the profiles observed to result from several processes: atmospheric deposition of Mn-containing particles, particle dissolution by photochemical reactions in surface waters, microbial oxidation that transforms Mn(II) in the water to MnO_x (solid) particles, incorporation of Mn in planktonic organisms (only a few percent of all particulate Mn), and particle settling. The high dissolved Mn concentrations in the top 40 m of the Sargasso Sea are attributed to *both* photoassisted dissolution (Mn oxide + organic reductants + photons) and light inhibition of microbial Mn(II) oxidation. We note that dissolved Mn decreases by about 75% between surface and 750-m depth. At a depth of 150 m the turnover time for conversion of dissolved Mn to MnO_x was computed to be about 30 days. (Bacterially mediated oxidation rates for this environment are given in Table 3.)

4.3. Pacific

Vertical profiles for manganese in the stratified central North Pacific at 28° N 155° W, measured in summer 1983, were reported by Bruland et

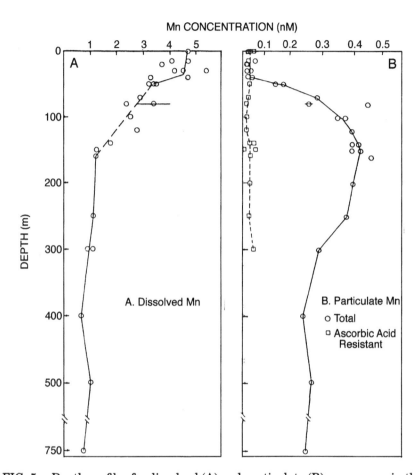

FIG. 5.   Depth profiles for dissolved (A) and particulate (B) manganese in the southwestern Sargasso Sea [60]. Ascorbic acid-resistant particles are distinguished from MnO particles readily dissolved by ascorbic acid. (Reprinted with permission from [60].)

al. [69], as shown in Fig. 6A and B. The concentration of dissolved manganese in the surface mixed layer attains a maximum of close to 1 nmol kg^{-1} (hereinafter nM), while the particulate Mn concentrations there are only 0.009 nM. In the summer season, there is a shallow (0–25 m), well-mixed, surface layer, underlain by stratified waters. The surface well-mixed layer bears an "aeolian imprint" of atmospheric input of

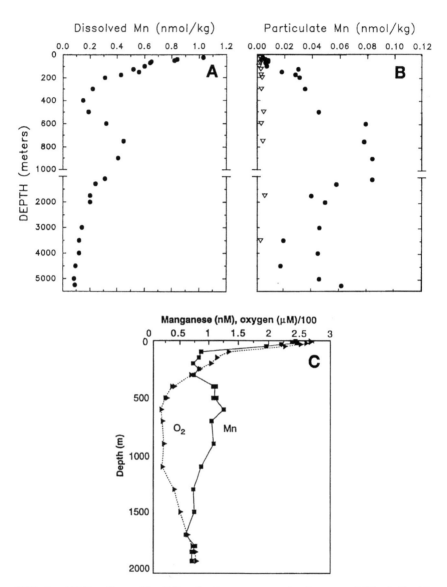

FIG. 6. (A) Depth profile of dissolved manganese in the central North Pacific Ocean [69]. (B) Depth profile of particulate manganese at the same location as in A. ∇ indicates particles resistant to dissolution by acid [69]. (C) Depth profiles for dissolved O₂ and dissolved Mn at a different station in the North Pacific [70]. (Reprinted with permission from [69] and [70].)

manganese that dissolves under the influence of chemical and photo-chemical reactions [69]. Figure 6A shows that dissolved Mn decreases progressively down to a depth of 400 m, then increases to a distinct maximum near 800 m, and from that point downward decreases pro-gressively by particle scavenging to less than 0.1 nM at 5000 m. As in the profile for the Sargasso Sea (Fig. 5), the ratio of dissolved to par-ticulate (acid-soluble) Mn is high. The surface layer particulate Mn of the North Pacific is found to be a factor of 3–4 *lower* than for the North Atlantic, reflecting differences in aeolian fluxes.

The profiles in Fig. 6 reflect similar processes of aeolian input, MnO_x reductive dissolution, and oxidative conversion of Mn(II) dis-cussed above and seen in the Sargasso Sea profile [60]. In the North Pacific ocean, a manganese residence time of ~100 years has been estimated for oxic intermediate and deep waters [69]. Bruland et al. [69] proposed that lateral mixing of dissolved Mn from waters in anoxic or suboxic environments, e.g., in coastal margin sediments, might account for observed dissolved Mn profile maxima in open-ocean water, such as is seen near 800 m in Fig. 6A. Lateral gradients, i.e., $d[Mn(II)]/dx$, between ocean margins and the deep ocean, if great enough, could transport Mn from coastal to deeper interior ocean waters.

Ocean profiles for dissolved Mn and dissolved O_2 measured in June 1991 at 35° 15′ N and 121° 52′ W, as presented by Johnson et al. [70], are shown in Fig. 6C. A "secondary Mn maximum" of dissolved Mn is observed over a range of depths within which $[O_2]$ concentrations are low, ~20 μM in comparison with surface O_2 concentrations. Three mech-anisms have been proposed to account for the profile maximum (1) *late-ral transport* of Mn from ocean margins of higher Mn to ocean interiors; (2) *equilibrium* with phases such as $Mn_3O_4(s)$ and MnOOH(s) under the conditions of low $[O_2]$ and low pH in deeper waters [36], and (3) a *kinetic* model balancing rates of reductive dissolution of MnO_x and release of Mn from decomposing biomass from the surface waters against rates of oxidative scavenging. The authors [70] propose a kinetic model in which the homogeneous path described in Eqs. (8) and (9) is invoked. The homogeneous rate expression [and heterogeneous ones such as Eqs. (12) and (13) also] account for effects of changing temperature, pH, and O_2 concentration with depth. A reasonable fit was obtained to the profile in Fig. 6C, if the vertical eddy diffusion influence on Mn(II) concentration change was included. The kinetic approach is appealing, but the information cost is high. Evidently, reliable information for rates of component processes already discussed above is needed and has to be applied for processes *throughout* the water column. The homogeneous expression for oxidation [Eq. (9)] employed [70] yields a pseudo-first-order rate constant k ~0.005 y^{-1} in the core of the O_2 minimum, and k ~0.05 y^{-1} at a depth of 2000 m. These results correspond to time scales for Mn scavenging of 200 and 20 years, respectively. Yeats and Strain [71], basing their deep-ocean model on fjord observations, estimated a deep-ocean scavenging time scale of 60 years.

5. FRESHWATERS

The processes the oceans disclose in their manganese profiles are also seen at play in lakes and deep rivers. The rate processes involved for producing and removing available Mn(II) in lakes, *mutatis mutandis*, are those relevant in ocean waters. Figure 7A shows a profile of dissolved Mn in Lake Bret measured in two different ways (one of them in situ) [72]. The consequences of stratification, with oxic surface water and anoxic or suboxic deep waters, are evident in the high dissolved Mn concentration of 7 μM below 15 m depth. Oxidative loss of Mn(II) dominates in the surface oxygenated waters. Reductive dissolution of MnO_x in anoxic waters and sediments dominates in the deep.

Striking profiles of dissolved Mn have been observed and interpreted quantitatively by Wehrli et al. [73] for the sediments and the immediately overlying waters of Lake Sempach, a highly eutrophic lake (Fig. 7B). Rates of Mn redox cycling in the deep waters ranged from ~0.5 to 5 mmol m^{-2} day^{-1}, and the half-life of Mn(II) during stratified periods averaged about 1.5 days, indicative of microbially mediated oxidative scavenging. The changing profiles with time reflect seasonal changes in the physical, chemical, and biological dynamics of the lake. The sediments are not at apparent steady state, unlike those of the slowly changing oceans. Consideration of sedimentation fluxes, particle resuspension, redox reactions, and vertical eddy diffusion provided a satisfying quantitative interpretation of the changing profiles with time.

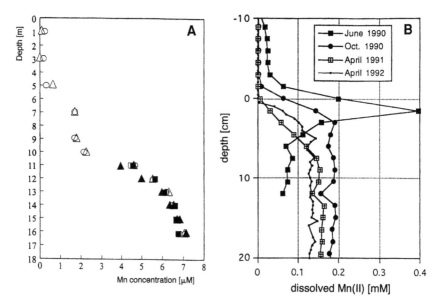

FIG. 7. (A) Depth profile for dissolved manganese in Lake Bret, Switzerland, August 1997 [72]. ■, Voltammetric in situ profiler, with square-wave anodic stripping voltammetry (SWASV); ▲, on-field (pumped) SWASV; □, inductively coupled plasma-atomic emission spectroscopy (ICP); △, ICP, 0.2-μm filtered samples; ○, ICP raw water samples. (B) Profiles of dissolved Mn(II) in sediments and overlying deep water of Lake Sempach, Switzerland [73]. (Reprinted with permission from [73].)

6. CONCLUDING REMARKS

6.1. Processes

In Fig. 8 a generalized view of processes is presented that may govern the distribution and availability of manganese in natural waters. The system illustrated is the ocean. Similar processes are at play in basins, fjords, stratified lakes, and deep estuaries. While the view in Fig. 8 remains a partial one, it may serve to illustrate the rich variety of processes and reactions that research into manganese chemistry in natural waters needs to continue to address. (As complex, if indeed not

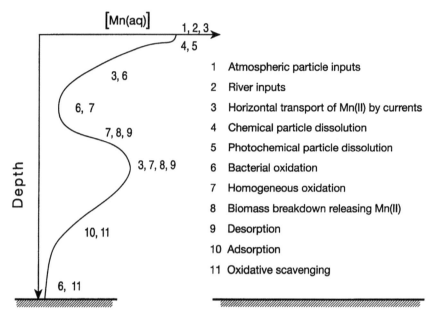

FIG. 8. A generalized illustrative profile for dissolved manganese in ocean waters. A number of important processes observed in ocean (and freshwater) environments are indicated.

more so, are the chemical and biological phenomena of sedimentary and soil environments.) Understanding of manganese distributions and dynamics in natural waters will continue to advance. In general, the rate of change of Mn(II) in water,

$$r_i = \left(\frac{d\,[\mathrm{Mn(II)}]}{dt}\right)$$

is described by $r_T = r_{hom,ox} + r_{het,ox} + r_{bact,ox} + r_{chem,red} + r_{photo,red} + r_{bact,red} + r_{biomass} + r_{adv} + r_{diff}$. Efforts are needed to consider those terms appropriate to each marine or freshwater environment.

6.2. Species

An overview of manganese speciation is presented in Fig. 9, with some indications of processes connecting species in solution and in precipi-

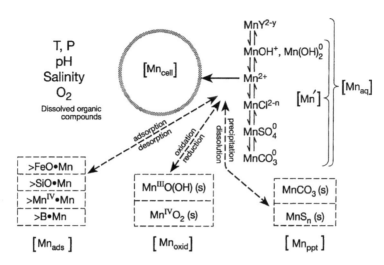

FIG. 9. Overview of manganese speciation in natural waters and some of the processes connecting dissolved, precipitated, and adsorbed forms.

tates or adsorbed forms. The pH, O_2, organic compounds (as reductants and potential ligands), and salinity (dissolved salts), in addition to temperature (T) and pressure (P), are key system parameters.

In the great majority of natural waters Mn^{2+} is the dominant species. In research on availability to phytoplankton, the quantity $[Mn']$, the Mn in water *not bound* to a strong complexing ligand is often the quantity of interest. Oceanic and estuarine diatom clones (*Thalassiosira oceanica* clone 13-1 and *T. pseudonana*, clone 3H) are reported by Sunda and Huntsman [74] to have $[Mn_{cell}]$ values in the range 3×10^{-5} to 5×10^{-4} mol L^{-1} *cell volume*, with diatom population growth rates saturating at about 4–5×10^{-4} mol L^{-1} *cell volume*. The Mn cell concentration was found to depend on *competition* between Mn^{2+} and Cu^{2+} ions in solution for a cell surface binding site. Thus, the availability of Mn(II) to the plankton cell depends not on Mn(II) speciation alone but on competition between metals:

$$MnX_{surface,cell} + Cu^{2+} \leftrightarrow CuX_{surface,cell} + Mn^{2+} \tag{18}$$

Thus, synergy and antagonism between a number of trace metals could prove very important in the oceans [75]. Cu^{2+} activity in seawater is thought to be regulated by strong organic ligand complexing; Mn^{2+}

forms less stable organic complexes than Cu(II) and Zn(II). Future developments in understanding Mn availability holds exciting prospects for multimetal, multiligand dynamics.

ACKNOWLEDGMENTS

The author expresses his heartfelt gratitude for the wise advice and challenging questions of his colleague and friend Professor Werner Stumm, who first introduced him to the chemistry of manganese in the aquatic environment, initiating "mein Leben mit Mangan." I wish to thank my Mn and Fe research "brothers and sisters in arms", Jessie Ho, Jack Smith, Frank Birkner, Halka Bilinski, François Morel, Michael Kessick, George Jackson, Jasenka Vuceta, Tom Holm, Jim Pankow, Windsor Sung, Lisa Anderson, Alan Stone, Simon Davies, Liyuan Liang, Yigal Erel, Michael Scott, Ken Klewicki, and Tom Lloyd, for joint efforts in learning about the aquatic chemistry of elements 25 and 26. Recent discussions on manganese research with Ken Bruland, Brad Tebo, Ken Johnson, Ken Coale, and Alan Stone were very helpful. Research support from the Mellon Foundation, the General Motors Research Foundation, and the U.S. National Science Foundation is gratefully acknowledged.

REFERENCES

1. J. Emsley, *The Elements*, Clarendon Press, Oxford, 1989.
2. P. A. Cox, *The Elements on Earth*, Oxford University Press, New York, 1995.
3. J. J. R. Fraústo da Silva and R. J. P. Williams, *The Biological Chemistry of the Elements*, Clarendon Press, Oxford, 1991.
4. W. Stumm and J. J. Morgan, *Aquatic Chemistry*, Wiley-Interscience, New York, 1996.
5. F. A. Cotton and G. Wilkinson, *Advanced Inorganic Chemistry*, Interscience, New York, 1972.
6. D. F. Shriver, P. W. Atkins, and C. H. Langford, *Inorganic Chemistry*, Freeman, New York, 1990.

7. C. R. Myers and K. H. Nealson, *Geochim. Cosmochim. Acta, 52,* 2927–2932 (1988).
8. S. Emerson, S. Kalhorn, L. Jacobs, B. M. Tebo, K. H. Nealson, and R. A. Rossen, *Geochim. Cosmochim. Acta, 46,* 1073–1079 (1982).
9. B. M. Tebo, W. C. Ghiorse, L. G. van Waasbergen, P. L. Siering, and R. Caspi in *Geomicrobiology* (J. F. Banfield and K. H. Nealson, eds.), Mineralogical Society of America, 1997, pp. 225–266.
10. E. V. Grill, *Geochim. Cosmochim. Acta, 46,* 2435–2446 (1982).
11. U. Von Stackelberg, in *Manganese Mineralization: Geochemistry and Mineralogy of Terrestrial and Marine Deposits* (K. Nicholson, J. R. Hein, B. Bühn, and S. Dasgupta, eds.), The Geological Society, London, 1997, pp. 153–176.
12. J. R. Hein, A. Koschinsky, P. Halbach, F. T. Mannheim, M. Bau, J. K. Kang, and N. Lubick, in *Manganese Mineralization: Geochemistry and Mineralogy of Terrestrial and Marine Deposits* (K. Nicholson, J. R. Hein, B. Bühn, and S. Dasgupta, eds.), The Geological Society, London, 1997, pp. 123–138.
13. J. M. Edmond, C. Measures, R. E. McDuff, L. H. Chan, R. Collier, B. Grant, L. I. Gordon, and J. B. Corliss, *Earth Planet. Sci. Lett., 46,* 1–18 (1979).
14. J. M. Edmond, C. Measures, B. Mangum, B. Grant, F. R. Sclater, R. Collier, A. Hudson, L. I. Gordon, and J. B. Corliss, *Earth Planet. Sci. Lett., 46,* 19–30 (1979).
15. K. L. Von Damm, J. M. Edmond, B. Grant, C. I. Measures, B. Walden, and R. F. Weiss, *Geochim. Cosmochim. Acta, 49,* 2197–2200 (1985).
16. K. L. Von Damm, J. M. Edmond, C. I. Measures, and B. Grant, *Geochim. Cosmochim. Acta, 49,* 2221–2237.
17. R. M. Garrels and F. T. Mackenzie, *Evolution of Sedimentary Rocks,* Norton, New York, 1971, p. 16f.
18. J. M. Martin and M. Maybeck, *Mar. Chem., 7,* 173–206 (1979).
19. J. R. Donat and K. W. Bruland, in *Trace Elements in Natural Waters* (B. Salbu and E. Steinnes, eds.), CRC Press, Boca Raton, 1995, pp. 247–282.
20. D. S. Cronan in *The Sea* (E. D. Goldberg, ed.), Wiley-Interscience, New York, 1974, pp. 491–536.
21. B. L. Lewis and W. M. Landing, *Deep-Sea Res., 38,* Suppl. 2, S773–S803 (1991).

22. M. L. Bender, G. P. Klinkhammer, and D. W. Spencer, *Deep-Sea Res.*, *24*, 799–812 (1977).

23. Y. Erel and J. J. Morgan, *Geochim. Cosmochim. Acta*, *55*, 1807–1813 (1991).

24. H. D. Holland, *The Chemical Evolution of the Atmosphere and Oceans*, Princeton Univ. Press, Princeton, 1984.

25. R. Osterberg, *Nature*, *249*, 382–383 (1974).

26. W. M. Landing and B. L. Lewis, in *Black Sea Oceanography* (E. Izdar and J. W. Murray, eds.), Kluwer Academic, Dordrecht, 1991, pp. 125–160.

27. M. Whitfield and D. R. Turner, *Nature*, *278*, 132–137 (1979).

28. V. L. Pecoraro, *Manganese Redox Enzymes*, VCH, New York, 1992, p. v.

29. J. W. Murray, L. S. Balestrieri, and B. Paul, *Geochim. Cosmochim. Acta*, *48*, 1237–1247 (1984).

30. R. G. Burns and V. M. Burns, in *Marine Minerals* (R. G. Burns, ed.), Mineralogical Society of America, Washington, D.C., 1979, pp. 1–46.

31. A. Manceau and J. M. Combes, *Phys. Chem. Minerals*, *15*, 283–295 (1988).

32. R. Hypolito, R. Giovanoli, V. Valarelli, and S. Andrade, *An. Acad. Bras. Ci.*, *65*, 377–387 (1993).

33. J. W. Murray, J. G. Dillard, R. Giovanoli, H. Moers, and W. Stumm, *Geochim. Cosmochim. Acta*, *49*, 463–470 (1985).

34. J. D. Hem and C. J. Lind, *Geochim. Cosmochim. Acta*, *47*, 2037–2046 (1983).

35. M. Kessick and J. J. Morgan, *Environ. Sci. Technol.*, *9*, 157–159 (1975).

36. L. M. Gramm-Osipov, in *Manganese Mineralization: Geochemistry and Mineralogy of Terrestrial and Marine Deposits* (K. Nicholson, J. R. Hein, B. Bühn, and S. Dasgupta, eds.), The Geological Society, London, 1997, pp. 301–308.

37. J. E. Kostka, G. W. Luther III, and K. H. Nealson, *Geochim. Cosmochim. Acta*, *59*, 885–894 (1995).

38. J. K. Klewicki and J. J. Morgan, *Environ. Sci. Technol.*, *32*, 2916–2922 (1998).

39. M. D. Aitken and R. L. Irvine, *Archiv. Biochem. Biophys.*, *276*, 405–414 (1990).

40. D. R. Turner, M. Whitfield, and A. G. Dickson, *Geochim. Cosmochim. Acta*, *45*, 855–881 (1981).

41. R. Carpenter, *Geochim. Cosmochim. Acta*, *47*, 875 (1983).

42. R. H. Byrne, L. R. Kump, and K. J. Cantrell, *Mar. Chem.*, *25*, 163–181 (1988).

43. E. D. Goldberg, in *The Sea* (M. N. Hill, ed.), Wiley-Interscience, New York, 1963, p. 3f.

44. J. D. Hem, *Chemical Equilibria and the Rates of Manganese Oxidation*, U.S. Geol. Survey Water Supply Paper 1667A, 1963.

45. J. J. Morgan and W. Stumm, The Role of Multivalent Metal Oxides in Limnological Transformations, As Exemplified by Iron and Manganese. *Proc. 2nd Int. Water Poll. Res. Conf.* (Tokyo), Pergamon, Oxford; 1965, pp. 103–131.

46. J. J. Morgan, in *Principles and Applications in Water Chemistry* (S. Faust and J. V. Hunter, eds.), John Wiley, New York, 1967, p. 606f.

47. D. Diem and W. Stumm, *Geochim. Cosmochim. Acta*, *48*, 151–173 (1984).

48. S. H. R. Davies and J. J. Morgan, *J. Colloid Inter. Sci.*, *129*, 63–77 (1989).

49. P. J. Von Langen, K. S. Johnson, K. H. Coale, and V. A. Elrod, *Geochim. Cosmochim. Acta*, *61*, 4945–4954 (1997).

50. P. G. Brewer, in *Chemical Oceanography* (J. P. Riley and G. Skirrow, eds.), Academic Press, New York, 1975, p. 465f.

51. W. Sung and J. J. Morgan, *Geochim. Cosmochim. Acta*, *45*, 2377–2383 (1981).

52. S. H. R. Davies, *Mn(II) Oxidation in the Presence of Metal Oxides*, Thesis, California Institute of Technology, 1985.

53. S. H. R. Davies, in *Geochemical Processes at Mineral Surfaces* (J. A. Davis and K. F. Hayes, eds.), American Chemical Society, Washington, D.C., 1986, p. 490f.

54. D. Hastings and S. Emerson, *Geochim. Cosmochim. Acta*, *50*, 1819–1824 (1986).

55. B. M. Tebo and S. Emerson, *Biogeochemistry*, *2*, 149–161 (1986).

56. P. W. L. Vojak, C. Edwards, and M. V. Jones, *Estuarine Coastal Shelf Sci.*, *20*, 661–671 (1985).

57. W. G. Sunda and S. A. Huntsman, *Limnol. Oceanogr.*, *32*, 552–564 (1987).

58. W. G. Sunda and S. A. Huntsman, *Limnol. Oceanogr.*, *35*, 325–338 (1990).

59. J. W. Moffett and J. Ho, *Geochim. Cosmochim. Acta*, *60*, 3415–3424 (1996).

60. W. G. Sunda and S. A. Huntsman, *Deep-Sea Res.*, *35*, 1297–1317 (1988).

61. J. P. Cowen, G. J. Massoth, and R. A. Feely, *Deep-Sea Res.*, *37*, 1619–1637 (1990).

62. K. W. Mandernack and B. M. Tebo, *Geochim. Cosmochim. Acta*, *57*, 3907–3923 (1993).

63. B. M. Tebo, *Deep-Sea Res.*, *38*, Suppl. 2, S883–S905 (1991).

64. A. T. Stone and J. J. Morgan, *Environ. Sci. Technol.*, *18*, 617–624 (1984).

65. W. G. Sunda and D. J. Kieber, *Nature*, *367*, 62–64 (1994).

66. T. D. Waite and R. Szymczak, *J. Geophys. Res.*, *98*, 2361–2369 (1993).

67. K. H. Nealson, C. R. Myers, and B. B. Wimpee, *Deep-Sea Res.*, *38*, Suppl. 2, S907–S920 (1991).

68. Y. Nozaki, *EoS, Trans. Am. Geophys. Union*, *78*, 221 (1997).

69. K. W. Bruland, K. J. Orians, and J. P. Cowen, *Geochim. Cosmochim. Acta*, *58*, 3171–3182 (1994).

70. K. S. Johnson, K. H. Coale, W. M. Berelson, and M. Gordon, *Geochim. Cosmochim. Acta*, *60*, 1291–1299 (1996).

71. P. A. Yeats and P. M. Strain, *Estuarine Coastal Shelf Sci.*, *31*, 11–24 (1990).

72. M.-L. Tercier-Waeber, C. Belmond-Hebert, and J. Buffle, *Environ. Sci. Technol.*, *32*, 1515–1521 (1998).

73. B. Wehrli, G. Friedl, and A. Manceau, in *Aquatic Chemistry* (C. P. Huang, C. R. O'Melia, and J. J. Morgan, eds.), American Chemical Society, Washington, D.C., 1995, pp. 111–134.

74. W. G. Sunda and S. A. Huntsman, *Limnol. Oceanogr.*, *28*, 924–934 (1983).

75. K. W. Bruland, J. R. Donat, and D. A. Hutchins, *Limnol. Oceanogr.*, *36*, 1555–1577 (1991).

2

Manganese Transport in Microorganisms

Valeria Cizewski Culotta

Departments of Environmental Health Sciences
and Biochemistry, Johns Hopkins University
School of Public Health, 615 N. Wolfe Street,
Baltimore, MD 21205, USA

1. INTRODUCTION AND OVERVIEW

As is the case with all living organisms, microorganisms require trace levels of manganese for survival. The list of enzymes that rely on manganese for activity is numerous. Manganese is utilized by certain oxygen-consuming organisms as the cofactor for the antioxidant defense enzymes catalase and superoxide dismutase. Photosynthetic bacteria employ manganese in oxygen evolution processes, and manganese-dependent enzymes have been implicated in diverse metabolic pathways including DNA synthesis, sugar metabolism, and protein modification by glycosylation. The number of manganese-dependent enzymes utilized by microorganisms is far too extensive for inclusion in this chapter focusing on metal transport. Yet a detailed presentation of a subset of such enzymes can be found elsewhere in this volume of *Metal Ions in Biological Systems*.

Because manganese performs so many vital cellular functions, all organisms have evolved with specialized systems devoted to the uptake and acquisition of this trace metal. Accumulation of manganese must also fall under tight control, since the metal is potentially toxic. Therefore, in many instances the uptake of manganese is regulated by the bioavailability of the metal. In this chapter, examples will be provided for both bacterial and fungal manganese transporters that are activated or repressed in response to metal ion availability. In certain cases, the molecular basis of this regulation is understood, and both transcriptional and posttranslational levels of control are evident.

In addition to the uptake of manganese across the cell surface, this metal needs to be transported within the cell lumen, particularly in the case of eukaryotes where the cell is compartmentalized into specialized organelles. Using the fungi *Saccharomyces cerevisiae* as a model, several intracellular membrane-bound proteins have been identified that participate in the partitioning of the metal between organelle and cytosolic compartments.

The genes and proteins that function in the microbial uptake and intracellular trafficking of metal ions are just now beginning to be unraveled. In many instances, information on manganese uptake is restricted to literature on the biochemistry of the transport process, where the relevant genes and proteins remain enigmatic. Therefore, this chapter will begin with a historical perspective regarding the biochemistry of manganese transport in microbes, followed by an in-depth overview of the limited cases in which the manganese transport process has been characterized at the molecular level.

2. BIOCHEMICAL STUDIES IN BACTERIA

From 1970 to the mid-1980s, a number of manganese transport systems were reported for gram-negative and gram-positive bacteria. The following represents an overview of those manganese transport systems that have been well characterized at the biochemical level in whole cells and/or isolated membranes.

2.1. *Bacillus subtilis*

Bacillus subtilis is highly dependent on manganese for sporulation, and studies in the Silver laboratory have demonstrated that manganese uptake in this organism is regulated by changes in life cycle and in metal bioavailability (reviewed in [1]). Under conditions of manganese starvation, *B. subtilis* develops a strong capacity for manganese uptake and cells rapidly accumulate the metal upon supplementation of manganese to the growth medium [2]. The metal hyperaccumulates and, in response, manganese uptake is subsequently depressed to maintain proper manganese homeostasis [2]. When exposed to physiological levels of manganese, a constant rate of metal uptake was observed during logarithmic growth of *B. subtilis*, which was repressed during approach to stationary phase. Upon sporulation, a second phase of manganese accumulation was induced [3]. Under all of these conditions, manganese uptake showed energy and temperature dependence, and the variations in metal accumulation that accommodated changes in growth phase or metal status reflected alterations in V_{max}, rather than K_m, of uptake [2,3]. Hence, a single regulatable transport system has been implicated. The same saturable manganese transporter has been examined in vitro in isolated membranes [4]. This transporter is not inhibited by calcium or by magnesium [4], yet appears to be the primary route of cadmium uptake in *B. subtilis* [5].

Although the mechanism underlying the regulation of manganese transport in *Bacillus* is not completely understood, recent work in the laboratory of Helmann suggests the involvement of a "manganese regulon" [6]. Helmann has discovered MntR, a putative regulator of manganese transport that responds to changes in manganese bioavailability. Possible targets for regulation by MntR include a member of the Nramp family of metal transporters [7] and a putative ABC metal transport protein [6,8].

2.2. *Escherichia coli*

Work in the laboratory of Silver additionally led to the identification of an active transport system for manganese in *Escherichia coli*. As is the case with *B. subtilis*, manganese uptake in this organism is energy- and temperature-dependent and is not inhibited by calcium or magnesium, although a slight inhibition was observed with iron and cobalt [9,10].

2.3. *Staphylococcus aureus*

Studies by Silver on cadmium accumulation in *S. aureus* led to the characterization of a manganese transporter in this organism. In iso-

lated membrane vesicles or in whole cells, an energy-dependent manganese uptake system was evaluated that was effectively competed by
cadmium, but not zinc, ions [11,12]. Hence, as is the case with *B. subtilis*,
the *S. aureus* manganese transporter is the principal route of cadmium
exposure.

2.4. *Lactobacillus plantarum*

Lactic acid bacteria accumulate remarkably high concentrations of
manganese. *Lactobacillus plantarum* accumulates 30–35 mM concentrations of manganese [13]. Since manganese can act as a scavenger of
superoxide, the extraordinarily high level of manganese accumulated
in *L. plantarum* bypasses the requirement for a superoxide dismutase
[14,15]. Studies by Archibald and Duong have revealed a specific active
transport system for manganese in *L. plantarum* that is driven by a
membrane proton gradient [16]. Interestingly, the calculated K_m for manganese uptake was comparable to that observed for *E. coli*, *S. aureus*,
and *B. subtilis*; however, in accordance with the high demand for manganese in *L. plantarum*, the velocity of uptake was orders of magnitude
higher than other bacterial systems characterized [16]. As is the case
with *S. aureus* and *B. subtilis*, cadmium uptake in *L. plantarum* involves the manganese transporter. Uptake of both cadmium and manganese is induced by metal starvation, suggesting the existence of a
regulatory feedback loop for control of manganese transport [16].

3. GENES CONTROLLING MANGANESE ACCUMULATION IN BACTERIA

3.1. *Synechocystis*

The unicellular cyanobacterium *Synechocystis* 6803 utilizes a tetra-
manganese cluster to evolve molecular oxygen during photosynthetic
growth. In a screen for photosynthetic mutants of *Synechocystis*,
Pakrasi and co-workers identified the MntABC manganese transporter
complex that shows significant homology to polypeptide components of
the ABC superfamily of transporter proteins [17]. MntA appears to
represent the ATP-binding cytoplasmic protein; MntB is a possible

integral membrane protein, and MntC may be the periplasmic component that captures the metal. Together, these three subunits form the
manganese permease at the cell surface [17]. Deletion of this transporter resulted in a growth defect that was readily rescued upon supplementation of micromolar concentrations of manganese, suggesting the
existence of a second transporter for manganese [18]. Unlike the
MntABC manganese transporter that is competed by cadmium, zinc,
and cobalt, this second transporter appears to be specific for manganese. Interestingly, these two transporters are regulated differentially by manganese availability. The MntABC transporter is induced
under manganese starvation conditions whereas the second high-
affinity transporter is induced by micromolar concentrations of the
metal [18]. Currently, there are no reports pertaining to the identification of this second transporter or the trans-acting regulator of manganese transport in *Synechocystis*.

3.2. *Streptococcus*

Streptococci represent important human pathogens. Virulence factors
for *Streptococcus* include members of the ABC superfamily of metal
transporters. In *S. pneumoniae*, Claverys and colleagues discovered the
adc operon that encodes a zinc-transporting ATPase and the *psaA*
operon that encodes an ABC transporter for manganese [19]. Similar to
the *mntABC* operon of *Synechocystis*, the *adc* and *psa* clusters of *Streptococcus* encode an ATP-binding protein, a transmembrane protein and
an additional component that may be a lipoprotein [19]. More recently,
a similar ABC transporter for manganese was described for *S. gordonii*,
encoded by the *sca* operon [20]. Kolenbrander and colleagues noted that
the ScaA transporter acts on both zinc and manganese, but not on other
metals such as copper and magnesium. Furthermore, this ABC transporter for manganese is induced under metal starvation conditions [20].
In both *S. gordonii* and *S. pneumoniae*, deletion of the manganese
transporters resulted in growth arrest, and the *psa* gene cluster has
been shown to be important for virulence [19]. The essential role of
manganese in the pathogenicity of *Streptococcus* is not completely understood, but may reflect the protective antioxidant effect of this metal
when the organism switches from a predominantly anaerobic niche to

the oxygen-rich environment of the oral cavity [19]. In any case, agents that specifically target ABC manganese transporters represent potential therapeutic avenues for the treatment of infections from *Streptococcus*.

3.3. *Mycobacterium*

Mycobacterium tuberculosis and *M. leprae* are life-threatening pathogens in humans. The pathogenicity of these organisms depends in part on their ability to multiply within host macrophages. Susceptibility to infection from *Mycobacterium* has been associated with the mammalian metal transporter Nramp (*n*atural *r*esistance *a*ssociated *m*acrophage *p*rotein), which is localized in the phagosomes of macrophages [21–26]. Mammalian Nramp1 is believed to deprive the mycobacterium of the redox-active metals iron and manganese, as part of the oxygen radical defense against these pathogens [27]. Recently, it was proposed by Agranoff and Krishna that *Mycobacterium* may counteract this process through the action of bacterial encoded Nramp transporters [28]. Indeed, a putative "Mramp" transporter has been identified in *M. tuberculosis* through analysis of the genome sequence. A model has been put forth in which bacterial Mramp acts to supply the mycobacteria with phagosomal manganese and/or iron, while mammalian Nramp operates to remove these ions from the organelle [28]. This model is illustrated in Fig. 1. Parasite pathogenicity may be strongly influenced by the effective balance of these two metal transporters. The precise contribution of *Mycobacterium* Mramp to manganese transport and virulence awaits further investigation.

4. GENES CONTROLLING MANGANESE ACCUMULATION IN YEAST

As is the case with bacteria, the unicellular eukaryote *Saccharomyces cerevisiae* relies on manganese for growth. Essential roles for the metal include antioxidant defense, protein processing in the mitochondria, protein glycosylation in the secretory pathway, and cell division. Anal-

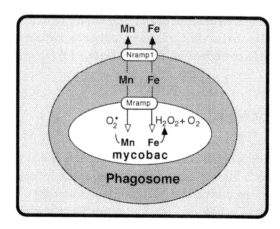

FIG. 1. Possible role of Nramp transporters in resistance to infection from mycobacterium. Shown is a cartoon of a macrophage cell with intracellular phagosome harboring a mycobacterium ("mycobac"). According to the model of Agranoff and Krishna [28], the phagosome Nramp1 transporter depletes the organelle of manganese and perhaps iron atoms as well, while a newly defined Nramp homolog in *M. tuberculosis* "Mramp" works in opposite to restore these metals to the phagosome. The redox-active metals may protect the parasite by scavenging superoxide, as shown.

ysis of yeast mutants defective in any one of these four cellular functions has led to the identification of genes controlling the uptake and intracellular trafficking of manganese ions. The characterization of these genes will be described in some detail herein.

4.1. The Smf1p Metal Transporter

The acquisition of manganese in yeast cells involves the action of Smf1p, a member of the Nramp family of metal transporters. Smf1p was originally identified as one of two genes that when overexpressed would suppress a manganese-dependent defect in processing of mitochondrial proteins [29]. Subsequently, Supek and colleagues identified Smf1p as a high-affinity transporter for manganese [30]. Like all members of the Nramp family of metal transporters, Smf1p contains 12 transmembrane (TM) spanning domains and a consensus transporter signature sequence found in a predicted cytosolic loop between TM8 and TM9 [7].

Members of the Nramp family have been found in diverse eukaryotes and in bacteria [7]. The baker's yeast contains three Nramp members: Smf1p, Smf2p, and Smf3p [7]. Like Smf1p, Smf2p contributes to cellular accumulation of manganese [30], whereas the function of Smf3p has not been determined. The role of the mammalian and fungal Nramp proteins is indeed conserved, as Pinner et al. have demonstrated that mammalian Nramp2 can complement the manganese starvation phenotype of a yeast mutant lacking Smf1p and Smf2p [31].

We identified Smf1p in a screen for genes responsible for suppressing oxidative damage in yeast cells lacking superoxide dismutase 1 (SOD1) [30]. *sod1* mutants are extremely sensitive to oxygen toxicity and rely on the redox activity of manganese ions to support aerobic growth [32]. We noted that a mutation in the *S. cerevisiae* BSD2 gene (*b*ypass *S*OD1 *d*efect) would overcome all of the oxidative damage of an *sod1* mutant by enhancing cellular accumulation of manganese [33]. Manganese is believed to essentially act as a mimic for SOD1 by neutralizing reactive oxygen species [13,15,34]. Our subsequent studies demonstrated that Bsd2p itself is not a manganese transporter but acts indirectly at a distance to downregulate the uptake of manganese from the cell surface [33]. Through a gene cloning strategy, we identified Smf1p as the target of Bsd2p action [33]. In wild-type cells, Bsd2p stifles Smf1p and the cells accumulate little manganese, but in *bsd2* mutants, Smf1p is activated, and the cells accumulate high levels of the metal [33]. The regulation of Smf1p by Bsd2p and manganese ions will be the subject of discussion in Sec. 4.3 below.

Smf1p is not specific for manganese. When this transporter is activated by *bsd2* mutations, the cells hyperaccumulate copper and cadmium ions, as well as manganese [33]. This broad specificity for metals is not unique to yeast Nramp. Mammalian Nramp2 (also known as DCT1) transports diverse metals, including the essential ions manganese, iron, zinc, and copper and the nonessential metals cadmium and lead [35].

4.2. The Smf2p Metal Transporter

Overall, Smf1p and Smf2p share nearly 49% identity at the amino acid level. However, identity is restricted to the hydrophobic domains, whereas the hydrophilic regions are not well conserved. Like Smf1p, overexpression of Smf2p can suppress a manganese-dependent step in mitochondrial protein processing [29], suggesting that Smf2p can also act on manganese. We found that Smf2p can additionally contribute to cellular accumulation of cadmium and copper and, like Smf1p, Smf2p falls under negative regulation of Bsd2p [36]. Together these findings suggest that Smf1p and Smf2p are redundant metal transporters. However, several lines of evidence argue against this notion. First, although both transporters act on manganese, copper, and cadmium, the consequences of metal accumulation are different. Only manganese accumulation by Smf1p can suppress oxidative damage in yeast lacking SOD1, and only copper and cadmium accumulation by Smf1p leads to metal toxicity [30]. Second, Smf2p contributes to cobalt accumulation, but Smf1p does not [30]. Third, we find that these transporters localize to distinct cellular compartments. Smf1p can be found at the cell surface, whereas Smf2p is confined to intracellular vesicles [36]. Therefore, we conclude that the action of Smf1p leads to the direct uptake of metals from the growth medium into a soluble, perhaps cytosolic compartment where the metal is prone to cause toxicity and mimic the actions of cytosolic SOD1. In comparison, the metal transported by Smf2p may be sequestered in intracellular vesicles.

4.3.   Regulation of Smf1p and Smf2p

The Bsd2p regulator of Smf1p and Smf2p is localized in the endoplasmic reticulum (ER) [30]. We found that a deletion of *BSD2* leads to hyperaccumulation of the Smf1 and Smf2 polypeptides without affecting mRNA levels. *BSD2* does not control these transporters at the transcriptional level but rather at the levels of protein stability and protein sorting through the secretory pathway [37]. Under normal growth conditions, Smf1p and Smf2p move directly from the Golgi to the vacuole where these metal transporters are degraded by vacuolar proteases. This trafficking to the vacuole is dependent on the presence of Bsd2p in the ER [37]. However, in *bsd2* mutants, the proteins fail to arrive at the vacuole and the bulk of Smf1p and Smf2p remain within compartments of the secretory pathway. In the case of Smf1p, a small fraction of the transporter can also be found at the cell surface, which is presumably responsible for the hyperaccumulation of metals in strains lacking Bsd2p [37].

Interestingly, Smf1p and Smf2p are also regulated by the availability of manganese in the growth medium [37]. When manganese is abundant, Smf1p and Smf2p are targeted to the vacuole for degradation in a Bsd2p-dependent manner. However, when cells are starved for manganese, these Nramp transporters fail to arrive at the vacuole. The bulk of Smf1p instead moves to the cell surface, while Smf2p remains at an intracellular location [36,37]. The downregulation of Smf1p and Smf2p is specific for manganese ions. A slight effect was observed with iron treatment, but supplementation with copper, zinc, and cobalt failed to induce the degradation of the Nramp transporters by vacuolar proteases [36,37].

Although the precise mechanism by which metals and Bsd2p regulate Smf1 is unknown, our recent evidence invokes a model in which the fate of Smf1p is dictated by conformational changes in the transporter protein (Fig. 2). By site-directed mutagenesis, we noted that only an active Smf1p transporter is regulated by Bsd2p and manganese ions. Mutations directed at either the well-conserved TM4 or the transport consensus sequence of Smf1p (i.e., G190A and G424A) abolished transport activity. These nonfunctional Smf1p molecules also failed to arrive at the vacuole in response to manganese ions and Bsd2p [38]. Therefore, transporter competence is necessary for regulation of Smf1p by Bsd2p and manganese ions. A second class of Smf1p mutants were identified (i.e., Q419A and E423A) that are wild type for manganese transport and regulation by Bsd2p; however, these mutants did not respond to changes in manganese availability. These "nonresponsive" mutants of Smf1p appear frozen in a conformation that is always recognized by Bsd2p for degradation in the vacuole, regardless of the metal ion status [38].

Together, these findings have led us to develop a two-step model for the regulation of Smf1p at the level of protein sorting (Fig. 2). Under physiological conditions when manganese is abundant, the transporter maintains an active conformation that is recognized by Bsd2p for targeting to the vacuole. The binding of manganese ions directly to the transporter may be responsible for inducing this conformation. The nonfunctional mutants of Smf1p cannot adopt this manganese-dependent conformation and therefore escape vacuolar degradation. Yet failure to

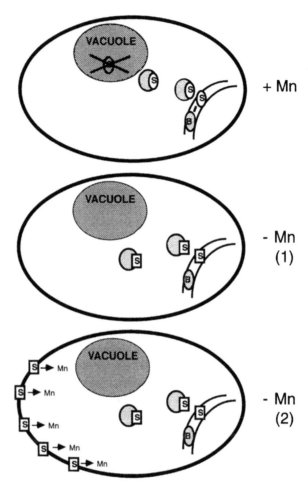

FIG. 2.   Regulation of yeast Smf1p by manganese ions. Shown is a model for
how the Nramp transporter Smf1p may be regulated at the level of protein
sorting. In the presence of manganese (+Mn), Smf1p adopts an active conformation (oval-shaped) that is recognized by Bsd2p in the endoplasmic reticulum for
trafficking to the vacuole where Smf1p is subsequently degraded. When cells are
starved for metals, Smf1p is proposed to adopt a unique conformation (rectangu-
lar) that escapes recognition by Bsd2p and fails to arrive at the vacuole (−Mn,
1). In a second step (−Mn, 2), this conformation of Smf1p signals movement of
the transporter to the cell surface where manganese uptake occurs.

arrive at the vacuole is not sufficient to direct Smf1p to the cell surface, since the bulk of this transporter remains at an intracellular location in *bsd2* mutants. A second step in Smf1p regulation must ensue, in which transporter conformation unique to the metal starvation state (e.g., an apo Smf1p) is recognized by the sorting machinery for plasma membrane localization. Both the nonfunctional and nonresponsive classes of Smf1p mutants appear incapable of adopting the conformation needed for movement to the cell surface (Fig. 2).

Regardless of the precise mechanism, the regulation of Smf1p by manganese ions is novel. Other metal transporters that have been investigated in yeast (e.g., Ctr1p for copper, Ztr1p for zinc, Ftr1p for iron) are primarily regulated at the transcriptional level by metal ion status [39–43]. There is some evidence for control of Ctr1p and Ztr1p by protein degradation, but this is only induced by toxic concentrations of the metal [44,45]. The tight control of Smf1p by physiological manganese may be particularly important for this transporter that recognizes both essential (e.g., manganese) and nonessential (e.g., cadmium) metal ions. When manganese ions are in ample supply, the bulk of Smf1p is degraded in the vacuole to prevent cellular accumulation of toxic metal ions. However, when cells are starved for manganese, the protein is rapidly directed to the cell surface where metal uptake can occur. In this manner, the cell can rapidly respond to changes in manganese ion status without the need for new protein synthesis.

5. GENES CONTROLLING THE INTRACELLULAR TRANSPORT AND TRAFFICKING OF MANGANESE IONS IN YEAST

In an eukaryotic organism such as *S. cerevisiae*, the compartmentalization of the cell by intracellular membranes poses a problem to nutrient trafficking. Metal ions such as manganese must be widely distributed within the cell for the activation of enzymes at diverse cellular locations. This problem in part has been solved by the evolution of intracellular transporters or trafficking proteins that ensure the proper partitioning of the metal ion. Genetic studies in yeast have led to the identification of numerous proteins of this type that effectively manage

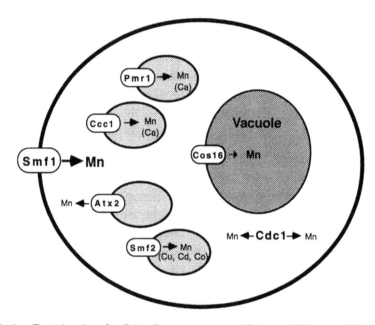

FIG. 3. Proteins involved in the transport and intracellular trafficking of manganese ions in yeast. Shown is a cartoon proposing the action of manganese homeostasis proteins in yeast (for detailed explanation, see text). Light-colored circles represent Golgi-like vesicles where the corresponding proteins were found to reside. Arrows indicate the proposed directions of manganese transport, consistent with genetic studies. However, biochemical studies are required to verify this directionality in the case of Atx2, Smf2, Ccc1, and Cos16. Indicated in parentheses are other ions thought to serve as substrates for the proposed manganese transport systems.

the homeostasis of manganese. The proposed action of these proteins is summarized in Fig. 3.

5.1. Pmr1p: A Manganese-Transporting ATPase in the Golgi

Pmr1p was originally identified as a calcium-transporting P-type ATPase confined to the Golgi [46,47]. We serendipitously isolated Pmr1p as a manganese homeostasis protein that can have a major impact on resistance to oxidative stress. In a search for mutational suppressors of

SOD1 deficiency, we identified mutations in *PMR1* that overcome all of the oxidative damage associated with loss of SOD1 [48]. Inactivation of Pmr1p also caused cells to hyperaccumulate toxic levels of manganese, predominantly in the cytosolic compartment of the cell [48,49]. This accumulation of manganese in the cytosol was responsible for suppressing the oxidative damage associated with loss of SOD1. Pmr1p is now described as the calcium and manganese transporting ATPase confined to the Golgi [50]. This action of Pmr1p is critical for the processing of proteins since a variety of Golgi glycosidases that decorate proteins with complex sugars require manganese as a cofactor [51–57]. As such, yeast cells lacking Pmr1p have a severe defect in protein processing and secretion [47,50].

An apparent communication exists between Pmr1p in the Golgi and Smf1p at the cell surface. A mutation in *PMR1* triggers activation of Smf1p in an attempt to correct the manganese-deficient state of the Golgi. Accordingly, cells containing a mutation in both *PMR1* and *SMF1* are inviable unless grown in the presence of high manganese [58]. The mechanism by which loss of Pmr1p activates Smf1p is not known but does not involve an increase in Smf1 polypeptide levels, as we have seen with Bsd2p regulation of Smf1p [59].

5.2. Ccc1p: A Golgi-Localized Manganese Homeostasis Protein

In an attempt to identify genes that mimic the action of Pmr1p, we isolated *CCC1*, previously shown by Fu et al. to encode a calcium-trafficking protein [60]. We find that, as is the case with Pmr1p, Ccc2p acts on both calcium and manganese to sequester these ions in Golgi-like vesicles [32]; a similar notion has been proposed by Cyert and colleagues [61]. Pmr1p and Ccc2p appear to act synergistically to remove manganese ions from the cytosol. In fact, overexpression of either protein is lethal to cells lacking SOD1, due to depletion of essential cytosolic manganese that helps combat oxidative damage [32]. Yet unlike Pmr1p, defects in Ccc2p fail to activate Smf1p, and also do not impinge on protein processing and secretion [32]. Apparently, Pmr1p and Ccc2p operate at distinct locations of the secretory pathway to partition manganese ions.

5.3. Atx2p: A Golgi-Localized Antagonizer of Pmr1p

ATX2 was isolated in a screen for yeast genes that when overexpressed suppress the oxidative damage associated with loss of SOD1 [62]. The gene was found to encode a Golgi-localized membrane protein that acts in maintaining cytosolic pools of manganese [62]. In essence, Atx2p functions opposite to Pmr1p. While Pmr1p depletes cytosolic manganese, Atx2p helps ensure that cytosolic manganese is adequately maintained.

Although Pmr1p clearly functions to pump manganese ions into the Golgi, the precise role of Atx2p and Ccc2p in metal partitioning is unknown. These two proteins exhibit no homology to known metal transporters. At the present time, we cannot exclude the possibility that Atx2p and Ccc2p are not themselves transporters, but rather regulators of manganese transport and trafficking, as is the case with Bsd2p.

5.4. Cdc1p: A Regulator of Cytosolic Manganese

The *CDC1* gene is essential for yeast viability and was originally assumed to play a vital role in the yeast cell cycle or cell division process [63]. The first clue that *CDC1* is in fact a manganese homeostasis gene stemmed from studies by Loukin and Kung, where a conditional growth defect of a *cdc1* temperature-sensitive (ts) mutant was rescued by manganese supplementation to the growth medium [64]. Supek et al. noted that a *cdc1* ts mutant is sensitive to metal chelators, and could be rescued by overproduction of the manganese transporter, Smf1p [27]. Most recently, a careful analysis by Paidhungat and Garrett revealed that Cdc1p is not directly involved in the cell cycle but rather functions to maintain cytosolic pools of manganese that are essential for division and growth of the yeast cell [58]. The exact role of Cdc1p in cytosolic manganese homeostasis is unknown, but the noted absence of potential membrane-spanning domains strongly indicates that the protein is not a metal transporter [58]. Instead, Cdc1p may represent a cytosolic carrier for manganese or a regulator of other factors that control the transport and intracellular trafficking of this ion.

5.5. Cos16p: A Putative Vacuolar Transporter for Manganese

In a screen for mutational suppressors of the *cdc1* growth defect, Paid-hungat and Garrett isolated a number of genes involved in vacuolar function [65]. The yeast vacuole plays a key role in manganese se-questration and storage [66]. Hence, disruption of vacuole biogenesis is expected to increase the availability of the metal. One of the genes identified was *COS16*, which encodes a membrane protein that localizes to the vacuole [65]. A deletion of *COS16* in combination with a mutation if *PMR1* resulted in severe hypersensitivity to manganese toxicity [65]. Both genes are proposed to participate in the sequestration of intra-cellular manganese. While Pmr1p pumps manganese into the Golgi [47,50], Cos16p has been proposed to sequester manganese in the vac-uole [65]. The precise role of Cos16p in vacuolar transport of manganese has not yet been established.

6. CONCLUSIONS AND DIRECTIONS FOR THE FUTURE

Manganese clearly plays an essential role in a host of cellular processes, and both eukaryotes and prokaryotes have evolved with transport mechanisms that ensure proper acquisition of the metal. Because the ion is potentially toxic and because nonessential metals are often "hitch-hikers" of the transport systems, transporters for manganese are typically regulated in accordance with the bioavailability of the metal ion. In all of the systems described herein for which regulated man-ganese transport has been demonstrated, the uptake of manganese from the environment is activated under conditions of metal starvation and repressed when manganese is abundant.

Although a number of manganese transport systems have been biochemically defined in bacteria, limited information is available on the genes and proteins involved. The years ahead promise to provide new insight into this area through the continual release of genome sequence information. It is expected that much homology will be shared between bacterial and eukaryotic transporters for manganese. Indeed, the manganese transport proteins identified thus far in bacteria are members of large families of transporters common to eukaryotes and prokaryotes, e.g., the ABC-type transporters and the Nramp metal transport proteins. P-type ATPase transporters for manganese are also expected to be revealed, as such proteins play well-documented roles in the bacterial acquisition or extrusion of cadmium, copper, and zinc ions (reviewed in [28]).

Multiple genes involved in the transport and trafficking of manganese ions have been identified for yeast; however, we have just begun to scratch the surface on our understanding of how this ion is handled in a compartmentalized eukaryotic cell. For example, how is manganese transported to the mitochondria for activation of proteins such as SOD2? What roles do the Cdc1, Atx2, and Ccc1 proteins play in the intracellular trafficking of manganese? Furthermore, are there intracellular escort proteins for this metal? Recently, a new family of proteins, termed metallochaperones, have been discovered that function in the cytosolic trafficking of copper ions to distinct cellular targets [67–72]. It is expected that a similar class of metallochaperones will emerge that specifically carry manganese ions to the multiple manganese-requiring enzymes residing at diverse cellular locations.

ACKNOWLEDGMENTS

Many of the findings presented here on yeast manganese homeostasis genes were supported by the Johns Hopkins University Center for Environmental Health Sciences and by NIH Grant ES 08996 (to V. C. C.). Deep gratitude is extended to Drs. S. Garrett, J. Helmann, and H. Pakrasi for personal communications.

ABBREVIATIONS

ATP   adenosine 5'-triphosphate
ER   endoplasmic reticulum
Nramp   *n*atural *r*esistance *a*ssociated *m*acrophage *p*rotein
SOD   superoxide dismutase

TM   transmembrane
ts   temperature-sensitive

REFERENCES

1. S. Silver and P. Jasper, in *Microorganisms and Minerals* (E. D. Weinberg, ed.), Marcel Dekker, New York, 1977.
2. S. Fisher, L. Buxbaum, K. Toth, E. Eisenstadt, and S. Silver, *J. Bacteriol.*, *113*, 1373–1380 (1973).
3. E. Eisenstadt, S. Fisher, C. L. Der, and S. Silver, *J. Bacteriol.*, *113*, 1363–1372 (1973).
4. P. Bhattacharyya, *J. Bacteriol.*, *123*, 123–127 (1975).
5. R. A. Laddaga, R. Bessen, and S. Silver, *J. Bacteriol.*, *162*, 1106–1110 (1985).
6. J. D. Helmann, *personal communications*.
7. M. Cellier, G. Prive, A. Belouchi, T. Kwan, V. Rodrigues, W. Chia, and P. Gros, *Proc. Natl. Acad. Sci. USA*, *92*, 10089–10093 (1995).
8. C. A. Doige and G. F. L. Ames, *Annu. Rev. Microbiol.*, *47*, 291–319 (1993).
9. S. Silver, P. Johnseine, and K. King, *J. Bacteriol.*, *104*, 1299–1306 (1970).
10. S. Silver and M. L. Kralovic, *Biochem. Biophys. Res. Commun.*, *34*, 640–645 (1969).
11. R. D. Perry and S. Silver, *J. Bacteriol.*, *150*, 973–976 (1982).
12. Z. Tynecka, Z. Gos, and J. Zajac, *J. Bacteriol.*, *147*, 305–312 (1981).
13. F. S. Archibald and I. Fridovich, *J. Bacteriol.*, *146*, 928–936 (1981).
14. F. S. Archibald and I. J. Fridovich, *J. Bacteriol.*, *145*, 422–451 (1981).
15. F. S. Archibald and I. Fridovich, *Arch. Biochem. Biophys.*, *214*, 452–463 (1982).
16. F. S. Archibald and M. N. Duong, *J. Bacteriol.*, *158*, 1–8 (1984).
17. H. B. Pakrasi and V. V. Bartsevich, *EMBO J.*, *14*, 1845–1853 (1995).
18. V. V. Bartsevich and H. B. Pakrasi, *J. Biol. Chem.*, *271*, 26957–26061 (1996).

19. A. Dintilhac, G. Alloing, C. Granadel, and J. P. Claverys, *Mol. Microbiol.*, *25*, 727–739 (1997).

20. P. E. Kolenbrander, R. N. Andersen, R. A. Baker, and H. F. Jenkinson, *J. Bacteriol.*, *180*, 290–295 (1998).

21. M. Cellier, A. Belouchi, and P. Gros, *Trends Genet.*, *12*, 201–204 (1996).

22. G. Govoni, S. M. Vidal, S. Gauthier, E. Skamene, D. Malo, and P. Gros, *Infect. Immun.*, *64*, 2923–2929 (1996).

23. G. Govoni and P. Gros, *Inflamm. Res.*, *47*, 277–284 (1998).

24. S. Gruenheid, E. Pinner, M. Desjardins, and P. Gros, *J. Exp. Med.*, *185*, 717–730 (1997).

25. S. M. Vidal, D. Malo, K. Vogan, E. Skamene, and P. Gros, *Cell*, *73*, 469–485 (1993).

26. P. G. Atkinson, J. M. Blackwell, and C. H. Barton, *Biochem. J.*, *325*, 779–786 (1997).

27. F. Supek, L. Supekova, H. Nelson, and N. Nelson, *Proc. Natl. Acad. Sci. USA*, *93*, 5105–5110 (1996).

28. D. D. Agranoff and S. Krishna, *Mol. Microb.*, *28*, 403–412 (1998).

29. A. H. West, D. J. Clark, J. Martin, W. Neupert, F. U. Hart, and A. L. Horwich, *J. Biol. Chem.*, *267*, 24625–24633 (1992).

30. X. F. Liu, F. Supek, N. Nelson, and V. C. Culotta, *J. Biol. Chem.*, *272*, 11763–11769 (1997).

31. E. Pinner, S. Gruenheid, M. Raymond, and P. Gros, *J. Biol. Chem.*, *272*, 28933–28938 (1997).

32. P. J. Lapinskas, S. J. Lin, and V. C. Culotta, *Mol. Microbiol.*, *21*, 519–528 (1996).

33. X. F. Liu and V. C. Culotta, *Mol. Cell. Biol.*, *14*, 7037–7045 (1994).

34. K. M. Faulker, I. Stefan, I. Liochev, and I. Fridovich, *J. Biol. Chem.*, *269*, 23471–23476 (1994).

35. H. Gunshin, B. Mackenzie, U. V. Berger, Y. Gushin, M. F. Romero, W. F. Boron, S. Nussberger, J. L. Gollan, and M. A. Hediger, *Nature*, *388*, 482–488 (1997).

36. X. F. Liu and V. C. Culotta, *submitted* (1999).

37. X. F. Liu and V. C. Culotta, *J. Biol Chem.*, *274*, 4863–4868 (1999).

38. X. F. Liu and V. C. Culotta, *submitted* (1999).

39. H. Zhao and D. Eide, *Proc. Natl. Acad. Sci. USA*, *93*, 2454–2458 (1996).

40. H. Zhao and D. Eide, *Mol. Cell. Biol.*, *17*, 5044–5052 (1997).

41. Y. Y. Iwai, M. Serpe, D. Haile, W. Yang, D. J. Kosman, R. D. Klausner, and A. Dancis, *J. Biol. Chem.*, *272*, 17711–17718 (1997).

42. R. Stearman, D. Yuan, Y. Yamaguchi-Iwan, R. D. Klausner, and A. Dancis, *Science*, *271*, 1552–1557 (1996).

43. Y. Yamaguchi-Iwai, R. Stearman, A. Dancis, and R. D. Klausner, *EMBO J.*, *15*, 3377–3384 (1996).

44. C. E. Ooi, E. Rabinovich, A. Dancis, J. S. Bonifacino, and R. D. Klausner, *EMBO J.*, *15*, 3515–3523 (1996).

45. R. S. Gitan, H. Lou, J. Rodgers, M. Broderius, and D. Eide, *J. Biol. Chem.*, *273*, 28617–28624 (1998).

46. A. Antebi and G. R. Fink, *Mol. Biol. Cell*, *3*, 633–654 (1992).

47. H. K. Rudolph, A. Antebi, G. R. Fink, C. M. Buckley, T. E. Dorman, J. LeVitre, L. S. Davidow, J. I. Mao, and D. T. Moir, *Cell*, *58*, 133–145 (1989).

48. P. J. Lapinskas, K. W. Cunningham, X. F. Liu, G. R. Fink, and V. C. Culotta, *Mol. Cell. Biol.*, *15*, 1382–1388 (1995).

49. P. J. Lapinskas. Characterization of genes involved in the homeostasis of oxygen free radicals and metal ions in *Saccharomyces cerevisiae*, PhD dissertation, Johns Hopkins University, 1995.

50. G. Durr, J. Strayle, R. Plemper, S. Elbs, S. K. Klee, P. Catty, D. H. Wolf, and H. K. Rudolph, *Mol. Biol. Cell*, *9*, 1149–1162 (1998).

51. H. Coste, M. B. Martel, G. Azzar, and R. Got, *Biochim. Biophys. Acta*, *814*, 1–7 (1985).

52. A. Haselbeck and R. Schekman, *Proc. Natl. Acad. Sci. USA*, *83*, 2017–2021 (1986).

53. R. Kaufman, M. Swaroop, and P. Murtha-Riel, *Biochemistry*, *33*, 9813–9819 (1994).

54. N. J. Kuhn, S. Ward, and W. S. Leong, *Eur. J. Biochem.*, *195*, 243–250 (1991).

55. T. Nakajima and C. E. Ballou, *Proc. Natl. Acad. Sci. USA*, *72*, 3912–3916 (1975).

56. A. J. Parodi, *J. Biol. Chem.*, *254*, 8343–8352 (1979).

57. B. P. Ram and D. D. Munjal, *CRC Crit. Rev. Biochem.*, *17*, 257–311 (1985).

58. M. Paidhungat and S. Garrett, *Genetics*, *148*, 1777–1786 (1998).

59. X. F. Liu and V. C. Culotta, *unpublished observations*.

60. D. Fu, T. J. Beeler, and T. M. Dunn, *Yeast*, *10*, 515–521 (1994).

61. T. Pozos, I. Sekler, and M. S. Cyert, *Mol. Cell. Biol.*, *16*, 3730–3741 (1996).

62. S. J. Lin and V. C. Culotta, *Mol. Cell. Biol.*, *16*, 6303–6312 (1996).

63. L. Hartwell, J. Culotti, and B. J. Reid, *Genetics*, *74*, 267–286 (1970).

64. S. Loukin and C. Kung, *J. Cell Biol.*, *131*, 1025–1037 (1995).

65. M. Paidhungat and S. Garrett, *Genetics*, *148*, 1787–1798 (1998).

66. L. A. Okorokov, L. P. Lichko, V. M. Kadomtseva, V. P. Kholodenko, V. T. Titovsky, and I. S. Kulaev, *Eur. J. Biochem.*, *75*, 373–377 (1977).

67. J. S. Valentine and E. B. Gralla, *Science*, *278*, 817–818 (1997).

68. S. J. Lin, R. Pufahl, A. Dancis, T. V. O'Halloran, and V. C. Culotta, *J. Biol. Chem.*, *272*, 9215–9220 (1997).

69. V. C. Culotta, L. Klomp, J. Strain, R. Casareno, B. Krems, and J. D. Gitlin, *J. Biol. Chem.*, *272*, 23469–23472 (1997).

70. R. Pufahl, C. Singer, K. L. Peariso, S. J. Lin, P. Schmidt, C. Fahrni, V. C. Culotta, J. E. Penner-Hahn, and T. V. O'Halloran, *Science*, *278*, 853–856 (1997).

71. T. D. Rae, P. J. Schmidt, R. A. Pufahl, V. C. Culotta, and T. V. O'Halloran, *Science*, *in press* (1999).

72. D. M. Glerum, A. Shtanko, and A. Tzagoloff, *J. Biol. Chem.*, *271*, 14504–14509 (1996).

3

Manganese Uptake and Transport in Plants

Zdenko Rengel

Soil Science and Plant Nutrition, Faculty of
Agriculture, The University of Western Australia,
Nedlands WA 6907, Australia

1. INTRODUCTION

Manganese is the eleventh most common element in the earth's crust, with an average concentration of total Mn of 900 mg kg^{-1} [1]. Soils known to cause Mn deficiency to susceptible crops are usually impoverished siliceous and calcareous sandy soils of neutral or alkaline pH that favor chemical and microbial oxidation and immobilization of plant-available Mn^{2+}. However, even these soils contain large reserves of total Mn relative to those removed in crop harvests. Therefore, resulting Mn deficiency of susceptible crops is due to insufficient availability of soil Mn to plants rather than an absolute shortage of soil Mn. Discussion on soil biogeochemistry of Mn is beyond the scope of this chapter; the reader is referred to other sources [2–5]. While Mn availability can range from deficiency to sufficiency to toxicity, this chapter will concentrate on uptake and translocation of Mn in deficient and sufficient conditions. Various other aspects of Mn nutrition can be found elsewhere [6–9].

The variation of Mn concentration in plant tissue can be enormous: in a survey of native species in southwestern Australia, a range from 4 µg Mn g^{-1} dry matter (in *Oxylobium capitatum*, family Fabaceae) to 2180 µg Mn g^{-1} dry matter (in *Phyla nodiflora*, family Verbenaceae) was found [10] (see also [11] for crop and pasture plants). In contrast, the standard figure for sufficient tissue Mn to allow 90% of the maximum growth is 50 µg Mn g^{-1} dry matter [12] or 25–35 µg g^{-1} dry matter [6], and can be as low as 11 µg Mn g^{-1} dry matter for the youngest emerged blades of *Triticum aestivum* [13]. So some plant species have the capacity to take up Mn at high rates, apparently higher than their physiological requirement. Mechanisms underlying these high uptake rates become especially puzzling when species like *Banksia attenuata* and a number of species from the family Proteaceae accumulate Mn to over 300 μg g^{-1} dry matter while growing on soil that is considered deficient in plant-available Mn ($<$2 μg Mn g^{-1} soil in the DTPA extract) [10]. Although it appears likely that capacity of these plants to accumulate Mn is linked to proteoid (cluster) roots that Proteaceae species produce, the exact mechanism remains to be elucidated. However, there is no doubt that chemistry and biology of rhizosphere have a significant influence on plant availability and hence uptake of Mn.

2. AVAILABILITY OF MANGANESE IN THE RHIZOSPHERE

Plant growth is dependent on the availability of water and nutrients and microbial activity in the rhizosphere, which is defined as the soil-root interface consisting of a soil layer varying in thickness between 0.1 and up to a few millimeters depending on the length of root hairs. An exception appears to be *Lupinus angustifolius* with the rhizosphere up to 18 mm in diameter under some conditions [14]. Availability of nutrients in the rhizosphere is controlled by the combined effects of soil properties, plant characteristics, and the interactions of plant roots with microorganisms and the surrounding soil [15].

2.1. Rhizosphere Chemistry

The availability of Mn to plants depends on its oxidation state: the oxidized form (Mn^{4+}) is not available to plants, while the reduced form (Mn^{2+}) is. Generally, oxidation reactions are predominantly biological, while reduction may be either biological or chemical in nature (cf. [16]). When oxygen is depleted from the growing medium, changes in the redox potential occur; in such a case, NO_3^-, Mn, and Fe serve as alternative electron acceptors for microbial respiration and are transformed into reduced ionic species. This process increases the solubility and availability of Mn and Fe.

The chemistry of Mn in soils of high pH where differences in availability of Mn occur is not clear at present. In aerated soils, Mn^{2+}

concentration in soil solution should theoretically decrease 100-fold for every unit of pH increase [1]. However, with various organic compounds capable of complexing Mn and changing solubility equilibria, a decrease in Mn^{2+} concentration with an increase in pH is not that severe (e.g., 5- to 10-fold decrease for a 0.5-unit pH increase [17]). The complexity of the relationship between Mn concentration in soil solution and pH was illustrated by Rule and Graham [18] who used ^{54}Mn to determine soil Mn pools. With an increase in pH, soil Mn pools under *Trifolium repens* actually increased, while pools in soils planted to *Festuca elatior* decreased. So soil supply of Mn is a complex variable that depends not only on soil chemistry but on plant responses as well as the activity of microorganisms.

Exudation of H^+ and organic acids can lower the pH of alkaline soils and thus increase micronutrient availability [19,20]. Since availability of Mn is low at neutral to alkaline pH, acidification of rhizosphere has an important role in mobilizing soil Mn [21]. The pH changes in rhizosphere depend on the buffering capacity of soils, bulk soil pH, nitrogen sources, and other factors ([22] and references therein).

The nature and activity of root exudate components that might be involved in mobilization of Mn are still unclear [9]. Both root and microbial cells exuded a low molecular weight substance that either mobilized Mn in the rhizosphere and/or facilitated transport across the root-cell plasma membrane [23]. The importance of organic acids (e.g., malic and citric) [24] remains unclear because their effectiveness in forming stable complexes with micronutrients is low at high pH [25,26], where Mn deficiency usually occurs. Further research on root exudates effective in mobilizing Mn from the high-pH substrates is warranted.

2.2. Microflora

Organic and inorganic compounds released from roots can stimulate microbial activity in the rhizosphere because the rhizosphere microorganisms derive energy from root exudates and secretions, sloughed-off cells, and other root debris [27]. Bacteria directly supported by root exudates may have a biomass of up to 36% of root dry weight in sand cultures [28]. The significance of microflora in micronutrient uptake, however, is not clear, even though Mn-transforming microbes may have an important role in Mn nutrition of plants, at least on soils with deficient or marginal availability of Mn [16,29,30].

Microorganisms which oxidize Mn [31] will decrease its availability to plants. Indeed, up to 10-fold greater numbers of Mn-oxidizing bacteria (and fewer Mn reducers) have been found on the roots of *Glycine max* in Mn-deficient patches of the crop than on plants from outside these patches [32]. The ratio between Mn-oxidizing and Mn-reducing bacteria may determine the availability of soil Mn to plants. Altering that ratio by inoculating wheat roots with Mn-reducing bacteria might increase Mn uptake and improve growth in Mn-deficient soil [33]. Inoculation of a Mn-deficient soil with the Mn-reducing fluorescent pseudomonad strain 2-79 increased Mn uptake by *Triticum aestivum* [34] and *G. max* [32]. Production of root exudates that are toxic to Mn-oxidizing microorganisms in the rhizosphere also increased Mn availability [35].

While mycorrhizal colonization may be beneficial to the host plant in terms of increased capacity to take up P, Zn, Cu, and some other nutrients, such colonization is generally associated with impaired, rather than improved, Mn nutrition [36,37]. The impairment is brought about by increased ratio of Mn-oxidizing to Mn-reducing microorganisms in the rhizosphere [38].

Comprehensive studies of microbe/plant/micronutrient interactions in soil will improve our understanding of the complex phenomena influencing growth of plants in environments with low availability of Mn and other micronutrients. This knowledge will allow integration of abiotic (soil chemistry, water, etc.) and biotic factors (plants, microorganisms, etc.) into a dynamic agricultural ecosystem and will improve our efforts toward conservation of native flora, including reintroduction of threatened native species into natural habitats.

3. UPTAKE OF MANGANESE BY PLANT CELLS

As Clarkson [39] pointed out in his review more than 10 years ago, the steady stream of research papers dealing with kinetics of Mn uptake and transport was dated in 1960s and since then has almost disappeared. So, while the knowledge on ion transport across plasma membranes as well as kinetics of uptake and transport is expanding tremendously for most nutrients, little is known about Mn. One possible reason for such a situation is that a requirement for Mn in tissue is quite small, despite relatively large tissue concentrations of Mn [6,39]. In addition, the role of free ionic Mn has not yet been described convincingly; there are only a few enzymes that have an absolute requirement for Mn to function properly [7].

Various methods have been used in studying Mn uptake into plant cells. The most frequently used method employs labeled isotope ^{54}Mn (e.g. [23,40–46]). The method that measures proton nuclear magnetic resonance (NMR) relaxation of water [47,48] relies on the interaction between paramagnetic metal cations (Mn^{2+}, Cu^{2+}, Ni^{2+}, Co^{2+}, Fe^{2+}, Fe^{3+}) and the resonating water molecules. In addition, electron paramagnetic resonance (EPR) spectroscopy analysis can be used to quantify the amount of Mn as well as its form in the cytoplasm [49].

Concentration of Mn in soil solution may range from 0.18 to 790 μM [1], even though in soils with poor availability of Mn it can be as low as 0.07 μM [50]. In comparison, the concentration of Mn used in nutrient solutions was frequently around 1 μM, while in some uptake studies concentrations of Mn as high as 1000 μM (e.g. [51]) or even 10 mM [52] have been used, with an obvious question mark as for the applicability of these results to the soil-grown plants.

Recently developed techniques of growing plants in chelator-buffered nutrient solutions [53–57] allowed for a major step forward in studying plant-micronutrient relationships at realistically low ionic activities of micronutrient cations that can constantly be maintained (i.e., buffered) around plant roots, thus mimicking the situation occurring in a soil. Chelator-buffered nutrient solutions have been used to study deficiencies of various micronutrients, including Mn [57,58], because the micronutrient stress of varying severity can be imposed in a predictable and reproducible manner. The calculated Mn^{2+} ionic activity sufficient for optimal growth of *Hordeum vulgare* plants was -8.3 [(as log (Mn^{2+})] (i.e., equivalent to around 5.0 nM Mn^{2+} activity in solutions with 0.4 μM concentration of total Mn) [57].

Plants growing in managed or natural landscapes take up Mn from the soil solution. Since soil solution contains ionic and chelated forms of Mn, Barber [1] has suggested that both forms can be taken up by plants. However, experimental evidence on this point is meager; if anything, it points to the differential kinetics of uptake of the two Mn forms. Free Mn^{2+} was taken up across the root-cell plasma membrane up to 50 times faster than the MnEDTA complex, even when all Mn was supplied as MnEDTA [23] (Table 1). Of course, from such double-labeled experiments ([54]Mn and ^{14}C-labeled EDTA), the ratio of the two labels in tissue could not be used to ascertain whether EDTA was transported across the plasma membrane as a complex with Mn or as Mn-independent moiety.

The proportion of Mn that is complexed may be important [59],

TABLE 1

An Average Uptake Rate of Mn by Various Higher Plant Species as Dependent on Plant Age, Length of the Uptake Period, Microorganisms, Genotype, Plant Age or Supply of Si, Mn, Zn, or P

Plant species	Solution Mn concentration (μM)	Mn uptake rate (μmol g^{-1} root DW day^{-1})	Ref.
Trifolium repens	0.09	0.3–0.8	[72]
Lolium perenne	0.09	0.06–5.0	[72]
Lolium multiflorum	5.5	0.001–0.2	[164]
Hordeum vulgare	100	370[a]	[73]
	20–10000	29–680[a]	[52]
	3.6	1.3–5.9[a]	[39]
	2 MnEDTA	0.2–4.5[a]	[23]
	20	4.7–25	[23]
Zea mays	3.6	2.4–5.3[a]	[40]
Triticum aestivum	0.2–1 MnHEDTA	0.4–7.2[a]	[45]
	0.2–1 MnHEDTA	0.2–7.7[a]	[46]
	1 MnHEDTA	0.5–1.1	[56]
	1 MnHEDTA	0.7–2.6	[80]
	1 MnHEDTA	0.3–2.6	[165]
	0–300 mg Mn/kg soil	0.01–0.1	[166]

[a]Fresh root weight = dry root weight × 15.

together with the nutritional status of plants: under nutrient deficiency, chelation of Mn with EDTA (up to 98% of Mn present in the chelated form) has actually increased Mn uptake [60]. Increased complexation of Mn with EDTA in the nutrient solution (around 45% of total Mn present as a complex) increased accumulation of Mn in *H. vulgare* [59], indicating that not only Mn^{2+} but the MnEDTA complex as well can be taken up across the plasma membrane.

Clarkson [39] concluded that the reduced form of Mn was present in soil solution bathing the root cell plasma membrane, therefore obviating the need for action of the plasma membrane-embedded ferric reductase. However, later research [61] clearly showed that the plasma membrane reductase of *Pisum sativum* and *G. max* effectively reduced Mn^{3+} to Mn^{2+}; this reduction was increased more than 10-fold under Fe deficiency that stimulated reductase activity. Unfortunately, *P. sativum* and *G. max* plants in that study were not exposed to Mn deficiency to test whether it would enhance reductase activity. However, in a different study [62], Mn deficiency did not increase activity of ferric reductase in *P. sativum*. In addition, Mn deficiency did not induce ferric reductase in the wild-type *Arabidopsis thaliana* plants [63]. In contrast, the *A. thaliana man1* mutant, which accumulates up to 7.5 times more Mn than the wild-type plants grown under the same conditions, has constitutively overexpressed ferric reductase (up to 20-fold greater activity compared to the wild type) regardless of the level of Mn supply [63]. Induction of ferric reductase by subjecting *Phaseolus vulgaris* plants to Fe deficiency also increased uptake of Mn [64].

Although there is a relative paucity of information regarding kinetics and regulation of Mn uptake by intact higher plants grown at realistically low Mn concentrations, numerous reports testify to Mn uptake being intensively studied in lower plants (algae, yeasts, etc.). In these plants, transport of Mn from the external medium across the plasma membrane has frequently been studied together with the transport to cell organelles (e.g., Mn transport into Golgi bodies in *Saccharomyces cerevisiae* cells occurs via Ca^{2+}-ATPase [65]). These relatively simple experimental systems are also useful in research aimed at cloning membrane transporters of Mn and other nutrients.

The *SMF1* gene codes for the plasma membrane proteins involved in transport of Mn in *S. cerevisiae* [66,67]. The *S. cerevisiae SMF1* gene is homologous to the *NRAMP2* gene that encodes the mammalian macrophage membrane protein, while the *OsNramp* genes in *Oryza sativa* encode a membrane protein that shares high homology in the hydrophobic membrane-spanning region with the *NRAMP* genes [68]; therefore, the three genes from the *O. sativa OsNramp* family may be the first Mn membrane transporters cloned from the higher plants.

Ion channels embedded in the root-cell plasma membrane, even when selective for ions other than Mn, can still facilitate uptake of Mn (e.g., the Ca^{2+}-selective ion channel from the wheat plasma membrane [69]). Such an uptake may decrease the flux of the ion for which the channel is selective (e.g., Mn^{2+} decreased Ca^{2+} uptake through the Ca^{2+}-selective channel in the *Zea mays* plasma membrane by 70% [70]), probably because of binding of Mn^{2+} to the Ca^{2+} binding site on the apoplasmic side of the channel [71].

3.1. Uptake Kinetics

In his review in 1988, Clarkson [39] pointed out that most literature concerning uptake and translocation of Mn by higher plants was rather old at the time and expressed hope that his review and the International Mn Symposium (held in Adelaide in 1988) will kick-start interest in the research on Mn. Unfortunately, after more than a decade since Clarkson's assessment that we have only old literature on kinetics of Mn uptake, the statement is still accurate.

With old literature on kinetics of nutrient uptake where unphysiologically high concentrations of nutrients, including Mn, were used in solution, one should keep in mind that technical capabilities to conduct experiments with realistically low concentrations of micronutrients in solution was not always there. Flowing nutrient solution systems were available in a relatively few laboratories (e.g. [72]) (Table 2). In addition, an absence of readily available and user-friendly computer models for calculating ionic speciation in complex solutions was hindering usage of low-concentration nutrient solutions.

The relationship between increasing solution concentrations of Mn and the rate of uptake follows a saturable curve [39,43,73]. However, using realistically low Mn activities in the chelate-buffered nutrient solution, Webb et al. [57] obtained a linear relationship between *ionic activity* of Mn^{2+} in solution and the Mn accumulation rate in *H.*

TABLE 2

Kinetic Parameters of the Mn Uptake Process (I_{max} = maximal net influx, K_m = Michaelis-Menten constant) in Various Lower and Higher Plants as Influenced by Various Experimental Conditions

Plant species	Solution Mn (μM)	High-affinity uptake		Low-affinity uptake		Ref.
		I_{max} (μmol g^{-1} DW h^{-1})	K_m (μM)	I_{max} (μmol g^{-1} DW h^{-1})	K_m (μM)	
Saccharomyces cerevisiae	0.025–200[a]	40 × 10^{-6}	0.3	690 × 10^{-6}	62	[41]
Chlorella salina	1–100	0.006[b]	2	1.0[b]	760	[42]
Candida utilis	0.01	0.06	0.02			[44]
Zea mays	1.5–6			40–302[c]	4.4–11	[43]
Hordeum vulgare	10–20000			720	400	[73]

[a]Range of concentrations in solution was 0.05–1 μM or high- and 5–200 μM for low-affinity uptake. I_{max} was expressed as μmol h^{-1} per 10^6 cells.
[b]I_{max} expressed as μmol h^{-1} per 10^6 cells.
[c]I_{max} expressed as μmol g^{-1} root dry weight h^{-1}. Protein was assumed to represent 22.5% of dry weight of roots.

vulgare. Given the fact that the relationship between ion concentration and ionic activity in complex nutrient solutions would in itself be a saturable one, it appears likely that results from older literature would be closer to a linear rather than to a saturable relationship if Mn supply to plant roots was expressed as ionic activity rather than concentration.

Initial uptake of Mn is rapid and represents uptake into the apoplasm of root cells; this fraction has a half-time of 8 min [74]. The fraction that represents uptake into the cytosol may be the one that Munns et al. [75] have identified as having the half-time of up to 2 h. The fraction with a longer half-time (up to 28 h) is likely to represent the vacuolar fraction [74,75].

Estimates of K_m for low-affinity Mn uptake by roots range between 4 and 400 μM (Table 2), which are relatively high concentrations in comparison with those in the soil solution, thus indicating that uptake of Mn from most soils should be linear [1]. The calculated supply of Mn from soil by mass flow and root interception was indeed linearly related to the measured total Mn accumulation by species with vastly different types of the root system (*Lactuca sativa*, *Lycopersicon esculentum*, *Triticum aestivum*, and *G. max* [76]).

3.2. Regulation of Uptake

Energy dependence of Mn uptake has been shown in a number of lower and higher plant species [42,44,47,48,73], but it is likely to be due to an indirect energy requirement that powers H^+-ATPase and allows maintenance of electrochemical potential difference across the plasma membrane, which then drives the uptake of cations into the negatively charged cytoplasm.

Deficiency of one micronutrient could substantially facilitate uptake of one or more other micronutrients [77]. The compensatory absorption of micronutrients under deficiency stress has been reported between Mn and Cu or Zn [78,79]; between Zn and Fe, Mn, or Cu [56, 80,81]; and between Fe and Mn [82–84] (but see [39] for different results).

Zinc deficiency can enhance Mn uptake in various plant species [56,80,85–88], with Mn concentration increasing more in shoots than in

roots [81] and even reaching toxic levels [89]. These effects of Zn deficiency are likely to be due to impaired selectivity of the root-cell plasma
membrane as a consequence of oxidation of sulfhydryl groups in the
plasma-membrane-embedded polypeptides [90].

Uptake of Mn by Z. mays [47] and H. vulgare roots [91] was
inhibited by increasing activity of H^+ in the solution. Similarly, progressively decreasing competition with H^+ in the chelator-buffered nutrient solutions of increasing pH resulted in an increase in Mn absorption by plants of H. vulgare genotypes [58]. However, in soil-grown
plants, increasing pH (thus decreasing H^+ activity) usually has an effect of decreasing Mn accumulation (e.g. [92]) because of pH-dependent
conversions of Mn into plant-unavailable forms (see [93]).

Uptake of Mn is generally sensitive to inhibition by other divalent
cations, with different cations showing differential inhibitory capacity
(from strong to none) depending on the experimental conditions and the
plant species studied. Increasing intracellular Mg concentrations in
S. cerevisiae decreased Mn uptake, probably due to Mg-related changes
in the transporter activity [94]. Moreover, Mg in the external medium
competitively inhibited both the high- and low-affinity Mn transport
across the plasma membrane of S. cerevisiae [41] and Chlorella salina
[42]. Other divalent cations in the external medium (e.g., Zn and Co, but
not Cd) inhibited only high-affinity Mn uptake by S. cerevisiae [41]. In
contrast, increasing Cd concentrations in the external medium displaced Mn from the root tissue and thus decreased Mn accumulation in
intact P. sativum [95] and T. repens plants [96]. Application of Fe to G.
max also decreased Mn accumulation in plants [97].

Manganese passes through the cytoplasm relatively quickly and
accumulates in the vacuole [47,48,51]. A ^{31}P-NMR study showed that
Z. mays root cells maintain low cytosolic Mn^{2+} concentration, with the
nonequilibrium distribution between cytosol and the vacuole, where
vacuole acted as a sink for Mn^{2+} [51]. These results indicate that transport of Mn^{2+} from the cytosol into the vacuole is energy demanding. The
^{31}P-NMR technique should be used in more studies to elucidate distribution of Mn^{2+} among intracellular pools under a variety of conditions.
Also, a possibility should be explored that there is active sequestration
of Mn^{2+} out of the cytosol and into the external medium via some form
of the plasma-membrane-embedded efflux pump akin to Ca^{2+}-ATPase.

4. TRANSPORT OF MANGANESE IN XYLEM AND PHLOEM

4.1. Long-Distance Transport of Manganese

Both xylem and phloem sap can be effectively collected from *Lupinus* species (see [98]), allowing for a number of studies of the long-distance transport of nutrients in these species (e.g. [99–102]). *Ricinus communis* has also been an excellent model plant for studying phloem transport because seedling is supplied with all nutrients via basipetal phloem flow during the first week; therefore, the phloem sap can be collected from a cut in the hook region (e.g. [103–106]) (Table 3).

Transport rates of Mn are from 41 to 51 nmol g^{-1} root dry weight per day in the xylem sap of *Lycopersicon esculentum* [107] and from 1 to 3 nmol per day in the phloem sap of *R. communis* [105]. Manganese concentration in the xylem sap can be as high as 1.2 mM and in the phloem sap up to 0.91 mM (Table 3). However, in rare instances when both the xylem and the phloem sap were collected from the same plant, there was significantly higher Mn concentration in the phloem than in the xylem [99,108]. This conflicts the general assessment that Mn is only partially mobile in the phloem (see below), even though a possibility cannot be excluded that higher phloem than xylem Mn concentrations may be specific to *Lupinus albus* and *Lupinus angustifolius* used in the study by Pate [108] and Hocking and colleagues [99].

A diurnal rhythm in xylem transport as well as in concentration of nutrients in the xylem sap has been clearly established [109]. Manganese concentration in the xylem sap also follows the diurnal rhythm: in *L. angustifolius* it varies from 6 μM at dawn to 2 μM at dusk on the same day [110]. Despite some reports to the contrary, it has been accepted that calculations by White et al. [111], with about 60% of Mn present in the xylem sap as divalent ion and only 40% complexed with citric and malic acid, represent a good generalization. It is also worth mentioning that citrate and malate as well as the complexing agent EDTA added to the growth medium did not influence xylem transport of Mn toward developing *Triticum aestivum* grains [112].

Proteinogenic amino acids did not bind Mn and other micronutrients in the phloem sap, thus not contributing significantly to their

TABLE 3

Concentrations of Mn in the Xylem and Phloem Saps
of Various Plant Species

Plant species	Growth medium	Xylem sap	Phloem sap	Ref.
		Mn concentration (μM)		
L. albus	na	11	26	[108]
	Sand culture	50	230	[167]
	0.002–9.1	2–750	20–910	[99]
	4.5	11–16	36–65	[100]
L. angustifolius	na	7	11	[108]
	0.002–9.1	1–510	10–620	[99]
Brassica oleracea	1.8	0.8–14	1.5–9	[120]
var. _italica_	Soil	135–1150	93	[168]
Nicotiana glauca	Soil	4	16	[169]
Spartium junceum	Soil	1	18	[167]
Helianthus annuus	5.5–470	20–1200		[170]
	2.5	70		[171]
Glycine max	1	7–10		[111]
Lycopersicon	4.5	15–56		[107]
esculentum	10	160–2260[a]		[172]
	1	5–7		[111]
Cucumis sativus	3	5–12		[173]
Coffea arabica	Soil	5–14		[174]
Vitis vinifera	Soil	7–10		[175]
Vitis rotundifolia	Soil	33–36		[176]
	Soil	28–84		[177]
	Soil	198–213		[178]
Ricinus communis	0		12	[105]
	Soil		9	[103]
	Soil		13	[104]
Arenga saccharifera	na		18	[179]
Yucca flaccida	Soil		9	[180]

na, information not available.
[a]Mn toxicity treatment.

phloem transport in *R. communis* [105], while peptides did bind some Mn in the phloem sap of that species [106]. In contrast, nicotianamine (NA), a nonproteinogenic amino acid, so far found in all plants, has been suggested as the endogenous chelator required for the transport of heavy metals within plants [113]. Concentration of NA in the phloem sap was estimated at around 200 μM for *R. communis* [113], thus being in the same range as many divalent micronutrient cations in the phloem sap. A constant stoichiometric ratio of NA and micronutrients was found in the *R. communis* phloem sap [105]. Manganese is a good candidate for transport in the Mn-NA complex because such complex is relatively stable at slightly alkaline pH values predominating in the phloem sap [105,114]. However, NA does not appear to be important in Mn translocation in *Lycopersicon esculentum* [107].

Most micronutrients, including Mn, are considered partially mobile in the phloem [8,45,46,77,115–119] depending on the stage of growth and other factors. Loneragan [117] calculated that Mn concentration in phloem would have to be between 25 and 100 μM to sustain the minimally required levels of 10–20 μg Mn g^{-1} dry weight in developing grains. However, Mn concentration in the phloem is frequently lower than that (ranging from 2 to 910 μM, but in most plants being below 20 μM [117]) (Table 3), indicating that the capacity of phloem to supply enough Mn to grain may often be limiting. However, Hocking et al. [99] reported that 80–90% of Mn in *Lupinus* grain was supplied via the phloem. Similarly, Shelp [120] concluded that the phloem contributes a significant proportion of Mn transported toward *Brassica oleracea* var. *italica* inflorescences (Table 3). Obviously, mechanisms that increase loading of Mn into the phloem would be crucial to increasing Mn supply to developing grain.

Root-supplied Mn was exported from the labeled root quickly: around a half hour after exposure, labeled Mn was detected in shoots of *Avena sativa* [75] and *T. aestivum* [45]. Manganese supplied via roots during the vegetative period was distributed among various parts of the *T. aestivum* plant based on the prior Mn status, with proportionally more Mn going to the older leaves in Mn-deficient and into younger leaves in Mn-sufficient plants [45]. Differences in the leaf transpiration rates as well as in the general metabolic rate might have contributed to such a pattern of Mn distribution.

Manganese supplied via roots during the grain development in *T.*

aestivum was not transported to the leaves, but instead accumulated in shoot (up to 2 weeks after anthesis) and was transported directly to the ear in more advanced stages of grain development [46]. Similarly, the stem served as a temporary Mn storage in *L. angustifolius* [115]. Such storage of Mn in shoots or stems of various plant species may be an important mechanisms of maintaining Mn in plant parts from which it can be relatively easily remobilized in the xylem for transport toward developing grain (as opposed to storage of Mn in leaves where remobilization would have to be via the phloem and, as such, has not been shown to occur in the case of Mn) [117,118,121]. Mechanisms allowing selective transport of Mn in the xylem sap (e.g., toward the ear in *T. aestivum* or the inflorescence in *L. angustifolius*, but not toward leaves whose xylem pathways branch out of the main veins leading upward toward fruiting bodies) is not understood at present.

Substantial transfer of Mn (about 60% of total transported from the root exposed to labeled Mn) occurred across a root system of *T. aestivum* when the entire root system was deficient in Mn, suggesting that Mn is mobile in the root phloem [45]. Similar results were obtained in *Solanum tuberosum*, where Mn was transported into nontranspiring tubers in the phloem [122]. In contrast, only a minute fraction of Mn exported from labeled roots of *Trifolium subterraneum* (0.5% of the total exported [121]) and *H. vulgare* [123] ended up in the nonlabeled part of the root system, probably because the split-root method (−Mn and +Mn) by which plants were pregrown in both of these studies might have left the −Mn part of the root system with impaired function, if not functionless (see [45]).

Manganese applied to leaves can be translocated out of leaves in the phloem sap (e.g., *A. sativa* [124], *G. max* [125], *Z. mays* [126]). However, calculations showed that foliarly-applied Mn would be transported to roots in the phloem sap at a rate insufficient to maintain vigorous root growth, at least in *T. aestivum* and *T. subterraneum* grown in the split-root system [117].

4.2. Remobilization

Although a small proportion of Mn externally applied to leaves can be translocated out of treated leaves (from 1% of the applied amount in *Z. mays* [126] to 10% in *A. sativa* [124]), Mn that accumulated in leaves in a physiological way via the xylem sap does not appear to be amenable to remobilization in most plant species [117]. In addition, Mn does not move out of senescing leaves of *T. subterraneum* [121] and *L. angustifolius* [115]. An absence of Mn remobilization from leaves would indicate that Mn is present in insoluble complexes; in contrast, Mn can be leached out of leaves by water [115,127]. Further research on chemical forms and compartmentation of Mn in leaf tissues and cells is warranted.

There are differences among species and genotypes within species in the capacity to remobilize Mn from leaves and other organs. *Lupinus albus* can remobilize some Mn from leaves, while *T. subterraneum* [121,127], *L. angustifolius* [128], and *G. max* cannot [129]. In contrast to leaves, remobilization of Mn from *L. angustifolius* stems [115] and *T. aestivum* shoots and roots [46,118] enhanced grain loading of Mn substantially. Manganese in petioles of *L. angustifolius* may also be remobilized [115], but the size of that Mn pool is too small to contribute to grain nutrition in a major way.

The majority of Mn from vegetative tissues of *T. aestivum* was remobilized within the first 2 weeks following anthesis. However, Mn was only remobilized from tissues with a direct xylem connection to the ear (i.e., the roots and the shoot) and not from leaves, thus indicating poor mobility of Mn in the leaf phloem. Such remobilization was greater under Mn deficiency than under Mn sufficiency [118]. In contrast, Hocking [130] did not observe any remobilization of Mn from leaves and shoots of field-grown *T. aestivum*, but he did not study remobilization from roots. Other species can also remobilize Mn from roots (*A. sativa* [75], *T. subterraneum* [127], and *L. angustifolius* [115]).

Little research was done on remobilization of Mn from various grain parts during germination. Moussavi-Nik et al. [131] measured remobilization of Mn from the grain coat and the endosperm of germinating *Triticum aestivum* grains. Remobilized Mn was directed mostly to roots during the first 3 days after commencement of imbibition and to both roots and shoots in the later stages. Grain coat represented the largest store of Mn and was depleted by 30–55%, depending on the genotype [131]. This relatively inefficient remobilization of Mn from the grain coat indicates that loading of Mn into pericarp of the developing grain [132,133], i.e., future grain coat of the mature grain, represents a somewhat wasteful process.

Although the stem in *L. angustifolius* [115] and the shoot in *T.*

aestivum during early stages of grain development [46] can represent stores of Mn for later transport into developing grain, it is not known where in the stem/shoot Mn is stored and which mechanisms allow for this reversible loading of Mn into the stem/shoot cells. It has also been suggested that the pod walls in *Lupinus* can represent stores of Mn for developing grain [99], but comprehensive research on that topic has not been carried out so far.

5. LOADING OF MANGANESE INTO DEVELOPING GRAIN

Mineral nutrient reserves in the grain must be adequate to sustain growth until the root system can take over the nutrient supply function [134]. Mineral nutrient content of grain also determines the quality of grain [119]. There is no better example than *L. angustifolius* where grain with low Mn concentration splits (with cotyledons or embryo protruding through the grain coat [135], thus reducing its commercial value as well as severely diminishing capacity of such grain to germinate [136,137]). A different species of the same genus, *L. albus*, never suffers from the split-grain disorder. *Lupinus albus* does form cluster roots that solubilize plant-unavailable Mn dioxide into plant-available Mn forms [138] and therefore accumulates more Mn than *L. angustifolius*, a species that does not form cluster roots [139,140]. However, grain Mn content in *L. albus* is almost an order of magnitude greater than in *L. angustifolius*, clearly indicating that the difference in grain Mn content is due to differences in mechanisms of remobilization, transport, and/or loading rather than just due to differences in capacity of these two lupin species to take up Mn from soil.

Large grain reserves of Mn are important for crops grown on soils that are deficient in Mn [98,141–143]. During germination and early growth in the Mn-deficient soil, high Mn content in grain will ensure better seedling vigor, higher tolerance to soilborne root and crown diseases, faster canopy development, better weed control, and higher yield potential (cf. [93,144,145]).

Loading of Mn into developing grain does not passively follow accumulation of assimilates; in contrast, there are Mn-specific processes involved in loading into, and translocation within, grain tissues. These processes have been deciphered recently for *T. aestivum* [46, 132,133,146–148], while only little work was done on other species (e.g., *G. max* [149]).

Phloem transport of Mn appears to be important in loading Mn into developing grains of *L. angustifolius* and *L. albus*, the two species with a close relationship between Mn concentration in grains and Mn concentration in the phloem sap collected from pods [98,99,115]. In contrast, Mn transported in the xylem toward developing *T. aestivum* grains was not loaded into the phloem within the peduncle or the rachis, but reached the floret via the xylem instead [46,150]. As much as 75% of Mn that had been transported toward the developing *T. aestivum* grain ended up in transpiring floral structures (palea, lemma, and glumes) [146] and was not retranslocated from them into the grain, thus depriving the mature grain of a major portion of Mn that was potentially available for loading [118]. It therefore appears that utilization of Mn in the grain-loading process in *T. aestivum* is fairly poor. A relatively small proportion of Mn remaining after most of it got partitioned into palea, lemma, and glumes (i.e., the proportion of Mn that was destined to enter the grain) was taken up by transfer cells in the xylem discontinuity of the grain stalk (for anatomy of the spikelet, see [151]) and was transferred to the grain vascular system [146,147], with transport across the plasma membrane into the phloem being a limiting step. Thereafter, Mn was transferred from the crease phloem into the vascular system of the pericarp before being transported relatively slowly to the embryo region, with only a little going to endosperm [133,146]. Indeed, the embryo of the mature *T. aestivum* grain has up to 50-fold higher concentration of Mn than the endosperm [131,152–155], which is important in grain germination and seedling establishment [131, 141–143].

Transport pathways within the developing *T. aestivum* grain were not the same for sucrose and Mn: sucrose moved laterally out of the crease vascular system into the endosperm cavity and was subsequently taken up and stored in the endosperm. In contrast, Mn was retained within the inner and outer pericarp initially and was then transported slowly to grain parts, mostly to the embryo, during grain maturation [132,133].

The loading rate and the amount of Mn loaded into developing

T. aestivum grain and the observed patterns of distribution within the grain are controlled by prior accumulation of Mn (sink strength) [148]. Increasing Mn concentration in the external medium resulted in a saturable, rather than linear, increase in Mn loading into developing grains, probably because of saturation of membrane transporters [132]. In field studies, concentration of Mn in cereal grain increased with an increase in Mn fertilization [156], but the nature of the relationship could not be ascertained. When Mn concentration in developing *T. aestivum* grain reached potentially toxic concentrations, further Mn loading in the grain was severely reduced [148].

6. GENOTYPIC DIFFERENCES IN MANGANESE UPTAKE AND UTILIZATION

On Mn-deficient soils, Mn fertilizers have a remarkably low residual value (they are quickly converted to the plant-unavailable forms) making them unsuitable for correction of deficiency. An alternative strategy of correcting problems associated with Mn-deficient soils is to breed crop cultivars for greater tolerance to this soil condition. Genotypic differences in tolerance to Mn-deficient soils have been recognized since the deficiency itself was first identified in the 1920s; it has been reported widely that such differences are, at least partly, under genetic control and could therefore be exploited in plant breeding [34,93,144]. A genotype tolerant to Mn deficiency, in an agronomic sense, is one that is able to grow and yield well without added Mn fertilizer in a soil that is limiting in available Mn for another, standard, genotype. Genotypes tolerant to Mn deficiency are usually able to extract more Mn from these "deficient" soils [34,93].

Differential tolerance to Mn deficiency can only be demonstrated with plants growing in soil; in nutrient solution both tolerant and sensitive *H. vulgare* genotypes grow and take up Mn at a similar rate regardless of Mn supply [157]. These results indicate specific rhizosphere processes and/or microbial dynamics in the rhizosphere are involved. The putative mechanisms of tolerance to Mn deficiency may rely on greater root excretion of various substances into the rhizosphere (H^+, reductants, chelating ligands, microbial suppressants/stimulants) to mobilize insoluble and plant-unavailable Mn.

Different plant species [158,159] and genotypes within a species [160,161] differentially influence the quantitative and qualitative composition of microbial populations in the rhizosphere. Therefore, rhizosphere microorganisms may have a role in the expression of genotypic differences in tolerance to Mn deficiency. Timonin [161] found greater numbers of Mn-oxidizing microbes in the rhizosphere of oat cultivars sensitive to Mn deficiency than in the tolerant ones and concluded that this was the basis of genotypic differences in Mn uptake. Similarly, the rhizosphere of Aroona wheat, tolerant to Mn deficiency, contained more Mn reducers under Mn-deficient than under control conditions, while some other wheat genotypes tolerant to Mn deficiency (e.g., C8MM) did not show such a response [162], indicating that mechanisms of tolerance to Mn deficiency in these two genotypes are not the same. Under Mn-deficient conditions, genotypes sensitive to Mn deficiency did not have an increase in the ratio of Mn reducers to Mn oxidizers in the rhizosphere that would be comparable to that in genotypes tolerant to Mn deficiency [162,163].

The genetic control of tolerance to Mn deficiency may be expressed through the qualitative and/or quantitative composition of root exudates encouraging a more favorable balance of Mn reducers to Mn oxidizers in the rhizosphere [163]. The experimental data on that topic are eagerly awaited.

7. CONCLUSIONS

Manganese is taken up from the root medium either as divalent cation or in a complex form. The uptake process is dependent on the electrochemical gradient across the root-cell plasma membrane created by energy-consuming H^+-ATPase. Uptake kinetics ranges from linear to saturable and may include low- and high-affinity plasma membrane transport, depending on the experimental system. The physiological requirement for Mn is low, and uptake capacity exceeds that requirement by up to several orders of magnitude, indicating a poor regulation of Mn uptake. Manganese is freely mobile in the xylem sap, while mobility in the phloem sap depends on the type and age of the plant part. Remobilization from leaves ranges from small to none, while remobilization from roots and stems or shoots may contribute to loading into developing grain substantially. In some plant species studied, Mn is transported toward developing grains in phloem (e.g., *L. angustifolius* and *L. albus*), while in other species the xylem is the most important pathway (*T. aestivum*). Rates and pathways for translocation of Mn within tissues of the developing grain have been deciphered so far only for *T. aestivum*. Genotypes of crop species differ in capacity to mobilize Mn in the rhizosphere and take it up. Physiological mechanisms underlying genotypic differences in tolerance to Mn deficiency are not known at present.

ACKNOWLEDGMENT

The research in the author's laboratory was funded by the Australian Research Council.

ABBREVIATIONS

DTPA   diethylene triamine-N,N,N',N'',N''-pentaacetate
DW   dry weight
EDTA   ethylenediamine-N,N,N',N'-tetraacetate
EPR   electron paramagnetic resonance
NA   nicotianamide
NMR   nuclear magnetic resonance

REFERENCES

1. S. A. Barber, *Soil Nutrient Bioavailability: A Mechanistic Approach*, 2nd ed. John Wiley and Sons, New York, 1995.
2. R. J. Bartlett, in *Manganese in Soils and Plants* (R. D. Graham, R. J. Hannam, and N. C. Uren, eds.), Kluwer Academic, Dordrecht, 1985, pp. 59–73.
3. W. A. Norvell, in *Manganese in Soils and Plants* (R. D. Graham, R. J. Hannam, and N. C. Uren, eds.), Kluwer Academic, Dordrecht, 1988, pp. 37–58.

4. N. C. Uren, *J. Plant Nutr.*, *12*, 173–185 (1989).

5. N. C. Uren and H. M. Reisenauer, *Adv. Plant Nutr.*, *3*, 79–114 (1988).

6. M. J. Mukhopadhyay and A. Sharma, *Bot. Rev.*, *57*, 117–149 (1991).

7. H. Marschner, *Mineral Nutrition of Higher Plants*, 2nd ed. Academic Press, London, 1995.

8. R. M. Welch, *Crit. Rev. Plant Sci.*, *14*, 49–82 (1995).

9. Z. Rengel, in *Mineral Nutrition of Crops: Mechanisms and Implications* (Z. Rengel, ed.), Haworth Press, New York, 1999, pp. 227–265.

10. W. Foulds, *New Phytol.*, *125*, 529–546 (1993).

11. J. S. Gladstones and J. F. Loneragan, in *Proc. 11 Int. Grassland Cong.*, Brisbane, Australia, 1970, pp. 350–354.

12. E. Epstein, *Mineral Nutrition of Plants: Principles and Perspectives*, John Wiley and Sons, New York, 1972.

13. R. D. Graham, W. J. Davies, and J. S. Ascher, *Aust. J. Agric. Res.*, *36*, 145–155 (1985).

14. C. G. Papavizas and C. B. Davey, *Plant and Soil*, *14*, 215–236 (1961).

15. G. D. Bowen and A. D. Rovira, in *Roots: The Hidden Half* (Y. Waisel, A. Eshel, and U. Kafkafi, eds.), Marcel Dekker, New York, 1992, pp. 641–669.

16. W. C. Ghiorse, In *Manganese in Soils and Plants* (R. D. Graham, R. J. Hannam, and N. C. Uren, eds.), Kluwer Academic, Dordrecht, 1988, pp. 75–85.

17. D. Neilsen, G. H. Neilsen, A. H. Sinclair and D. J. Linehan, *Plant and Soil*, *145*, 45–50 (1992).

18. J. H. Rule and E. R. Graham, *Soil Sci. Soc. Am. J.*, *40*, 853–857 (1976).

19. S. C. Jarvis and D. J. Hatch, *Ann. Bot.*, *55*, 41–51 (1985).

20. B. Dinkelaker, C. Hengeler and H. Marschner, *Bot. Acta*, *108*, 183–200 (1995).

21. H. Marschner, V. Römheld, W. J. Horst, and P. Martin, *Z. Pflanzenernähr. Bodenkd.*, *149*, 441–456 (1986).

22. Y. Tong, Z. Rengel, and R. D. Graham, *Ann. Bot.*, *79*, 53–58 (1997).

23. D. A. Barber and R. B. Lee, *New Phytol.*, *73*, 97–106 (1974).

24. G. H. Godo and H. M. Reisenauer, *Soil Sci. Soc. Am. J.*, *44*, 993–995 (1980).

25. D. L. Jones and P. R. Darrah, *Plant and Soil*, *166*, 247–257 (1994).

26. D. L. Jones, A. C. Edwards, K. Donachie, and P. R. Darrah, *Plant and Soil*, *158*, 183–192 (1994).

27. J. M. Lynch and J. M. Whipps, *Plant and Soil*, *129*, 1–10 (1990).

28. J. M. Whipps and J. M. Lynch, *New Phytol.*, *95*, 605–623 (1983).

29. S. M. Bromfield and D. J. David, *Soil Biol. Biochem.*, *8*, 37–43 (1976).

30. P. B. Tinker, *Plant and Soil*, *76*, 77–91 (1984).

31. S. M. Bromfield, *Plant and Soil*, *49*, 23–39 (1979).

32. D. M. Huber and T. S. McCay-Buis, *Plant Dis.*, *77*, 437–447 (1993).

33. P. Marschner, J. S. Ascher, and R. D. Graham, *Biol. Fertil. Soils*, *12*, 33–38 (1991).

34. R. D. Graham, in *Manganese in Soils and Plants* (R. D. Graham, R. J. Hannam, and N. C. Uren, eds.), Kluwer Academic, Dordrecht, 1988, pp. 261–276.

35. M. I. Timonin, in *Microbiology and Soil Fertility* (C. M. Gilmore and O. N. Allen, eds.), Oregon State Univ. Press, Corvallis, 1965, pp. 135–138.

36. L. K. Abbott, A. D. Robson, and M. A. Scheltema, *Crit. Rev. Biotechnol.*, *15*, 213–228 (1995).

37. K. Posta, H. Marschner, and V. Römheld, *Mycorrhiza*, *5*, 119–124 (1994).

38. S. K. Kothari, H. Marschner, and V. Römheld, *New Phytol.*, *117*, 649–655 (1991).

39. D. T. Clarkson, in *Manganese in Soils and Plants* (R. D. Graham, R. J. Hannam, and N. C. Uren, eds.), Kluwer Academic, Dordrecht, 1988, pp. 101–111.

40. B. Ferguson and D. T. Clarkson, *New Phytol.*, *75*, 69–79 (1975).

41. G. M. Gadd and O. S. Laurence, *Microbiology*, *142*, 1159–1167 (1996).

42. G. W. Garnham, G. A. Codd, and G. M. Gadd, *Appl. Microbiol. Biotechnol.*, *37*, 270–276 (1992).

43. S. Landi and F. Fagioli, *J. Plant Nutr.*, 6, 957–970 (1983).

44. M. J. Parkin and I. S. Ross, *J. Gen. Microbiol.*, 132, 2155–2160 (1986).

45. J. N. Pearson and Z. Rengel, *J. Exp. Bot.*, 46, 833–839 (1995).

46. J. N. Pearson and Z. Rengel, *J. Exp. Bot.*, 46, 841–845 (1995).

47. S. Ratkovic and Z. Vucinic, *Plant Physiol. Biochem.*, 28, 617–622 (1990).

48. C. Roby, R. Bligny, R. Douce, S. I. Tu, and P. E. Pfeffer, *Biochemical J.*, 252, 401–408 (1988).

49. C. Farcasanu, N. Ohta, and T. Miyakawa, *Biosci. Biotechnol. Biochem.*, 60, 468–471 (1996).

50. D. J. Linehan, A. H. Sinclair, and A. C. Mitchell, *J. Soil Sci.*, 40, 103–115 (1989).

51. H. Quiquampoix, B. C. Loughman, and R. G. Ratcliffe, *J. Exp. Bot.*, 44, 1819–1827 (1993).

52. E. V. Maas, D. P. Moore, and B. J. Mason, *Plant Physiol.*, 44, 796–800 (1969).

53. R. L. Chaney, P. F. Bell, and B. A. Coulombe, *Hort. Sci.*, 24, 565–572 (1989).

54. W. A. Norvell and R. M. Welch, *Plant Physiol.*, 101, 619–625 (1993).

55. D. R. Parker, R. L. Chaney, and W. A. Norvell, in *Chemical Equilibrium and Reaction Models* (R. H. Loeppert, A. P. Schwab, and S. Goldberg, eds.), Soil Science Society of America and American Society of Agronomy, Madison, WI, 1995, pp. 163–200.

56. Z. Rengel and R. D. Graham, *Plant and Soil*, 176, 317–324 (1995).

57. M. J. Webb, W. A. Norvell, R. M. Welch, and R. D. Graham, *Plant and Soil*, 153, 195–205 (1993).

58. C. Huang, M. J. Webb, and R. D. Graham, *Plant and Soil*, 155/156, 437–440 (1993).

59. S. H. Laurie, N. P. Tancock, S. P. McGrath, and J. R. Sanders, *Plant Sci.*, 109, 231–235 (1995).

60. S. H. Laurie, N. P. Tancock, S. P. McGrath, and J. R. Sanders, *J. Exp. Bot.*, 42, 509–513 (1991).

61. W. A. Norvell, R. M. Welch, M. L. Adams, and L. V. Kochian, *Plant and Soil*, 155/156, 123–126 (1993).

62. C. K. Cohen, W. A. Norvell, and L. V. Kochian, *Plant Physiol.*, *114*, 1061–1069 (1997).

63. E. Delhaize, *Plant Physiol.*, *111*, 849–855 (1996).

64. A. L. Fleming, *J. Plant Nutr.*, *12*, 715–732 (1989).

65. G. Duerr, J. Strayle, R. Plemper, S. Elbs, S. K. Klee, P. Catty, D. H. Wolf, and H. K. Rudolph, *Mol. Biol. Cell*, *9*, 1149–1162 (1998).

66. E. Pinner, S. Grünheid, M. Raymond, and P. Gros, *J. Biol. Chem.*, *272*, 28933–28938 (1997).

67. F. Supek, L. Supekova, H. Nelson, and N. Nelson, *Proc. Natl. Acad. Sci. USA*, *93*, 5105–5110 (1996).

68. A. Belouchi, T. Kwan, and P. Gros, *Plant Mol. Biol.*, *33*, 1085–1092 (1997).

69. M. Piñeros and M. Tester, *Planta*, *195*, 478–488 (1995).

70. J. Marshall, A. Corzo, R. A. Leigh, and D. Sanders, *Plant J.*, *5*, 683–694 (1994).

71. K. S. Shumaker and H. Sze, *J. Biol. Chem.*, *261*, 12172–12178 (1986).

72. S. C. Jarvis and L. H. P. Jones, *Plant and Soil*, *99*, 231–240 (1987).

73. E. V. Maas, D. P. Moore, and B. J. Mason, *Plant Physiol.*, *43*, 527–530 (1968).

74. E. R. Page and J. Dainty, *J. Exp. Bot.*, *15*, 428–443 (1964).

75. D. N. Munns, L. Jacobsen, and C. M. Johnson, *Plant and Soil*, *19*, 193–204 (1963).

76. E. H. Halstead, S. A. Barber, D. D. Warncke, and J. Bole, *Soil Sci. Soc. Am. Proc.*, *32*, 69–72 (1968).

77. L. V. Kochian, in *Micronutrients in Agriculture*, 2nd ed. (J. J. Mortvedt, F. R. Cox, L. M. Shuman, and R. M. Welch, eds.), Soil Sci. Soc. Am., Madison, WI, 1991, pp. 229–296.

78. L. Del Río, F. Sevilla, M. Gomez, J. Yanez, and J. Lopéz-Gorgé, *Planta*, *140*, 221–225 (1978).

79. S. J. Harrison, N. W. Lepp, and D. A. Phipps, *Z. Pflanzenphysiol.*, *109*, 285–289 (1983).

80. Z. Rengel and R. D. Graham, *J. Exp. Bot.*, *47*, 217–226 (1996).

81. Z. Rengel, V. Römheld, and H. Marschner, *J. Plant Physiol.*, *152*, 433–438 (1998).

82. J. C. Brown and R. A. Olsen, *J. Plant Nutr.*, 2, 661–682 (1980).

83. I. Iturbe-Ormaetxe, J. F. Moran, C. Arrese-Igor, Y. Gogorcena, R. V. Klucas, and M. Becana, *Plant Cell Environ.*, 18, 421–429 (1995).

84. R. M. Welch, W. A. Norvell, S. C. Schaefer, J. E. Shaff, and L. V. Kochian, *Planta*, 190, 555–561 (1993).

85. R. D. Graham, R. M. Welch, D. L. Grunes, E. E. Cary, and W. A. Norvell, *Soil Sci. Soc. Am. J.*, 51, 652–657 (1987).

86. D. Gries, S. Brunn, D. E. Crowley, and D. R. Parker, *Plant and Soil*, 172, 299–308 (1995).

87. D. R. Parker, *Soil Sci. Soc. Am. J.*, 61, 167–176 (1997).

88. R. M. Welch and W. A. Norvell, *Plant Physiol.*, 101, 627–631 (1993).

89. K. Ohki, *Agron. J.*, 69, 969–974 (1977).

90. Z. Rengel, *Physiol. Plant.*, 95, 604–612 (1995).

91. D. R. R. Malkanthi, M. Moritsugu, and K. Yokoyama, *Soil Sci. Plant Nutr.*, 41, 253–262 (1995).

92. N. K. Fageria, F. J. P. Zimmermann, and V. C. Baligar, *J. Plant Nutr.*, 18, 2519–2532 (1995).

93. Z. Rengel, J. F. Pedler, and R. D. Graham, in *Biochemistry of Metal Micronutrients in the Rhizosphere* (J. A. Manthey, D. E. Crowley, and D. G. Luster, eds.), Lewis Publishers/CRC Press, Boca Raton, FL, 1994, pp. 125–145.

94. K. J. Blackwell, J. M. Tobin, and S. V. Avery, *Appl. Microbiol. Biotechnol.*, 47, 180–184 (1997).

95. L. E. Hernandez, R. Carpena Ruiz, and A. Garate, *J. Plant Nutr.*, 19, 1581–1598 (1996).

96. X. Yang, V. C. Baligar, D. C. Martens, and R. B. Clark, *J. Plant Nutr.*, 19, 265–279 (1996).

97. S. Roomizadeh and N. Karimian, *J. Plant Nutr.*, 19, 397–406 (1996).

98. N. Longnecker, R. Brennan, and A. Robson, in *Lupins as Crop Plants: Biology, Production and Utilization* (J. S. Gladstones, C. A. Atkins, and J. Hamblin, eds.), CAB International, Wallingford, UK, 1998, pp. 121–148.

99. P. J. Hocking, J. S. Pate, S. C. Wee, and A. J. McComb, *Ann. Bot.*, 41, 677–688 (1977).

100. P. J. Hocking and J. S. Pate, *Aust. J. Agric. Res.*, *29*, 267–280 (1978).

101. W. D. Jeschke, C. A. Atkins, and J. S. Pate, *J. Plant Physiol.*, *117*, 319–330 (1985).

102. J. S. Pate, J. Kuo, and P. J. Hocking, *Aust. J. Plant Physiol.*, *5*, 321–326 (1978).

103. S. M. Hall and D. A. Baker, *Planta*, *106*, 131–140 (1972).

104. P. J. Hocking, *Ann. Bot.*, *49*, 51–62 (1982).

105. I. Schmidke and U. W. Stephan, *Physiol. Plant.*, *95*, 147–153 (1995).

106. B. J. Van Goor and D. Wiersma, *Physiol. Plant.*, *36*, 213–216 (1976).

107. A. Pich and G. Scholz, *J. Exp. Bot.*, *47*, 41–47 (1996).

108. J. S. Pate, in *Encyclopedia of Plant Physiology*, Vol. 1 (M. H. Zimmermann and J. A. Milburn, eds.), Springer-Verlag, New York, 1975, pp. 451–473.

109. U. Schurr, *Trends Plant Sci.*, *3*, 293–298 (1998).

110. P. J. Hocking, J. S. Pate, C. A. Atkins, and P. J. Sharkey, *Ann. Bot.*, *42*, 1277–1290 (1978).

111. M. C. White, A. M. Decker, and R. L. Chaney, *Plant Physiol.*, *67*, 292–300 (1981).

112. J. N. Pearson, Z. Rengel, C. F. Jenner, and R. D. Graham, *Physiol. Plant.*, *98*, 229–234 (1996).

113. U. W. Stephan and G. Scholz, *Physiol. Plant.*, *88*, 522–529 (1993).

114. U. W. Stephan, I. Schmidke, V. W. Stephan, and G. Scholz, *Biometals*, *9*, 84–90 (1996).

115. R. J. Hannam, R. D. Graham, and J. L. Riggs, *Ann. Bot.*, *56*, 821–834 (1985).

116. S. Kannan, *Crit. Rev. Plant Sci.*, *4*, 341–375 (1987).

117. J. F. Loneragan, in *Manganese in Soils and Plants* (R. D. Graham, R. J. Hannam, and N. C. Uren, eds.), Kluwer Academic, Dordrecht, 1988, pp. 113–124.

118. J. N. Pearson and Z. Rengel, *J. Exp. Bot.*, *45*, 1829–1835 (1994).

119. R. M. Welch, *Adv. Plant Nutr.*, *2*, 205–247 (1986).

120. B. J. Shelp, *J. Exp. Bot.*, *38*, 1619–1636 (1987).

121. R. O. Nable and J. F. Loneragan, *Aust. J. Plant Physiol.*, *11*, 113–118 (1984).

122. D. P. Nelson, W. L. Pan, and V. R. Franceschi, *J. Exp. Bot.*, *41*, 1143–1148 (1990).

123. C. H. Henkens and E. Jongman, *Neth. J. Agric. Sci.*, *13*, 392–407 (1965).

124. P. B. Vose, *J. Exp. Bot.*, *14*, 448–457 (1963).

125. K. Ohki, *Agron. J.*, *68*, 861–864 (1976).

126. F. K. El Baz, P. Maier, A. H. Wissemeier, and W. J. Horst, *Z. Pflanzenernähr. Bodenkd.*, *153*, 279–282 (1990).

127. R. O. Nable and J. F. Loneragan, *Aust. J. Plant Physiol.*, *11*, 101–111 (1984).

128. P. F. Reay, *Ann. Bot.*, *59*, 219–226 (1987).

129. J. B. Drossopoulos, D. L. Bouranis, and B. D. Bairaktari, *J. Plant Nutr.*, *17*, 1017–1035 (1994).

130. P. J. Hocking, *J. Plant Nutr.*, *17*, 1289–1308 (1994).

131. M. Moussavi-Nik, Z. Rengel, N. J. Pearson, and G. Hollamby, *Plant and Soil*, *197*, 271–280 (1997).

132. J. N. Pearson, C. F. Jenner, Z. Rengel, and R. D. Graham, *Physiol. Plant.*, *97*, 332–338 (1996).

133. J. N. Pearson, Z. Rengel, C. F. Jenner, and R. D. Graham, *Aust. J. Plant Physiol.*, *25*, 139–144 (1998).

134. C. J. Asher, in *Crop Establishment Problems in Queensland: Recognition, Research and Resolution* (I. M. Wood, W. H. Hazard, and F. R. From, eds.), Aust. Inst. Agric. Sci., Brisbane, 1987, pp. 88–106.

135. G. H. Walton, *Aust. J. Agric. Res.*, *29*, 1177–1189 (1978).

136. J. Crosbie, N. E. Longnecker, and A. D. Robson, *Aust. J. Agric. Res.*, *45*, 1469–1482 (1994).

137. N. Longnecker, J. Crosbie, F. Davies, and A. Robson, *Crop Sci.*, *36*, 355–361 (1996).

138. W. K. Gardner, D. G. Parbery, and D. A. Barber, *Plant and Soil*, *68*, 19–32 (1982).

139. J. S. Gladstones, *Aust. J. Exp. Agric. Anim. Husb.*, *2*, 213–220 (1962).

140. C. L. White, A. D. Robson, and H. M. Fisher, *Aust. J. Agric. Res.*, *32*, 47–59 (1981).

141. N. E. Longnecker, N. E. Marcar, and R. D. Graham, *Aust. J. Agric. Res.*, *42*, 1065–1074 (1991).

142. N. E. Marcar and R. D. Graham, *Plant and Soil*, *96*, 165–174 (1986).

143. M. Moussavi-Nik, Z. Rengel, G. J. Hollamby, and J. S. Ascher, in *Plant Nutrition for Sustainable Food Production and Environment* (T. Ando, K. Fujita, T. Mae, H. Matsumoto, S. Mori, and J. Sekiya, eds.), Kluwer Academic, Dordrecht, 1997, pp. 267–268.

144. Z. Rengel, R. D. Graham, and J. F. Pedler, *Plant and Soil*, *151*, 255–263 (1993).

145. Z. Rengel, G. Batten, and D. Crowley, *Field Crops Res.*, *60*, 28–40 (1999).

146. J. N. Pearson, Z. Rengel, C. F. Jenner, and R. D. Graham, *Physiol. Plant.*, *95*, 449–455 (1995).

147. J. N. Pearson, C. F. Jenner, Z. Rengel, and R. D. Graham, *Physiol. Plant.*, *97*, 332–338 (1996).

148. J. N. Pearson, Z. Rengel, and R. D. Graham, *J. Plant Nutr.*, *22*, in press (1999).

149. J. A. Laszlo, *J. Plant Nutr.*, *13*, 231–248 (1990).

150. T. Herren and U. Feller, *J. Plant Nutr.*, *17*, 1587–1598 (1994).

151. T. P. O'Brien, M. E. Sammut, J. W. Lee, and M. G. Smart, *Aust. J. Plant Physiol.*, *12*, 487–511 (1985).

152. J. N. A. Lott and E. Spitzer, *Plant Physiol.*, *66*, 494–499 (1980).

153. A. P. Mazzolini, C. K. Pallaghy, and G. J. F. Legge, *New Phytol.*, *100*, 483–509 (1985).

154. K. Tanaka, T. Yoshida, and Z. Kasai, *Soil Sci. Plant Nutr.*, *20*, 87–91 (1974).

155. T. Wada and J. N. A. Lott, *Can. J. Bot.*, *75*, 1137–1147 (1997).

156. J. S. Ascher, R. D. Graham, D. E. Elliott, J. M. Scott, and R. S. Jessop, in *Wheat in Heat-Stressed Environments: Irrigated, Dry Areas and Rice-Farming Systems* (D. A. Saunders and G. P. Hettel, eds.), CIMMYT, Mexico, D.F., 1994, pp. 297–308.

157. C. Huang, M. J. Webb, and R. D. Graham, *J. Plant Nutr.*, *17*, 83–95 (1994).

158. P. Lemanceau, T. Corberand, L. Gardan, X. Latour, G. Laguerre, J. M. Boeufgras, and C. Alabouvette, *Appl. Environ. Microbiol.*, *61*, 1004–1012 (1995).

159. W. Wiehe and G. Hoflich, *Microbiol. Res.*, *150*, 201–206 (1995).

160. R. Khanna, S. Chandra, and K. K. Khanna, *Biological Memoirs*, *19*, 111–121 (1993).

161. M. I. Timonin, *Soil Sci. Soc. Am. Proc.*, *11*, 284–292 (1946).

162. Z. Rengel, R. Guterridge, P. Hirsch, and D. Hornby, *Plant and Soil*, *183*, 269–277 (1996).

163. Z. Rengel, *Plant and Soil*, *196*, 255–260 (1997).

164. Z. Rengel and D. L. Robinson, *Commun. Soil Sci. Plant Anal.*, *20*, 253–269 (1989).

165. Z. Rengel and M. S. Wheal, *J. Exp. Bot.*, *48*, 927–934 (1997).

166. Z. Rengel and R. D. Graham, in *Plant Nutrition—From Genetic Engineering to Field Practice* (N. J. Barrow, ed.), Kluwer Academic, Dordrecht, 1993, pp. 685–688.

167. J. S. Pate, P. J. Sharkey, and O. A. M. Lewis, *Planta*, *122*, 11–26 (1975).

168. B. J. Shelp and L. Liu, *Plant and Soil*, *140*, 151–155 (1992).

169. P. J. Hocking, *Ann. Bot.*, *45*, 633–643 (1980).

170. R. D. Graham, *Plant Cell Environ.*, *2*, 139–143 (1979).

171. T. Gollan, U. Schurr, and E. D. Schulze, *Plant Cell Environ.*, *15*, 551–559 (1992).

172. J. Le Bot, E. A. Kirkby, and M. L. Van Beusichem, *J. Plant Nutr.*, *13*, 513–526 (1990).

173. P. Zornoza and O. Carpena, *J. Plant Nutr.*, *19*, 469–480 (1996).

174. M. Bundt, S. Kretzschmar, W. Zech, and W. Wilcke, *Plant and Soil*, *197*, 157–166 (1997).

175. J. A. Campbell and S. Strother, *J. Plant Nutr.*, *19*, 867–879 (1996).

176. P. C. Andersen and B. V. Brodbeck, *Am. J. Enol. Vitic.*, *40*, 155–160 (1989).

177. P. C. Andersen and B. V. Brodbeck, *Physiol. Plant.*, *75*, 63–70 (1989).

178. P. C. Andersen and B. V. Brodbeck, *Am. J. Enol. Vitic.*, *42*, 245–251 (1991).

179. P. M. L. Tammes, *Acta Bot. Neerl.*, *7*, 233–234 (1958).

180. P. M. L. Tammes and J. Van Die, *Acta Bot. Neerl.*, *13*, 76–83 (1964).

4

Manganese Metabolism in Animals and Humans Including the Toxicity of Manganese

Carl L. Keen, Jodi L. Ensunsa,
and Michael S. Clegg

Department of Nutrition, University of California
at Davis, Davis, CA 95616, USA

1. INTRODUCTION

Manganese, the twelfth most abundant element in the biosphere, has been recognized since the Roman Empire; its name is thought to be derived from a Greek word for *magic*. That manganese in excess can be harmful to humans has been recognized since 1837, when Couper [1] reported that the chronic inhalation of high amounts of manganese oxide could result in neurological damage. That a deficit of this element could result in pathology in mammals was shown in 1931 by Kemmerer and co-workers when they reported that dietary manganese deficiency in the rat resulted in impaired growth [2]. That manganese deficiency could result in biochemical abnormalities in humans was first shown by Doisy in 1972 [3]. In this chapter, we will briefly summarize some of the literature related to manganese nutrition, toxicology, and metabolism in humans and experimental animals. Based on space constraints, review articles rather than original sources will be cited in many cases; the reader is directed to these reviews for the original citations and for an expanded discussion of the topics.

2. CHEMICAL AND PHYSICAL PROPERTIES

Manganese is a transition element located in group 7 (formerly VIIA) of the periodic table. It can exist in 11 oxidation states from -3 to $+7$. The most common valences are $+2$, $+4$, and $+7$, with the $+2$ valence found in most biological systems. In addition to the common salts (e.g., sulfates, chlorides, etc.), important manganese organometal compounds include the gasoline antiknock agent, methylcyclopentadienyl manganese tricarbonyl (MMT), and manganese ethylenebisdithiocarbamate, a fungicide. Manganese is also widely used as an oxidizing agent, in fertilizers and in dry cell batteries, and to form alloys with iron, aluminum, bronze, nickel-silver, and nickel-chromium [4].

The solution chemistry of manganese is relatively simple. The aqua ion is resistant to oxidation in acidic and neutral solutions. It does not begin to hydrolyze until pH 10, and as a consequence free Mn^{2+} can be present in neutral solutions at high concentrations [5]. Divalent manganese (Mn^{2+}) is a d^5 ion and typically forms high spin complexes lacking crystal field stabilization energies. The above properties, along with its rather large ionic radius and small charge/radius ratio, result in manganese forming relatively weak complexes with many ligands compared to other first-row divalent ions such as Ni^{2+} and Cu^{2+}. Free Mn^{2+} has a strong isotropic electron paramagnetic resonance (EPR) signal that can be used to assess its concentration in the micromolar range [6]. Mn^{3+} is also crucial in biological systems, as it is the oxidative state of manganese in superoxide dismutase and the form in which transferrin binds manganese.

3. ANALYSIS

While manganese is widely distributed in the biosphere, it is present in only trace concentrations in animal tissues. Serum concentrations are typically less than 10 nM, while tissue concentrations are generally less than 4 μM [7]. During the collection and handling of tissues, considerable care must be taken to minimize contamination given the comparably high environmental levels of manganese. Common analytical methods that can sensitively measure manganese (18 nmol/L) include neutron activation analysis, X-ray fluorescence, proton-induced X-ray emission, inductively coupled plasma (ICP) emission, EPR, and flameless atomic absorption spectrophotometry (FAAS). The most common methods currently employed to measure manganese in biological samples are ICP and FAAS, although the use of magnetic resonance imaging (MRI) to detect high concentrations of manganese is increasing. All of the methods, except EPR, measure the total concentration of manganese in the sample. EPR allows selective measurement of bound vs. free manganese.

4. PHYSIOLOGICAL ROLE

4.1. Tissue and Cellular Concentrations

There is little variation among species with regard to tissue manganese concentrations, reflecting in part the absence of manganese storage proteins. The average human body contains between 200 and 400 μmol of manganese, which is distributed uniformly throughout the body [7]. Tissues with high levels of mitochondria tend to have high manganese concentrations, as the concentration of manganese in mitochondria is higher than in cytoplasm. Hair can accumulate high amounts of manganese, and it has been suggested that hair manganese concentration can reflect manganese status [8], although this is an area of debate. Pigmented structures such as retina, dark skin, and melanin granules contain high concentrations of manganese. Bone, liver, pancreas, and kidney typically have higher concentrations of manganese (20–50 nmol/g) than other tissues. Brain, heart, lung, and muscle typically contain <20 nmol Mn/g; blood and serum concentrations are on the order of 200 and 20 nmol/L, respectively [8]. Bone can account for up to 25% of total body manganese because of its mass; however, bone manganese concentrations are not homeostatically controlled, and bone manganese is not readily mobilizable. In contrast to several other essential trace elements (e.g., zinc, copper, iron), the fetus does not accumulate manganese stores before birth, and fetal tissue concentrations are markedly less than adult concentrations. That manganese is not significantly accrued during the prenatal period can be attributed in part to the lack of storage proteins and the late ontogenic expression of many of the manganese-containing enzymes. Given that breast milk manganese concentrations can be very low (<10 nmol/L), it might be reasonable to assume that manganese deficiency would be a common finding in infants; however, as is discussed below, this has not been found to be the case.

4.2. Absorption, Transport, and Storage

Manganese absorption is thought to occur throughout the small intestine. The efficiency of manganese absorption is typically reported to be low, and it is not thought to be under homeostatic controls that are specific for manganese. For adult humans, manganese absorption has been reported to typically range from 2% to 15% when [54]Mn-labeled test meals are used and 25% when balance studies are conducted [9–11]. However, the absorption can be considerably higher (>30%) when iron is low in the diet or if the individual is anemic [9]. The above observation suggests that manganese and iron can share a common transport site or ligand(s) in the gut. Consistent with this concept, it has been reported that manganese may be transported via the DCT-1 pathway [12].

Using the Caco-2 cell line, Leblondel and Allain [13] have recently reported that under steady-state conditions the transport characteristics of manganese exhibit two components, a saturable (V_{max} = 3.70 ± 0.07 nmol/cm^2/h, K_m = 32.2 ± 3.4 μM) and a nonsaturable (slope 1.4 ± 0.2 × 10^{-6} cm^{-2}/h) pathway, which presumably reflect transcellular (carrier-mediated) and paracellular (diffusional) pathways, respectively. The above report is consistent with the idea that manganese can be transported via the DCT-1 pathway.

Manganese retention from human milk and infant formula is particularly high during infancy [14], and it has been suggested that infants may be particularly sensitive to the development of manganese toxicosis [15]. However, as is discussed below, cases of manganese toxicity in infants are rare.

The higher retention of manganese in young animals relative to adult animals reflects in part an immaturity of manganese excretion pathways during the neonatal period, and the very low tissue concentrations in infants, which dictate a positive uptake of manganese as the ontogenic expression of several manganese metalloenzymes occurs during early infancy [7].

High amounts of dietary calcium, phosphorus, fiber, and phytate can increase the requirement for dietary manganese, presumably due to the formation of poorly absorbed insoluble manganese complexes in the intestinal tract [16]. While the above interaction can be demonstrated in metabolic studies, the practical significance of these dietary factors with regard to human manganese requirements is an issue of considerable debate. A low fractional absorption of manganese from soy formula has been related to its high phytate content, and the dephytinization of soy formula with microbial phytase has been reported to increase fractional manganese absorption by twofold [9]. While the above change in absorption is impressive, the human health implications of such a change have yet to be resolved.

Manganese absorbed from the gastrointestinal tract enters the portal blood where it may either remain free or bind to α_2-macroglobulin, which is rapidly taken up by the liver. A small fraction (typically <10%) enters the systemic circulation where it can be oxidized to Mn^{3+} and bound to transferrin [17,18]. The factors governing the oxidation rate of manganese and its subsequent binding to transferrin are a subject of debate.

Manganese uptake by the liver has been reported to be through a unidirectional saturable process, with properties of passive transport [19]. Once manganese enters the liver, it can enter one of several pools. A high percentage of manganese enters the lysosome pool, from which it is transferred to the bile canaliculus. This is a rapid pathway, as evidenced by the observation that up to 50% of manganese absorbed either from the diet or from an intravenous injection may be recovered in the feces within 24 h. A second pool of manganese is associated with the mitochondria; the uptake and release of manganese by mitochondria is thought to be linked to calcium flux, and manganese may move through calcium channels. A third pool of manganese is found in the nuclear fraction of the cell; the role(s) of this pool is poorly understood. A fourth pool is incorporated into, or associated with, newly synthesized manganese proteins. Manganese can influence numerous metabolic pathways by binding to manganese-activated enzymes, ATP, and select membrane binding sites. A fifth pool is free Mn^{2+}; fluctuations in this pool can represent an important regulation of cellular metabolic control in a manner analogous to free Ca^{2+} and Mg^{2+} [19,20]. For example, manganese can block glucose-induced insulin release in pancreatic cells by altering cellular calcium fluxes, and manganese can augment contractions in smooth muscle by a mechanism similar to that of calcium [21,22].

The mechanism(s) by which manganese is transported to, and taken up by, extrahepatic tissues has not been firmly identified. Within the plasma pool, a high fraction of manganese is associated with transferrin, and it has been suggested that this is a major transport protein for the element [17,18]. Consistent with this, manganese metabolism has been reported to be abnormal in the Belgrade rat, an animal characterized by defects in transferrin metabolism [23]. In contrast to the above, Malecki et al. [24] have recently reported that whole-body [54]Mn kinetics are similar in mice with normal and very low levels of transferrin. This finding suggests that transferrin does not play an essential role in manganese uptake by extrahepatic tissues. The observation that manganese uptake by extrahepatic tissues is not increased under conditions of manganese deficiency [25] suggests the lack of a specific inducible manganese transport protein in either the plasma pool or in cell membranes.

Changes in the levels of adrenal, pancreatic, and pituitary-gonadal axis hormones can affect tissue manganese concentrations [26]; however, it is unclear as to whether hormone-induced changes in tissue manganese concentrations are due to direct alterations in the cellular uptake or release of manganese, vs. changes in the production of select manganese-activated enzymes or manganese metalloenzymes. For example, in diabetes, liver and kidney manganese concentrations can be grossly elevated; however, this is thought to be due to increases in tissue arginase (a manganese metalloenzyme) activity, rather than a change in the insulin regulation of manganese transport or tissue manganese uptake [27].

4.3. Metabolic Function and Essentiality

Manganese functions as a constituent of metalloenzymes and as an enzyme activator. Manganese-containing enzymes include arginase, pyruvate carboxylase, and manganese-superoxide dismutase (MnSOD). Arginase, a cytosolic enzyme responsible for urea formation, contains 4 mol Mn^{2+} per mol of enzyme [8]. It has been found that manganese binding by arginase is critical for the pH sensing function of this enzyme in the ornithine cycle, suggesting that manganese may play a role in pH regulation [28]. The activity of arginase can be sharply reduced in manganese-deficient animals, and this can represent a functional challenge (see below).

Pyruvate carboxylase, the enzyme that catalyzes the first step of carbohydrate synthesis from pyruvate, contains 4 mol Mn^{2+} per mol of enzyme [8]. As is discussed below, the activity of this enzyme is only marginally influenced by dietary manganese intake.

MnSOD catalyzes the disproportionation of $O_2^{\bullet-}$ to H_2O_2 and O_2.

The essential role of MnSOD in the free radical defense system has been elegantly demonstrated by MnSOD knockout models. Mice that are null for MnSOD die within the first few weeks of life with a dilated cardiomyopathy, accumulation of lipid in liver and skeletal muscle, and metabolic acidosis [29]. Similarly, mice that are heterozygous for the MnSOD gene show a 50% decrease in liver MnSOD activity and extensive tissue oxidative damage [30]. In contrast to the above, transgenic animals that overexpress MnSOD are characterized by improved resistance to numerous stressors including alcohol, ozone, tumor necrosis factor-α (TNF-α), and irradiation [31,32]. As would be predicted from the above, in the normal animal, exposure to stressors that induce the production of reactive oxygen species (e.g., alcohol, TNF-α, ozone, etc.) typically results in an increase in MnSOD activity in target tissues [33,34]. Importantly, the activity of MnSOD can also be affected by the manganese status of the animal; the functional significance of manganese deficiency-associated reductions in tissue MnSOD activity is discussed below.

For manganese-activated reactions, the metal can act by binding either to the substrate (such as ATP) or directly to the protein, resulting in conformational changes. In contrast to the relatively few manganese metalloenzymes, there are a large number of manganese-activated enzymes, including hydrolases, kinases, decarboxylases, and transferases [7]. Manganese activation of these enzymes can occur as a direct result of the metal binding to the protein, causing a conformational change, or by binding to the substrate, such as ATP. Many of these metal activations are nonspecific in that other metal ions, particularly Mg^{2+}, can replace Mn^{2+}. An exception to this nonspecific manganese activation of enzymes is the manganese-specific activation of glycosyltransferases. Several manganese deficiency-induced pathologies have been attributed to a low activity of these enzymes [35,36]. A second example of an enzyme that may be specifically activated by manganese is phosphoenolpyruvate carboxykinase (PEPCK), the enzyme that catalyzes the conversion of oxaloacetate to phosphoenolpyruvate, GDP, and CO_2. Although low activities of PEPCK can occur in manganese-deficient animals [37], the functional significance of this is not clear.

A third example of a manganese-activated enzyme is glutamine synthetase. This enzyme, found in high concentrations in the brain, catalyzes the reaction NH_3 + glutamate + ATP $\rightarrow$ glutamine + ADP +

P_i. Brain glutamine synthetase activity can be normal even in severely manganese-deficient animals, suggesting that the enzyme either has a high priority for manganese or that magnesium can act as a substitute when manganese is lacking [38].

4.4. Homeostasis

While tissue manganese concentrations typically fall within a narrow range, well-defined homeostatic control mechanisms for this element have not been elucidated. Thus the cellular concentration of manganese is primarily determined by the level of expression of manganese-activated enzymes and manganese metalloproteins. The lack of a clearly identified manganese storage protein stands in marked contrast to the case for zinc, copper, and iron. However, the apparent lack of manganese storage proteins may provide one explanation as to why genetic causes of mammalian manganese toxicity have not been identified to date. The lack of robust homeostatic controls for manganese suggests that under normal environmental circumstances animals are not typically exposed to prolonged periods of either manganese deficiency or manganese toxicity, or that if they are exposed to an excess, tissue pathology occurs relatively late in life.

5. MANGANESE DEFICIENCY

5.1. Experimental Animals

Signs of manganese deficiency have been induced in numerous species including rats, mice, pigs, chickens, and cattle. Significantly, while it has often been argued that manganese deficiency is difficult to induce, cases of manganese deficiency in chickens and cattle have been reported to occur even under nonexperimental conditions [8,39,40]. Typical signs of manganese deficiency include impaired growth, skeletal abnormalities, impaired reproductive performance, congenital ataxia, and defects in lipid, carbohydrate, and protein metabolism. Some of the biochemical defects that contribute to the above deficiency signs are considered below.

One of the major effects of manganese deficiency during early development is on the skeleton. In rats and mice, a deficit of manganese during the early postnatal period can result in a syndrome characterized by a shortening of the radius, ulna, tibia, and fibula; a curvature of the spine; and a localized dysplasia of the tibial epiphysis [8]. In cattle, manganese deficiency has been reported to result in a dwarf-like appearance, joint laxity, domed forehead, and growth plate abnormalities including irregularly aligned and short columns of chondrocytes [39,40]. Finally, in chickens and other birds, manganese deficiency can result in perosis, a disorder which is characterized by shortened and thickened limbs, curvature of the spine, and swollen and enlarged joints [8]. The above bone abnormalities have been largely attributed to abnormal cartilage and bone matrix formation secondary to a reduction in the production of stable proteoglycans. The reduction in proteoglycan content and stability is attributed to reductions in the activity of manganese-activated glycosyltransferases [8]. In addition to low glycosyltransferase activity, manganese deficiency can result in impaired osteoblast and osteoclast activities [41], and in abnormal growth factor metabolism [42]. In this regard, it has been demonstrated that manganese deficiency results in decreased circulating insulin-like growth factor-1 (IGF-1) concentrations. This mitogenic factor has a defined role in growth, and in bone and glucose metabolism. Thus it is reasonable to speculate that abnormal rates of bone growth, and remodeling, may also contribute to the occurrence of some of the bone deformities observed in manganese-deficient animals.

A striking defect that can be associated with prenatal manganese deficiency is a congenital irreversible ataxia, which is characterized by a lack of equilibrium and retraction of the head. The ataxia occurs as a result of an impaired development of the otoliths, i.e., calcified structures in the inner ear that are essential for righting reflexes. Similar to the bone abnormalities described above, the major biochemical defect thought to contribute to the occurrence of abnormal otoliths in manganese-deficient animals is low activity of manganese-activated glycosyltransferases [8]. It is worth noting that two genetic models for ataxia—the pallid mouse and the screwneck mink—are responsive to high levels of dietary manganese. When the diet of the pregnant pallid mouse (or screwneck mink) contains a control level of manganese, the offspring typically expresses an ataxia. However, if the mother's diet is supplemented with high levels of manganese, the phenotypic expression of ataxia is prevented [8,43]. While the most dramatic phenotype of the pallid and screwneck gene is ataxia, both mutants also show coat color defects which are responsive to manganese supplementation [8,43]. The above observation would seem to indicate that the gene defect in both species involves a manganese transport or binding ligand that is independent of glycosyltransferase. Recent reports that the pallid mouse may have utility as a model for emphysema [44,45] should provide an impetus for the increased characterization of these manganese-responsive genes at the molecular level.

In addition to skeletal and inner ear lesions, manganese deficiency can result in numerous ultrastructural abnormalities in multiple tissues. In young animals, manganese deficiency can result in pancreatic pathology, with deficient animals showing severe hypoplasia of all cellular components [46]. In cardiac and hepatic tissue, and in the retina, manganese deficiency can trigger ultrastructural changes that include alterations in the integrity of cell membranes, swollen and irregular endoplasmic reticulum, and elongated mitochondria with stacked cristae [34,47,48]. The above membrane defects are thought to be due in part to excessive oxidative damage secondary to reductions in tissue MnSOD activity. Consistent with this are observations that an early effect of manganese deficiency can be a reduction in MnSOD activity that is accompanied by evidence of increased lipid peroxidation rates [34,49]. Furthermore, the retinal degeneration observed in the WBN/Kob rat (a mutant strain characterized by low retinal SOD levels) is similar to that observed in the manganese-deficient rat [47,50]. Finally, manganese-deficient animals have been shown to have an increased sensitivity to insults such as ozone and alcohol which produce oxidative stress [34,51] in a manner analogous to that observed for MnSOD knockout models [52,53]. These studies underscore the pivotal role MnSOD plays in protecting the mitochondria from oxidative events arising in the cytosol and/or within the mitochondria itself. In regard to the latter, MnSOD, along with mitochondrial pore-forming proteins such as BCL-2, protects the mitochondrial membrane potential by sequestering leaking radicals derived from inefficient coupling of the electron transport system during mitochondrial respiration [54,55]. Using overexpression systems, investigators have shown that MnSOD blocks apoptosis mediated by cytokines such as TNF-α. Thus, MnSOD affords the cell protection against both receptor- and non-receptor-mediated apoptotic signals.

Abnormal lipid metabolism is another characteristic of manganese deficiency. In rats and mice, chronic manganese deficiency can result in lipid accumulation in the liver and in the peritoneal cavity as well as hypocholesterolemia and low high-density lipoprotein concentrations [8]. The mechanisms underlying the increased fat deposition have not been identified; however, abnormal lipoprotein metabolism has been reported to be a consequence of manganese deficiency in some species, although this is highly strain-dependent [56–58]. Deficient animals can also be characterized by a shift to smaller plasma high-density lipoprotein particles, lower high-density lipoprotein apolipoprotein E (apo E) concentrations, and higher apo C concentrations [57].

Manganese-deficient animals can be characterized by numerous abnormalities in carbohydrate metabolism. As could be predicted by the extensive pancreatic pathology that can be present in these animals (see above), these animals can be characterized by low insulin production and a diabetic-type condition [59]. Interestingly, while some of the reduction in insulin production may be linked to a reduction in pancreatic cell mass, manganese also appears to have a direct role in insulin release from the β cell. It has been suggested that this occurs in part through an interaction with calcium [60,61]. Insulin release from islets isolated from manganese-deficient rats has also been shown to be impaired using both glucose and arachidonic acid as stimuli [60]. The above observation is important as it suggests that the manganese-deficient cells have at least two sites of aberrant signal transduction. In addition to defects in insulin release, manganese-deficient animals can have low insulin mRNA levels [60]; it is not known if the low levels are the consequence of decreased transcription or enhanced insulin mRNA turnover. Similarly, it is not known whether the changes in mRNA levels are a direct or an indirect effect of low cellular manganese concentrations. The observation that the regulation of the expression of other pancreatic genes, such as amylase, can also be influenced by dietary manganese [62] suggests that some of the effects may be indirect. Finally, manganese deficiency results in decreased circulating IGF-1. This hormone, acting through its own receptor, has been shown to mimic insulin effects on glucose metabolism [63]. Hence, the compound effect of decreased circulating insulin and IGF-1 may explain the elevated circulating glucose concentrations typical of manganese-deficient animals.

Compounding the defects in insulin metabolism, gluconeogenesis can be affected by manganese deficiency. Pyruvate carboxylase and PEPCK both require manganese for optimal function, with pyruvate carboxylase a manganese metalloenzyme and PEPCK a manganese-activated enzyme. While pyruvate carboxylase activity is not significantly reduced in manganese-deficient animals, PEPCK activity can be [37]. The observation that gluconeogenesis and PEPCK activity can be reduced in the deficient animal is consistent with the observation that the activation of PEPCK during gluconeogenesis requires a significant shift in intracellular manganese pools [6]. While the above changes in glucose metabolism can often be detected in manganese-deficient animals, it should be emphasized that these perturbations are often not robust. Thus their functional significance for the health of the animal can be questioned. Future work aimed at defining the influence of severe manganese deficiency on glucose homeostasis in the neonate may be particularly enlightening in this regard, as there is an as-of-yet unexplained high mortality rate in manganese-deficient animals during the first few days of life [8].

An important biochemical abnormality in manganese-deficient animals can be marked reductions (>50%) in liver arginase activity. While arginase is not typically considered to be a rate-limiting enzyme for urea synthesis, manganese-deficient animals have been shown to be characterized by higher than normal levels of plasma ammonia [62]. While the magnitude of the increase in ammonia in the above report was not severe, high mortality rates have been observed in manganese-deficient rats under conditions of high gluconeogenic demand [51].

5.2. Humans

That a condition of manganese deficiency could arise in a human subject due to dietary means was first suggested by Doisy in 1972 [3] (Table 1). This investigator reported a case of a subject who developed abnormal lipid metabolism, and a redding of hair, after the long-term consumption of a purified diet in which manganese had been inadvertently omitted. While this report elicited considerable comment, it was not

TABLE 1

Selected Cases of Suspected Human Manganese Deficiency

Observation	Authors/Ref.
Accidental Mn deficiency in a male subject	Doisy, 1972 [3]
Epileptics have low blood Mn	Papavasiliou et al., 1979 [68]
A link between Mseleni's disease and Mn deficiency	Fincham et al., 1981 [66]
Low blood Mn in non–head injury epileptics	Carl et al., 1986 [69]
Experimental Mn deficiency in male subjects	Friedman et al., 1987 [64]
Skin lesions and bone abnormalities due to Mn deficiency in an infant on long-term TPN	Norose and Arai, 1987 [65]
Iron supplementation (60 mg/day for 125 days) resulted in reduced lymphocyte MnSOD activity in adult women	Davis and Greger, 1992 [79]
High percentage of postmenopausal women have low blood Mn; Mn supplementation enhanced bone mass gain	Strause et al., 1994 [67]

considered conclusive due to the uncontrolled nature of the study. In 1987, Friedman et al. [64] reported that signs of manganese deficiency (dermatitis and increases in serum calcium, phosphorus, and alkaline phosphatase) were observed in healthy male subjects fed manganese-deficient diets (0.1 mg Mn/day vs. 2–4 mg Mn/day for controls) for 39 days. Significantly, the clinical signs of the deficiency resolved rapidly upon reintroduction of manganese into the diet. A case of dietary manganese deficiency has also been reported by Norose and Arai [65], who describe skin lesions and potential bone abnormalities in an infant maintained on long-term total parenteral nutrition. Complementing the reports on dietary manganese deficiency in humans, several disease states including epilepsy, Mselini's disease, Down's syndrome, Perthes' disease, and osteoporosis have been reported to be characterized by evidence of low soft tissue or blood manganese concentrations [46,66]. Two of these diseases, epilepsy and osteoporosis, may merit special attention. In the case of osteoporosis, Strause and co-workers [67] have reported that a high percentage of postmenopausal women have very low blood manganese concentrations. In a provocative study, these investigators showed that the addition of manganese to a mineral supplement significantly enhanced bone mass gain in postmenopausal women involved in a clinical trial. While the above trial should not be overinterpreted, the results obtained with the human subjects are consistent with the experimental animal literature.

With respect to epilepsy, several authors have reported that blood manganese levels tend to be low in epileptics [68,69]. Significantly, the low values cannot be attributed to anticonvulsant use [70]. Furthermore, values are lower in subjects with epilepsy of unknown origin than in subjects with head trauma-induced epilepsy [69], suggesting a possible genetic cause. Consistent with the above idea, the genetically epilepsy-prone rat (GEPR) is characterized by low tissue manganese concentrations relative to its genetic control prior to the occurrence of its first seizure [71], and manganese-deficient rats show an increased susceptibility to electroshock-induced epilepsy [72]. The mechanism(s) underlying an increased risk for epilepsy under conditions of manganese deficiency has not been identified. While it has been postulated that severe manganese deficiency might result in a reduction in brain glutamine synthetase activity (a manganese-activated enzyme), this hypothesis has not received experimental support [38].

A third disease that has been investigated with respect to manganese therapy is diabetes. Rubenstein and co-workers in 1962 [73] reported a case in which a diabetic subject in South Africa responded to low doses of manganese (5–10 mg) with a sharp reduction in plasma glucose concentration. The subject was tested with manganese supplements due to his statement that a common folk remedy in his area for the treatment of "sweet urine disease" was an alfalfa tea, which proved to be rich in manganese. In a series of studies with ^{54}Mn, it was observed that the subject had a higher than normal urinary excretion of manganese. Consistent with the report by Rubenstein and co-workers [73], Hassanein et al. found that individuals with manganese toxicity can exhibit prolonged reactive hypoglycemia following the administration of intravenous glucose [74]. Others have found high doses of manganese to act in an insulin-mimetic manner in rabbits [75,76]. While the above reports appear promising, particularly when combined with the known effects of manganese deficiency on insulin and glucose metabolism in experimental animals, it must be noted that in a study of six diabetic and seven nondiabetic subjects, manganese doses up to 10 mg had no effect on blood glucose levels [77]. While it is tempting to advocate large clinical trials of manganese supplementation in osteoporotics, epileptics, and diabetics, considerable risks can be associated with the excessive use of manganese supplements (see below).

In light of the above discussion, it is worth asking the question of whether dietary manganese intake by human populations is on the low or high side. While dietary intakes will clearly vary considerably across different geographic areas and across different dietary patterns, intakes are thought to be on the marginal side in many populations [78]. Significantly, even modest levels of iron supplementation (60 mg/day for 125 days) have been reported to result in reduced lymphocyte MnSOD activities in adult women [79]. Consistent with the above, Kuratko [80] has reported that in a rat model, modest levels of dietary iron supplementation (140 mg/kg) can result in reductions in MnSOD activity in colonic mucosa. This author suggested that a reduction in MnSOD activity could increase the risk for colonic cancer. While the functional significance of a modest reduction in tissue manganese concentrations with iron supplementation is a matter of debate, this is an area that demands further study.

6. MANGANESE TOXICITY

6.1. Experimental Animals

In domestic as well as experimental animals, the most commonly reported effect of dietary manganese toxicity is a secondary iron deficiency. As discussed above, the iron deficiency primarily arises as a consequence of a competitive inhibition between manganese and iron for common transport sites and ligands [8]. However, while relatively modest levels of iron supplementation can result in a reduction in manganese absorption, dietary manganese levels typically have to exceed 1000 μg/day prior to there being an effect on iron absorption. Diets containing in excess of 2000 μg Mn/g have been reported to cause signs of depressed growth, anorexia, and altered brain function and behavioral abnormalities in experimental animals [8,60]. In marked contrast to dietary manganese deficiency, dietary manganese toxicity is not associated with reproductive failure in experimental animals. While high levels of manganese have been reported to be teratogenic in mice, rats, rabbits, and hamsters [81], these reports have been limited to situations in which the dose was given by injection. It is important to also note that in the above cases the dose of manganese used was sufficient to induce signs of maternal toxicity; thus, the reported developmental toxic effects of manganese can be the result of secondary changes in maternal metabolism (i.e., elevated production of acute phase proteins, stress hormones, select cytokines, etc.), rather than due to a direct effect of manganese on the conceptus.

Acute manganese toxicity in experimental animals can result in marked abnormalities in carbohydrate metabolism. When adult rats are given an intraperitoneal injection of manganese (2.5 μg/kg BW), there is a rapid uptake of manganese by the pancreas, liver, and kidney. In the liver, one consequence of this is a rapid mobilization of liver glycogen stores, which contributes to a marked hyperglycemia in the injected animals. Concomitant with the above, insulin release from the pancreas is sharply reduced following acute manganese exposure. Presumably, this reduction in insulin output further contributes to the hyperglycemic condition. Within 2–4 h following the manganese injection, pancreatic and liver manganese concentrations decrease sharply to near-normal levels, and insulin is released from the pancreas. The amount of insulin released can be significant, and a condition of hypoglycemia will arise in some animals [82,83]. While the above effects can be dramatic, it is important to note that altered carbohydrate homeostasis has not been reported to be characteristic of dietary manganese toxicosis in experimental animals, nor is it a characteristic of human manganese toxicity.

Similar to humans (see below), chronic manganese toxicity in experimental animals can result in central nervous system pathology [84]. Nonhuman primates given multiple injections of manganese over a several week period can develop a parkinsonian syndrome characterized by bradykinesia, rigidity, and facial grimacing [85–87]. While multiple components of the brain are affected by manganese toxicosis, the globus pallidus and substantia nigra pars reticularis are particularly affected in primates [86–88]. Pappas and co-workers [89] reported that day 30 rat pups borne to dams who received water containing 10 mg/mL manganese throughout gestation and lactation had a thinning of the cerebral cortex; the mechanism(s) underlying this defect is unknown.

In rodent models, chronic manganese toxicosis has been shown to result in behavioral abnormalities. Rats treated with manganese (350 μg/kg BW) for 30 days showed an impaired ability to traverse a T maze compared to noninjected controls; the above behavioral abnormality was corrected following the cessation of the injections [90]. The authors of the above work suggested that the behavioral abnormalities noted in their study were secondary to manganese toxicity-induced changes in brain lipid metabolism.

An additional behavioral abnormality, which has been described by several investigators, is an increase in spontaneous activity [89]; again, the mechanisms underlying this effect of manganese toxicity have not been identified.

Several groups have argued that the central nervous system pathology associated with manganese toxicosis is largely due to manganese-induced cellular free radical damage [91,92]. The above hypothesis is based on the potent redox properties of manganese and the observation that in vitro manganese can act to oxidize numerous biomolecules [91–93]. However, in vivo, manganese appears to act as an antioxidant rather than a prooxidant [94]. That the extensive neurological damage associated with chronic manganese toxicosis is not primarily due to manganese-induced oxidative damage is supported by the recent observations of Brenneman et al. [95] that brain mitochondrial 8-hydroxy-2'-deoxyguanosine concentrations (a marker of DNA oxidative damage) are not elevated even in rats showing marked signs of manganese toxicosis. However, in contrast to the above, Ali et al. [96] have reported that acute manganese intoxication is associated with an increase in oxidative stress in rat caudate nucleus and hippocampus. Furthermore, Desole et al. [97] and Hirata et al. [98] have reported that manganese-induced oxidative stress can be sufficient to trigger the apoptopic pathway. While the observations on manganese-induced apoptosis are intriguing, it must be emphasized that to date this effect has only been observed in in vitro models.

Finally, Zheng et al. [99] have recently reported that both in vitro and in vivo, high levels of manganese can result in brain region-specific reductions in aconitase activity. These authors have argued that the reduction in aconitase activity is secondary to manganese-induced changes in iron metabolism. The authors also suggest that the reduction in aconitase activity is sufficient to result in a disruption in mitochondrial energy production. Given the critical role that aconitase plays in cellular iron metabolism, it is reasonable to speculate that several iron-dependent pathways could be negatively affected in the manganese-intoxicated animal.

6.2. Humans

In humans, manganese toxicity is recognized to be a serious health hazard, resulting in severe pathologies of the central nervous system. In its most severe forms, manganese toxicity can result in a syndrome characterized by severe psychiatric symptoms, including hyperirritability, violent acts, hallucinations, decreases of libido, and incoordination. If the exposure occurs for a long period of time, the toxicity can result in a permanent crippling of the extrapyramidal system, with symptoms reminiscent of Parkinson's disease [100] (Table 2). The term *manganese madness* (locura manganica) has been applied to the above symptoms of manganese toxicity [60]. While the majority of cases of manganese toxicity have been reported in individuals exposed to very high concentrations of airborne manganese (>5 mg/m^3; values that can occur in manganese mines and battery factories), subtle signs of manganese toxicity including delayed reaction time, impaired motor coordination, and impaired memory have been observed in workers exposed to airborne manganese concentrations less than 1 mg/m^3 [60,101]. In humans, manganese accumulation can be particularly pronounced in the nuclei of the basal ganglia, particularly the caudate, putamen, globus pallidus, subthalamic nucleus, and substantia nigra. To a significant extent, pathological changes in the brain primarily correspond to those areas that accumulate high levels of manganese [60]. As discussed above for experimental animals, the mechanisms underlying the neurotoxic effects of high levels of manganese in humans are poorly understood. The sensitivity of individuals to airborne manganese toxicity may reflect the fact that manganese can be transported directly

TABLE 2

Selected Cases of Human Manganese Toxicity

Observation	Authors/Ref.
Paralytic disease in workers in a pyrolusite mill	Couper, 1837 [1]
Neurological disorders due to Mn toxicity via contaminated water	Kawamura et al., 1941 [114]
Neurological disorders in Mn mine workers	Cotzias et al., 1968 [100]
Mn toxicity due to excessive oral Mn supplements	Banta and Markesbury, 1977 [113]
Pancreatitis due to Mn-contaminated dialysis fluid	Taylor and Price, 1982 [105]
Behavioral abnormalities due to high Mn in drinking water	Kondakis et al., 1989 [115]
Mn toxicity due to chronic TPN feeding	Fell et al., 1996 [11]
Elevated brain Mn caused by cirrhosis correlated with behavioral abnormalities	Spahr et al., 1996 [108]; Layrargues et al., 1998 [110]

from the respiratory tract to the brain. In addition to alveolar absorption into the bloodstream, it has been reported that significant amounts of manganese uptake may occur via the nasal mucosa, with direct olfactory axonal transport to the central nervous system [102]. Regrettably, the neurological damage in adults that occurs following chronic manganese intoxication can persist for years, even when the individual is removed from the high manganese environment [60,103]. The observation that the above occurs despite a normalization of tissue manganese concentrations [60,103] suggests that there is significant neuronal loss during the course of the toxicity. In contrast to the findings for adults, it was recently reported that neurological signs of manganese toxicity in children can resolve following the removal of the insult [104]. It is not clear if the difference between the experience for children and adults represents a difference in the length of the initial manganese exposure, or if it reflects an age-dependent change in susceptibility to manganese toxicity.

In addition to extensive neural damage, reproductive and immune system dysfunction, nephritis, testicular damage, pancreatitis, and hepatic damage can occur with manganese toxicity (Table 2), but the incidence of these disorders is not known [60,105]. Manganese is known to be mutagenic in nonmammalian systems, but mutagenicity has not been reported in mammalian systems [106]. High levels of dietary manganese have not been reported to be teratogenic in the absence of overt signs of maternal toxicity [81]. High levels of brain manganese have been reported in subjects with amyotrophic lateral sclerosis, and it has been suggested that this increase may contribute to the progression of the disease [107].

Manganese toxicity has also been reported to occur in individuals with impaired biliary function. For example, a variety of conditions causing cirrhosis result in elevated blood and brain manganese concentrations which have been correlated with the occurrence of behavioral abnormalities [108–110]. Several cases of manganese toxicity have also been reported to occur as a result of chronic total parenteral nutrition (TPN) feeding, where the TPN fluids contain high amounts of manganese [111,112]. Additionally, Banta and Markesbury [113] have reported a case of manganese toxicity occurring in an individual who consumed manganese supplements for several years (Table 2).

In contrast to the above, there are relatively few cases in the literature to suggest that high levels of dietary manganese result in toxicity syndromes. Kawamura et al. [114] reported that 25 cases of manganese toxicity, including 2 deaths, occurred in a village that consumed water from a well contaminated with manganese. The authors reported that the contamination (estimated at 28 mg Mn/L) was secondary to the disposal of dry-cell batteries. Interestingly, all of the reported cases involved adults, and children living in the area appeared unaffected. While the above report is intriguing, it is important to note that in the Kawamura study the actual intakes of manganese by the subjects were not documented, nor is there an extensive documentation of tissue manganese concentrations in the subjects. Thus, it is difficult to evaluate the extent to which the reported pathologies occur directly due to manganese, rather than a coordination of factors. More recently, Kondakis and co-workers [115] reported a high incidence of behavioral abnormalities in adult individuals living in areas in Greece exposed to high concentrations of manganese in drinking water (1.8–2.3 mg Mn/L), relative to individuals living in areas in which drinking water contained less than 0.075 mg Mn/L. However, while this paper has received considerable attention by regulatory agencies, there is a critical lack of information in the paper on the manganese intake by the two populations. In the absence of this information, the Kondakis report cannot be critically evaluated. It is important to note that in contrast to the Kondakis paper, Vieregge et al. [116] recently reported that individuals who consumed well water containing high levels of manganese for several years were neurologically normal. While a number of concerns have been expressed over the Kawamura and Kondakis reports, data from these papers were used in the establishment of the recent US EPA oral reference dose (RFD) for manganese. The RFD was set at 0.14 mg/kg/day for dietary sources. However, for nondietary sources (including water and soil), the RFD level was set at 0.05 mg/kg/day [117].

Finally, there has been concern recently that the risk for manganese toxicity may be increasing in some geographic areas because of the use of MMT in gasoline as an antiknock agent. However, there is little evidence that air, water, or food manganese concentrations have markedly increased in geographic areas in which this fuel additive has been used [101].

7. ASSESSMENT OF MANGANESE STATUS

Reliable biomarkers for the assessment of manganese status have yet to be identified [118]. In experimental animals, bone and select soft tissues (brain, liver, kidney, and pancreas) can reflect conditions of severe manganese toxicosis and manganese deficiency. However, neither bone nor soft tissue manganese analysis has been shown to be of value in identifying conditions of marginal manganese status [8,60]. Similarly, in humans, while soft tissue (brain and liver) manganese concentrations have been reported to be increased under conditions of severe toxicity, they have not been shown to be of value in identifying either marginal conditions of deficiency or toxicity [8,60]. Whole-blood manganese concentrations have been shown to be reflective of soft tissue manganese concentrations in rats; however, similar relationships have not been shown in humans [119], although the finding of grossly elevated blood manganese levels in humans has been associated with high brain manganese concentrations [108,109].

Serum and plasma manganese concentrations have been reported to be reduced in individuals fed low-manganese diets under controlled conditions [64], and low levels have also been reported in women given high levels of iron supplements [79]. Conversely, plasma manganese concentrations have been shown to be elevated in subjects given TPN solutions high in manganese content and in individuals with choleostatic liver disease [108,109,111,112]. While the above findings suggest that the measurement of blood and plasma manganese levels can be of value, it should be emphasized that there is a lack of clearly defined normative values for both plasma and blood manganese. Furthermore, there is a dearth of information on the influence of most disease states on the blood plasma concentration of manganese.

Lymphocyte and soft tissue MnSOD activity has been reported to be sensitive to dietary manganese intake [8,79,120]; however, MnSOD activity can also be influenced by a variety of factors that induce oxidative stress including ethanol, ozone, strenuous physical exercise, and high-fat diets [8,121–123]. Thus, this assay in isolation is of limited diagnostic value. As discussed above, in experimental animals the measurement of liver and kidney arginase activity can be of some value in the assessment of manganese status. However, the activity of this enzyme can be influenced by a number of other factors including diabetes and high-protein diets [8].

As a complement to the measurement of tissue manganese concentrations and the determination of the activities of select manganese enzymes, there are some signs of manganese deficiency and manganese toxicosis that can be tested for. As described above, typical signs of manganese deficiency include growth retardation, skeletal abnormalities, and some subtle metabolic changes (a diabetic-like glucose tolerance curve and changes in lipoprotein profiles); however, none of the above signs are robust or specific enough to be diagnostic. With respect to manganese toxicosis, the combined use of select neurofunctional tests and positron emission tomography (PET) and MRI techniques may be diagnostic for mild to severe manganese toxicity [108,109,124]. While it is relatively expensive, the use of MRI and PET to detect early evidence of brain manganese accumulation in individuals living in or around high-manganese environments may be of value. In addition, the use of MRI may be useful in the evaluation of patients with liver disease.

8. SUMMARY AND FUTURE DIRECTIONS

In contrast to other essential trace elements, the absorption of manganese is not well regulated, and there is little evidence of homeostatic mechanisms that directly regulate the uptake and efflux of manganese from the gut. Absorbed manganese primarily is transported via α-macroglobulin and transferrin; the ligand(s) that facilitates tissue uptake of manganese have yet to be identified, though transferrin is thought to participate in this function. Studies aimed at the identification of the ligands that influence extrahepatic tissue manganese uptake (particularly the brain) are urgently needed. In addition to the intestinal tract, significant amounts of manganese can be taken up via the respiratory tract, and manganese taken up through the nasal mucosa can be transported directly to the brain via olfactory axonal transport. Despite significant amounts of manganese in the environment, tissue concentrations of this element are typically low; these low concentrations in part reflect the lack of manganese storage proteins.

Fluctuations in the intracellular concentration of free Mn^{2+} can provide a regulatory role for some metabolic processes via the activation of select enzymes. While manganese deficiency is rare, spontaneous cases do arise in domestic animals and in avian species. The incidence of spontaneous manganese deficiency in humans is not known, but several disease states are characterized by low blood manganese concentrations. Studies aimed at an evaluation of the value of manganese supplementation in these diseases are needed. At the biochemical level, manganese deficiency is reflected by low tissue glycosyltransferase, MnSOD, and arginase activities. Manganese-deficient animals are characterized by connective tissue defects, behavioral abnormalities, and abnormalities in lipid and carbohydrate metabolism. A striking feature of severe manganese deficiency can be abnormal pancreatic function.

Manganese is required for normal brain function, and deficient animals may be characterized by an increased risk for epilepsy. Conversely, manganese toxicity can result in severe and persistent neurological damage. Manganese toxicity has been primarily reported to occur in individuals exposed to high levels of manganese in the air in the work environment; however, cases of manganese toxicosis due to excessive dietary exposure have been reported. In addition, manganese toxicity has been reported to be a common complication of liver disease, as manganese is primarily excreted through the bile. Given the persistent neurological damage that can arise as a consequence of chronic manganese toxicity, a better understanding of the biochemical lesions underlying the toxic effects of manganese is clearly needed. In a similar vein, improved biomarkers for the assessment of manganese status should be a research priority.

ACKNOWLEDGMENT

Some of the research described in Sec. 5.1 was supported by NIH-DK46178.

ABBREVIATIONS

ADP	adenosine 5'-diphosphate
Apo C	apolipoprotein C
Apo E	apolipoprotein E
ATP	adenosine 5'-triphosphate
BW	body weight
DCT-1	divalent cation transporter-1
EPR	electron paramagnetic resonance
FAAS	flameless atomic absorption spectrophotometry
GDP	guanosine 5'-diphosphate
GEPR	genetically epilepsy-prone rat
ICP	inductively coupled plasma
IGF-1	insulin-like growth factor-1
MMT	methylcyclopentadienyl manganese tricarbonyl

MnSOD   manganese-superoxide dismutase
MRI   magnetic resonance imaging
mRNA   messenger ribonucleic acid
PEPCK   phosphoenolpyruvate carboxykinase
PET   positron emission tomography
P_i inorganic phosphate
RFD   reference dose
TNF-α tumor necrosis factor-α
TPN   total parenteral nutrition
US EPA   United States Environmental Protection Agency

REFERENCES

1. J. Couper, *Br. Ann. Med. Pharm. Vital Statis. General Sci.*, *1*, 41–42 (1837).

2. A. R. Kemmerer, C. A. Elvehjem, and E. B. Hart, *Biol. Chem.*, *92*, 623–630 (1931).

3. E. Doisy, Jr., Micronutrient controls of biosynthesis of clotting proteins and cholesterol, *Trace Substances in Environmental Health, Vol. 6* (D. Hemphill, ed.), University of Missouri, Columbia, 1972, p. 193.

4. C. L. Keen and R. M. Leach, in *Handbook on Toxicity of Inorganic Compounds* (H. G. Seiler, H. Sigel, and A. Sigel, eds.), Marcel Dekker, New York, 1987, pp. 405–415.

5. F. A. Cotton and G. Wilkinson, in *Advanced Organic Chemistry*, 4th ed., Wiley-Interscience, New York, 1980.

6. D. E. Ash, in *Manganese in Metabolism and Enzyme Function* (V. L. Schramm and F. C. Wedler, eds.), Academic Press, New York, 1986, pp. 327–356.

7. C. L. Keen, B. Lönnerdal, and L. S. Hurley, Manganese, in *Biochemistry of the Essential Ultratrace Elements* (E. Frieden, ed.), Plenum Press, New York, 1984, pp. 89–132.

8. L. S. Hurley and C. L. Keen, Manganese, in *Trace Elements in Human Health and Animal Nutrition* (E. Underwood and E. Mertz, eds.), New York, Academic Press, 1987, pp. 185–223.

9. L. Davidsson, A. Almgren, M. A. Juillerat, and R. F. Hurrell, *Am. J. Clin. Nutr.*, *62*, 984–987 (1995).

10. J. H. Freeland-Graves, F. Behmardi, C. W. Bales, V. Dougherty, P. H. Lin, J. B. Crosby, and P. C. Trickett, *J. Nutr.*, *118*, 764–773 (1988).

11. P. E. Johnson, G. I. Lykken, and E. D. Korynta, *J. Nutr.*, *121*, 711–717 (1991).

12. H. Gunshin, B. Mackenzie, U. V. Berger, Y. Gunshin, M. F. Romero, W. F. Boron, S. Nussberger, J. L. Goloan, and M. A. Hediger, *Nature*, *388*(6641), 482–488 (1997).

13. G. Leblondel and P. Allain, *Biol. Trace Elem. Res.*, *67*, 13–28 (1999).

14. C. L. Keen, J. G. Bell, and B. Lönnerdal, *J. Nutr.*, *116*, 395–402 (1986).

15. B. Lönnerdal, Manganese in health and disease, in *Manganese Nutrition of Infants* (D. J. Klimis-Tavantzis, ed.), CRC Press, Boca Raton, FL, 1994, pp. 175–191.

16. L. Davidsson, A. Cederblad, B. Lönnerdal, and B. Sandstrom, *Am. J. Clin. Nutr.*, *54*, 1065–1070 (1991).

17. L. Davidsson, B. Lönnerdal, B. Sandstrom, K. Kunz, and C. L. Keen, *J. Nutr.*, *119*, 1461–1464 (1989).

18. J. W. Critchfield and C. L. Keen, *Metabolism*, *41*, 1087–1092 (1992).

19. V. L. Schramm and M. Brandt, *Fed. Proc.*, *45*, 2817–2820 (1986).

20. M. Korc, *Prog. Clin. Biol. Res.*, *380*, 235–255 (1993).

21. J. W. Finley, *Biol. Trace Elem. Res.*, *64*, 101–118 (1998).

22. T. Nasu and M. Sasaki, *J. Pharm. Pharmacol.*, *50*, 437–442 (1998).

23. A. C. Chua and E. H. Morgan, *J. Comp. Phys.*, *167*, 361–369 (1997).

24. E. A. Malecki, A. G. Devenyi, J. L. Beard, and J. R. Conor, *Biometab.*, *11*, 265–276 (1998).

25. C. L. Keen, S. Zidenberg-Cherr, and B. Lönnerdal, Dietary manganese toxicity and deficiency: Effects on cellular manganese metabolism, in *Nutritional Bioavailability of Manganese* (C. Kies, ed.), American Chemical Society, Washington, DC, 1987, p. 21.

26. M. L. Failla, Hormonal regulation of manganese metabolism, in *Manganese in Metabolism and Enzyme Function* (V. L. Schramm and F. C. Wedler, eds.), Academic Press, Orlando, FL, 1986, p. 93.

27. J. Y. Uriu-Hare, J. S. Stern, and C. L. Keen, *Diabetes*, *38*, 1282–1290 (1989).

28. J. J. Kuhn, S. Ward, M. Piponski, and T. W. Young, *Arch. Biochem. Biophys.*, *320*, 24–34 (1995).

29. B. H. Robinson, *J. Inher. Metab. Dis.*, *21*, 598–603 (1998).

30. M. D. Williams, H. Van Remmen, C. C. Conrad, T. T. Huang, C. J. Epstein, and A. Richardson, *J. Biol. Chem.*, *273*, 28510–28515 (1998).

31. Z. Chen, B. Siu, Y. S. Ho, R. Vincent, C. C. Chua, R. C. Hamdy, and B. H. Chua, *J. Mol. Cell. Cardiol.*, *30*, 2281–2289 (1998).

32. H. C. Yen, T. B. Oberley, C. G. Gairola, L. I. Szweda, and D. K. St. Clair, *Arch. Biochem. Biophys.*, *362*, 59–66 (1999).

33. C. L. Keen, T. Tamura, B. Lönnerdal, L. S. Hurley, and C. H. Halsted, *Am. J. Clin. Nutr.*, *41*, 929–932 (1985).

34. S. Zidenberg-Cherr and C. L. Keen, Essential trace elements in antioxidant processes, in *Trace Elements, Micronutrients, and Free Radicals* (I. E. Dreosti, ed.), Humana Press, Totowa, NJ, 1991, pp. 107–127.

35. A. C.-H. Liu, B. S. Heinrichs, and M. Leach, Jr., *Poult. Sci.*, *73*, 663–669 (1994).

36. P. Yang and D. J. Klimis-Tavantzis, *Biol. Trace Elem. Res.*, *64*, 275–288 (1998).

37. D. L. Baly, C. L. Keen, and L. S. Hurley, *J. Nutr.*, *115*, 872–879 (1985).

38. J. W. Critchfield, G. F. Carl, and C. L. Keen, *Epilepsy Res.*, *14*, 3–10 (1993).

39. C. E. Doige, H. G. G. Townsend, E. D. Janzen, and M. McGowen, *Vet. Pathol.*, *27*, 16–25 (1990).

40. G. P. Staley, J. J. van der Lugt, G. Axsel, and A. H. Loock, *J. South Afr. Vet. Assoc.*, *65*, 73–78 (1994).

41. L. Strause, P. Saltman, and J. Glowacki, *Calcif. Tissue Int.*, *41*, 145–150 (1987).

42. M. S. Clegg, S. M. Donovan, M. H. Monaco, D. L. Baly, J. L. Ensunsa, and C. L. Keen, *Proc. Soc. Exp. Biol. Med.*, *219*, 41–47 (1998).

43. L. Erway, L. S. Hurley, and A. Fraser, *Science*, *152*, 1766–1768 (1966).

44. M. Keil, G. Lungarella, E. Cavarra, P. van Even, and P. A. Martorana, *Lab. Inv.*, *74*, 353–362 (1996).

45. C. Gardi, E. Cavarra, P. Calzoni, P. Marcolongo, M. de Santi, P. A. Martorana, and G. Lungarella, *Biochem. J.*, *299*, 237–245 (1994).

46. C. L. Keen, S. Zidenberg-Cherr, and B. Lönnerdal, Nutritional and toxicological aspects of manganese intake: An overview, in *Risk Assessment of Essential Elements* (W. Mertz, C. O. Abernathy, and S. S. Olin, eds.), ILSI Press, Washington, DC, 1994, pp. 221–235.

47. H. Q. Gong and T. Amemiya, *Invest. Ophthalmol. Vis. Sci.*, *37*, 2200–2211 (1996).

48. S. Zidenberg-Cherr, C. L. Keen, and L. S. Hurley, *Biol. Trace Elem. Res.*, *7*, 31–48 (1985).

49. E. A. Malecki and J. L. Greger, *J. Nutr.*, *125*, 27–33 (1996).

50. T. Ogawa, A. Ohira, and T. Amemiya, *Curr. Eye Res.*, 1067–1073 (1998).

51. S. Zidenberg-Cherr, C. L. Keen, and L. S. Hurley, *J. Nutr.*, 2498–2504 (1983).

52. H. Van Remman, C. Salvador, H. Yang, T. T. Huang, C. J. Epstein, and A. Richardson, *Arch. Biochem. Biophys.*, *363*, 91–97 (1999).

53. K. Murakami, T. Kondo, M. Kawase, Y. Li, S. Sato, S. F. Chen, and P. H. Chan, *J. Neurosci.*, *18*, 205–213 (1998).

54. S. K. Manna, H. J. Zhang, T. Yan, L. W. Oberley, and B. B. Aggarwal, *J. Biol. Chem.*, *273*, 13245–13254 (1998).

55. J. J. Li and L. W. Oberley, *Cancer Res.*, *57*, 1991–1998 (1997).

56. J. Kawano, D. N. Ney, C. L. Keen, and B. O. Schneeman, *J. Nutr.*, *117*, 902–906 (1987).

57. P. N. Taylor, H. H. Patterson, and D. J. Klimis-Tavantzis, *J. Nutr. Biochem.*, *7*, 392–396 (1996).

58. D. J. Klimis-Tavantzis, P. N. Taylor, and I. Wolinsky, Manganese, lipid metabolism and atherosclerosis, in *Manganese in Health and Disease* (D. J. Klimis-Tavantzis, ed.), CRC Press, Boca Raton, FL, 1994, pp. 87–100.

59. D. L. Baly, D. L. Curry, C. L. Keen, and L. S. Hurley, *Endocrinology*, *116*, 1734–1740 (1985).

60. C. L. Keen, J. L. Ensunsa, M. H. Watson, D. L. Baly, S. M.

Donovan, M. Monaco, and M. S. Clegg, *Neurotoxicology*, *20*(2–3), 213–223 (1999).

61. D. L. Baly, I. Lee, and R. Doshi, *FEBS Lett.*, *239*, 55–58 (1988).

62. A. A. Brock, S. A. Chapman, E. A. Ulman, and G. F. Wu, *J. Nutr. (with erratum)*, *124*, 340–344 (1994).

63. G. Di Cola, M. H. Cool, and D. Accili, *J. Clin. Invest.*, *99*, 2538–2544 (1997).

64. B. J. Friedman, J. H. Freeland-Graves, C. W. Bales, F. Behmardi, R. L. Shorey-Kutschke, R. A. Willis, J. B. Crosby, P. C. Trickett, and S. D. Houston, *J. Nutr.*, *117*, 133–143 (1987).

65. N. Norose and K. Arai, *Jpn. J. Parent. Ent. Nutr.*, *9*, 978–981 (1987).

66. J. E. Finchan, S. J. van Rensburg, and W. F. O. Marasas, *South Afr. Med. J.*, *60*, 445–447 (1981).

67. L. Strause, P. Saltman, K. T. Smith, M. Bracker, and M. B. Andon, *J. Nutr.*, *124*, 1060–1064 (1994).

68. P. S. Papavasiliou, H. Kutt, S. T. Miller, V. Rosal, Y. Y. Wang, and R. B. Aronson, *Neurology*, *29*, 1466–1473 (1979).

69. G. F. Carl, C. L. Keen, B. B. Gallagher, M. S. Clegg, W. H. Littleton, D. B. Flannery, and L. S. Hurley, *Neurology*, *36*, 1584–1587 (1986).

70. J. W. Critchfield, F. G. Carl, and C. L. Keen, *Metabolism*, *42*, 907–910 (1993).

71. G. F. Carl, J. W. Critchfield, J. L. Thompson, G. L. Holmes, B. B. Gallagher, and C. L. Keen, *Epilepsia*, *31*, 247–252 (1990).

72. L. S. Hurley, D. E. Woolley, and P. S. Timiras, *Proc. Soc. Exp. Biol. Med.*, *106*, 343–346 (1961).

73. A. H. Rubenstein, N. W. Levin, and G. A. Elliott, *Lancet*, *2*, 1348–1351 (1962).

74. M. Hassanein, H. A. Ghaleb, E. A. Haroun, M. R. Hegazy, and M. A. H. Khayyal, *Br. J. Indust. Med.*, *23*, 67–70 (1966).

75. M. S. Akhtar, A. Qureshi, and J. Iqbal, *J. Pakistan Med. Assoc.*, *40*, 147–150 (1990).

76. M. S. Akhtar and J. Iqbal, *J. Ethnopharmacol.*, *31*, 49–57 (1991).

77. R. M. Walter, Jr., T. T. Aoki, and C. L. Keen, *J. Trace Elem. Exp. Med.*, *4*, 73–79 (1991).

78. F. A. Pennington and S. A. Schoen, *Int. J. Vit. Nutr. Res.*, *66*, 350–362 (1996).

79. C. D. Davis and J. L. Greger, *Am. J. Clin. Nutr.*, *49*, 747–752 (1992).

80. C. N. Kuratko, *Nutr. Cancer*, *28*, 36–40 (1997).

81. C. L. Keen, Teratogenic effects of essential metals: Deficiencies and excesses, in *Toxicology of Metals* (L. W. Chang, L. Magos, and T. Suzuki, eds.), CRC Press, Boca Raton, FL, 1996, pp. 977–1001.

82. D. L. Baly, B. Lönnerdal, and C. L. Keen, *Toxicol. Lett.*, *25*, 95–102 (1985).

83. C. L. Keen, D. L. Baly, and B. Lönnerdal, *Biol. Trace Elem. Res.*, *6*, 309–315 (1984).

84. M. C. Newland, *Neurotoxicology*, *20*(2–3), 415–432 (1999).

85. A. Pentschew, F. F. Ebner, and R. M. Kovatch, *J. Neuropathol. Exp. Neurol*, *22*, 488–499 (1963).

86. C. W. Olanow, P. F. Good, H. Shinotoh, K. A. Hewitt, F. Vingerhoets, B. J. Snow, M. F. Beal, D. B. Calne, and D. P. Perl, *Neurology*, *46*, 492–498 (1996).

87. M. D. Shinotoh, B. J. Snow, K. A. Hewitt, B. D. Pate, D. Doudet, R. Nugent, D. P. Perl, W. Olanow, and D. B. Calne, *Neurology*, *45*, 1199–1204 (1995).

88. M. C. Newland, T. L. Ceckler, J. H. Kordower, and B. Weiss, *Exp. Neurol.*, *106*, 251–258 (1987).

89. B. A. Pappas, D. Zhang, C. M. Davidson, T. Crowder, G. A. S. Park, and T. Fortin, *Neurotoxicol. Teratol.*, *19*, 17–25 (1997).

90. G. Oner and U. K. Senturk, *Food Chem. Toxicol.*, *33*, 559–563 (1995).

91. J. Donaldson, F. S. LaBella, and D. Gesser, *Neurotoxicology*, *2*, 53–64 (1980).

92. E. Heilbronn, H. Eriksson, and J. Hagglad, *Neurobehav. Toxicol. Teratol.*, *4*, 655–658 (1982).

93. W. N. Sloot, J. Korf, J. F. Koster, L. E. A. DeWit, and J. B. P. Gramsbergen, *Exp. Neurol.*, *138*, 235–245 (1996).

94. P. I. Oteiza, C. G. Fraga, and C. L. Keen, *Arch. Biochem. Biophys.*, *300*, 517–521 (1993).

95. K. A. Brenneman, R. C. Cattley, S. F. Ali, and D. C. Dorman, *Neurotoxicology*, *20*, 477–487 (1999).

96. S. F. Ali, H. M. Duhart, G. D. Newport, G. W. Lipe, and W. Slikker, *Neurodegeneration*, *4*, 329–334 (1995).

97. M. S. Desole, L. Sciola, M. R. Delogu, S. Sircana, R. Migheli, and E. Miele, *Neurochem. Intl.*, *31*(2), 169–176 (1997).

98. Y. Hirata, K. Adachi, and K. Kiuchi, *J. Neurochem.*, *71*, 1607–1615 (1998).

99. W. Zheng, S. Ren, and J. H. Graziano, *Brain Res.*, *799*, 334–342 (1998).

100. G. C. Cotzias, K. Horiuchi, S. Fuenzalida, and I. Mena, *Neurology*, *18*, 376–382 (1968).

101. J. M. Davis, *Environ. Health Perspect.*, *106*(Suppl. 1), 191–201 (1998).

102. A. Takeda, S. Ishiwatar, and S. Okada, *Brain Res.*, *811*, 147–151 (1998).

103. C.-C. Huang, N. S. Chu, C.-S. Lu, R.-S. Chen, and D. B. Calne, *Am. Acad. Neurol.*, *50*, 698–700 (1998).

104. Y. Kafritsa, J. Fell, S. Long, M. Bynevelt, W. Taylor, and P. Milla, *Arch. Dis. Child.*, *79*, 263–265 (1998).

105. P. A. Taylor and J. D. E. Price, *Can. Med. Assoc. J.*, *126*, 503–505 (1982).

106. M. Joardar and A. Sharma, *Mutat. Res.*, *240*, 159–163 (1990).

107. T. Kihira, M. Mukoyama, K. Ando, Y. Yase, and M. Yasui, *J. Neurosci.*, *98*, 251–258 (1990).

108. L. Spahr, R. F. Butterworth, S. Fontaine, L. Bui, G. Therrien, P. C. Milette, L. H. Lebrun, J. Zayed, A. Leblanc, and T. Pomier-Layrargues, *Hepatology*, *24*, 1116–1120 (1996).

109. R. A. Hauser, T. A. Zesiewicz, A. S. Rosemurgy, C. Martinez, and C. W. Olanow, *Ann. Neurol.*, *36*, 871–875 (1994).

110. G. P. Layrargues, C. Rose, L. Spahr, J. Zayed, L. Normandin, and R.F. Butterworth, *Metab. Brain Dis.*, *13*, 311–317 (1998).

111. J. M. Fell, A. P. Reynolds, N. Meadow, K. Khan, S. G. Long, G. Quaghebeur, W. J. Taylor, and P. J. Milla, *Lancet*, *347*(9010), 1218–1221 (1996).

112. R. Mehta and J. J. Reilly, *J. Parent. Ent. Nutr.*, *14*, 428–430 (1990).

113. R. G. Banta and W. R. Markesbury, *Neurology*, 27, 213–216 (1977).

114. R. Kawamura, H. Ikuta, S. Fuduzumi, R. Yamada, S. Tsubaki, T. Kodama, and S. Kurata, *Kisasato Arch. Exp. Med.*, 18, 145–169 (1941).

115. X. G. Kondakis, N. Makris, M. Leotsinidis, M. Prinous, and T. Papapetropoulos, *Arch. Environ. Health*, 44, 175–178 (1989).

116. P. Vieregge, B. Heinzow, G. Korf, H. M. Teichert, P. Scheifenbaum, and H. U. Mosingen, *Can. J. Neurol. Sci.*, 22, 286–289 (1995).

117. U.S. Environmental Protection Agency, Oral reference dose (RfD) for manganese, *IRIS (Integrated Risk Information System)*, 1995.

118. J. L. Greger, *Neurotoxicology*, 20(2–3), 205–212 (1999).

119. M. S. Clegg, B. Lönnerdal, L. S. Hurley, and C. L. Keen, *Anal. Chem.*, 157, 12–18 (1986).

120. G. DeRosa, C. L. Keen, R. M. Leach, and L. S. Hurley, *J. Nutr.*, 110, 795–804 (1980).

121. H. Ohno, S. Kayashima, N. Nagata, H. Yamashita, T. Ookawara, and N. Taniguchi, *Clin. Chim. Acta*, 215, 213–219 (1993).

122. A. C. Phylactos, L. S. Harbige, and M. A. Crawford, *Lipids*, 29, 111–115 (1994).

123. J. Thome, P. Foley, W. Gsell, E. Davids, N. Wodarz, G. A. Wiesbeck, J. Boning, and P. Riederer, *Alcohol and Alcoholism*, 32(1), 65–69 (1997).

124. Y. Kim, J.-W. Kim, K. Ito, H.-S. Lim, H.-K. Cheong, J. Y. Kim, Y. C. Shin, K. S. Kim, and Y. Moon, *Neurotoxicology*, 20(2–3), 249–252 (1999).

5

Interrelations Between Manganese and Other Metal Ions in Health and Disease

James C. K. Lai,[1] Margaret J. Minski,[2]
Alex W. K. Chan,[2] and Louis Lim[3]

[1]College of Pharmacy, Idaho State University,
Pocatello, ID 83209, USA

[2]Imperial College Reactor Centre, University of London,
Silwood Park, Ascot, Berkshire SL5 7PY, UK

[3]Institute of Neurology, University of London,
Queen Square, London WCIN 2NS, UK

1. INTRODUCTION

Ideally, if one can demonstrate directly the mechanisms that causally link the metabolism of manganese to those of other metals, then one can define the physiological and/or other situations or conditions that show *interdependence* between Mn and other metal ions. However, largely because of methodological limitations as well as limitations of experimental approaches, the data in the literature and those of ongoing studies are better or more accurately defined as depicting the *interrelations* between Mn and other metal ions [1–3]. This conceptual distinction should be borne in mind when one assesses the advances in the topic areas to be discussed in this chapter.

The scope of this chapter is limited to a discussion of the interrelations between Mn and other metal ions after chronic exposure of animals or humans to Mn because organ distributions of Mn usually reflect chronic rather than acute exposure.

2. INTERDEPENDENCE BETWEEN MANGANESE AND OTHER METALS IN ABSORPTION

2.1. Animal Models of Normal Absorption of Manganese and Other Metals

Since Mn is an essential trace metal, animal models of normal absorption of Mn and other metals involve the assessment of dietary intake of Mn (and other metals) with the amounts that are absorbed [4–6]. On the other hand, because Mn also occurs in air and in drinking water, some animal models address the absorption of this metal via the lungs and that absorbed from the drinking water [6]. (See also Chapter 4 in this volume.)

Intestinal Mn absorption is dependent on dietary iron. High dietary Fe leads to a lowering of Mn absorption whereas low dietary Fe results in enhanced Mn absorption [4–6]. Similarly, high dietary Mn leads to decreased Fe absorption [4,6]. Dietary copper also induces decreased Mn absorption [6,7]. Furthermore, addition of essential and nonessential trace metals to the drinking water of rats and mice can result in altered peripheral tissue accumulation of essential trace metals (including Mn) in those animals [8,9]: these observations suggest that Mn interacts with other trace metals in absorption and subsequent tissue distribution [1–3].

2.2. Animal Models of Manganese Toxicity and Absorption of Metals

Mn toxicity can arise from exposing the animals to the metal from different sources—air, water, and diet [1–6]. Consequently, the animal models that address dose–effect relationships in acute and chronic Mn toxicity include all three types of exposure routes. Furthermore, some of the animal models of chronic Mn toxicity involve exposing developing or aging animals to the metal [1–3,6].

3. INTERRELATIONS BETWEEN MANGANESE AND OTHER METALS IN PERIPHERAL ORGANS

3.1. Distributions of Manganese and Other Metals in Peripheral Organs

Once Mn and other metals enter the bloodstream, they distribute to different organs within the body. However, although plasma proteins act as the temporary and limited capacity reservoir for metals, the molecular mechanisms that control the organ distribution of metals in the circulation have not been fully elucidated [1–3,6]. Most of the data in the literature as well as those reported herein (Tables 1 and 2) are derived from analysis of steady-state organ contents of metals using sensitive analytical techniques. Some analytical techniques, e.g., instrumental neutron activation analysis (INAA), allow the near-simultaneous determinations of a large number of metals in a tissue sample, thus leading to the construct of matrices of metals in different organs [3,10–13]. In the absence of data from studies that directly show interdependence (as defined above), the matrices of metals in various organs in control and metal-treated animals provide the only data option for elucidating the interrelations between metals [3,10–13].

Among the various trace metals in organs, Fe shows the highest

TABLE 1

Effects of Chronic Manganese Treatment on Organ Distribution of Iron, Aluminum, and Zinc

Organ	Metal (μg/g)	Control	Group A	Mn-treated Group B	Group C
Heart	Fe	103 ± 11	93 ± 13	123 ± 13	99 ± 2
	Al	5.68 ± 0.08	4.04 ± 0.27	4.51 ± 0.46	5.07 ± 0.22
	Zn	16.05 ± 2.84	16.47 ± 1.32	16.77 ± 0.58	16.79 ± 1.42
Lung	Fe	140 ± 30	140 ± 40	240 ± 40*+	240 ± 20*+
	Al	3.98 ± 0.53	3.85 ± 0.99	3.80 ± 0.75	5.36 ± 0.85
	Zn	16.98 ± 3.26	15.99 ± 2.47	14.73 ± 1.24	13.44 ± 1.16
Kidney	Fe	100 ± 18	105 ± 13	153 ± 7*+	67 ± 5*+
	Al	4.13 ± 0.54	5.74 ± 1.10	5.97 ± 0.58	5.92 ± 0.88
	Zn	24.56 ± 4.17	22.85 ± 2.68	24.25 ± 1.39	21.76 ± 0.93
Spleen	Fe	1059 ± 253	1747 ± 255*	2985 ± 141*+	939 ± 94
	Al	7.17 ± 0.53	5.58 ± 0.87	9.21 ± 1.19*	6.28 ± 0.50
	Zn	17.34 ± 2.82	19.42 ± 2.04	21.00 ± 1.16	17.05 ± 1.16
Liver	Fe	280 ± 50	330 ± 50	410 ± 60*	270 ± 30
	Al	6.57 ± 0.65	6.74 ± 0.95	7.12 ± 0.59	5.50 ± 0.57
	Zn	41.13 ± 2.57	25.78 ± 2.28*	26.38 ± 1.65*	26.20 ± 1.93*

Values (in μg/g wet weight) are mean ± SD–derived 6–10 female rats. Statistical analysis of data was by ANOVA and post hoc Tukey test: $*p < 0.05$ vs. control; $**p < 0.01$ vs. control; $+p < 0.05$ vs. Group A. Wistar rats (MRC Porton strain) were exposed to manganese chloride (group A: 1 mg $MnCl_2 \cdot 4H_2O$ per mL of drinking water; group B: 10 mg $MnCl_2 \cdot 4H_2O$ per mL of drinking water; group C: 20 mg $MnCl_2 \cdot 4H_2O$ per mL of drinking water; control group given water without manganese addition) continuously throughout development until they were used for experiments at adulthood (120-day-old females) [1,3,12,13].

TABLE 2

Effects of Chronic Manganese Treatment on Organ Distribution
of Copper, Manganese, and Selenium

Organ	Metal (µg/g)	Control	Mn-treated		
			Group A	Group B	Group C
Heart	Cu	5.33 ± 1.62	5.33 ± 2.28	5.08 ± 0.43	6.24 ± 2.00
	Mn	0.32 ± 0.08	0.50 ± 0.09	0.72 ± 0.16*	1.76 ± 0.15**
	Se	0.39 ± 0.09	0.45 ± 0.09	0.35 ± 0.08	0.62 ± 0.16
Lung	Cu	2.53 ± 0.26	3.01 ± 0.73	5.23 ± 0.02*+	3.66 ± 0.57*
	Mn	0.20 ± 0.04	0.22 ± 0.05	0.23 ± 0.01	0.46 ± 0.18*
	Se	0.40 ± 0.08	0.39 ± 0.11	0.38 ± 0.01	0.61 ± 0.11*
Kidney	Cu	10.39 ± 2.06	15.55 ± 2.76*	16.55 ± 4.12*	12.13 ± 1.55
	Mn	0.78 ± 0.09	1.07 ± 0.17	1.83 ± 0.31*+	2.73 ± 0.18**+
	Se	1.54 ± 0.49	1.29 ± 0.39	0.61 ± 0.02*+	1.50 ± 0.15
Spleen	Cu	3.79 ± 0.22	2.14 ± 0.26*	2.52 ± 0.22*	2.24 ± 0.35*
	Mn	0.34 ± 0.06	0.46 ± 0.08	0.78 ± 0.09*	1.06 ± 0.09**+
	Se	0.72 ± 0.21	0.73 ± 0.15	0.56 ± 0.02	0.62 ± 0.04
Liver	Cu	5.41 ± 0.61	4.50 ± 0.44	3.84 ± 0.85	4.47 ± 0.96
	Mn	2.76 ± 0.20	2.85 ± 0.43	3.74 ± 0.44*	4.72 ± 0.53*+
	Se	1.26 ± 0.15	1.09 ± 0.27	1.24 ± 0.23	1.73 ± 0.22*+

Values (in µg/g wet weight) are mean ± SD–derived 6–10 female rats. Statistical analysis of data was by ANOVA and post hoc Tukey test: *$p < 0.05$ vs. control; **$p < 0.01$ vs. control; +$p < 0.05$ vs. Group A. Wistar rats (MRC Porton strain) were exposed to manganese chloride (group A: 1 mg $MnCl_2 \cdot 4H_2O$ per mL of drinking water; group B: 10 mg $MnCl_2 \cdot 4H_2O$ per mL of drinking water; group C: 20 mg $MnCl_2 \cdot 4H_2O$ per mL of drinking water; control group given water without manganese addition) continuously throughout development until they were used for experiments at adulthood (120-day-old females) [1,3,12,13].

levels (Tables 1–4) [13,14]. The relative abundance of trace metals in various peripheral organs reflects the storage capacities of the organs and the amounts of metal-binding macromolecules (e.g., proteins and nucleic acids) therein. The rank order of the relative abundance of trace metals in peripheral organs is: Fe $\gg$ Zn > Cu > Al > Mn > Se (Tables 1 and 2). The rank order of Fe level in peripheral organs is: spleen $\gg$ liver > lung > heart $\simeq$ kidney (Table 1). The rank order of Zn level is: liver $\gg$ kidney > spleen $\simeq$ lung $\simeq$ heart (Table 1). The rank order of Cu is: kidney $\gg$ liver $\simeq$ heart > spleen > lung. The rank order of Mn is: liver $\gg$ kidney $\gg$ spleen $\simeq$ heart > lung, whereas that for Se is: kidney $\geqslant$ liver > spleen > lung = heart (Table 2). On the other hand, the rank order of the nonessential metal Al is: spleen > liver > heart > kidney $\simeq$ lung (Table 1).

3.2. Organ-Specific Changes in Levels of Manganese and Other Metals in Development

For most trace metals, dramatic changes in their levels in peripheral tissues of the rat occur between day 10 and day 22/23 postnatal (i.e., weaning), presumably reflecting the onset of maturation of hepatic metal excretory system [6].

Table 3 shows the organ distribution of iron, aluminum, and zinc. In rat heart and spleen, Fe levels do not change in the first three postnatal weeks; then they rise significantly to adult level after weaning. In rat lung, Fe level doubles between day 10 and day 22 postnatal to attain adult level. Fe level in rat kidney is high in the first 10 days postnatal and thereafter sharply declines. Rat liver Fe level is triphasic, being high at day 5 postnatal, decreasing drastically between day 5 and day 10, and rising dramatically between weaning and day 120 postnatal.

In rat heart, lung, kidney, and liver, the trend for postnatal variation in their Zn levels is the same: their Zn levels rise between day 5 and day 10, decrease drastically between day 10 and weaning, and thereafter rise markedly to their adult levels. By contrast, rat spleen Zn level does not significantly vary during postnatal development.

The organ distribution of copper, manganese, and selenium is given in Table 4. Rat heart Cu level stays constant during the first three

TABLE 3

Organ Distribution of Iron, Aluminum, and Zinc During Postnatal Development

Organ	Metal (μg/g)	Postnatal age (days)			
		5	10	22/23	120
Heart	Fe	51 ± 5	48 ± 8	39 ± 12	100 ± 10
	Al	6.22 ± 0.78	2.99 ± 0.83*	3.51 ± 0.36*	5.68 ± 0.08
	Zn	11.12 ± 0.19	18.81 ± 3.43*	6.47 ± 0.55*+	16.05 ± 2.84*
Lung	Fe	74 ± 10	55 ± 6	140 ± 57	140 ± 30
	Al	5.48 ± 1.08	4.84 ± 1.00	3.82 ± 0.39	3.98 ± 0.53
	Zn	10.52 ± 0.71	15.07 ± 1.34*	8.33 ± 1.36	16.98 ± 3.26*
Kidney	Fe	45 ± 5	42 ± 18	19 ± 3*+	10 ± 2*+
	Al	5.49 ± 0.96	6.15 ± 1.10	5.24 ± 0.39	4.13 ± 0.55
	Zn	13.18 ± 1.60	19.05 ± 1.17*	8.69 ± 0.77*+	24.56 ± 4.16*
Spleen	Fe	110 ± 20	119 ± 17	82 ± 18	1060 ± 250*++
	Al	8.05 ± 0.46	3.89 ± 0.56*	8.48 ± 0.55*	7.17 ± 0.53
	Zn	15.14 ± 1.72	15.99 ± 1.57	10.95 ± 1.35	17.34 ± 2.82
Liver	Fe	222 ± 30	19 ± 3**	41 ± 11**	280 ± 50+
	Al	6.83 ± 0.54	7.12 ± 0.14	7.66 ± 0.98	6.57 ± 0.65
	Zn	41.33 ± 6.91	64.11 ± 7.39*	18.15 ± 2.23*+	41.13 ± 2.57+

Values (in μg/g wet weight) are mean ± SD–derived 6–10 female rats. Statistical analysis of data was by ANOVA and post hoc Tukey test: *$p < 0.05$ vs. day 5; **$p < 0.01$ vs. day 5; +$p < 0.05$ vs. day 10. ++$p < 0.05$ vs. other groups [12,21].

TABLE 4

Organ Distribution of Copper, Manganese, and Selenium During Postnatal Development

Organ	Metal (µg/g)	Postnatal age (days)			
		5	10	22/23	120
Heart	Cu	17.74 ± 1.67	16.15 ± 1.71	16.08 ± 1.69	5.33 ± 1.62+++
	Mn	1.97 ± 0.44	0.28 ± 0.02**	0.34 ± 0.02**	0.32 ± 0.09**
	Se	0.31 ± 0.06	0.71 ± 0.08*	0.21 ± 0.01*+	0.39 ± 0.09++
Lung	Cu	6.01 ± 0.83	2.27 ± 0.23**	12.10 ± 1.66***+	2.53 ± 0.26**
	Mn	0.62 ± 0.09	0.16 ± 0.02**	0.20 ± 0.03**	0.20 ± 0.04**
	Se	0.33 ± 0.07	0.13 ± 0.02*	0.25 ± 0.02+	0.40 ± 0.08+
Kidney	Cu	9.33 ± 0.76	3.13 ± 0.39**	11.80 ± 1.01+	10.39 ± 2.06+
	Mn	0.45 ± 0.07	0.49 ± 0.07	0.90 ± 0.05*+	0.78 ± 0.10*+
	Se	0.37 ± 0.03	0.60 ± 0.10*	0.44 ± 0.02*+	1.54 ± 0.50**++
Spleen	Cu	14.48 ± 2.01	4.79 ± 0.37+++	29.65 ± 3.25+++	3.79 ± 0.23+++
	Mn	0.53 ± 0.00	0.26 ± 0.05*	0.34 ± 0.02*	0.35 ± 0.06*
	Se	0.43 ± 0.04	0.90 ± 0.11**	0.41 ± 0.00+	0.72 ± 0.21*
Liver	Cu	29.52 ± 0.98	44.97 ± 8.21+++	13.98 ± 0.29+++	5.41 ± 0.61+++
	Mn	0.89 ± 0.21	0.94 ± 0.11	2.04 ± 0.30+++	2.76 ± 0.29+++
	Se	0.49 ± 0.06	0.55 ± 0.11	0.62 ± 0.06	1.26 ± 0.15+++

Values (in µg/g wet weight) are mean ± SD—derived 6–10 female rats. Statistical analysis of data was by ANOVA and post hoc Tukey test: $*p < 0.05$ vs. day 5; $**p < 0.01$ vs. day 5; $+p < 0.05$ vs. day 10; $++p < 0.05$ vs. day 10; $+++p < 0.05$ vs. all other groups [12,21].

weeks postnatal; thereafter, it decreases by 60% to the adult level. Rat lung and spleen Cu levels show the same trend during postnatal development: they decline between day 5 and day 10, then rise between day 10 and weaning, and decline again between weaning and adulthood. Rat kidney Cu level declines between day 5 and day 10, and rises to adult level between day 10 and weaning. Rat liver Cu is high at day 5, reaches a peak at day 10, and thereafter declines continually to adult level.

Mn levels in rat heart, lung, and spleen are high at day 5 postnatal; they then decrease and attain their adult levels between day 5 and day 10. On the other hand, Mn levels in rat kidney and liver are quite low up to day 10 postnatal; between day 10 and weaning, they rise and attain their adult levels.

Rat heart, kidney, and spleen Se levels increase between day 5 and day 10 postnatal, then decrease between day 10 and weaning, and increase thereafter to achieve their respective adult levels. Rat lung Se level decreases between day 5 and day 10 postnatal; it then rises gradually thereafter. Rat liver Se is practically unchanged from day 5 until weaning but doubles thereafter.

Being a nonessential metal for mammals, the organ-specific changes in Al level during postnatal development of the rat are quite different from those of the essential trace metals (e.g., Fe, Zn, Cu, Mn, Se) (compare data in Tables 3 and 4). Between day 5 and day 120 postnatal, rat lung, kidney, and liver Al levels are unchanged (Table 3). However, rat heart Al level decreases by 50% between day 5 and day 10 postnatal and rises after weaning to attain adult level (Table 3). Similar to that in heart, rat spleen Al level also decreases by 50% between day 5 and day 10 postnatal but doubles between day 10 and weaning to attain adult level (Table 3).

3.3.   Chronic Manganese Treatment Alters Distributions of Manganese and Other Metals in Organs

3.3.1.   Chronic Manganese Treatment Induces Organ-Specific Changes in Manganese and Other Metals in Suckling Rats

Employing the developmental rat model of chronic Mn exposure, Lai and co-workers have systematically investigated the organ distributions of several trace metals in suckling (i.e., 10 days old postnatal) and adult (120 days old postnatal) rats and the effects of Mn treatment (10 mg $MnCl_2 \cdot 4H_2O$/mL of drinking water) thereon [1,12,13]. The rats were exposed to Mn in utero via their mothers' circulation; postnatally, they were exposed to Mn via their mothers' milk. From around weaning (i.e., 21/22 days postnatal) onward, the rats were directly exposed to Mn in the drinking water. Their tissue levels of trace metals were determined using the sensitive technique of INAA [1,3,10,12].

In 10-day-old rats, chronic Mn exposure induces organ-specific changes in several trace metals, including Fe, Cu, Mn, and Al. In control, age-matched rats, the rank order of Fe distribution in various tissues is: spleen $\gg$ lung $\simeq$ heart $\simeq$ kidney $\gg$ liver (Table 3). In Mn-treated rats, Fe level is significantly increased in kidney (+238.1%), liver (+226.3%), heart (+64.6%), and spleen (+42.0%) but not in lung (Table 5). The rank order of organ distribution of Fe in Mn-treated, 10-day-old rats becomes spleen > kidney > heart > liver > lung.

In control 10-day-old rats, the rank order of Cu distribution is: liver $\gg$ heart > spleen > kidney > lung (Table 4). In Mn-treated,

TABLE 5

Effects of Chronic Manganese Treatment
on Organ Distribution of Iron, Aluminum,
Copper, and Manganese in 10-Day-Old Rats

Organ	Metal (% of control)			
	Fe	Al	Cu	Mn
Heart	+64.6*	+73.2*	−67.1*	+51.2*
Lung	NS	NS	NS	+132.1**
Kidney	+238.1*	NS	+74.7*	NS
Spleen	+42.0*	+136.0**	NS	+86.8*
Liver	+226.3*	NS	NS	+221.1**

NS, not significant.
Values are mean (expressed as % of corresponding control value)–derived 6–10 female rats. Statistical analysis of data was by ANOVA and post hoc Tukey test: *$p < 0.05$ vs. control; **$p < 0.01$ vs. control; + implies increase over control; − implies decrease over control [12,21].

10-day-old rats, Cu level is significantly decreased in heart (-67.1%) but increased in kidney ($+74.7\%$) (Table 5). The rank order of organ distribution of Cu in the Mn-treated, 10-day-old rats becomes liver $\gg$ spleen $\simeq$ kidney $>$ heart $>$ lung.

In control 10-day-old rats, the rank order of Mn distribution is: liver $\gg$ kidney $>$ heart $>$ spleen $>$ lung (Table 4). In Mn-treated, 10-day-old rats, Mn level is significantly increased in liver ($+221.1\%$), lung ($+132.1\%$), spleen ($+86.8\%$), and heart ($+51.2\%$) but not in kidney (Table 5). The rank order of organ distribution of Mn in those Mn-treated rats becomes liver $\gg$ kidney $>$ spleen $>$ heart $\simeq$ lung.

In control 10-day-old rats, the rank order of distribution of Al (a nonessential metal) is: liver $\simeq$ kidney $>$ lung $\simeq$ spleen $>$ heart. Mn-treatment results in significant increases in Al level only in spleen ($+136.0\%$) and heart ($+73.2\%$) (Table 5). The rank order of organ distribution of Al in Mn-treated, 10-day-old rats becomes spleen $>$ liver $\simeq$ kidney $>$ heart $\simeq$ lung.

In contrast to its effects on organ distributions of Fe, Cu, Mn, and Al, Mn treatment does not induce any significant changes in the organ distributions of Zn and Se in 10-day-old rats, nor does it alter the tissue contents of these two trace metals in those animals (data not shown).

3.3.2. Chronic Manganese Treatment Induces Organ-Specific Changes in Manganese and Other Metals in Adult Rats

In 120-day-old rats chronic Mn treatment induces differential, dose-dependent increases in Mn in peripheral organs (Table 2). Compared to Mn, the organ-specific changes induced by Mn treatment in the levels of other metals are less marked (Tables 1 and 2). However, despite the Mn-induced changes in the levels of several metals in peripheral organs, the rank orders of levels of metals among the organs are not significantly altered: these observations contrast with those detected in various brain regions where Mn treatment induces region-specific changes (see Sec. 4.3. below).

Chronic Mn treatment gives rise to dose-dependent increases in Mn in rat heart, kidney, spleen, and liver; by contrast, lung Mn is only significantly increased in rats treated with the highest Mn dose (Table 2).

Fe levels in rat spleen and lung are significantly increased when animals are treated with the lower two and the higher two Mn doses, respectively (Table 1). Liver Fe is only significantly increased in rats treated with the intermediate Mn dose whereas heart Fe is unaffected by the Mn treatment at the doses investigated (Table 1). On the other hand, kidney Fe is increased and decreased in rats treated with the intermediate and highest Mn dose, respectively (Table 1).

Chronic Mn treatment at all three doses induces a decrease in Zn only in liver (Table 1). On the other hand, the level of Al, a nonessential metal, is only significantly increased in spleen of rats treated with the intermediate Mn dose (Table 1).

Spleen Cu is decreased in rats treated with all three Mn doses whereas Cu levels in lung and kidney show trends of increases (Table 2). Neither heart Cu nor liver Cu is affected by Mn treatment at the doses investigated (Table 2).

Se levels in lung and liver are significantly increased in rats treated with the highest Mn dose; however, heart, spleen, and kidney Se levels are not affected by Mn treatment at the doses investigated (Table 2).

4. INTERRELATIONS BETWEEN MANGANESE AND OTHER METALS IN BRAIN

4.1. Blood–Brain Barrier Transfer of Manganese

Even though brain accumulation of Mn increases as a function of Mn intake, implying the occurrence of blood–brain transfer of this metal [1–3,12,13,15], the mechanisms of blood-brain transport of Mn have not been fully elucidated. The few studies available suggest that the blood–brain barrier transport of Mn can occur by (1) saturable, facilitated diffusion and nonfacilitated diffusion [17,18]; (2) active transport [19]; and (3) receptor-mediated endocytosis via binding to transferrin [16,20]. Moreover, there are indications that (1) the chemical and valency state of Mn, (2) its binding to transferrin, albumin and other plasma proteins, and (3) the presence of free and transferrin-bound Fe may play a regulatory role in the blood–brain barrier transfer of Mn [16–19]. However, which of the above transport mechanisms plays a more quantitatively important role and which of the factors controls such a mechanism remains to be resolved.

4.2.   Brain Regional Distributions of Manganese and Other Metals

Despite the fact that it is a trace metal, Fe level in brain approaches those of electrolytes such as calcium and magnesium [21]. Whole-brain levels of trace metals are in the order: Fe ≫ Zn ≫ Al ≫ Cu ≫ Se ≃ Mn [21]. However, most trace metals show region-specific changes during development resulting in each metal having its characteristic regional distribution in the adult brain. Moreover, in aging, brain levels of several metals (e.g., Ca, Fe, Cu, Mn, and Se) are also altered. (See Ref. 21 for a detailed discussion and additional references.)

     In adult rats, the brain regional distribution of Fe is different from those of several other metals (compare Tables 6–9). The Fe level is higher in hippocampus, hypothalamus, pons and medulla, and cerebellum than in midbrain, striatum, and cerebral cortex (Table 7). The Zn level is higher in hippocampus and cerebral cortex than in the other regions (Table 8). The level of Al in cerebral cortex is lower than those in other regions (Table 6). The Cu level is highest in hypothalamus, intermediate in striatum, midbrain, and cerebellum, but lowest in hippocampus, pons and medulla, and cerebral cortex (Table 7). The Se level is highest in hippocampus, midbrain, and hypothalamus, intermediate in cerebellum and cerebral cortex, but lowest in striatum and pons and medulla (Table 8). The Mn level is highest in midbrain, cerebellum, and pons and medulla, intermediate in cerebral cortex and hypothalamus, but lowest in striatum and hippocampus (Table 6).

     The distributions of electrolytes are also somewhat different from those of trace metals. In adult rats, the Ca level is lower in cerebral cortex and midbrain than in the other regions (Table 9). Similarly, the Mg level in cerebral cortex is lower than those in other regions (Table 9).

4.3.   Chronic Manganese Treatment Alters Brain Regional Distributions of Manganese and Other Metals

In the chronic rat model of Mn toxicity developed by Lai and co-workers [1,12,13], all regions show dose-dependent increases in Mn with the

TABLE 6

Effect of Chronic Manganese Treatment
on Brain Regional Distribution of Manganese and Aluminum

Brain region	Metal (μg/g)	Control	Group A	Mn-treated	
				Group B	Group C
MB	Mn	0.38 ± 0.01	0.64 ± 0.14*	1.35 ± 0.10***‡	1.33 ± 0.20***‡
	Al	10.53 ± 1.83	9.67 ± 0.41	9.09 ± 1.01	9.01 ± 0.00
CB	Mn	0.38 ± 0.05	0.51 ± 0.06*	0.94 ± 0.07***‡	1.04 ± 0.03***‡
	Al	10.03 ± 1.42	10.55 ± 4.15	8.59 ± 0.74	7.59 ± 0.96
PM	Mn	0.37 ± 0.12	0.44 ± 0.19	1.07 ± 0.22*‡	1.12 ± 0.10*‡
	Al	7.18 ± 2.43	7.26 ± 1.62	9.54 ± 0.99	8.65 ± 1.80
CC	Mn	0.34 ± 0.07	0.36 ± 0.09	0.61 ± 0.16*‡	0.88 ± 0.16*‡
	Al	7.00 ± 1.27	6.28 ± 1.98	6.28 ± 0.40	6.27 ± 0.47
HYP	Mn	0.300 ± 0.12	0.72 ± 0.20*	1.11 ± 0.21**	1.89 ± 0.12***‡
	Al	8.38 ± 1.50	16.38 ± 6.42	7.96 ± 1.08	7.12 ± 1.59
ST	Mn	0.24 ± 0.03	0.55 ± 0.01*	1.13 ± 0.24***‡	1.39 ± 0.24***‡
	Al	9.93 ± 1.73	11.75 ± 0.89	10.81 ± 2.56	8.66 ± 1.30
HIP	Mn	0.21 ± 0.04	0.37 ± 0.14	0.99 ± 0.11***‡	1.10 ± 0.22***‡
	Al	8.57 ± 1.94	9.38 ± 3.00	7.46 ± 1.45	6.17 ± 1.11

Values (in μg/g wet weight) are mean ± SD–derived 6–10 female rats. *$p < 0.05$ vs. control; **$p < 0.01$ vs. control; ‡$p < 0.05$ vs. Group A. Other details are the same as those in the legends to Table 1. Reprinted with permission from [1].

TABLE 7

Effects of Chronic Manganese Treatment
on Brain Regional Distribution of Iron and Copper

Brain region	Metal (μg/g)	Control	Group A	Mn-treated	
				Group B	Group C
HIP	Fe	32.0 ± 9.0	56.0 ± 26.0	48.0 ± 9.0*	26.0 ± 7.0
	Cu	4.19 ± 1.31	6.98 ± 1.97	7.82 ± 0.71*	7.65 ± 0.74*
HYP	Fe	29.0 ± 11.0	97.0 ± 33.0*	102.0 ± 11.0**	40.0 ± 9.0
	Cu	12.81 ± 0.66	14.89 ± 2.33	13.90 ± 1.37	11.59 ± 1.30
PM	Fe	29.0 ± 6.0	40.0 ± 7.0	56.0 ± 2.0*‡	25.0 ± 6.0
	Cu	3.90 ± 1.9	4.58 ± 1.71	7.06 ± 0.39*	7.58 ± 1.2*
CB	Fe	27.0 ± 8.0	43.0 ± 6.0*	61.0 ± 7.0*‡	29.0 ± 10.0
	Cu	5.61 ± 2.05	6.38 ± 2.10	6.63 ± 0.74	6.18 ± 0.39
MB	Fe	23.0 ± 4.0	32.0 ± 8.0	54.0 ± 7.0*	25.0 ± 5.0
	Cu	5.80 ± 2.0	7.71 ± 1.15	7.61 ± 0.51	8.18 ± 1.09
ST	Fe	19.0 ± 5.0	27.0 ± 6.0*	60.0 ± 4.0*‡	37.0 ± 8.0*
	Cu	7.00 ± 1.00	11.56 ± 0.19*	11.01 ± 1.03*	9.50 ± 1.16
CC	Fe	18.0 ± 2.0	21.0 ± 4.0	19.0 ± 8.0	13.0 ± 2.0*‡
	Cu	2.99 ± 0.57	3.16 ± 0.16	3.62 ± 0.20	3.67 ± 0.30

Values (in μg/g wet weight) are mean ± SD–derived 6–10 female rats. *$p < 0.05$ vs. control; **$p < 0.01$ vs. control; ‡$p < 0.05$ vs. Group A. Other details are the same as those in the legends to Table 1. Reprinted with permission from [1].

TABLE 8

Effects of Chronic Manganese Treatment
on Brain Regional Distribution of Zinc and Selenium

Brain region	Metal (μg/g)	Control	Mn-treated		
			Group A	Group B	Group C
HIP	Zn	15.84 ± 2.78	13.72 ± 0.46	17.59 ± 1.52	14.04 ± 1.87
	Se	0.67 ± 0.15	0.70 ± 0.11	0.67 ± 0.06	0.71 ± 0.15
CC	Zn	13.67 ± 1.46	15.31 ± 2.99	15.15 ± 2.08	14.17 ± 2.17
	Se	0.20 ± 0.06	0.56 ± 0.08*	0.18 ± 0.02	0.10 ± 0.02*‡
HYP	Zn	11.79 ± 1.27	18.55 ± 8.45	19.20 ± 0.88**	11.66 ± 2.66
	Se	0.45 ± 0.09	1.24 ± 0.11**	0.40 ± 0.04‡	0.88 ± 0.11*
CB	Zn	11.29 ± 2.24	13.75 ± 2.33	15.68 ± 1.23	10.75 ± 0.63
	Se	0.36 ± 0.14	0.64 ± 0.10	0.63 ± 0.05	0.75 ± 0.04*
ST	Zn	11.06 ± 1.75	15.18 ± 1.69	18.59 ± 1.78*	10.66 ± 1.57
	Se	0.11 ± 0.01	0.80 ± 0.16**	1.03 ± 0.21**	1.27 ± 0.14**†
MB	Zn	10.17 ± 1.13	12.48 ± 0.65	11.08 ± 0.55	9.64 ± 1.46
	Se	0.46 ± 0.02	0.67 ± 0.07*	0.68 ± 0.17*	0.78 ± 0.20*
PM	Zn	9.70 ± 1.73	10.41 ± 2.25	9.10 ± 0.62	7.26 ± 0.12
	Se	0.09 ± 0.00	0.45 ± 0.01**	0.47 ± 0.06**	0.84 ± 0.01**‡

Values (in μg/g wet weight) are mean ± SD–derived 6–10 female rats. $*p < 0.05$ vs. control; $**p < 0.01$ vs. control; $‡p < 0.05$ vs. Group A. Other details are the same as those in the legends to Table 1. Reprinted with permission from [1].

TABLE 9

Effects of Chronic Manganese Treatment on Brain Regional Distribution of Calcium and Magnesium

Brain region	Metal (mg/g)	Control	Mn-treated		
			Group A	Group B	Group C
HYP	Ca	0.14 ± 0.03	0.07 ± 0.01*	0.16 ± 0.01	0.10 ± 0.00
	Mg	0.24 ± 0.09	0.27 ± 0.09	0.25 ± 0.00	0.25 ± 0.15
HIP	Ca	0.13 ± 0.01	0.08 ± 0.02*	0.10 ± 0.01	0.09 ± 0.01
	Mg	0.32 ± 0.09	0.24 ± 0.08	0.21 ± 0.02	0.19 ± 0.02
CB	Ca	0.11 ± 0.01	0.08 ± 0.01*	0.09 ± 0.00*	0.06 ± 0.01*
	Mg	0.22 ± 0.02	0.22 ± 0.04	0.21 ± 0.02	0.19 ± 0.01
PM	Ca	0.10 ± 0.01	0.13 ± 0.02	0.19 ± 0.04*	0.11 ± 00.0
	Mg	0.26 ± 0.03	0.24 ± 0.07	0.22 ± 0.02	0.18 ± 0.03*
ST	Ca	0.08 ± 0.01	0.09 ± 0.01	0.12 ± 0.01	0.10 ± 0.02
	Mg	0.23 ± 0.04	0.26 ± 0.05	0.28 ± 0.08	0.23 ± 0.03
CC	Ca	0.08 ± 0.00	0.06 ± 0.01	0.08 ± 0.02	0.06 ± 0.00
	Mg	0.15 ± 0.03	0.15 ± 0.02	0.06 ± 0.01*‡	0.18 ± 0.02
MB	Ca	0.03 ± 0.01	0.06 ± 0.01*	0.08 ± 0.02**	0.08 ± 0.02**
	Mg	0.27 ± 0.02	0.21 ± 0.03	0.25 ± 0.02	0.20 ± 0.03

Values (in mg/g wet weight) are mean ± SD–derived 6–10 female rats. *$p < 0.05$ vs. control; **$p < 0.01$ vs. control; ‡$p < 0.05$ vs. Group A. Other details are the same as those in the legends to Table 1. Reprinted with permission from [1].

exception of cerebral cortex and hippocampus of rats treated with the lowest dose (Table 6). The dose-related increases in Mn are especially marked in hypothalamus, striatum, and hippocampus. Because of the large and dose-related increases in Mn in these three regions, the brain regional distribution patterns of Mn in the treated rats significantly shift away from the pattern detected in control animals, with the least changes being noted in cerebral cortex. Thus, those results (Table 6) are consistent with the hypothesis that chronic Mn treatment induces alterations of brain regional distribution of this metal [1,12,13]. Other workers have also noted similar findings. For example, employing a different rat model of Mn exposure [$MnCl_2 \cdot 4H_2O$ (3 mg/kg, i.p.) for 30 days], Scheuhammer and Cherian [23] also found increased accumulation of Mn in striatum, thalamus, and midbrain compared to other regions. Similarly, Chandra et al. [24] detected increased Mn in cerebral cortex, cerebellum, diencephalon, corpus striatum, midbrain, and pons but not in medulla oblongata of monkeys treated chronically with $MnCl_2 \cdot 4H_2O$ (20 mg/kg daily, orally for 18 months).

In Mn-treated rats, the largest increases in Fe level are noted in hypothalamus, striatum, and cerebellum (Table 7). In the developmental rat model of chronic and life-span Mn treatment of Lai et al. [1,12,13], the dose-related and region-selective Mn accumulation appears to influence the region-selective accumulation of Fe more so than those of the other metals investigated (compare Table 7 with Tables 8 and 9). Thus, the results (Tables 6–9) strongly suggest that, among the interactions in brain between Mn and other metals noted in Mn-treated rats, the interactions between brain Mn and brain Fe are most remarkable in that not only are such interactions noted in almost every brain region, they are also to some extent correlatable with the doses of Mn treatment (Table 7). For example, in Mn-treated rats, the largest increases in Fe level are found in hypothalamus, striatum, and cerebellum (Table 7); these are also the same regions that show highest accumulation of Mn (Table 6). Furthermore, in the Mn-treated rats, modest increases in Fe level are detected in hippocampus, pons and medulla, and midbrain (Table 7); similarly, these regions also accumulate significant amounts of Mn (Table 6). On the other hand, the interaction between Fe and Mn appears to differ in cerebral cortex as compared to those in other regions in that in rats treated with the lower two doses of Mn, Fe levels in cerebral cortex are unaffected whereas the Fe level in this region actually declines in rats treated with the highest Mn dose (Table 6). However, in sharp contrast with our results (Table 7), Scheuhammer and Cherian [23] did not detect significant changes in Fe content in any of the brain regions examined in a different rat model of chronic Mn treatment [$MnCl_2 \cdot 4H_2O$ (3 mg/kg, i.p.) for 30 days], although they did report a significant positive correlation between Mn and Fe distributions in control rats. Taken together, the results of Lai et al. [1,12,13] (Table 7) and those of Scheuhammer and Cherian [23] suggest that Mn and Fe interactions in brain regions in Mn-exposed rats may critically depend on the route of entry of Mn.

Mn treatment only at the intermediate dose (i.e., 10 mg $MnCl_2 \cdot 4H_2O$ per mL of drinking water) induces increases in Zn level in hypothalamus and striatum (Table 8). By contrast, Scheuhammer and Cherian [23] detected decreased Zn levels in certain brain regions in their rat model. Thus, taken together, the results from the studies of Lai et al. [1,12,13] (Table 8) and those of Scheuhammer and Cherian [23] suggest that the interactions between Mn and Zn in brain may vary depending on the route of administration of Mn.

The regional distribution of Al in Mn-treated rats is not significantly different from that in control rats (Table 6), suggesting that Mn, at the doses studied, does not interact with Al in the adult brain even though brain regional distribution of Al is affected by Mn treatment during postnatal development [2].

In Mn-treated rats, striatal Cu levels are increased in rats treated with the lower two Mn doses (Table 7). On the other hand, Cu levels in hippocampus and pons and medulla are increased in rats treated with the higher two Mn doses (Table 7). However, the regional distribution of Cu is not affected by the Mn treatment at the three doses studied (Table 7). Similar to the findings of Lai et al. [1,12,13] (Table 7), Scheuhammer and Cherian [23] also observed, in their rat model of chronic Mn exposure, increases in Cu in some of the brain regions they studied. On the other hand, Chandra et al. [24] only observed increased Cu levels in pons and medulla oblongata in monkeys treated with manganese chloride for 18 months.

In Mn-treated rats, the largest increases in Se level are noted in striatum and pons and medulla. As a result, the brain regional Se distribution is markedly altered, with striatum being the region showing the highest (rather than the lowest) Se level (Table 8). On the other hand, when compared to the corresponding level in control animals, Se level in cerebral cortex is increased in animals treated with the lowest Mn dose and decreased in animals treated with the highest Mn dose (Table 8). The Se level in hypothalamus is increased in rats treated with the lowest Mn dose, unchanged in rats treated with the intermediate Mn dose, and is increased in rats treated with the highest Mn dose (Table 8). Neither Scheuhammer and Cherian [23] nor Chandra et al. [24] reportedly studied the interactions between Mn and Se in brain in Mn exposure.

In Mn-treated rats, the Ca level in midbrain is markedly increased—more than doubled—in a dose-related manner (Table 9). On the other hand, the Ca level in cerebellum is decreased in a dose-related manner in the Mn-treated rats (Table 9). In their primate model of chronic Mn exposure, Chandra et al. [24] also noted decreases in Ca levels in pons, medulla oblongata, and corpus striatum. However, Scheuhammer and Cherian [23] have not reportedly studied Ca in the rat.

In rats treated with the highest Mn dose, Mg level is decreased in pons and medulla compared to corresponding level in control rats (Table 9): these data suggest that chronic Mn treatment does not markedly influence Mg distribution in the adult brain. By contrast, the brain regional distribution of Mg is known to be affected by chronic Mn treatment during postnatal development [12]. Neither Scheuhammer and Cherian [23] nor Chandra et al. [24] reportedly studied the interactions between Mn and Mg in brain in chronic Mn exposure.

4.4.   Cellular Uptake and Distribution of Manganese and Other Metals

Although primary neural cell cultures have been employed to investigate the cellular mechanisms of metal toxicity, interactions between Mn and other metals have only been studied to a very limited extent in these cells [22,25]. Chick cerebrocortical astrocytes in primary culture contain 100–200 μM Mn, Fe, Zn, and Cu but 7 mM Mg [26]. These astrocytes take up Mn(II) by facilitated diffusion; Mn(II) efflux from these cells is biphasic with a fast component releasing some 30–40% of total cellular Mn, and a slower component releasing the remainder of cellular Mn [27]. Both Ca(II) and Zn(II) inhibit but Cu(II) activates astrocytic Mn(II) uptake [27]. However, neither Zn(II) nor Cu(II) inhibits Mn(II) efflux from these cells [28,29].

Compared to its uptake in astrocytes [27–29], even less is known about Mn uptake in neurons. There is some evidence that Mn can enter neurons and astrocytes via agonist-activated divalent cation-permeable kainate receptors on these two cell types [30]. Axonal transport of Mn may mediate the intracerebral transfer of this metal; two such examples are anterograde axonal transport of Mn in the basal ganglia [31] and uptake of Mn into the olfactory receptor cells and its transfer along the primary olfactory neurons into the brain [32]. A third type of neuronal uptake of Mn can occur at nerve endings since isolated nerve ending particles (i.e., synaptosomes) can take up Ca; however, Mn uptake and release [33] by this route has not been systematically investigated [22,25]. Nevertheless, the physiological and quantitative importance of these neuronal Mn transport mechanisms is unknown and remains to be elucidated.

4.5. Subcellular Distributions of Manganese and Other Metals: Modulations by Chronic Manganese Treatment

Few studies have addressed the interrelations between metals at the subcellular level. By combining their INAA and subcellular fractionation techniques, Lai et al. [1–3,13,15,22] have systematically investigated the subcellular distributions of trace metals and electrolytes and the effects of chronic Mn treatment thereon.

Table 10 reports data of the effect of chronic Mn treatment on the subcellular distribution of trace metals and electrolytes. In control rat brain, Mn level is highest in mitochondria, capillaries, and cytosol; intermediate in microsomes and synaptosomes; and lowest in myelin and nuclei. The Fe level is higher in cytosol than in the other fractions. The Cu level is highest in cytosol and capillaries; intermediate in mitochondria, nuclei, and microsomes; and lowest in synaptosomes and nuclei. By contrast, the distribution of Zn has the following rank order:

capillaries > nuclei ≥ mitochondria ≥ cytosol ≥ myelin > synaptosomes. For the nonessential trace metal Al, the rank order of distribution differs yet again: synaptosomes = nuclei = mitochondria > myelin > capillaries > cytosol > microsomes. For Ca, the rank order of distribution is capillaries > mitochondria > cytosol = nuclei > synaptosomes > microsomes > myelin. On the other hand, for Mg the rank order of distribution is cytosol > synaptosomes > nuclei > microsomes > mitochondria = myelin > capillaries. Thus, these results are comparable to those reported by Rajan et al. [34] who had investigated five metals (Cu, Fe, Zn, Mg, Ca) in only three subcellular fractions (myelin, synaptosomes, mitochondria) derived from whole-brain and selected brain regions of normal rats.

Chronic Mn treatment in vivo gives rise to 93% increase in Mn in brain homogenate but does not markedly alter the relative distribution of this metal in various subcellular fractions. However, compared with respective control values, the largest increases in Mn are noted in nuclei (+122%), mitochondria (+70%), and synaptosomes (+60%). Consistent with the enhanced mitochondrial Mn accumulation upon chronic Mn exposure in vivo are the recent findings that Mn is sequestered by liver and brain mitochondria through the mitochondrial Ca uniporter [35,36]. Thus, such observations [1,35,36] suggest that mitochondria, synaptosomes, and nuclei may be subcellular targets for Mn neurotoxicity [2].

Chronic Mn treatment in vivo induces changes in the subcellular distributions of several trace metals and electrolytes. The Fe level is increased in nuclei but decreased in myelin and cytosol whereas the Cu level is markedly increased in synaptosomes and nuclei but decreased in capillaries. The Zn level is markedly increased in cytosol, nuclei, and mitochondria but the Mg level is significantly increased in nuclei, cytosol, and capillaries. The Al level is decreased in synaptosomes but increased in microsomes. The Ca level is slightly increased in synaptosomes and cytosol but decreased in capillaries. These observations (Table 10) strongly suggest that chronic Mn treatment not only influences the regional distributions of other metals in brain (Tables 6–9) but differentially alters the subcellular distributions of other metals and electrolytes [1]. However, the molecular mechanisms underlying the Mn–metal interactions remain to be elucidated.

TABLE 10

Effect of Chronic Manganese Treatment on Subcellular Distribution of Trace Metals and Electrolytes

Metal	Treatment	H	M	Syn	N	Mye	Cap	Mic	Cyto
Ca	C	0.70 ± 0.10	3.40 ± 0.40	1.68 ± 0.05	2.05 ± 0.41	0.60 ± 0.24	3.98 ± 0.28	0.94 ± 0.05	2.07 ± 0.10
	T	0.66 ± 0.08	3.88 ± 0.70	1.80 ± 0.05*	1.86 ± 0.40	0.54 ± 0.10	2.95 ± 0.27*	1.09 ± 0.07	2.98 ± 0.45*
Fe	C	0.32 ± 0.01	0.57 ± 0.07	0.60 ± 0.07	0.54 ± 0.05	0.49 ± 0.09	ND	ND	2.53 ± 0.20
	T	0.46 ± 0.12*	0.61 ± 0.06	0.51 ± 0.10	1.58 ± 0.25*	0.32 ± 0.01*	ND	ND	1.05 ± 0.49*
Mg	C	2.06 ± 0.50	1.11 ± 0.02	3.21 ± 0.25	2.81 ± 0.41	1.01 ± 0.49	0.85 ± 0.10	1.63 ± 0.80	5.30 ± 0.41
	T	1.89 ± 0.10	1.32 ± 0.08	2.94 ± 0.89	4.81 ± 0.55**	1.86 ± 0.65	2.61 ± 0.45**	2.87 ± 0.87	9.58 ± 0.85**
Al	C	40.20 ± 8.26	99.50 ± 19.70	100.0 ± 15.80	100.0 ± 25.9	72.26 ± 29.2	42.0 ± 8.20	25.92 ± 5.60	30.0 ± 2.94
	T	25.31 ± 6.4**	78.2 ± 27.9	37.5 ± 4.7**	99.0 ± 20.0	57.4 ± 22.0	55.14 ± 14.3	75.4 ± 13.4*	36.0 ± 3.8

Cu	C	62.8 ± 10.2	141.8 ± 16.7	47.7 ± 4.5	95.1 ± 9.5	40.5 ± 4.5	369.1 ± 81.0	80.3 ± 12.1	497.9 ± 181.5
	T	85.2 ± 5.2*	135.3 ± 35.3	81.1 ± 5.3**	192.2 ± 37.1	37.8 ± 3.4	180.3 ± 5.1**	70.0 ± 1.2	508.7 ± 142.5
Mn	C	3.95 ± 0.89	12.53 ± 1.32	8.00 ± 1.91	4.40 ± 0.65	4.64 ± 1.00	11.96 ± 1.60	8.45 ± 1.53	10.23 ± 2.85
	T	7.61 ± 1.50**	21.30 ± 1.84*	12.89 ± 2.24*	9.79 ± 0.74**	6.67 ± 0.90*	14.94 ± 1.28*	12.72 ± 3.0*	15.78 ± 2.84*
Zn	C	80.0 ± 10.0	235.0 ± 20.3	148.6 ± 10.3	238.5 ± 22.3	204.9 ± 49.0	525.6 ± 30.2	ND	229.9 ± 23.6
	T	557.0 ± 89.0**	304.8 ± 39.9*	121.8 ± 29.3	329.6 ± 48.9*	261.8 ± 50.0	587.3 ± 67.9	ND	572.0 ± 68.9**

Values (in µg/g protein for Al, Cu, Mn, and Zn; and in mg/g protein for Ca, Fe, and Mg) are mean ± SD of 3–5 experiments. In each experiment, hypothalamus, striatum, midbrain, and hippocampus from five adult rats were pooled for preparation of the homogenate, which was then employed for subcellular fractionation by the procedure of Lai and Clark (see Ref. 1 and details therein). The abbreviations are: H, homogenate; M, nonsynaptic mitochondria; Syn, synaptosomes; N, nuclei; Mye, myelin; Cap, capillaries; Mic, microsomes; Cyto, cytosol; and ND, not determined. Two groups of adult female rats were used: C, control rats (i.e., those not treated with Mn); T, rats were treated with 10 mg of $MnCl_2 \cdot 4H_2O$ (i.e., group B). *p < 0.05, and **p < 0.01 vs. corresponding values in control group.
Reprinted with permission from [1].

5. INTERRELATIONS BETWEEN MANGANESE AND OTHER METALS IN BRAIN IN HUMAN HEALTH AND DISEASES

5.1. Neurodegenerative Diseases

The selective vulnerability of cells and organelles in brain to oxidative injury mediated by transition metals has been proposed as one of the major pathogenetic mechanisms of neurodegenerative diseases (see Refs. 37–40 for a detailed discussion and additional references). The relevance to this proposed mechanism of the interrelations between Mn and other metals in several neurological diseases is discussed below.

5.1.1. Alzheimer's Disease

Few studies have addressed the role of Mn in the pathophysiology and/ or pathogenesis of Alzheimer's disease (AD). An early study on one patient with an extrapyramidal syndrome and dementia (which was confirmed with brain biopsy in which neuritic plaques and neurofibrill-ary tangles typical of AD were found) reported increased and toxic Mn levels in brain, serum, hair, and feces [41]. High brain levels of Ca and Al were found in several cases of Japanese amyotropic lateral sclerosis (ALS) and AD and Guam Parkinson's disease (PD) with a significant positive correlation between Ca and Al and/or between Ca and Mn [42]. Thus, both studies [41,42] implicate Mn in AD; however, a subsequent, more detailed INAA study of various regions of aging and AD brains revealed that the grand mean for brain Mn was higher in AD brains than in adult control brains although that difference did not reach statistical significance [43]. Hershey et al. [44] did not find any relation-ship between Mn, Al, As, or Pb levels in cerebrospinal fluid (CSF) in AD or other dementing diseases; however, Basun et al. reported increases in plasma Al, Cd, Hg, and Se but decreases in plasma Mn and Fe in AD patients and the plasma levels of Mn and Fe were related to changes in behavior of patients [45]. Thus, results of the studies discussed above [41–46] suggest that Mn may interact with the metabolism of other metals in AD.

Fe is known to interact with Mn in brain (see above); thus, it is not surprising that in AD the brain metabolism of Fe is disturbed. As determined by INAA, Fe is elevated in multiple regions of the AD brain [47]. Moreover, Fe in the cores and rims of senile plaques of amygdala of AD patients is elevated compared to that in the neuropil of this region in AD patients [48]. These observations are of interest because Fe (like Cu and Zn) can accelerate aggregation of β-amyloid peptide [48], which may be associated with plaque formation, a neuropathological hallmark of AD. The latter conclusion is consistent with the observation that neuritic plaques and the surrounding cells contain high levels of stainable Fe [49]. These observations (and others) led Connor to propose that in the AD brain increased Fe accumulation in the presence of decreased transferrin, together with the lack of compensatory increase in ferritin production, may induce excess free radical production and hence oxidative brain damage [49].

In addition to Fe, Zn, and Al, Hg levels are also increased in different regions of the AD brain [47,48], although their high variability precludes the differences between values in AD and control brains from attaining statistical significance. All of the metals mentioned above (i.e., Fe, Zn, Al, Cu) have been proposed to be responsible for inducing cell death in the AD brain due to (1) formation of reactive oxygen species, (2) other metal-mediated cytotoxic effects, or (3) a combination of both (1) and (2) [2,21,39,40,49].

5.1.2. Parkinson's Disease

Even though several transition metals, including Mn, have been implicated in the free radical-mediated neuronal cell death in neurodegenerative diseases (see above), few studies have determined the brain levels of Mn in Parkinson's disease (PD) [50–52]. (Nevertheless, chronic Mn toxicity in humans shows signs and symptoms that are reminiscent of those found in PD and dystonia. See the next two sections for further discussion.) An early study of one case, which revealed increased brain, serum, hair, urine, and feces levels of Mn associated with an extrapyramidal syndrome and dementia, suggests that parkinsonian signs and symptoms are related to excess accumulation of Mn in brain [41]. Two subsequent studies of PD patients [51,52] indicate, in most brain regions investigated, Mn is not significantly different from those in control subjects, with the exception of a small decrease (20%) noted in the medial putamen [52].

Substantia nigra and the pigment neuromelanin isolated therefrom contain large amounts of Mn, Fe, Zn, Pb, and Cu [54] and some
workers have found increased Fe and Zn in substantia nigra of PD
patients [52]. Taken together, such findings [52,54] suggest that heavy
metals in neuromelanin may interact with each other.

Some but not all authors have found a consistent increase in Fe in
substantia nigra of PD patients relative to that in control subjects (see
Ref. 40 for a detailed discussion and additional references) and this
increase is associated with decreases in ferritin and Cu but increases in
Zn in this region [53]. Moreover, there is some evidence that Fe and Al
accumulate in neuromelanin granules in substantia nigra of PD patients [40,41]. The latter observations prompted some authors to suggest that the accumulation of Fe and other metals in neuromelanin of
PD substantia nigra promotes oxidative stress [40,41].

5.1.3. Chronic Manganese Toxicity

Chronic Mn toxicity in humans, as shown by miners exposed to this
metal, is characterized by signs and symptoms reminiscent of those of
PD and dystonia [1,12,13,22]. Other studies suggest that pathological
changes in chronic Mn intoxication are more pronounced in globus pallidus than in substantia nigra (see Ref. 41 and references therein). Moreover, Mn intoxication has been detected in chronic liver disease (see Sec.
5.2.2 below). The available evidence implicates the dysfunction of the
central dopaminergic system in chronic Mn toxicity although the molecular mechanisms underlying this dysfunction are unclear [1,41].

Notwithstanding that few studies on human Mn toxicity have
addressed this issue, investigations employing animal models of chronic
Mn toxicity strongly suggest that tissue Mn accumulation in chronic
Mn toxicity interact with the metabolism of other trace metals and
electrolytes (see Tables 1–10 and Secs. 2–4 above).

5.2. Other Neurological/Neuropsychiatric Syndromes

5.2.1. Other Neurological Syndromes

Evidence is accumulating that in neurological diseases other than AD
and PD brain metabolism of Mn and other metals may also be dis-

turbed. Pick's disease is associated with increases in brain Mn, Fe, and Na and decreases in brain Cr and Se [55]. In ALS brain, levels of Al and Ca are elevated with a positive correlation between Ca and Al and between Ca and Mg [42]. These data also suggest that Mn may interact with the brain metabolism of other metals in Pick's disease and in ALS although additional studies are needed to better define the underlying mechanism(s).

5.2.2. Chronic Hepatic Encephalopathy

Early studies suggested that in some metabolic encephalopathies brain metabolism of metals is disturbed [56–59]. In dialysis encephalopathy [57], chronic renal failure without dialysis [57], and hepatic coma [58], brain Al is elevated; this increased brain Al may be one pathophysiological factor underlying these metabolic encephalopathies since Al is neurotoxic [59].

Recent studies implicate Mn having a role in the pathogenesis of portal-systemic encephalopathy [56]. In patients with chronic liver diseases, blood and brain Mn levels are elevated and are associated with a pallidal signal hyperintensity on T_1-weighted magnetic resonance imaging (MRI) [56]. Mn content detected in globus pallidus of cirrhotic patients who had died in hepatic coma shows two- to sevenfold increases [56]. The MRI signal intensity correlates with blood Mn and with the extrapyramidal symptoms found in most of the cirrhotic patients [56]. Liver transplantation eliminates the extrapyramidal symptoms and the normalization of the pallidal MRI signal [56]. However, portosystemic shunting leads to accumulation of Mn in brain, especially in basal ganglia, and the appearance of some symptoms of cognitive and motor dysfunction [56]. Based on the results of studies using animals models (see Secs. 2–4 above), one may propose that, in addition to increased brain Mn being a contributing factor to the development of cognitive and motor dysfunction in patients with chronic hepatic encephalopathy, the interactions between brain Mn and other trace metals and electrolytes may also be contributing factors in the pathogenesis of hepatic coma [1]. Nevertheless, additional studies are required to test this hypothesis and to further elucidate the underlying molecular mechanisms [1].

6. CONCLUSIONS AND PROSPECTS FOR FUTURE STUDIES

This chapter highlights the advances in our understanding of the interrelations between Mn and other metal ions in brain and peripheral organs derived from studies employing animal models. It also discusses the interrelations between Mn and other metal ions in human health and diseases, especially diseases affecting the central nervous system. Because of recent advances in molecular biological and cell biological studies of metal metabolism [1,7,49], the field is ready to address more mechanistic issues underlying the interdependence between Mn and other metal ions.

ACKNOWLEDGMENTS

The authors acknowledge the encouragement and support of the late Professor Alan N. Davison. The authors thank Professor John B. Clark for his interests and encouragement. J. C. K. Lai wishes to thank Dean Barbara Wells and Dr. Chris Daniels for their interests and continued support. These studies were supported, in part, by the Worshipful Company of Pewterers, London, U.K. (J. C. K. Lai), the Brain Research Trust (L. Lim), University of London Research Funds (M. J. Minski and A. W. K. Chan), a State Board of Education, Idaho grant (J. C. K. Lai), and an ISU University Research Committee grant (J. C. K. Lai).

ABBREVIATIONS

AD	Alzheimer's disease
ALS	amyotropic lateral sclerosis
CB	cerebellum
CC	cerebral cortex
CSF	cerebrospinal fluid
HIP	hippocampus
HYP	hypothalamus

INAA   instrumental neutron activation analysis
MB   midbrain
MRI   magnetic resonance imaging
PD   Parkinson's disease
PM   pons and medulla
ST   striatum

REFERENCES

1. J. C. K. Lai, M. J. Minski, A. W. K. Chan, T. K. C. Leung, and L. Lim, *Neurotoxicol.*, *20*, 433–444 (1999).

2. J. C. K. Lai, A. W. K. Chan, M. J. Minski, and L. Lim, in *Mineral and Metal Neurotoxicology* (M. Yasui, K. Ota, M. J. Strong, and M. A. Verity, eds.), CRC Press, Boca Raton, FL, 1997, pp. 297–303.

3. J. C. K. Lai, A. W. K. Chan, M. J. Minski, T. K. C. Leung, L. Lim, and A. N. Davison, in *Metal Ions in Neurology and Psychiatry* (S. Gabay, J. Harris, and B. T. Ho, eds.), Alan Liss, New York, 1985, pp. 323–343.

4. M. Diez-Ewald, L. R. Weintraub, and W. H. Crosby, *Proc. Soc. Exp. Biol. Med.*, *129*, 448–451 (1968).

5. C. D. Davis, T. L. Wolf, and J. L. Greger, *J. Nutr.*, *122*, 1300–1308 (1992).

6. *Draft Toxicological Profile for Manganese*, U.S. Department of Health and Human Services, Public Health Service, Agency for Toxic Substances and Disease Registry, 1997, pp. 92–93.

7. P. E. Johnson, and E. D. Korynta, *Proc. Soc. Exp. Biol. Med.*, *199*, 470–480 (1992).

8. H. A. Schroeder, and A. P. Nason, *J. Nutr.*, *104*, 167–178 (1974).

9. H. A. Schroeder, and A. P. Nason, *J. Nutr.*, *106*, 198–203 (1976).

10. A. W. K. Chan, M. J. Minski, and J. C. K. Lai, *J. Neurosci. Methods*, 7, 317–328 (1983).

11. E.-L. Lakomaa, in *Metal Ions in Neurology and Psychiatry* (S. Gabay, J. Harris, and B. T. Ho, eds.), Alan Liss, New York, 1985, pp. 303–322.

12. A. W. K. Chan, M. J. Minski, L. Lim, and J. C. K. Lai, *Metab. Brain Dis.*, 7, 21–33 (1992).

13. P. Du, C. R. Buerstatte, A. W. K. Chan, M. J. Minski, L. Bennett, and J. C. K. Lai, *Conference Proceedings of 1997 Conference on Hazardous Wastes and Materials*, Pocatello, Idaho, pp. 1–14.

14. E. J. Underwood, *Trace Elements in Human and Animal Nutrition*, 4th ed., Academic Press, New York, 1977.

15. J. C. K. Lai, in *Handbook on Metal-Ligand Interactions in Biological Fluids*, Vol. 2 (G. Berthon, ed.), Marcel Dekker, New York, 1995, pp. 146–152.

16. M. Aschner and J. L. Aschner, *Brain Res. Bull.*, *24*, 857–860 (1990).

17. V. A. Murphy, K. C. Wadhwani, Q. R. Smith, and S. I. Rapoport, *J. Neurochem.*, *57*, 948–954 (1991).

18. K. C. Wadhwani, V. A. Murphy, Q. R. Smith, and S. I. Rapoport, *Am. J. Physiol.*, *262* (2 Pt 2), R284–R288 (1992).

19. O. Rabin, L. Hegedus, J. M. Bourre, and Q. R. Smith, *J. Neurochem.*, *61*, 509–517 (1993).

20. M. Aschner and M. Gannon, *Brain Res. Bull.*, *33*, 345–349 (1994).

21. J. C. K. Lai, A. W. K. Chan, M. J. Minski, and L. Lim, in *Metal Ions in Neurology and Psychiatry* (S. Gabay, J. Harris, and B. T. Ho, eds.), Alan Liss, New York, 1985, pp. 49–67.

22. J. C. K. Lai, T. K. C. Leung, and L. Lim, in *Metal Ions in Neurology and Psychiatry* (S. Gabay, J. Harris, and B. T. Ho, eds.), Alan Liss, New York, 1985, pp. 177–197.

23. A. M. Scheuhammer and M. G. Cherian, *Toxicol. Appl. Pharmacol.*, *61*, 227–233 (1981).

24. S. V. Chandra, R. S. Srivastava, and G. S. Shukla, *Toxicol. Lett.*, *4*, 189–192 (1979).

25. J. C. K. Lai, P. C. L. Wong, and L. Lim, in *Neural Membranes* (G. Y. Sun, N. Bazan, J.-Y. Wu, G. Porcellati, and A. Y. Sun, eds.), Humana Press, Clifton Heights, NJ, 1983, pp. 355–374.

26. G. Tholey, M. Ledig, P. Mandel, L. Sargentini, A. H. Frivold, M. Leroy, A. A. Grippo, and F. C. Wedler, *Neurochem. Res.*, *13*, 45–50 (1988).

27. F. C. Wedler, B. W. Ley, and A. A. Grippo, *Neurochem. Res.*, *14*, 1129–1135 (1989).

28. F. C. Wedler and B. W. Ley, *Neurochem. Res.*, *15*, 1221–1228 (1990).

29. F. C. Wedler, in *Progress in Medicinal Chemistry*, Vol. 30 (G. P. Ellis and D. K. Luscombe, eds.), Elsevier, Amsterdam, 1993, pp. 89–133.

30. R. M. Pruss, R. L. Akeson, M. M. Racke, and J. L. Wilburn, *Neuron*, 7, 509–518 (1991).

31. W. N. Sloot and J. B. Gramsbergen, *Brain Res.*, 657, 124–132 (1994).

32. H. Tjalve, C. Mejare, and K. Borg-Neczak, *Pharmacol. Toxicol.*, 77, 23–31 (1995).

33. A. Takeda, S. Ishiwatari, and S. Oada, *Brain Res.*, 811, 147–151 (1998).

34. K. S. Rajan, R. W. Colburn, and J. M. Davis, *Life Sci.*, 18, 423–432 (1976).

35. C. E. Gavin, K. K. Gunter, and T. E. Gunter, *Biochem. J.*, 266, 329–334 (1990).

36. C. E. Gavin, K. K. Gunter, and T. E. Gunter, *Toxicol. Appl. Pharmacol.*, 115, 1–5 (1992).

37. S. J. Robb-Gaspers and J. R. Connor, in *Metals and Oxidative Damage in Neurological Disorders* (J. R. Connor, ed.), Plenum Press, New York, 1997, pp. 341–355.

38. M. P. Mattson, in *Int. Rev. Neurobiol.*, Vol. 42 (R. J. Bradley, R. A. Harris, and P. Jenner, eds.), Academic Press, San Diego, 1998, pp. 103–168.

39. L. A. Shinobu and M. F. Beal, in *Metals and Oxidative Damage in Neurological Disorders* (J. R. Connor, ed.), Plenum Press, New York, 1997, pp. 237–275.

40. W. R. Markesbery and J. M. Carney, *Brain Pathol.*, 9, 133–146 (1999).

41. R. G. Banta and W. R. Markesbery, *Neurology*, 27, 213–216 (1977).

42. F. Yosimasu, M. Yasui, Y. Yase, S. Iwata, D. C. Gajdusek, C. J. Gibbs, Jr., and K. M. Chen, *Folia Psychiatr. Neurol. Jpn.*, 34, 75–82 (1980).

43. W. R. Markesbery, W. D. Ehmann, T. I. Hossain, and M. Alauddin, *Neurotoxicology*, 5, 49–57 (1984).

44. C. O. Hershey, L. A. Hershey, A. Varnes, S. D. Vibhakar, P. Lavin, and W. H. Strain, *Neurology*, 33, 1350–1353 (1983).

45. H. Basun, L. G. Forssell, L. Wetterberg, and B. Winblad, *J. Neural Transm. Park. Dis. Dement. Sect.*, 3, 231–258 (1991).

46. W. D. Ehmann, W. R. Markesbery, M. Alauddin, T. I. Hossain, and E. H. Brubaker, *Neurotoxicology*, 7, 195–206 (1986).

47. C. R. Cornett, W. R. Markesbery, and W. D. Ehmann, *Neurotoxicology*, *19*, 339–345 (1998).

48. M. A. Lovell, J. D. Robertson, W. J. Teesdale, J. L. Campbell, and W. R. Markesbery, *J. Neurol. Sci.*, *158*, 47–52 (1998).

49. J. R. Connor, in *Metals and Oxidative Damage in Neurological Disorders* (J. R. Connor, ed.), Plenum Press, New York, 1997, pp. 23–39.

50. P. F. Good, D. P. Perl, and C. W. Olanow, in *Metals and Oxidative Damage in Neurological Disorders* (J. R. Connor, ed.), Plenum Press, New York, 1997, pp. 277–294.

51. N. A. Larsen, H. Pakkenberg, E. Damsgaard, K. Heydorn, and S. Wold, *J. Neurol. Sci.*, *51*, 437–446 (1981).

52. D. T. Dexter, F. R. Wells, A. J. Lees, F. Agid, P. Jenner, and C. D. Marsden, *J. Neurochem.*, *52*, 1830–1836 (1989).

53. D. T. Dexter, A. Carayon, F. Javoy-Agid, Y. Agid, F. R. Wells, S. E. Daniel, A. J. Lees, P. Jenner, and C. D. Marsden, *Brain*, *114*, 1953–1975 (1991).

54. L. Zecca and H. M. Swartz, *J. Neural Transm. Park. Dis. Dement. Sect.*, *5*, 203–213 (1993).

55. W. D. Ehmann, M. Alauddin, T. I. Hossain, and W. R. Markesbery, *Ann. Neurol.*, *15*, 102–104 (1984).

56. G. Pomier Layrargues, C. Rose, L. Spahr, J. Zayed, L. Normandin, and R. F. Butterworth, *Metab. Brain Dis.*, *13*, 311–318 (1998).

57. A. C. Alfrey, *Neurotoxicology*, *1*, 43–53 (1980).

58. A. I. Arieff, J. C. Cooper, D. Armstrong, and V. C. Lagarowitz, *Ann. Intern. Med.*, *90*, 741–747 (1979).

59. J. C. K. Lai and J. P. Blass, *J. Neurochem.*, *42*, 438–446 (1984).

6

The Use of Manganese as a Probe for Elucidating the Role of Magnesium Ions in Ribozymes

Andrew L. Feig*

Department of Chemistry and Biochemistry, University of Colorado, Campus Box 215, Boulder, CO 80309, USA

---

*Present affiliation: Department of Chemistry, Indiana University, Bloomington, IN 47405, USA

1.   INTRODUCTION

1.1.   Metal Ions in Ribozyme Biochemistry

Catalytic RNAs or ribozymes are polynucleotides capable of carrying
out a chemical reaction. In their natural context, most ribozymes act on
themselves in an autolytic manner. RNase P, a ribozyme that processes
pre-tRNAs, is a notable exception in that its natural behavior is catalytic [1,2]. By engineering the sequence appropriately, most ribozymes
have been converted into true catalysts in vitro, capable of acting on an
independent substrate molecule [3]. Ribozymes vary greatly in their
size and complexity. The smallest reported ribozyme is just three nucleotides in length [4], whereas other ribozymes have minimal sequences hundreds of nucleotides long. Several of the more commonly
studied small ribozymes ($\leq$100 nt) include hammerhead ribozyme, hepatitis δ virus ribozyme, hairpin ribozyme, and *Neurospora* VS ribozyme.
The class of large ribozymes includes group I intron, group II intron,
and RNase P. Reviews of general ribozyme biochemistry are available in
a number of recent sources [5–8] and will not be discussed in detail
here. Instead, this chapter will focus on the experiments that use the
special properties of Mn^{2+} as a probe for the Mg^{2+} binding sites on
ribozymes. These methods include phosphorothioate rescue, X-ray crystallography, electron paramagnetic resonance (EPR), and nuclear magnetic resonance (NMR). Most of the examples cited will revolve around

the hammerhead ribozyme, as this small catalytic motif has been studied extensively by these methods. This system shows the utility of these techniques as well as their limitations.

A common denominator among ribozymes is the requirement for a globular structure that positions the catalytically important functional groups into an active site. In this regard, RNA enzymes are very similar to their protein counterparts. The anionic nature of the phosphodiester backbone, however, imposes significant constraints on the folding of the molecule. To bring the charged backbone into a compact form electrostatic repulsion must be overcome. Therefore, RNA folding is extremely dependent on the ionic environment of the solution. Metal ions play two general roles in the folding process. Through nonspecific binding, the ions screen electrostatic repulsion and form an "ionic core" [9] which acts to stabilize the folded structure in a manner analogous to the hydrophobic core of a protein. Discrete metal-binding events also help to nucleate the folding process by creating regions of local structure around which the rest of the molecule can organize. Divalent metal ions are sufficiently important for RNA folding that many studies use the addition or removal of these ions to initiate the process [10–14].

Many articles in the literature discuss the idea that metal ions participate directly in the chemical step of ribozyme cleavage reactions [15,16]. This hypothesis derives from the observation that these catalysts are inactive without Mg^{2+} or a suitable substitute. Such evidence is insufficient to establish this requirement, as a similar dependence would result were Mg^{2+} required for the formation of a critical structural element. In the case of the hairpin ribozyme, Co(NH$_3$)$_6^{3+}$ experiments showed that outer-sphere metal binding was sufficient to induce cleavage, supporting the idea that the ions play a primarily structural role [17–19]. Recently, the observation that high concentrations of monovalent ions can support activity for several ribozymes also questioned the obligatory requirement of Mg^{2+} in the activity of small ribozymes [20]. Such data are interesting in that they make us think seriously about how the ions behave, but their relevance to the conditions observed within a biological context is minimal. One must therefore phrase the question relative to normal ribozyme physiology. Do Mg^{2+} ions facilitate the chemical step of these reactions or are they present merely to mediate the structures necessary for catalysis?

1.2.   Metal Ion Specificity in Ribozymes

As a polyelectrolyte, RNAs will condense cations to their surface, even
in their denatured state [21,22]. Because of this property, given the
appropriate conditions, almost any metal ion can be induced to bind an
RNA molecule. This aspect of metal binding is nonspecific and is not
likely to represent accurately the interactions with a native or folded
ribozyme. It is therefore important to study metal binding under conditions where the RNA maintains its appropriate tertiary structure. In
most cases, this caveat will require that a folding agent be present, the
nature of which will be dependent on the RNA in question.

In vivo, Mg^{2+} is the dominant ionic species that binds RNA due to
its high cellular concentration. The total Mg^{2+} concentration is approximately 30 mM in mammalian cells, the majority of which is bound to
cellular ligands. Only 0.5–1 mM is free in solution [23]. Because of this
high cellular concentration, there is little evolutionary pressure for
Mg^{2+} binding sites to be particularly tight. Mg^{2+} therefore binds to
RNAs weakly (high µM affinities are common), and the bound ions
exchange rapidly with those free in solution. This phenomenon con-
trasts with most metalloprotein systems where metal binding sites
with submicromolar affinities are common [23].

Another difficulty in studying metal-RNA interactions is that each
ribozyme will bind a multitude of ions, approximately one for every two
nucleotides under low ionic strength conditions [24]. This value corresponds with electroneutrality for the RNA-metal complex. The real
task, therefore, is to identify sites where highly specific binding occurs.
These sites might indicate important structural interactions required
for the overall fold or identify ions that play a role in the catalytic
function. It is the task of the experimentalist to isolate and study these
unique metal binding sites despite the multitude of additional electrostatic interactions.

Whereas it is easy to make such a statement, this goal is quite
difficult to achieve in laboratory and is currently one of the major
challenges in the field. Only a few studies have measured the affinities
for a series of ions at a discrete ribozyme site. One site is on the
hammerhead ribozyme [25] and another the group I intron [26]. In both
cases, the affinity for the site varies as a function of Z^2/r of the ion. This

charge/radial function is also related to the hydration enthalpy of the ion [27] and thus may reflect the ease with which the RNA can induce partial dehydration of the ion in preparation for inner-sphere coordination. Probing of additional sites will help determine if this relationship is general or only pertains to a small subset of the interactions.

1.3. The Ability of Mn^{2+} to Substitute for Mg^{2+} in Ribozymes

In many ribozyme systems, in vitro studies have shown that Mn^{2+} can support catalytic activity when added in concentrations comparable to that of Mg^{2+} [28–30]. In each case, the K_m^{Mg} is similar to K_m^{Mn}. The cellular concentration of Mn^{2+}, however, is significantly lower than that of Mg^{2+}. As a result, the sites would contain Mg^{2+} under physiological conditions. The fact that this type of substitution retains normal functionality allows the use of Mn^{2+} as a probe for Mg^{2+} binding. At high concentrations, Mn^{2+} can sometimes inhibit the activity of certain ribozymes [29]. In these cases, it is likely that Mn^{2+} binding induces the formation of alternative, inactive conformations of the RNA.

The substitution of Mg^{2+} for Mn^{2+} works so well due to the similarity of their physical properties (Table 1). The most important issue is

TABLE 1

Comparison of the Physical Properties
of Mg^{2+} and Mn^{2+}

Physical property	Mg^{2+}	Mn^{2+}
Hydration number	6	6
Ionic radius (Å)[a]	0.72	0.67
ΔH_{hyd} (kJ/mol)[a]	-1922.1	-1845.6
Water exchange rate (s^{-1})[a]	$\approx 10^6$	2.1×10^7
pK_a of aqua ion[a]	11.42	10.6
Absolute hardness η[b]	47.59	9.02
Absolute electronegativity χ[b]	32.55	24.66

[a]Data from [97].
[b]Data from [98].

probably the similarity in ionic radius and charge, both of which play a critical role in metal binding to a rigidly defined site. The pK_a values of the aqua ions are slightly different, with the Mn^{2+} ion being a bit more acidic. This property results in a greater amount of the monohydroxide species $[M(H_2O)_5(OH)]^+$ being present at a given pH. As a result, Mn^{2+} often stimulates hydrolysis reactions dependent on the availability of a general base more efficiently than Mg^{2+}. Documentation of this behavior is extensive for the hammerhead ribozyme [31–35]. The result of this ΔpK_a is that Mn^{2+}-promoted ribozyme cleavage occurs more rapidly ($\approx$ 20-fold) than that in the presence of Mg^{2+}. The dependence of the cleavage rate on the nature of the metal cofactor [36] argues for the ions being directly involved in the cleavage chemistry under these conditions rather than simply assuming a structural role.

2.   USE OF Mn^{2+} IN BIOCHEMICAL STUDIES OF PHOSPHOROTHIOATE-CONTAINING RIBOZYMES

2.1.   What Are Phosphorothioate Modified RNAs?

One of the most common methods of locating metal binding sites in ribozymes is by a phosphorothioate rescue experiment. Figure 1 shows the structures of the different phosphorothioate linkages, each of which has one or more of the phosphoryl oxygen atoms replaced by a sulfur. Five types of phosphorothioates have been used in ribozymes studies: 3'-bridging [37–39], 5'-bridging [32,34], R_p-nonbridging [40,41], S_p-nonbridging [40,41], and the phosphorodithioate [42,43]. These experiments have involved a variety of different ribozymes including the hammerhead [31,32,35,41,44–49], the hairpin [50], the hepatitis δ virus [51–53], the *Neurospora* VS ribozyme [54], the group I intron [39,55–57], the group II intron [58,59], and RNase P [60–63]. In each case, the phosphorothioate modification causes no change in activity at most positions. At certain sites, however, the phosphorothioate linkage leads to reduced reaction rates in the presence of Mg^{2+} alone. For a subset of these modified ribozymes, addition of Mn^{2+} or Cd^{2+} restores activity. The most common interpretation of these data is that an interaction exists between a metal ion and the modified atom.

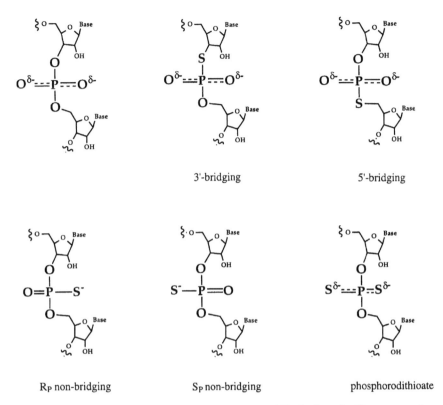

FIG. 1.   Diagram of the sulfur-containing modified phosphodiester species used in rescue experiments involving Mn^{2+} and ribozymes.

Although phosphorothioates are conservative mutations, local structural perturbations might result. Therefore, cautious interpretation of these experiments is important. Several significant physical differences exist between the phosphorothioate and the typical phosphodiester moiety. The first obvious difference is that two of the derivatives contain chiral centers. In most ribozymes, the two isomers exhibit radically different behavior at the key sites. The second difference relates to the charge distribution around the phosphate group. In the case of the parent phosphate, the nonbridging oxygens carry approximately equal charges, calculated to be approximately −0.4 [64]. In the case of the phosphorothioate, this balanced distribution is disrupted.

The bulk of the negative charge resides on the sulfur atom ($\approx$ -0.8), leaving what is formally a P-O double bond to the other nonbridging site [64]. The third difference relates to a geometric issue. Because of the larger radius of sulfur as compared to oxygen, the P-S bond distance is significantly longer than the corresponding P-O bond. This shift is about 0.3 Å [64] , but in certain instances may be sufficient to misalign important structural elements and result in reduced activity.

The widespread usage of phosphorothioate chemistry is due to their ease of incorporation into RNA oligonucleotides. In the case of the R_p phosphorothioate, in vitro transcription in the presence of NTP-α-S yields the desired material [44,65]. This method has the disadvantage, however, of creating a pool of molecules substituted at all or a subset of the positions, depending on the ratio of NTP/NTP-α-S used in the reaction. Site-specific incorporation of the phosphorothioate makes the data more easily interpreted and therefore is preferable to the ensemble experiments. Several sulfurizing reagents compatible with standard phosphoramidite chemistry are available [40,66–69]. This method produces a mixture of the R_p and S_p isomers that then require separation, usually by high-performance liquid chromatography (HPLC) [41]. For short oligos ($n \leqslant 20$), these separations are relatively straightforward, but the separations occasionally prove to be problematic for longer RNAs. The literature on the chemistry of bridging phosphorothioates is much more scarce due in part to the greater difficulty of synthesizing the necessary precursors as well as the lower stability of the final oligonucleotide product.

2.2. Manganese to the Rescue!

As mentioned above, when incorporated at specific positions in either the ribozyme or substrate oligonucleotide, a phosphorothioate linkage can cause a loss of ribozyme activity in the presence of Mg^{2+}. This loss of activity, or thio effect, is the ratio of the rates under standard Mg^{2+} conditions [see Eq. (1) below]. Rescue describes the recovery of that activity upon addition of a second metal ion, usually a softer ion such as Mn^{2+} or Cd^{2+}. It is also generally discussed in terms of the ratio of the rate constants as shown in Eq. (2) where k_{thio}^{Mg} and k_{thio}^{Mn} are the rates of the phosphorothioate modified ribozyme in Mg^{2+} and Mn^{2+}, respectively. This method accounts for the fact that the rate of many ribozymes depends on the identity of the metal ion cofactor used in the reaction ($k_{oxy}^{Mn}/k_{oxy}^{Mg} \neq 1$). Many of the early studies that probed phosphorothioate rescue simply replaced the Mg^{2+} ions in the reaction with Mn^{2+} at the same concentration. Recent studies have shown better rescue when addition of Mn^{2+} or Cd^{2+} occurs in the presence of a high background of Mg^{2+} [46], in which case k_{thio}^{Mn} more formally refers to k_{thio}^{Mn+Mg}. These conditions isolate the effects of the metal at the phosphorothioate substitution by allowing Mg^{2+} to bind at all other positions. It is therefore easier to interpret the results and decreases the likelihood that nonnative conformations affect the experiment.

$$\text{Thio effect} = \frac{k_{native}}{k_{modified}} \tag{1}$$

$$\text{Rescue} = \frac{k_{thio}^{Mn}}{k_{thio}^{Mg}} \tag{2}$$

The basic principle of the rescue experiment relates to hard-soft acid-base theory and the ability of metal ion cofactors to discriminate between oxygen and sulfur ligands. Quantitative application of this theory to metal binding by ATP analogs containing phosphorothioate linkages showed that the modification disfavors Mg^{2+} binding whereas it left Mn^{2+} binding virtually unaffected [70]. Consequently, sulfur incorporation yields a specificity switch. An extension of these studies probed AMP derivatives that are potentially more relevant to the binding modes observed in ribozyme biochemistry [71]. Cd^{2+} shows an even greater specificity shift than Mn^{2+}. The enhanced specificity implies the potential for achieving greater rescue with less thiophilic metal present. The use of Cd^{2+} can be problematic, however, due to its propensity to chelate to the N7 positions of the purine bases and thus induce nonnative conformations. Therefore, Mg^{2+} should always be present during Cd^{2+} rescue experiments.

The most extensive collection of phosphorothioate data is available for the hammerhead ribozyme. These data exemplify the utility of these experiments in understanding the role of the Mg^{2+} metal ions in ribozyme systems. Phosphorothioate substitutions were incorporated at every site around the core of the ribozyme [44,72,73]. Only four of these sites show significant thio effects (Fig. 2). For several positions,

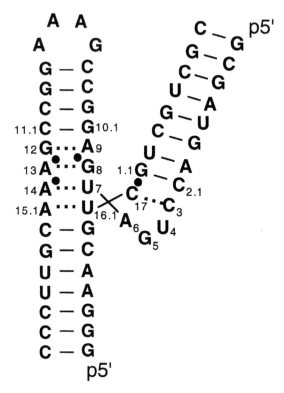

FIG. 2.   Schematic diagram of hammerhead ribozyme 16 (HH16) showing the standard numbering scheme [100]. Cleavage occurs between residues 17 and 1.1. The four sites indicated by the solid circles (p1.1, p9, p13, and p14) show significant thio effects. Note that the phosphate associated with the A13 sits above the base in the schematic diagram, whereas the one associated with A9 lies below it due to the tetraloop that reverses the direction of the phosphodiester backbone.

including the cleavage site, thio effects were reported in several hammerhead constructs (Table 2). The extent of Mn^{2+} or Cd^{2+} rescue has varied greatly leading to a variety of interpretations of these data. Recent experiments using Cd^{2+} in the presence of Mg^{2+} [45,46] showed dramatically improved rescue relative to earlier studies using Mn^{2+} alone [32,41,44]. Under these conditions, significantly lower concentrations of Cd^{2+} achieved complete rescue and thus the second ion did not affect the rate of the unmodified ribozyme.

TABLE 2

Hammerhead Ribozyme Phosphorothioate Effects

Hammerhead	Modification site	Rescue metal	R$_P$ isomer		S$_P$ isomer		Ref.
			Thio effect	Rescue	Thio effect	Rescue	
HH8	p1.1	Cd^{2+}/Mg^{2+}	18,000	2000	0.9	1	[46]
HH16	p9	Cd^{2+}/Mg^{2+}	500	8500	1.1	5	[45]
HHα1	p9	Cd^{2+}/Mg^{2+}	13	150	0.7	n.d.	[73]
HHα1	p13	Cd^{2+}/Mg^{2+}	1600[a]	1	a	1	[73]
HHα1	p14	Cd^{2+}/Mg^{2+}	10,000[a]	1	a	1	[73]
HH10	p1.1	Mn^{2+}	50	~12	n.d.	n.d.	[28]
R37	p1.1	Mn^{2+}	33	~4	2	n.d.	[41]
CL-2,4	p1.1	n.d.	55	n.d.	0.4	n.d.	[49]
R32	p1.1	Mn^{2+}	540	5.8	29	14	[31,32]
HH3	p1.1	Mn^{2+}	1000	530	1	1	[72]
R34	p1.1	Hg^{2+}/Mg^{2+}	25	9	2	1	[99]

[a]Isomeric separation was not possible, so the experiment looked at the R$_P$/S$_P$ mixture in a biphasic kinetic reaction. The fast phase presumably corresponds to the S$_P$ isomer and the slow phase the R$_P$ material. n.d. = not determined.

2.3.   Is Recruitment a Serious Problem?

Recruitment refers to the idea that incorporation of the modified phosphodiester linkage into a ribozyme creates a specific metal binding site
where one did not exist in the original molecule. This argument is
difficult to refute. The strongest evidence against recruitment comes
from the structural experiments on the hammerhead described below.
In several cases, the sites predicted to involve metal-phosphate interactions from the biochemical studies appeared independently as metal
binding sites in structural studies. Furthermore, hammerhead ribozymes that contain a phosphorodithioate linkage at the cleavage site
are active in Mg^{2+} alone [74]. This result contradicts the axiom that if
one sulfur atom causes recruitment, the presence of two sulfurs should
enhance the effect.

3.   USE OF Mn^{2+} IN CRYSTALLOGRAPHIC
EXPERIMENTS TO FIND Mg^{2+} BINDING SITES

3.1.   Why Is Mn^{2+} Used as a Substitute for Mg^{2+}?

Hydrated Mg^{2+} ions are difficult to detect unambiguously in X-ray
crystallographic studies of RNA molecules. The origin of this problem
derives from Mg^{2+} ions having just 10 electrons, 2 more than the water
molecules that typically make up 30–70% of the crystal lattice. X-ray
diffraction experiments rely on the electron cloud for detection, so this
small difference complicates the assignment. A further difficulty is that
the buffer solutions often also contain sodium or potassium. To build an
accurate model, one must be able to distinguish these ions from one
another. Additional ambiguity results from disorder of the ions within a
binding site, causing the density to appear more diffuse and sometimes
disappear entirely from the electron density map.
     When the structure of tRNA was originally determined, several
excellent criteria assisted in the identification of the bound metal ions
[75,76]. These criteria included angular and distance constraints on the
coordination geometry of the ion. The main idea was that Mg^{2+} should
appear with approximately octahedral geometry and contain seven

distinct electron density features (i.e., the Mg^{2+} ion and the six water molecules bound in the inner coordination shell). An inner-sphere contact to a ligand provided by the RNA could substitute for any individual water molecule. The distance of the typical metal-water bond length distinguished sodium and magnesium from one another, but this feature is less reliable at the modest resolutions of most of the current RNA structures. Further complication of these bond length comparisons results from the possibility that one or more of the water ligands might be deprotonated and therefore exhibit a different geometric constraint. These criteria for defining metal binding sites in RNA crystal structures remain the most rigorous that have been used.

One extremely useful method for identifying metal binding sites that circumvents the requirement for high-resolution data relies on the substitution of Mn^{2+} for Mg^{2+}. This substitution is advantageous for two reasons. First, the ion has significantly more electron density than Mg^{2+}, making it more easily observed in the map. Second, Mn^{2+} has an absorption edge at 1.8961 Å, a wavelength that is easily accessible at many synchrotron facilities. This physical property allows the collection of anomalous scattering data that assist in determining the location of the Mn^{2+} ion(s) [77].

3.2. Will Mn^{2+} Bind at the Same Site(s) as Mg^{2+}?

One of the primary questions asked during Mn^{2+} substitution experiments is whether it accurately identifies Mg^{2+} binding sites. In the hammerhead ribozyme crystal structures, it was possible to identify both Mn^{2+} and Mg^{2+} binding sites [78–80]. The Mn^{2+} data confirmed the locations and the assignments of peaks previously identified as potential Mg^{2+} ions. Overlaying the structural models (Fig. 3A) shows that three of the Mn^{2+} electron density peaks colocalize with Mg^{2+} binding sites within 3 Å. In a fourth site the Mn^{2+} and Mg^{2+} ions are about 7 Å apart but bind to the same residues of the RNA.

It is instructive to focus on two of the actual detailed sites because it clearly identifies the limitations of the experiment. The site near to G5 shows that Mg^{2+} and Mn^{2+} both bind, but do so approximately 2 Å apart (Fig. 3B). These ions bind adjacent to the Watson-Crick face of the guanine base. The modest resolution limits precluded observation of

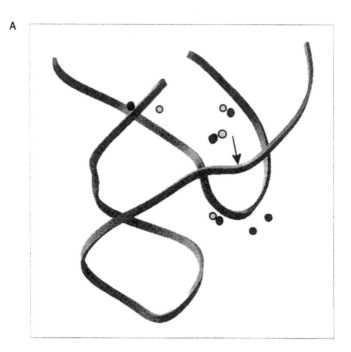

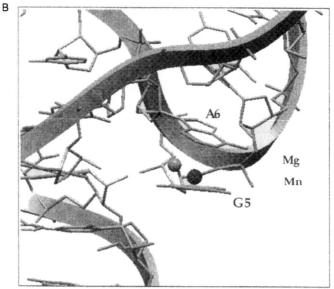

FIG. 3. (A) Superposition of the crystallographically observed Mg^{2+} (light gray) and Mn^{2+} (dark gray) binding sites on the ribbon diagram of the hammerhead ribozyme crystal structure. The cleavage site is marked by the arrow. (B) Expanded view of the G5 metal binding site. (Adapted with permission from [24]).

the water ligands, but it would be impossible to simultaneously bind Mn^{2+} and Mg^{2+} in their respective positions. Consequently, these ions bind to a single site. The different binding modes of Mn^{2+} and Mg^{2+} are apparent at the p9 site of the hammerhead where the ions bind ≈6.8 Å apart. This movement reflects a shift from an inner-sphere binding mode in the case of the Mn^{2+} ion to an outer-sphere interaction for Mg^{2+}. The Mn^{2+} ion binds to the pro-S_P phosphate oxygen of p9 and the N7 of G10.1. The related Mg^{2+} ion interacts via an outer-sphere binding mode to the pro-R_P oxygen of the same phosphate and to the keto oxygen (O6) of that guanine. The pro-R_P oxygen at p9, was originally identified through phosphorothioate experiments as being a metal binding site [44] and the crystallographic studies confirmed the result. The shift in the binding sites between Mg^{2+} and Mn^{2+} at p9 is not particularly surprising considering the ligand preferences of the ions. The N7 position of adenine and guanine bases readily binds a variety of metal ions including Mn^{2+}. It is unclear at present why certain sites are not observed in both the Mg^{2+} and Mn^{2+} experiments. It is possible that the extra Mn^{2+} sites are positions of greater disorder for the Mg^{2+} and thus the residual electron density simply does not meet the criteria required for the assignment.

Currently, most metal binding sites observed in RNA crystal structures are at lower resolution than their protein counterparts. In most cases, the water molecules that comprise part or all of the ligand sphere are implicit rather than directly observed. The availability of high-resolution RNA structures will eventually alleviate part of this problem, but ambiguities will likely remain. Many Mg^{2+}-RNA interactions have lower affinities than the equivalent protein sites. This weaker binding translates to structural disorder and therefore difficulty associating the electron density peaks with the ion and its coordinated water molecules. Therefore, other methods must complement the crystallographic studies to obtain detailed pictures of the coordination environment of these ions.

4. USE OF Mn²⁺ IN MAGNETIC RESONANCE EXPERIMENTS TO STUDY METAL BINDING SITES

Magnetic resonance techniques provide a powerful set of methods for probing metal binding sites on ribozymes. The majority of the published studies have used NMR [81-83], but recently a number of EPR experiments have been reported as well [84]. Clearly, future work will use more of these methods. These two sets of techniques complement each other since they fundamentally probe the metal binding site from opposite directions and have different experimental limitations. In both cases, substitution of Mn^{2+} for the native Mg^{2+} in the binding site is advantageous.

Typical EPR titration cannot provide direct information regarding the location of the metal binding sites on the RNA molecule. Instead, it is a powerful method for measuring binding affinities, analogous to one used to study Mn^{2+} binding to proteins [85]. The experiment works because free Mn^{2+} provides the typical six-line Mn^{2+} signal. Upon binding to the RNA, the room temperature signal of the bound Mn^{2+} broadens beyond our ability to observe it. An approximation of the number of metal binding sites and their average affinities results from the integration of the signals and subsequent fitting of the titration profile. This method generally assumes noncooperative behavior although cooperative models are available.

In the case of the hammerhead ribozyme [84], EPR studies in the presence of 100 mM NaCl found 3–4 Mn^{2+} ions bind with an affinity of approximately 4 μM. An additional 5 ions bind with an affinity of 400–500 μM. In the presence of 1 M NaCl, all but one of these Mn^{2+} ions is displaced. These results imply the presence of one highly specific binding site with the other sites being only modestly selective. The authors speculated that the high-specificity site might be either that near G5 or p9, but left the localization of the site to future studies. The authors compared the activity profile of the hammerhead in Mn^{2+} with their binding results (Fig. 4). The overlay clearly shows that the 4 tightly bound Mn^{2+} ions are insufficient to generate the active ribozyme and that at least one of the more weakly bound ions participates in the formation of the transition state. It is therefore difficult to understand the role of these tight Mn^{2+} ions. This result is likely to remain a mystery until the locations of the ions are known.

NMR experiments approach the issue of metal binding from the opposite perspective of the EPR experiments just discussed. Instead of viewing the Mn^{2+} ion itself, these experiments rely on the effect of the paramagnetic ion on the RNA. When Mn^{2+} binding occurs, nearby resonances become broadened due to an increase in the nuclear spin

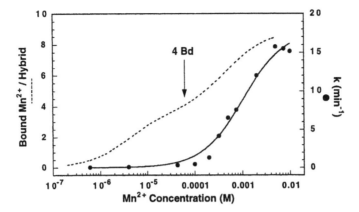

FIG. 4. Results of the Mn^{2+} EPR titration with the hammerhead ribozyme showing the binding isotherm (dashed line) superimposed on an activity profile (solid line). (Reprinted with permission from [84].)

relaxation rate. The increase in relaxation rate is proportional to r^{-6}, where r is the distance between the Mn^{2+} ion and the observed nucleus, as well as the occupancy of the site [86]. When high concentrations of Mn^{2+} ions are present in RNA samples, usually all resonances broaden due to nonspecific binding. Site-specific binding, on the other hand, selectively broadens those resonances in the vicinity of the paramagnetic ion. The size limitations on typical solution NMR studies make it impossible to study most intact ribozymes, although two small catalytic RNAs were probed in this manner [83,87]. For larger systems, it is common to characterize small fragments with the idea that these domains fold into independent units [81]. This method works well for sites created by local interactions but will be insensitive to sites created by the convergence of disparate elements from the RNA structure.

G·U wobble base pairs are present in the active sites of several ribozymes [88–90] and are also recognition elements in certain tRNAs [91–93]. The unique functionalities presented into the major (G-O6, G-N7, and U-O4) and minor (G-N2) grooves by this noncanonical interaction help to form the recognition sites. The distortions around the wobble base also locally increase the calculated electrostatic potential of the RNA helix [94], stabilizing metal binding and increasing the overall affinity. NMR studies have been instrumental in the develop-

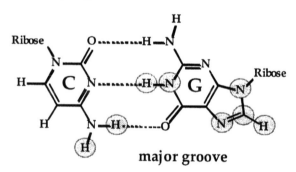

FIG. 5.   Binding of the Mn²⁺ ions occurs near G•U, AU and CG base pairs in the P1 helix. Gray shaded nuclei are affected by the paramagnetic ion upon binding. The localization of the effects indicates that the ion binds within the major groove of the RNA helix. (Modified with permission from [81].)

ment of the concept that these wobble sites may act through the generation of a specific metal ion interaction [81,82,95,96].

The Mn^{2+} binding site best characterized by NMR comes from a
fragment of the group I self-splicing introns containing a conserved G•U
at the splice site of these ribozymes [81]. The results of this study
showed the presence of two independent Mn^{2+} binding sites, one of
which is next to the G•U base pair. By comparing the broadening pattern of the nearby resonances, the authors were able to establish that
Mn^{2+} binds in the major groove at this site (Fig. 5). Whereas the
paramagnetic NMR experiment located the binding site, it could not
directly address the question of the ligands that bind the metal ion. A
helix containing tandem G•U pairs has also been studied by NMR, but
$[Co(NH_3)_6]^{3+}$ was used as the $Mg(H_2O)_6^{2+}$ surrogate [96]. In this case,
the metal-RNA interaction was through N7 and O6 positions of the
guanines. The O4 keto oxygen of uridine is also in the major groove, but
it does not appear to participate in the binding in this case.

The major obstacle in Mn^{2+} NMR experiments can be the limited
specificity of the sites. NMR studies of Mn^{2+} binding to the hammerhead ribozyme [87] found that substoichiometric concentrations of
Mn^{2+} broadened all ³¹P NMR signals rather than just those around a
specific site. A single resonance broadened first, but it was impossible to
measure the binding affinity by using this methodology. Incorporation
of ¹⁷O into the nonbridging positions of the phosphate allowed the
assignment of this resonance as that of A_{13}. The same resonance
broadens and shifts upfield upon addition of Mg^{2+}. From titrations and
line shape analysis, the Mg^{2+} affinity was measured at 550–570 μM
[87]. Based on the NMR experiments, this is the first metal binding site
populated, but the affinity differs significantly from those determined
by EPR [84]. The source of this discrepancy is currently unknown but
may relate to the substitution of Mn^{2+} for Mg^{2+}.

5. CONCLUSIONS

Mn^{2+} substitution for Mg^{2+} ions in ribozyme systems has provided
significant insights into the chemistry of these novel catalysts. The
ability to make this substitution is predicated on the fact that Mn^{2+} ions

support ribozyme catalysis in most systems. Moreover, Mn^{2+} confers the ability to probe for specific metal-phosphate interactions through phosphorothioate rescue experiments. The total substitution of Mn^{2+} for Mg^{2+} used in many of these experiments is in hindsight probably a poor approach due to the potential to induce alternate conformations of the RNA. Instead, the doped addition of Mn^{2+} in a background of Mg^{2+} should be considered a better methodology.

The paramagnetic and anomalous scattering properties of the Mn^{2+} ion have been utilized in a relatively small set of cases aimed at identifying the location and affinities of Mg^{2+} binding sites. The continued use of these methods will further expand our understanding of metal-RNA interactions. In localization studies, however, there will always be a concern that the substitution has shifted the observed binding mode. The method allows observation of the low-resolution site, but the specifics of the Mg^{2+} binding geometry must be inferred cautiously from Mn^{2+} data. Furthermore, the apparent affinities for Mn^{2+} and Mg^{2+} measured by biophysical approaches may have significant systematic differences as evidenced by the recent NMR and EPR experiments. Finally, it should be recognized that Mn^{2+} substitution for Mg^{2+} is only one of the possible replacements that provides a spectroscopic handle for the observation of metal binding to the RNA. The greatest understanding of these interactions will result from application of the broad array of tools available to probe these sites.

ACKNOWLEDGMENTS

This work has been supported in part by a grant from the Colorado RNA Center. I would also like to thank E. Jabri and K. Kossen for their comments on this manuscript prior to publication and V. DeRose and A. Pardi for providing preprints of their work.

ABBREVIATIONS

AMP	adenosine 5'-monophosphate
ATP	adenosine 5'-triphosphate

EPR	electron paramagnetic resonance
HPLC	high-performance liquid chromatography
RNA	ribonucleic acid
NMR	nuclear magnetic resonance
nt	nucleotide
NTP	nucleotide 5'-triphosphate
RNase P	ribonuclease P
tRNA	transfer ribonucleic acid
VS ribozyme	Varkud satellite ribozyme

REFERENCES

1. M. E. Harris, D. N. Frank, and N. R. Pace, in *RNA Structure and Function* (R. W. Simons and M. Grunberg-Manago, eds.), Cold Spring Harbor Laboratory Press, Cold Spring Harbor, NY, 1998, pp. 309–337.

2. S. Altman, M. F. B. Baer, H. Gold, C. Guerrier-Takada, L. A. Kirsebom, N. Lumelsky, and K. Peck, *Gene*, *82*, 63–64 (1989).

3. O. Uhlenbeck, *Nature*, *328*, 596–600 (1987).

4. S. Kazakov and S. Altman, *Proc. Natl. Acad. Sci. USA*, *89*, 7939–7943 (1992).

5. R. G. Kuimelis and L. W. McLaughlin, *Chem. Rev.*, *98*, 1027–1044 (1998).

6. R. Gesteland, T. Cech, and J. Atkins, eds., *The RNA World*. Cold Spring Harbor Laboratory, Cold Spring Harbor, NY, 1998.

7. R. Simons and M. Grunberg-Manago, eds., *RNA Structure and Function*. Cold Spring Harbor Laboratories, Cold Spring Harbor, NY, 1998.

8. F. Eckstein and D. M. J. Lilley, eds., *Catalytic RNA*, Vol. 10. Springer-Verlag, Berlin, 1997.

9. J. H. Cate, R. L. Hanna, and J. A. Doudna, *Nature Struct. Biol.*, *4*, 553–558 (1997).

10. R. J. Cain and G. D. Glick, *Biochemistry*, *37*, 1456–1464 (1998).

11. B. Sclavi, M. Sullivan, M. R. Chance, M. Brenowitz, and S. A. Woodson, *Science*, *279*, 1940–1943 (1998).

12. P. P. Zarrinkar and J. R. Williamson, *Science*, *263*, 918–924 (1994).

13. J. A. Doudna and E. A. Doherty, *Fold. Des.*, *2*, R65–R70 (1997).

14. T. Pan and T. R. Sosnick, *Nature Struct. Biol.*, *4*, 931– 938 (1997).

15. M. Yarus, *FASEB J.*, *7*, 31–39 (1993).

16. A. M. Pyle, in *Interactions of Metal Ions with Nucleotides, Nucleic Acids, and Their Constituents, Metal Ions in Biological Systems*, *Vol. 32* (A. Sigel and H. Sigel, eds.), Marcel Dekker, New York, 1996, pp. 479–520.

17. S. Nesbitt, L. A. Hegg, and M. J. Fedor, *Chem. Biol.*, *4*, 619–630 (1997).

18. A. Hampel and J. A. Cowan, *Chem. Biol.*, *4*, 513–517 (1997).

19. K. J. Young, F. Gill, and J. A. Grasby, *Nucl. Acids Res.*, *25*, 3760–3766 (1997).

20. J. B. Murray, A. A. Seyhan, N. G. Walter, J. M. Burke, and W. G. Scott, *Chem. Biol.*, *5*, 587–595 (1998).

21. C. F. Anderson and M. T. Record, Jr., *Annu. Rev. Phys. Chem.*, *46*, 657–700 (1995).

22. M. T. Record, Jr., T. M. Lohman, and P. de Haseth, *J. Mol. Biol.*, *107*, 145–158 (1976).

23. J. A. Cowan, *Chem. Rev.*, *98*, 1067–1088 (1998).

24. A. L. Feig and O. C. Uhlenbeck, in *The RNA World* (R. Gesteland, T. Cech, and J. Atkins, eds.), Cold Spring Harbor Laboratory, Cold Spring Harbor, NY, 1998.

25. A. L. Feig, M. Panek, W. D. Horrocks, Jr., and O. C. Uhlenbeck, *Chem. Biol.*, in press (1999).

26. S. Basu, R. P. Rambo, J. Strauss-Soukup, J. H. Cate, A. R. Ferre-D'Amare, S. A. Strobel, and J. A. Doudna, *Nature Struct. Biol.*, *5*, 986–992 (1998).

27. D. E. Draper and V. K. Misra, *Nature Struct. Biol.*, *5*, 927–930 (1998).

28. S. C. Dahm and O. C. Uhlenbeck, *Biochemistry*, *30*, 9464–9469 (1991).

29. C. A. Grosshans and T. R. Cech, *Biochemistry*, *28*, 6888–6894 (1989).

30. Y.-A. Suh, P. K. R. Kumar, K. Taira, and S. Nishikawa, *Nucl. Acids Res.*, *21*, 3277–3280 (1993).

31. D.-M. Zhou, Q.-C. He, J.-M. Zhou, and K. Taira, *FEBS Lett.*, *431*, 154–160 (1998).

32. D.-M. Zhou, P. K. R. Kumar, L.-H. Zhang, and K. Taira, *J. Am. Chem. Soc.*, *118*, 8969–8970 (1996).

33. D.-M. Zhou and K. Taira, *Chem. Rev.*, *98*, 991–1026 (1998).

34. D. M. Zhou, L. H. Zhang, and K. Taira, *Proc. Natl. Acad. Sci. USA*, *94*, 14343–14348 (1997).

35. D.-M. Zhou, N. Usman, F. E. Wincott, J. Matulic-Adamic, M. Orita, L.-H. Zhang, M. Komiyama, P. K. R. Kumar, and K. Taira, *J. Am. Chem. Soc.*, *118*, 5862–5866 (1996).

36. S. C. Dahm, W. B. Derrick, and O. C. Uhlenbeck, *Biochemistry*, *32*, 13040–13045 (1993).

37. S. Sun, A. Yoshida, and J. A. Piccirilli, *RNA*, *3*, 1352–1363 (1997).

38. L. B. Weinstein, D. J. Earnshaw, R. Cosstick, and T. R. Cech, *J. Am. Chem. Soc.*, *118*, 10341–10350 (1996).

39. L. B. Weinstein, B. C. N. M. Jones, R. Cosstick, and T. R. Cech, *Nature*, *388*, 805–808 (1997).

40. F. Eckstein, *Oligonucleotides and Analogues: A Practical Approach* (D. Rickwood and B. D. Hames, eds.), The Practical Approach Series, IRL, Oxford, 1991.

41. G. Slim and M. J. Gait, *Nucl. Acids Res.*, *19*, 1183–1188 (1991).

42. P. H. Seeberger, P. N. Jorgensen, D. M. Bankaitis-Davis, G. Beaton, and M. H. Caruthers, *J. Am. Chem. Soc.*, *118*, 9562–9566 (1996).

43. W. Derrick and O. C. Uhlenbeck, in preparation (1999).

44. D. E. Ruffner and O. C. Uhlenbeck, *Nucl. Acids Res.*, *18*, 6025–6029 (1990).

45. A. Peracchi, L. Beigelman, E. C. Scott, O. C. Uhlenbeck, and D. Herschlag, *J. Biol. Chem.*, *272*, 26822–26826 (1997).

46. E. C. Scott and O. C. Uhlenbeck, *Nucl. Acids Res.*, *27*, 479–484 (1999).

47. O. Heidenreich, F. Benseler, A. Fahrenholz, and F. Eckstein, *J. Biol. Chem.*, *269*, 2131–2138 (1994).

48. R. G. Kuimelis and L. W. McLaughlin, *J. Am. Chem. Soc.*, *117*, 11019–11020 (1995).

49. M. Koizumi and E. Ohtsuka, *Biochemistry*, *30*, 5145–5150 (1991).

50. B. M. Chowrira and J. M. Burke, *Nucl. Acids Res.*, *20*, 2835–2840 (1992).

51. Y.-H. Jeoung, P. K. R. Kumar, Y.-A. Suh, K. Taira, and S. Nishikawa, *Nucl. Acids Res.*, *22*, 3722–3727 (1994).

52. N. S. Prabhu, G. Dinter-Gottlieb, and P. A. Gottlieb, *Nucl. Acids Res.*, *25*, 5119–5124 (1997).

53. H. Fauzi, J. Kawakami, F. Nishikawa, and S. Nishikawa, *Nucl. Acids Res.*, *25*, 3124–3130 (1997).

54. V. D. Sood, T. L. Beattie, and R. A. Collins, *J. Mol. Biol.*, *282*, 741–750 (1998).

55. R. B. Waring, *Nucl. Acids Res.*, *17*, 10281–10293 (1989).

56. J. A. Piccirilli, J. S. Vyle, M. H. Caruthers, and T. R. Cech, *Nature*, *361*, 85–88 (1993).

57. E. L. Christian and M. Yarus, *Biochemistry*, *32*, 4475–4480 (1993).

58. G. Chanfreau and A. Jacquier, *Science*, *266*, 1383–1387 (1994).

59. M. Podar, P. S. Perlman, and R. A. Padgett, *Mol. Cell. Biol.*, *15*, 4466–4478 (1995).

60. F. Conrad, A. Hanne, R. K. Gaur, and G. Krupp, *Nucl. Acids Res.*, *23*, 1845–1853 (1995).

61. M. E. Harris and N. R. Pace, *RNA*, *1*, 210–218 (1995).

62. J. M. Warnecke, J. P. Furste, W. D. Hardt, V. A. Erdmann, and R. K. Hartmann, *Proc. Natl. Acad. Sci. USA*, *93*, 8924–8928 (1996).

63. W. D. Hardt, J. M. Warnecke, V. A. Erdmann, and R. K. Hartmann, *EMBO J.*, *14*, 2935–2944 (1995).

64. P. A. Frey and R. D. Sammons, *Science*, *228*, 541–545 (1985).

65. F. Eckstein and G. Gish, *Trends in Biol. Sci.*, *14*, 97–100 (1989).

66. R. P. Iyer, L. R. Phillips, W. Egan, J. B. Regan, and S. L. Beaucage, *J. Org. Chem.*, *55*, 4693–4699 (1990).

67. M. Y.-X. Ma, J. C. Dignam, G. W. Fong, L. Li, S. H. Gray, B. Jacob-Samuel, and S. T. George, *Nucl. Acids Res.*, *25*, 3590–3593 (1997).

68. Q. Xu, K. Musier-Forsyth, R. P. Hammer, and G. Barany, *Nucl. Acids Res.*, *24*, 1602–1607 (1996).

69. Q. Xu, G. Barany, R. P. Hammer, and K. Musier-Forsyth, *Nucl. Acids Res.*, *24*, 3643–3644 (1996).

70. V. L. Pecoraro, J. D. Hermes, and W. W. Cleland, *Biochemistry*, *23*, 5262–5271 (1984).

71. R. K. O. Sigel, B. Song, and H. Sigel, *J. Am. Chem. Soc.*, *119*, 744–755 (1997).

72. R. Knöll, R. Bald, and J. P. Fürste, *RNA*, *3*, 132–140 (1997).

73. E. C. Scott, Ph.D. thesis, University of Colorado (1997).

74. W. Derrick, Ph.D. thesis, University of Colorado (1999).

75. A. Jack, J. E. Ladner, D. Rhodes, R. S. Brown, and A. Klug, *J. Mol. Biol.*, *111*, 315–328 (1977).

76. S. R. Holbrook, J. L. Sussman, R. W. Warrant, G. M. Church, and S.-H. Kim, *Nucl. Acids Res.*, *4*, 2811–2820 (1977).

77. J. P. Glusker and K. N. Trueblood, *Crystal Structure Analysis*. Oxford University Press, New York, 1985.

78. W. G. Scott, J. T. Finch, and A. Klug, *Cell*, *81*, 991–1002 (1995).

79. H. W. Pley, K. M. Flaherty, and D. B. McKay, *Nature*, *372*, 68–74 (1994).

80. W. G. Scott, J. B. Murray, J. R. P. Arnold, B. L. Stoddard, and A. Klug, *Science*, *274*, 2065–2069 (1996).

81. F. H. T. Allain and G. Varani, *Nucl. Acids Res.*, *23*, 341–350 (1995).

82. G. Ott, L. Arnold, and S. Limmer, *Nucl. Acids Res.*, *21*, 5859–5864 (1993).

83. M. Vogtherr and S. Limmer, *FEBS Lett.*, *433*, 301–306 (1998).

84. T. E. Horton, D. R. Clardy, and V. J. DeRose, *Biochemistry*, *37*, 18094–18101 (1998).

85. A.-Y. M. Woody, S. S. Eaton, P. A. Osumi-Davis, and R. W. Woody, *Biochemistry*, *35*, 144–152 (1996).

86. I. Bertini and C. Luchinat, *NMR of Paramagnetic Molecules in Biological Systems* (A. B. P. Lever and H. B. Gray, eds.), Physical Bioinorganic Chemistry Series, Benjamin/Cummings, Menlo Park, 1986, Vol. 3.

87. M. R. Hansen, J.-P. Simorre, P. Hanson, V. Mokler, L. Bellon, L. Beigelman, and A. Pardi, *RNA* (submitted for publication) (1999).

88. B. B. Konforti, D. L. Abramovitz, C. M. Duarte, A. Karpeisky, L. Beigelman, and A. M. Pyle, *Mol. Cell*, *1*, 433–441 (1998).

89. A. T. Perrotta and M. D. Been, *Nucl. Acids Res.*, *24*, 1314–1421 (1996).

90. D. S. Knitt, G. J. Narlikar, and D. Herschlag, *Biochemistry*, *33*, 13864–13879 (1994).

91. W. H. McClain and K. Foss, *Science*, *240*, 793–796 (1988).

92. Y.-M. Hou and P. R. Schimmel, *Nature*, *333*, 140–145 (1988).

93. K. Musier-Forsyth, N. Usman, S. Scaringe, J. A. Doudna, R. Green, and P. Schimmel, *Science*, *253*, 784–786 (1991).

94. J. H. Cate and J. A. Doudna, *Structure*, *4*, 1221–1229 (1996).

95. S. Limmer, H.-P. Hofmann, G. Ott, and M. Sprinzl, *Proc. Natl. Acad. Sci. USA*, *90*, 6199–6202 (1993).

96. J. S. Kieft and I. Tinoco, Jr., *Structure*, *5*, 713–721 (1997).

97. D. T. Richens, *The Chemistry of Aqua Ions*, John Wiley and Sons, New York, 1997.

98. R. G. Pearson, *Inorg. Chem.*, *278*, 734–740 (1988).

99. L. A. Cunningham, J. Li, and Y. Lu, *J. Am. Chem. Soc.*, *20*, 4518–4519 (1997).

100. K. J. Hertel, A. Pardi, O. C. Uhlenbeck, M. Koizumi, E. Ohtsuka, S. Uesugi, R. Cedergren, F. Eckstein, W. L. Gerlach, R. Hodgson, and R. H. Symons, *Nucl. Acids Res.*, *20*, 3252 (1992).

7

Mn²⁺ as a Probe of Divalent Metal Ion Binding and Function in Enzymes and Other Proteins

George H. Reed and Russell R. Poyner

Institute for Enzyme Research and Department of Biochemistry, University of Wisconsin, Madison, WI 53705, USA

1. INTRODUCTION AND OVERVIEW

Advances in structural and mechanistic work on proteins has provided insight into the roles of metal ions in the diverse biological functions of proteins [1]. Structural issues in this broad category of metal ion-protein complexes have been approached successfully by methods such as X-ray crystallography. Spectroscopic approaches used in modern inorganic chemistry [2] (e.g., NMR, EPR, CD, MCD, EXAFS, IR, and resonance Raman), however, continue to provide a means to obtain information regarding structure and function of metal ion-protein complexes, albeit on a less global scale than that provided by crystallographic methods. These spectroscopic methods also provide an independent way for corroboration of results from other structural investigations. The spectroscopic approaches have been aided by advances in instrumentation and methodologies that allow more detailed interpretations—in many cases at atomic resolution.

The natural functions of various forms of manganese are discussed in several chapters of this volume. Many aspects of Mn in biological complexes have been covered in excellent reviews and monographs [3–11]. A substantial fraction of metal ion-dependent proteins normally function with colorless, diamagnetic metal ions such as Mg^{2+} or Ca^{2+} or Zn^{2+}. Replacement of these spectroscopically silent metal ions with ions having more favorable spectroscopic properties is a well-established strategy for biophysical research. The purpose of this chapter is to survey applications of divalent manganese primarily as a surrogate metal ion in spectroscopic studies of the roles of divalent cations in the biological functions of enzymes and other proteins.

2. SURVEY OF COORDINATION PROPERTIES AND TENDENCIES

The most stable state of Mn in aqueous media is the divalent cation, and higher oxidation states of Mn are typically strong oxidants. The redox potential of the Mn^{3+}/Mn^{2+} couple is ~1.5 V. Solutions of Mn^{2+} lacking some complexing agent are susceptible to air oxidation at neutral and higher pH values. Mn^{3+} may be further oxidized to Mn^{4+} or may undergo disproportionation to a Mn(II)-Mn(IV) species. Oxidation of Mn^{2+} under these conditions is apparent from the development of a brown precipitate.

The Mn^{3+} is the resting state of the Mn-metallo enzyme, superoxide disumutase (SOD) from bacteria and mitochondria [12]. The means by which the protein stabilizes the 3+ oxidation state has been of considerable interest. The X-ray structure of the enzyme from *Thermus thermophilus* shows that the Mn center has a five-coordinate, trigonal bipyramidal geometry [13]. Recent results from site directed mutagenesis of human MnSOD provide some interesting information on the role of nearby residues in stabilizing the Mn^{3+} state in the wild-type enzyme [14]. Higher oxidation states of Mn are important in several of the natural biological functions of the element; however, the focus of this chapter is on the manganous ion.

Mn^{2+} is a hard Lewis acid—a property shared by the more common biological cofactor, Mg^{2+}. Both of these hard Lewis acids prefer ligands in the hard Lewis base category (e.g., ligands with O or N donor moieties). There are, however, examples of Mn^{2+} coordination to softer Lewis bases (e.g., S) [15–17]. A further example of Mn^{2+} binding to a soft Lewis base, S^{2-}, is evidenced by formation of the insoluble sulfide, MnS. Despite some differences in ionic radii (Mn^{2+} $r = 0.97$ Å; Mg^{2+} $r = 0.86$ Å) and electrophilic properties, the two ions have similar coordination chemistry with respect to preferred coordination geometry, stability of their complexes with complexing agents, and ligand exchange rates. The similarities in coordination properties in vitro do not, however, carry over to living organisms which distinguish between Mg^{2+} and Mn^{2+} efficiently [4]. The mechanisms by which the ions are distinguished by biological systems is still considered somewhat enigmatic. It has been suggested that the higher oxidation states available to Mn^{2+} provide a means for biological selectivity [4,18]. However, selectivity in binding based on ionic radius of the metal ion [19–21] is perhaps an equally plausible means by which carriers distinguish between Mg^{2+} and Mn^{2+}.

Mn^{2+} is more electrophilic than Mg^{2+} as evidenced by the pK_a values of water bound to the ions, 10.1 and 11.4, respectively. Stabilities of Mn^{2+} complexes with many complexing agents [22], especially biologically relevant ligands containing phosphate and carboxylate functional groups, are typically slightly greater than those of Mg^{2+}. The greater stabilities of Mn^{2+} complexes relative to those of Mg^{2+} probably contribute to the slightly lower turnover numbers often observed for enzymes assayed with Mn^{2+} in place of Mg^{2+}. The relatively common occurrence of rate-limiting product release in enzymic catalysis [23] reinforces the conjecture that product release is likely slower in complexes of Mn^{2+}. In aqueous media, six is the most common coordination number of both ions. Thus, in most properties that can be construed as important for maintenance of structure and function, Mn^{2+} is perhaps the least perturbing substitute for Mg^{2+} within the family of divalent cations.

As indicated earlier, a major reason to employ Mn^{2+} as a surrogate cation in studies of enzymes and other proteins is to take advantage of its spectroscopic properties. The ground state electronic configuration of Mn^{2+} is $3d^5$, and, with few exceptions, the ion exhibits a high-spin, S = 5/2 ground state. In the gas phase the designation of this electronic configuration is ^6S, which indicates a spherical distribution of charge around the ion, and a spin multiplicity [S(S + 1)] of six. The spherical distribution of 3d electrons is distorted in condensed phases wherein ligands attach at specific points. In most cases, however, the S-state properties of the free ion are largely preserved in condensed phases. The spin and parity forbidden $3d \rightarrow 3d$ electronic transitions have low extinction coefficients ($\varepsilon < 0.05$ M^{-1} cm^{-1}) [24], and dilute solutions of manganous complexes are therefore virtually colorless. The electron paramagnetic resonance absorption from the five unpaired electrons, however, provides a means to probe the environment of the ion in macromolecular complexes such as occur in enzymes and other proteins.

3.   CW EPR PROPERTIES

3.1.   Description and Analysis of Spectra

A distinguishing feature of S-state ions such as Mn^{2+} is that of long-lived electron spin states which yield sharp EPR signals which are readily observable at room temperature. Thus, for most complexes of Mn^{2+}, EPR spectra can be obtained from samples in the solution phase. Despite the relative ease of recording EPR spectra of Mn^{2+}, analysis of the spectra is somewhat more complicated than for ions that have fewer unpaired electrons. The six possible orientations of the Mn^{2+} electron spin ($M_s = \pm 5/2, \pm 3/2, \pm 1/2$) in an external magnetic field yield five fully allowed ($\Delta M_s = \pm 1$) EPR fine structure transitions. The S = 5/2 spin property of Mn^{2+} is further complicated by the I = 5/2 nuclear spin of ^{55}Mn (100% natural abundance). The hyperfine interaction between the electron spin and the nuclear spin splits all of the energy levels into six sublevels corresponding to the six possible orientations of the ^{55}Mn nuclear spin. This sextet splitting is the EPR signature of mononuclear Mn sites. The combination of the electron spin of 5/2 and the nuclear spin of 5/2 leads to 36 energy levels and 30 fully allowed ($\Delta M_s = \pm 1$, $\Delta m_I = 0$) transitions. Resolution of all 30 allowed transitions is realized in some situations—most notably in studies of Mn^{2+}-doped single crystals. In unordered solids and in macromolecular complexes in solution, the strong orientation dependence of all but the central ($M_s\ -1/2 \to 1/2$) fine structure transition renders this transition the dominant signal in the standard first-derivative display of EPR spectra.

3.2.   Spin Hamiltonian

A completely rigorous analysis of EPR spectra of Mn^{2+} complexes is not always necessary in order to use the information provided in the spectra. A basic understanding of the origins of the various signals does, however, provide a level of confidence that is useful, e.g., in identifying the presence of contributions from more than a single species. The spectra are normally interpreted in terms of a spin Hamiltonian, and several detailed descriptions of the spin Hamiltonian of Mn^{2+} are available [7,25,26]. A simplified Hamiltonian is given by Eq. (1):

$$\mathcal{H}s = g\beta H_o S_z + A\vec{I}\cdot\vec{S} + \vec{S}\cdot\mathbf{D}\cdot\vec{S} + \mathcal{H}_{SH} \tag{1}$$

where the first term is the Zeeman interaction of the unpaired electrons with the laboratory field, H_o, the second term is the ^{55}Mn hyperfine interaction, the third term is the zero field splitting (zfs) interaction, and $\mathcal{H}_{SH}$ represents superhyperfine interactions with magnetically active nuclei on ligands. The simplifications that have been incorporated into Eq. (1) are as follows: (1) The Zeeman interaction has been simplified to reflect the magnetic field along the z axis and the nearly isotropic g tensor typical of Mn^{2+}. (2) The hyperfine interaction is written as a scalar coupling. (3) The nuclear Zeeman and nuclear quadrupole interaction terms have been omitted. (4) The small cubic zero field splitting term has also been omitted. The hyperfine interaction is usually isotropic because of the approximately spherical distribution of unpaired electrons about the nucleus. The major effect of the nuclear Zeeman term is to produce some forbidden ($\Delta M_s = \pm 1$, $\Delta m_I \neq 0$) transitions that are most conspicuous in spectra obtained at the standard X-band microwave frequency (9 GHz). The nuclear quadrupole term typically contributes negligibly—another "bonus" from the S-state properties of the ion.

The zfs interaction, $\vec{S}\cdot\mathbf{D}\cdot\vec{S}$, is the major source of anisotropy (orientation dependence) in the EPR spectra. This interaction is brought about by asymmetries in the electronic environment which lift the degeneracy of the three Kramer's doublets, $M_s = \pm 1/2$, $\pm 3/2$, $\pm 5/2$, in the absence of an externally applied field. The zfs typically has unique values for each type of coordination site being probed, and this term therefore endows the EPR spectra with features that are characteristic of a particular coordination environment. Unfortunately, it is not yet feasible to use the zfs terms to draw detailed conclusions about the detailed make-up of the binding site such as the identity of ligands. It is, however, relatively safe to infer that if there is a significant change in the spectrum resulting from addition of an exogenous ligand to a Mn^{2+} complex with a protein, then the ligand binding has altered the coordination sphere of Mn^{2+} [27,28].

The tensor describing the zfs interaction, $\mathbf{D}$, is traceless and therefore has a zero isotropic average as, for example, occurs in liquid solution upon rotation of a small complex. The requirements with respect to the rates of molecular rotation sufficient to erase the effects of the anisotropies due to the zfs are, however, difficult to realize for complexes that have even modest dimensions. For larger complexes, such as those with proteins, molecular rotation is largely ineffective in averaging the zfs anisotropy, and the spectra are powder-like even in the liquid state [7]. The traceless property of the tensor, **D**, also means that the tensor can be specified by just two parameters, the axial, D, and rhombic, E, zfs terms. The extent of rhombicity is measured by $|E/D|$, which varies between 0 (uniaxial) and 1/3 (maximally rhombic). The positions of the outer fine structure transitions are influenced in first order by the zfs, whereas the influence of the zfs on the position of the central fine structure transition appears only in second and higher orders. Hence, in a powder spectrum, the intensities of the outer fine structure transitions are distributed over a range of magnetic field leaving the relatively unperturbed central fine structure transition as the dominant source of signal. The second-order effects of zfs on the central fine structure transition can be used to determine the magnitudes of the zfs parameters, D and E [7,29,30]. The high electron spin and nuclear spin multiplicities of Mn^{2+} make it expeditious to use approximate expressions derived from applications of perturbation theory to calculate energy levels for spectral simulations [29,31]. This is especially true for powder spectra wherein energy levels need to be evaluated for many different molecular orientations with respect to the laboratory axis system. Simulations using the expressions from perturbation calculations are reasonably successful in reproducing the experimental spectra obtained at higher microwave frequencies such as Q band (35 GHz) because the assumptions regarding the relative magnitudes of the terms in Eq. (1) are better at higher magnetic field strengths. Simulations involving diagonalization of the full Hamiltonian have been demonstrated [32]. It is also noteworthy that the zfs and Zeeman interaction terms in Eq. (1) are expressed in different coordinate frames—the lab frame (Zeeman) and a molecular frame (zfs). Details of the rotations necessary to bring the terms into a common frame of reference are given elsewhere [7,29,31,33]. Examples of different symmetries are given in Fig. 1. The magnitudes of the zfs terms for Mn^{2+} are typically much smaller than those for high spin Fe^{3+} which has the same S = 5/2 spin state [25,26].

The last term in Eq. (1), $\mathcal{H}_{SH}$, represents contributions to the energy from the superhyperfine coupling between the unpaired elec-

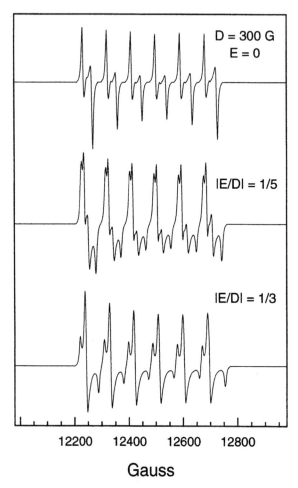

FIG. 1.   Powder pattern simulations of the M_s $-1/2 \rightarrow 1/2$ fine structure transition of Mn^{2+} at Q band (35 GHz) illustrating the axial symmetry and two degrees of rhombic symmetry. For each spectrum D = 300 G, and E or E/D is indicated in the figure. Forbidden transitions have been suppressed in the output. A Lorentzian linewidth of 5 G and a ^{55}Mn hyperfine splitting constant of 90 G were used in the simulations. Spectra were calculated correct to third order using the expression provided by Markham et al. [29].

trons on Mn^{2+} and nuclear spins located on ligand groups. The magnitudes of ligand superhyperfine splittings are typically less than the intrinsic line widths of EPR signals in spectra of Mn^{2+} complexes, and the splittings are therefore unresolved in the CW EPR spectra except in some well-ordered doped crystals. The superhyperfine coupling interaction, however, provides a direct means of identifying ligands [34]. Some strategies for extracting this information are discussed in a subsequent section.

3.3. Exchange Interactions

A significant number of enzymes are now known to have binuclear centers of divalent metal ions as cofactors [10]. For binuclear complexes of Mn^{2+}, another term is included in the Hamiltonian to account for the interaction between the unpaired electrons in the two ions. Thus, a term of the form $J\vec{S}_1 \cdot \vec{S}_2$ is necessary to account for the scalar part of this spin-spin interaction. The exchange interaction may contain anisotropic terms—the anisotropic exchange and antisymmetric exchange [35]. The zfs term also becomes more complex because it now includes the dipole-dipole interaction between the two ions, contributions from the asymmetry at each site, and the anisotropic parts of the exchange interaction [26]. The presence of exchange interactions in spectra of Mn^{2+} is accompanied by the appearance of multiline patterns for the ^{55}Mn hyperfine splitting wherein separation of the hyperfine lines is ~1/2 that typical for a mononuclear site. In most cases, the electron spin-spin interaction is mediated through bridging ligands and is therefore a form of superexchange. The interaction is typically antiferromagnetic in such cases [36]. There are several excellent sources of information on the exchange interaction [25,26,35,36].

3.4. Experimental Considerations

The ease with which the robust sextet EPR spectrum of $Mn^{II}(H_2O)_6$ is obtained from dilute solutions of Mn^{2+} salts is somewhat deceptive with regard to the relative difficulties that are encountered in obtaining spectra of Mn^{2+} complexes with proteins. The high symmetry of $Mn^{II}(H_2O)_6$

and its rapid molecular tumbling in solution contribute to an isotropic situation wherein the five fine structure transitions are degenerate and are superimposed within the [55]Mn sextet hyperfine pattern. These isotropic conditions are voided upon complexation of Mn^{2+} with a protein, leaving the central fine structure transition as the dominant EPR signal in the region near $g2$. This same region of the spectrum is occupied by the isotropic signals of $Mn^{II}(H_2O)_6$, and the signals from the latter need to be suppressed in order to observe signals from the bound form of the ion. Concentrations of protein, Mn^{2+}, and other ligands need to be manipulated in a manner consistent with the equilibrium constants of the complexes to maximize the concentration of the bound ion and lower the concentration of $Mn^{II}(H_2O)_6$ to eliminate its contribution to the spectrum. The EPR properties of the bound ion such as the intrinsic linewidths of the signals and the zfs anisotropy are somewhat unique to each complex, so it is difficult to establish firm guidelines with respect to the concentration of bound Mn^{2+} required to produce a usable spectrum. Generally, however, bound Mn^{2+} in the range of 300–500 µM will give adequate S/N, if $[Mn^{II}(H_2O)_6]$ is 10–50 times smaller. It is obvious that tight binding (e.g., dissociation constants in the µM to tens of µM region) of Mn^{2+} to the protein is a distinct advantage. The ability to concentrate the protein to concentrations of the order of mM is also a positive asset.

The second-order influences of the zfs interaction on the central fine structure transition are diminished at the higher magnetic field strengths employed in high-frequency EPR spectrometers. Thus, spectra are simplified substantially at Q band and higher microwave frequencies [7]. The simplifications largely offset the increased difficulties in sampling encountered at the higher operating frequencies. Applications of very high frequency spectrometers (>90 GHz) [37,38] can be useful, although spectra at Q band are usually adequate for most circumstances.

4. LIGAND SUPERHYPERFINE SPLITTINGS AND STRUCTURE DETERMINATIONS

Identification of ligands is a major step in understanding how metal ions are bound in active sites of enzymes and in binding sites of other proteins. The superhyperfine coupling between unpaired electrons of a paramagnetic ion and nuclear spins on ligands establishes the connection between ligand and metal ion in an unambiguous fashion [39]. The difficulty associated with this information for complexes of Mn^{2+} is that the superhyperfine splitting from nuclear spins on ligands is typically smaller than the intrinsic line width of the EPR signals. The superhyperfine splitting is therefore unresolved in the CW EPR spectra, although the splitting does contribute to an inhomogeneous broadening of the signals. In many cases of Mn^{2+}-ligand superhyperfine coupling, observation is perhaps better suited for more advanced EPR methods such as ENDOR or ESEEM. There are, however, some instances wherein divalent metal ions bind to a protein as a complex with a ligand (such as a nucleotide or other metabolite) or the ligand attaches to the metal ion-protein complex. These situations open up opportunities to label the ligand with a magnetically active isotope, such as ^{17}O, and to observe the effects of superhyperfine coupling on the linewidths of the CW EPR signals. Isotopic enrichment of specific residues in proteins has also been demonstrated using a ^{17}O-enriched amino acid in an efficient expression system [38].

4.1. Analysis of CW Spectra for Superhyperfine Interactions with ^{17}O

The intrinsic linewidths of EPR signals in Q-band spectra of Mn^{2+} complexes with proteins typically range from ~5 G to >20 G. These linewidths are greater than any reported superhyperfine splitting constants for Mn^{2+} with the exception of ^{19}F [39]. Hence, the superhyperfine splitting is unresolved in the EPR signals. The unresolved splitting, however, contributes to an inhomogeneous broadening of the EPR signals [40]. The linewidth observed, ΔH_{obs}, in the presence of unresolved coupling is approximately:

$$\Delta H_{obs} = [\Delta H_i^2 + \Delta H_{SH}^2]^{1/2} \tag{2}$$

where ΔH_i is the linewidth in the absence of unresolved splitting and ΔH_{SH} is the width of the superhyperfine splitting manifold. The width of the superhyperfine splitting manifold depends on the multiplicity of the nuclear spin. For example, ^{17}O ($I = 5/2$) produces a sextet splitting for which the overall width is 5 times the superhyperfine splitting constant

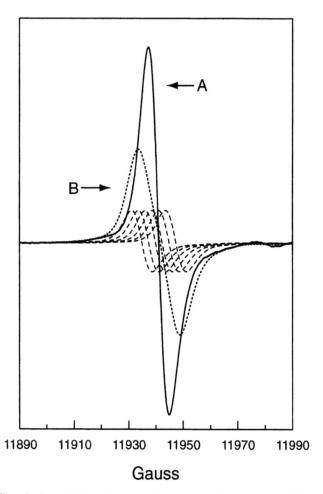

FIG. 2.   Simulation of the influence of unresolved hyperfine splitting ($I = 5/2$)
on the linewidth of an EPR signal whenever the hyperfine splitting constant is
smaller than the intrinsic linewidth of the signal. Curve A is the signal without
hyperfine splitting. The dashed curves show the subspectra representing the
individual hyperfine lines. Curve B is the sum of the dashed curve or the
inhomogeneously broadened signal. This situation would apply if there were
one ^{17}O nucleus coupled and if the isotopic enrichment in ^{17}O were 100%.
Experimental spectra for isotopic enrichments less than 100% would be a
weighted sum of curves A and B.

of 2–3 G. The consequences of this splitting on the linewidth and amplitude of an EPR signal are illustrated in Fig. 2. The patterns become wider and contain more transitions for cases where two or more ^{17}O nuclei are coupled to Mn^{2+} [41]. Inhomogeneous broadening due to superhyperfine coupling from ligands enriched in ^{17}O is apparent in the EPR signals from the enriched samples as illustrated in Fig. 3. The extent of broadening depends on the number of coordination sites occupied by the labeled ligand, the intrinsic width of the signal in the corresponding unlabeled sample, and the isotopic enrichment of the label [34].

4.2. Ligand Counting Methods

In most cases, one or more solvent molecules are in the first coordination sphere of the metal ion. The number of solvent ligands can be determined quantitatively by an analysis of the EPR signals from samples prepared in normal water and in water enriched in $H_2^{17}O$ [34,42]. The spectrum observed in water enriched in ^{17}O is a superposition of signals from Mn^{2+} having nonmagnetic isotopes (^{16}O, ^{18}O) of O bound— a signal that is identical in line shape to that obtained from the sample in normal water—and broader signals corresponding to Mn^{2+} coupled to one or more ^{17}O nuclear spins. The distribution of species depends on the isotopic enrichment of the water and the number of sites for water ligands in the complex. The fraction, F_{nonmag}, of the sample that has exclusively nonmagnetic isotopes of O as ligands is:

$$F_{nonmag} = [\text{atom fraction } (^{16}O + {}^{18}O)]^n \qquad (3)$$

where n is the number of water molecules in the coordination sphere. For example, if the water is 40% in ^{17}O, then Eq. (3) indicates that $F_{nonmag} = 0.6; 0.36; 0.22; 0.13$ for one, two, three, and four water ligands, respectively. If one subtracts 60% of the spectrum of the unlabeled sample from the spectrum of the enriched sample and there are two or more sites for water, then the difference spectrum contains the negative image of the former (Fig. 3). It is important to note that this method is a straightforward subtraction of spectra that does not require any knowledge of the magnitude of the superhyperfine splitting constant or assumptions regarding the line shape of the signals. This method has

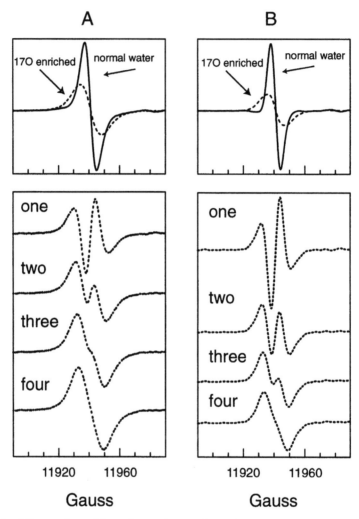

FIG. 3.   Illustration of the subtraction method of counting water ligands. Just
one of the six ^{55}Mn hyperfine components is shown. Column A shows the signals
obtained in normal water and in 41% $H_2{}^{17}O$. The dotted curves show the difference spectra obtained with one, two, three, and four water ligands. Column B
shows the same data after resolution enhancement of the experimentally observed spectra. The model of four water ligands gives the best fit to the data.

worked exceptionally well for counting water ligands in different types of Mn^{2+} complexes with proteins.

Equation (2) indicates that unresolved superhyperfine splitting is most easily discerned when the natural linewidths of the EPR signals, ΔH_i, is small. Fourier transform-based resolution enhancement (RE) techniques allow the detection of unresolved superhyperfine splitting in broader signals whenever the spectra can be collected with relatively high S/N ratios [41,43]. In the specific case of the $Mn^{II}GDP$ complex with ras p21 (a GTPase that is important in signal transduction), RE of the signals of samples in ^{17}O-enriched water allows one to visualize the superposition of the sharp signal from the fraction of the sample that has only nonmagnetic isotopes of O as ligands on the broader signals from the various ^{17}O-coordinated species (Fig. 4) [41].

4.3. Stereochemistry and Coordination Schemes

In some ligands, such as nucleotides, coordination of different donor atoms to the metal ion leads to different stereochemistry for the complex. The diastereotopic positions in the triphosphate chain of nucleoside triphosphates are labeled in Scheme 1.

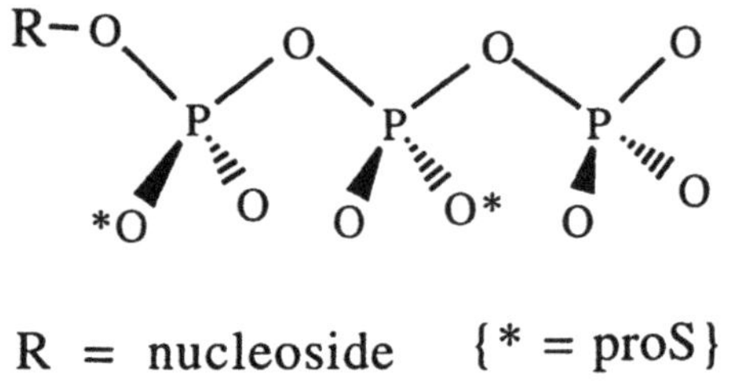

R = nucleoside   {* = proS}

SCHEME 1

Neglecting the possibility for attachment of a metal ion to two oxygens from any of the three phosphate groups, there are still 17 different isomers of metal-nucleoside complexes. The regio- and stereochemistry of metal coordination to nucleotides at the active sites of enzymes has been probed using nucleoside phosphorothioate analogs wherein one of the diastereotopic oxygen atoms in the polyphosphate chain is replaced by a sulfur [44,45]. Questions about the regiochemis-

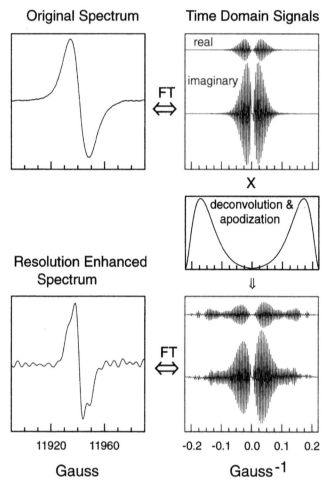

FIG 4.   Resolution enhancement of one of the ^{55}Mn hyperfine components of
the Q-band EPR spectrum of the complex of Mn^{II}GDP with ras p21 in water
containing up to 40 atom% ^{17}O. A cosine ("Hanning") window function was used
for apodization [83].

try of coordination [21,34,46–49] and of the stereochemical configurations [50–52] of Mn^{2+}-nucleotide complexes have also been approached using ^{17}O-labeled forms of the nucleotides and of nucleoside phosphorothioate analogs [17]. The results from these studies show that coordination of Mn^{2+} to the β- and γ-phosphate moieties of nucleoside triphosphates occurs in some proteins [48,49,53,54] whereas α,β,γ-tridentate coordination occurs with creatine kinase [46], pyruvate kinase [21], and 3-phosphoglycerate kinase [47,55]. Proteins that are members of the "P-loop" superfamily [56] appear to bind the β,γ-bidentate form of the metal-nucleotide complex. Binding of a second divalent cation [42] and simultaneous coordination of ligands from amino acid side chains [41,48,49] among the group of nucleotide-binding proteins provide interesting variations in the mode of metal-nucleotide binding. In virtually all of the enzymic reactions of metal-nucleotide complexes, the metal ion is an essential cofactor. It is clear that the shape and positions of the polyphosphate chain are determined by the mode of coordination of the metal ion. The positive charge of the metal ion is, no doubt, also a factor in the reactivity of the phosphate groups, although it is difficult to separate the structural influences from the electronic influences.

The inhomogeneous broadening from ligands enriched in ^{17}O has been used to establish direct coordination of Mn^{2+} to the inhibitor, oxalate, in complexes with pyruvate kinase [42] and pyruvate-phosphate dikinase [57]. The methods have also been applied to a determination of the mode of coordination of the inhibitor of enolase, phosphonoacetohydroxamate, to two metal ions in the active site [58]. The hydration status of Mn^{2+} bound to the fosfomycin resistance protein, FosA, has been determined by EPR [28].

4.4.   Other Nuclear Spins

Substitution of ^{2}H for ^{1}H can influence CW EPR signals of Mn^{2+} complexes with proteins. Protons from water ligands and from side chain ligands such as Ser and Thr are close to Mn^{2+} and their superhyperfine splitting contributes to the linewidth of the EPR signals. In the case of a protein such as ras p21 where several water molecules coordinate to Mn^{2+}, there is a significant decrease in the linewidths of signals from samples made up in ^{2}H$_2$O [41]. Detection of superhyperfine splitting from other nuclear spins, such as ^{31}P, ^{14}N, ^{15}N, and ^{13}C, is normally too small to be a significant contributor to the linewidths of CW EPR signals of Mn^{2+} in protein complexes. For these nuclei, the CW EPR signals serve as "carriers" for application of more specialized methods, such as ENDOR and ESEEM spectroscopy.

5.   ENDOR AND ESEEM METHODS

The complementary techniques of ENDOR and ESEEM spectroscopy are well suited to the task of detecting superhyperfine couplings that are too weak to result in resolved splitting in CW EPR spectra [59,60]. For applications to complexes of Mn^{2+}, the electron spin relaxation rates must be slowed by carrying out measurements near 4 K. In the ESEEM measurement, microwave pulses are used to generate a train of electron spin-echoes [61,62]. Weak superhyperfine couplings interfere with the coherent formation of the echoes such that the amplitudes of the echoes are modulated by the precession frequencies of the nuclear spins. The modulation frequencies carry the information on the super-hyperfine frequencies and Larmor frequencies of the coupled nuclei [60,61]. In the various forms of ENDOR, radiofrequency radiation is used to stimulate NMR transitions that are detected by EPR [59,60,63]. These methods offer the potential to detect superhyperfine coupling from nuclear spins of coordinated atoms and from spins that are slightly further from Mn^{2+}. Both methods offer far greater resolution of electron spin-nuclear spin coupling than can be achieved with conventional CW EPR. In most cases, an ability to deliver isotopic substitutions selectively greatly simplifies assignments and interpretation of the signals obtained by ESEEM and ENDOR.

The ESEEM method has been used to probe Mn^{2+} binding sites in several enzymes and other proteins [64–70]. The depths of echo modulations produced by a given nuclear spin depend on several variables [71,72], and an inability to detect modulations from nuclear spins is not necessarily an interpretable result. Instruments that can be operated at more than one microwave frequency are useful in circumventing some of these limitations. The basic theory [71] has been elaborated to account for the high electron spin multiplicity of Mn^{2+} [73].

The ENDOR method applied to Mn^{2+} complexes with proteins has also been demonstrated [74]. One can anticipate that pulsed ENDOR methods and higher frequency ENDOR spectrometers [59] will enjoy success in probing binding sites of Mn^{2+} in proteins.

6. ELECTRON SPIN-SPIN COUPLING AND MULTINUCLEAR METAL CENTERS

EPR methods including ENDOR and ESEEM with Mn^{2+} have been useful in characterizing the binuclear metal centers in several enzymes and proteins [10,21,51,58,75–81]. Hybrid centers, wherein one of the two sites is populated by a diamagnetic partner, allow one to characterize the remaining Mn^{2+} site using the conventional strategies for a mononuclear site [21,42,51,58,76]. Whenever both sites are populated by Mn^{2+}, the proximity of the two cations normally results in a strong exchange (superexchange) interaction. The strong exchange interaction couples the electron spins of the individual ions into a manifold of integer spin states—$S = 0, 1, 2, 3, 4, 5$. Transitions within the individual S states give rise to EPR signals. These signals are distinguished from signals due to Mn^{2+} in a mononuclear site by a ~45 G spacing of the ^{55}Mn hyperfine lines [26,36].

The energies of the S states depend on the magnitude of the exchange coupling constant J according to the Lande interval rule [26]. For antiferromagnetic coupling, the relative energies of the $S = 0, 1, 2, 3, 4, 5$, levels are 0, J, $3J$, $6J$, $10J$, and $15J$, respectively. For values of J typical of binuclear Mn^{2+} centers, several of the S states are thermally populated even at temperatures near 4 K, and an analysis of the temperature dependence of the EPR spectra can be used to determine the magnitude of J. One approach to a determination of J is to identify a feature in the EPR spectrum that arises from a particular S state and analyze the temperature dependence of the intensity of the feature using a Boltzmann function [36]. Another approach is feasible using the technique of singular value decomposition (SVD) [82]. The SVD approach also gives the spectra contributed by the individual S states. There are several examples of the use of SVD to analyze the exchange coupling in binuclear Mn^{2+} centers [77,80,81].

ACKNOWLEDGMENT

Work from the authors' laboratory that is cited in this chapter was supported by NIH Grant GM35752.

ABBREVIATIONS

CD	circular dichroism
CW EPR	continuous wave electron paramagnetic resonance
ENDOR	electron nuclear double resonance
EPR	electron paramagnetic resonance
ESEEM	electron spin echo envelope modulation
EXAFS	extended X-ray absorption fine structure
GDP	guanosine diphosphate
GTPase	guanosine triphosphatase
IR	infrared
MCD	magnetic circular dichroism
NMR	nuclear magnetic resonance
RE	resolution enhancement
S/N	signal-to-noise ratio
SOD	superoxide dismutase
SVD	singular value decomposition
zfs	zero-field splitting

REFERENCES

1. R. H. Holm, P. Kennepohl, and E. I. Solomon, *Chem. Rev.*, *96*, 2239–2314 (1996).
2. E. A. V. Ebsworth, D. W. H. Rankin, and S. Cradock, *Structural Methods in Inorganic Chemistry*, 2nd ed., Blackwell Scientific, Oxford, 1991.
3. W. M. Coleman and L. T. Taylor, *Coord. Chem. Rev.*, *32*, 1–31 (1980).
4. G. C. Cotzias, *Fed. Proc.*, *20*, 98–103 (1961).

5. G. R. Lawrence and D. T. Sawyer, *Coord. Chem. Rev.*, *27*, 173–193 (1978).

6. A. R. McEuen, *Inorg. Biochem.*, *3*, 314–343 (1982).

7. G. H. Reed and G. D. Markham, *Biol. Magn. Res.*, *6*, 73–142 (1984).

8. K. Sauer, *Acc. Chem. Res.*, *13*, 249–256 (1980).

9. V. L. Schramm and F. C. Wedler, eds., *Manganese in Metabolism and Enzyme Function*, Academic Press, Orlando, 1986.

10. G. C. Dismukes, *Chem. Rev.*, *96*, 2909–2926 (1996).

11. V. K. Yachandra, K. Sauer, and M. P. Klein, *Chem. Rev.*, *96*, 2927–2950 (1996).

12. W. F. Beyer, Jr., and I. Fridovich, in *Manganese in Metabolism and Enzyme Function* (V. L. Schramm and F. C. Wedler, eds.), Academic Press, Orlando, 1986, pp. 193–219.

13. W. C. Stallings, K. A. Pattridge, R. K. Strong, and M. L. Ludwig, *J. Biol. Chem.*, *260*, 16424–16432 (1985).

14. Y. Hsieh, Y. Guan, C. Tu, P. J. Bratt, A. Amgerhofer, J. R. Lepock, M. J. Hickey, J. A. Tainer, H. S. Nick, and D. N. Silverman, *Biochemistry*, *37*, 4731–4739 (1998).

15. D. Leussing and T. N. Tisher, *J. Am. Chem. Soc.*, *83*, 65–70 (1961).

16. R. K. Boggess, J. R. Absher, S. Morelen, L. T. Taylor, and J. W. Hughes, *Inorg. Chem.*, *22*, 1273–1279 (1983).

17. G. W. Smithers, R. D. Sammons, P. J. Goodhart, R. LoBrutto, and G. H. Reed, *Biochemistry*, *28*, 1597–1604 (1989).

18. R. M. Leach and M. S. Lilburn, *World Rev. Nutr. Diet.*, *32*, 123–134 (1978).

19. D. O. Foster, H. A. Lardy, P. D. Ray, and J. B. Johnston, *Biochemistry*, *6*, 2120–2128 (1967).

20. Y. H. Baek and T. Nowak, *Arch. Biochem. Biophys.*, *217*, 491–497 (1982).

21. J. L. Buchbinder and G. H. Reed, *Biochemistry*, *29*, 1799–1806 (1990).

22. L. G. Sillén and A. E. Martell, *Stability Constants*, Chem. Soc. Spec. Publ. No. 17, London, 1964.

23. W. W. Cleland, *Acc. Chem. Res.*, *8*, 145–151 (1975).

24. F. A. Cotton and G. Wilkinson, *Advanced Inorganic Chemistry*, Wiley Interscience, New York, 1962.

25. A. Abragam and B. Bleaney, *Electron Paramagnetic Resonance of Transition Ions*, Clarendon, Oxford, 1970.

26. W. Weltner, Jr., *Magnetic Atoms and Molecules*, Dover, New York, 1983.

27. A. K. Whiting, Y. R. Boldt, M. P. Hendrich, L. P. Wackett, and L. Que, Jr., *Biochemistry*, 35, 160–170 (1996).

28. B. A. Bernat, L. T. Laughlin, and R. N. Armstrong, *Biochemistry*, 36, 3050–3055 (1997).

29. G. D. Markham, B. D. Nageswara Rao, and G. H. Reed, *J. Magn. Reson.*, 33, 595–602 (1979).

30. P. C. Taylor, J. F. Baugher, and H. M. Kriz, *Chem. Rev.*, 75, 203–240 (1975).

31. E. Meirovitch and R. Poupko, *J. Phys. Chem.*, 82, 1920–1925 (1978).

32. A. R. Coffino and J. Peisach, *J. Magn. Reson. B*, 111, 127–134 (1996).

33. P. L. Nordio, *General magnetic resonance theory*, in *Spin Labeling Theory and Applications* (L. J. Berliner, ed.), Academic Press, New York, 1976, pp. 5–52.

34. G. H. Reed and T. S. Leyh, *Biochemistry*, 19, 5472 (1980).

35. A. Bencini and D. Gatteschi, *EPR of Exchange Coupled Systems*, Springer-Verlag, Berlin, 1990.

36. J. Owen and E. A. Harris, in *Electron Paramagnetic Resonance* (S. Geschwind, ed.), Plenum Press, New York, 1972.

37. B. F. Bellew, C. J. Halkides, G. J. Gerfen, R. G. Griffin, and D. J. Singel, *Biochemistry*, 35, 12186–12193 (1996).

38. C. J. Halkides, B. F. Bellew, G. J. Gerfen, C. T. Farrar, P. H. Carter, B. Ruo, D. A. Evans, R. G. Griffin, and D. J. Singel, *Biochemistry*, 35, 12194–12200 (1996).

39. B. A. Goodman and J. B. Raynor, *Adv. Inorg. Radiochem.*, 13, 135–62 (1970).

40. J. R. Norris, R. A. Uphaus, H. L. Crespi, and J. J. Katz, *Proc. Natl. Acad. Sci. USA*, 68, 625 (1971).

41. D. G. Latwesen, M. Poe, J. S. Leigh, and G. H. Reed, *Biochemistry*, *31*, 4946–4950 (1992).

42. D. T. Lodato and G. H. Reed, *Biochemistry*, *26*, 2243–2250 (1987).

43. J. K. Kauppinen, D. J. Moffatt, H. H. Mantsch, and D. G. Cameron, *Appl. Spectrosc.*, *35*, 271–276 (1981).

44. M. Cohn, *Acc. Chem. Res.*, *15*, 326–332 (1982).

45. F. Eckstein, *Annu. Rev. Biochem.*, 54, 367–402 (1985).

46. T. S. Leyh, P. J. Goodhart, A. C. Nguyen, G. L. Kenyon, and G. H. Reed, *Biochemistry*, *24*, 308–316 (1985).

47. J. M. Moore and G. H. Reed, *Biochemistry*, *24*, 5328–5333 (1985).

48. J. F. Eccleston, M. R. Webb, D. E. Ash, and G. H. Reed, *J. Biol. Chem.*, *256*, 10774–10777 (1981).

49. M. R. Webb, D. E. Ash, T. S. Leyh, D. R. Trentham, and G. H. Reed, *J. Biol. Chem.*, *257*, 3068–3072 (1982).

50. T. S. Leyh, R. D. Sammons, P. A. Frey, and G. H. Reed, *J. Biol. Chem.*, *257*, 15047–15053 (1982).

51. J. L. Buchbinder, J. Baraniak, P. A. Frey, and G. H. Reed, *Biochemistry*, *32*, 14111–14116 (1993).

52. P. A. Frey, R. Iyengar, G. W. Smithers, and G. H. Reed, in *Biophosphates and Their Analogues—Synthesis, Structure, Metabolism and Activity* (S. Bruzik and W. J. Stec, eds.), Elsevier, Amsterdam, 1987, pp. 267–278.

53. G. W. Smithers, M. Poe, D. G. Latwesen, and G. H. Reed, *Arch. Biochem. Biophys.*, *280*, 416–420 (1990).

54. L. R. Olsen and G. H. Reed, *Arch. Biochem. Biophys.*, *304*, 242–247 (1993).

55. G. H. Reed, *Biochem. Soc. Trans.*, *13*, 567–571 (1985).

56. J. E. Walker, M. Saraste, J. M. Runswick, and N. J. Gay, *EMBO J.*, *1*, 945–951 (1982).

57. J. L. Kofron, D. E. Ash, and G. H. Reed, *Biochemistry*, *27*, 4781–4787 (1988).

58. R. R. Poyner and G. H. Reed, *Biochemistry*, *31*, 7166–7173 (1992).

59. B. M. Hoffman, V. J. DeRose, P. E. Doan, R. J. Bubriel, A. L. P. Houseman, and J. Telser, *Biol. Magn. Reson.*, *13*, 151–218 (1993).

60. H. Thomann and M. Bernardo, *Biol. Magn. Reson.*, *13*, 275–322 (1993).

61. W. B. Mims and J. Peisach, *Biol. Magn. Reson.*, *3*, 213–263 (1981).

62. J. R. Norris, M. C. Thrunauer, and M. K. Bowman, *Adv. Biol. Med. Phys.*, *17*, 365–416 (1980).

63. C. P. Scholes, in *Multiple Electron Paramagnetic Resonance Spectroscopy* (M. M. Dorio and J. H. Freed, eds.), Plenum Press, New York, 1979.

64. P. A. Tipton and J. Peisach, *Biochemistry*, *30*, 739–744 (1991).

65. R. LoBrutto, G. W. Smithers, G. H. Reed, W. H. Orme-Johnson, S. L. Tan, and J. S. Leigh, *Biochemistry*, *25*, 5654–5660 (1986).

66. C. J. Halkides, C. T. Farrar, R. G. Larsen, A. G. Redfield, and D. J. Singel, *Biochemistry*, *33*, 4019–4035 (1994).

67. M. P. Espe, J. P. Hosler, S. Ferguson-Miller, G. T. Babcock, and J. McCracken, *Biochemistry*, *34*, 7593–7602 (1995).

68. C. T. Farrar, C. J. Halkides, and D. J. Singel, *Structure*, *5*, 1055–1066 (1997).

69. C. Buy, G. Girault, and J. L. Zimmermann, *Biochemistry*, *35*, 9880–9891 (1996).

70. P. A. Tipton, T. P. Quinn, J. Peisach, and P. F. Cook, *Protein Sci.*, *5*, 1648–1654 (1996).

71. W. B. Mims, *Phys. Rev.*, *B6*, 3543–3546 (1972).

72. A. Lai, H. L. Flanagan, and D. J. Singel, *J. Chem. Phys.*, *89*, 7161–7166 (1988).

73. R. G. Larsen, C. J. Halkides, and D. J. Singel, *J. Chem. Phys.*, *98*, 6704–6721 (1993).

74. X. Tan, R. R. Poyner, G. H. Reed, and C. P. Scholes, *Biochemistry*, *32*, 7799–7810 (1993).

75. G. D. Markham, *J. Biol. Chem.*, *256*, 1903–1909 (1981).

76. R. Bogumil, R. Kappl, J. Hüttermann, and H. Witzel, *Biochemistry*, *36*, 2345–2352 (1997).

77. A. E. Meier, M. M. Whittaker, and J. W. Whittaker, *Biochemistry*, *35*, 348–360 (1996).

78. S. Kangulov, M. Sivaraja, V. V. Barynin, and G. C. Dismukes, *Biochemistry*, *32*, 4912–4924 (1993).

79. A. Ivancich, V. V. Barynin, and J. L. Zimmermann, *Biochemistry*, *34*, 6628–6639 (1995).

80. S. Kangulov, P. J. Pessiki, V. V. Barynin, D. E. Ash, and G. C. Dismukes, *Biochemistry*, *34*, 2015–2025 (1995).

81. B. S. Antharavally, R. R. Poyner, and P. W. Ludden, *J. Am. Chem. Soc.*, *120*, 8897–8898 (1998).

82. R. W. Hendler and R. I. Shrager, *J. Biochem. Biophys. Methods.*, *28*, 1–33 (1994).

83. W. H. Press, B. P. Flannery, S. A. Teukolsky, and W. T. Vettering, *Numerical Recipes*, Cambridge University Press, New York, 1989, p. 425.

8

Enzymes and Proteins Containing Manganese: An Overview

*James D. Crowley, Deborah A. Traynor,
and David C. Weatherburn**

School of Chemical and Physical Sciences,
Victoria University of Wellington, P. O. Box 600,
Wellington, New Zealand

---

*Address correspondence to this author.

1. INTRODUCTION

This chapter provides an overview of manganese-containing and manganese-dependent proteins and enzymes with an emphasis on molecules in which the metal ion binding site is well characterized. If the protein or enzyme is considered in other chapters of this volume then only a brief mention will be made of the molecule in this chapter. Where possible, references are selected from the literature since 1990. Books and review articles which cover the earlier literature are available [1–10]. Because of space limitations we have cited only a limited number of references. We wish to acknowledge the important contributions of other investigators whose work we have not cited. References to their work can be found in the cited publications.

1.1 Manganese Coordination Chemistry

The aqueous chemistry of manganese with particular relevance to biological systems has been reviewed by a number of authors [8,9,11]. Mn^{n+} in biological systems adopts a range of coordination environments and may occur in the II, III, or IV oxidation states. Because Mn^{2+} is EPR-active it has been used as a probe of the metal binding site in many studies of Mg^{2+}- and Ca^{2+}-containing enzymes and this is a focus of Chap. 7 of this volume [12].

Mn^{2+} has a high-spin d^5 electron configuration. It has no coordination geometry preferences and forms relatively weak complexes with ligands, in general stronger than Ca^{2+} and Mg^{2+} but weaker than the other transition metal ions. Mn^{2+} prefers hard oxygen donor atoms to the softer nitrogen or sulfur donors and the coordination environment of Mn^{2+} in all structurally characterized proteins contains oxygen donors. There are some enzymes that contain one or two imidazole nitrogens bound to Mn^{2+} but there are still no structurally characterized examples of Mn^{2+} bound to cysteine or methionine sulfur atoms. One finds reference to Mn^{2+} being thiophilic and compared to Mg^{2+} this is true, but compared to the later first-row transition metals, Mn^{2+} has a low affinity for sulfur donors. Mn^{3+} should have an even lower affinity for sulfur. Mn^{3+} complexes are usually distorted octahedral species that would be expected to form more thermodynamically stable complexes than their Mn^{2+} counterparts. However, little information about their relative stability is available.

Both $Mn(H_2O)_6^{2+}$ and $Mn(H_2O)_6^{3+}$ ions are labile. This has important consequences in the isolation and characterization of enzymes containing manganese. The lability of Mn^{2+} and the lack of thermodynamic stability of its complexes can result in the complete loss of Mn^{2+} in the isolation procedure of an enzyme and as a consequence the enzyme must be reactivated by the addition of Mn^{2+} once isolated. Mn^{3+}-containing proteins are frequently isolated containing manganese but the manganese content is often substoichiometric.

The coordination chemistry of Mn^{4+} is dominated by octahedral coordination and a tendency to form polynuclear mixed-valence [Mn(III)/Mn(IV)] complexes with μ_2-oxo ligands. Although Mn(IV) with a d^3 electron configuration would be expected to be inert, the mixed-valence clusters are labile probably due to rapid electron delocalization within the cluster.

Mn^{2+} can replace Mg^{2+} [13], Ca^{2+} [14], Zn^{2+} [15,16], Fe^{2+} [17], Ni^{2+} [18], and Co^{2+} [19] in the active sites of enzymes and many of these substituted enzymes are functional with Mn^{2+} in the active site. The most studied of these replacement reactions is the replacement of Mg^{2+} and the observed effects are different with different enzymes. An increase or decrease in reaction rate may be observed; the enzyme can become less specific in its reaction and in some cases the stoichiometry of metal binding is different [20]. For example, exonuclease III, a DNA repair enzyme, binds two Mn^{2+} ions in solution but only one Mg^{2+} or Ca^{2+} ion under the same conditions [2]. The X-ray structure of this enzyme shows only one Mn^{2+} ion bound [21] presumably because of the crystallization conditions employed. Mn^{2+} substitution for another metal can produce structural changes in the active site of the enzyme that result in inactivation [14,15,22].

Labile metal ions such as Mn^{2+}, Mg^{2+}, and Ca^{2+} in a metalloprotein are in dynamic equilibrium with the metal ions in their environment and the metal ion bound to the protein will be dependent on the metal ion concentration in the immediate environment of the protein and the relative affinity of the protein for metal ions. The concentration of Mn^{2+} in most cells under physiological conditions is not known but is usually thought to be in the micromolar range. This is much smaller than the intracellular concentration of Mg^{2+} (~0.5 mM), so that Mg^{2+} has a large concentration advantage that usually outweighs the thermodynamic advantage of Mn^{2+}. However, some compartments in a cell can have a quite different chemical environment from other parts of the cell and some organisms may accumulate much higher concentrations of manganese than normal. *Lactobacillus plantarum* has an intracellular concentration of Mn^{2+} of 0.025 M [1]. *Micrococcus radiodurans*, a radiation-resistant bacterium that has developed a very efficient DNA excision/repair system, accumulates Mn^{2+} to an extent that there is one Mn^{2+} ion per 10 nucleotide bases present in the cell [23]. The extrapallial fluid of the mussel *Pinna nobilis* contains 0.11 mM Mn^{2+} (five orders of magnitude greater than the concentration in seawater) mostly bound to a low molecular weight polypeptide [24] and the byssal threads from freshwater mussels have manganese concentrations 30- to 100-fold higher than those from lake water mussels [25].

A particular reaction in one species may be catalyzed by an enzyme containing a particular metal and by an enzyme containing a different metal in another species. Well-known examples include ribonucleotide reductase (Fe, Co, and Mn), superoxide dismutase (Cu, Zn, Fe, Mn, and Ni), and catalase (Fe and Mn), but there are probably other unrecognized examples. It has been reported that the enzymes present in the mammalian brain are more likely to be Mn^{2+}-dependent than similar Mg^{2+}-dependent enzymes in other organs from the same animal, such as glutamine synthetase [26], aminopeptidase [27], ATPase [28], and adenylate cyclase [29]. These factors make it difficult to decide in many cases whether a particular enzyme is Mn-activated or not. Our resolution of this difficulty is discussed below.

1.2. Manganese as an Oxidizing/Reducing Agent

The $Mn(H_2O)_6^{3+}$ ion is a powerful oxidizing agent, $E^0 = +1.51$ V. The Mn(III)/Mn(II) redox potential is, however, highly dependent on the coordination sphere of the metal ion. Binding nitrogen to Mn(III) lowers the reduction potential of the Mn(III) complex and carboxylate ligands have the same, although smaller, effect. Experience with simple inorganic complexes suggests that five- and seven-coordinate Mn(II) complexes are more difficult than octahedral complexes to oxidize to Mn(III). The behavior of Mn bound to proteins is consistent with the behavior of the simple complexes; Mn(III) in enzymes such as catalase and superoxide dismutase is bound to two or more histidine moieties although the coordination sphere is not always octahedral. The Mn(II) ion in manganese-dependent peroxidase, which is oxidized to Mn(III), has a coordination sphere comprising two water molecules, a propionate from the heme group, and three carboxylate residues [30].

One of the most remarkable features of manganese-dependent enzymes is their very wide range of functionality illustrated by the enzymes listed in Table 1 and discussed below. Table 1 lists those enzymes that are reported to be Mn-dependent but that are currently structurally uncharacterized and that are not discussed elsewhere in this chapter. In constructing Table 1 we have been mindful of the relative affinities of proteins for metal ions and (when available) the reported relative reactivity of the metalloenzyme when it contains Mn^{2+}

and Mg^{2+}. There are numerous reports of enzymes activated by these two metals with the Mn^{2+}-substituted form being more active at a lower concentration of metal ion. We have not included such enzymes in Table 1 unless the activity is approximately an order of magnitude higher with Mn^{2+} and the activity is maximal at less than 1 mM Mn^{2+}. There are exceptions to this rule, however, and the cited reference will probably explain why the particular example has been included.

2. OXIDOREDUCTASES

Manganese is a cofactor in a number of proteins that are involved in biological oxidation reduction processes. Many of these proteins are among the best characterized of the manganese-containing enzymes and are the subject of separate chapters in this volume. Most catechol dioxygenases, EC 1.13.11.1, are iron enzymes, but several bacterial enzymes are manganese-dependent and these are reviewed in Chap. 15 [185]. Manganese-dependent ribonucleotide reductase, EC 1.17.4.1, was previously believed to contain a binuclear manganese active site, but it now appears that the enzyme from *Corynebacterium ammoniagenes* has a mononuclear manganese active site [186]. Manganese-containing ribonucleotide reductase is discussed in Ref. 187. Manganese superoxide dismutase, EC 1.15.1.1, is described in Chap. 18 [188] and bacterial manganese catalase, EC 1.11.1.6, which contains a binuclear manganese active site, is discussed in Chap. 16 [189]. Manganese-dependent peroxidases, EC 1.11.1.13, which are used by white-rot fungi to degrade lignin in wood, are described in Chap. 17 [190]. The tetranuclear manganese cluster at the heart of Photosystem II, which is responsible for the evolution of oxygen from photosynthetic organisms, is described in Chaps. 19 and 20 of this volume [191,192].

2.1. Oxidases

2.1.1. Amine Oxidase

A copper-containing amine oxidase, EC 1.4.3.6, that catalyzes the oxidation of amines to the corresponding aldehyde and ammonia has been

TABLE 1

Enyzmes Containing Manganese Not Discussed Elsewhere in This Chapter

Enzyme	EC number	Source	Ref.
D-Arabitol dehydrogenase	1.1.1.11	*Galdiera sulphuraria*	[31]
Lactate dehydrogenase	1.1.1.27	*Lactobacillus*	[1]
Malic enzyme	1.1.1.40	Liver	[32]
6-Phosphogluconate dehydrogenase	1.1.1.43	*Zymomonas mobilis*	[33]
Dimethylmalate dehydrogenase	1.1.1.84	*Pseudomonas*	[34]
Tartrate dehydrogenase	1.1.1.93	*P. putida*	[35]
20α-Hydroxysteroid dehydrogenase	1.1.1.149	*Clostridium scindes*	[36]
Malolactic enzyme	1.1.1.–	*Lactobacillus*	[37]
4-Hydroxymandelate oxidase	1.1.3.19	*P. convexa*	[38]
2-Oxoglutarate dehydrogenase	1.2.4.2	Heart	[39]
Cucurbitacin B Δ^{23} reductase	1.3.1.5	*Cucurbita maxima*	[40]
Thiosulfate oxidase	1.8.99.–	*Thiobacillus versutus*	[41,42]
2-Aminophenol oxidase	1.10.3.4	*Pycnoporus coccineus*	[43]
Polyphenol oxidase	1.10.3.1	Litchi	[44]
Peanut peroxidase	1.11.–	Peanut	[45]
Lipoxygenase	1.13.11.12	*Gaumannomyces graminis*	[46,47]
Chlorocatechol dehydrogenase	1.13.11.–	*Rhodococcus erythropolis*	[48]
Phloroglucinol oxidase	1.–	Cabbage	[49]

Protein	EC number	Source	Reference
S-Adenosyl-L-methionine sialate-8-O-methyl-transferase	2.1.1.6	Asterias rubens	[50]
γ-Glutamyl transpeptidase	2.3.2.2	Actinobacillus actinomycetemcomitans	[51]
Chitin synthetase	2.4.1.16	Entamoeba invadens	[52]
UDP-Glucuronyltransferase	2.4.1.17	Mammals	[53]
β-1,4-Galactosyltransferase	2.4.1.22	Mammals	[54]
Galactosyltransferase	2.4.1.38	Mammals	[55]
UDP-GalNAc-polypeptide N-acetylgalactosaminyl-transferase	2.4.1.41	Mammals	[56]
UDP-Galactose-GM2 ganglioside β-1-3 galactosyltransferase	2.4.1.62	Chicken brain	[57]
UDP-Glucose-collagen glucosyltransferase	2.4.1.66	Chicken embryos	[58]
UDP-Glucose-ceramide glucosyltransferase	2.4.1.80	Golgi apparatus	[59]
Globoside α-N-acetyl galactosaminyltransferase	2.4.1.88	Mammals	[60]
N-Acetyllactosamine synthetase	2.4.1.90	Mammals	[61]
β-1,6-N-Acetylglucosaminyltransferase	2.4.1.102	Plants	[62]
UDP-Glc:protein transglucosylase	2.4.1.112	Potato	[63]
Dolichyldiphosphooligosaccharide protein glycotransferase	2.4.1.119	Mammals	[64]
Galactinol synthase	2.4.1.123	Kidney bean, zucchini	[65]
UDP Gal:N-Acetyl-D-glucosamine-β-(1,4)galactosyltransferase	2.4.1.124	Ehrlich ascites tumor cells	[66]
UDP-Gal:β-D-Gal(1,4)-D-GlcNAc α-(1,3)-galactosyl-transferase	2.4.1.124	Ehrlich ascites tumor cells	[67]

TABLE 1

Continued

Enzyme	EC number	Source	Ref.
Galactosylgalactosylxylosyl-protein 3β-galactosyl-transferase	2.4.1.135	Bovine serum	[53]
N-Acetylglucosaminyldiphosphodolichol N-acetyl-β-glucosaminidase	2.4.1.141	*Tritrichomonas foetus*	[68]
α-1,3-Mannosyl-glycoprotein β-1,4-N-acetylglucos-aminyltransferase	2.4.1.145	Cattle, rat	[69,70]
Acetylgalactosaminyl-O-glycosylglycoprotein β-1,3-N-acetylglucosaminyltransferase	2.4.1.147	Pig, rat	[71]
(GlcNAc β 1-6)GalNAc-R (GlcNAc to Gal) β1,3-N-acetylglucosaminyltransferase	2.4.1.149	Pig	[72]
UDP-GalNAc:NeuAc α-2,3 Gal β-R-(GalNAc to Gal)β-1,4-N-acetylgalactosaminyltransferase	2.4.1.165	Human	[73]
Lactosylceramide 1,3-N-acetyl-β-D-glucosaminyltransferase	2.4.1.206	Rat	[74]
UDP-GlcNAcGal-β-(1-4) GlcNAc-β-(1-3)N-acetylglycosaminyltransferase	2.4.1._	Human	[75]
β-1,4,N-Acetylgalactosaminyltransferase	2.4.1._	Pig	[76]

β-1,2-Mannosyltransferase	2.4.1.-	*E. coli*	[77]
α-1,3-Mannosyltransferase	2.4.1.-	*E. coli*	[78]
α-1,6-Mannosyltransferase	2.4.1.-	*Candida albicans, E. coli*	[79]
N-Acetyl-α-galactosaminidase	2.4.1.-	*Tritrichomonas foetus*	[68]
UDP-GlcNAc-GlcNAc-β-1,6 (GlcNAc-β-1→2)-Man-α-1-]R[GlcNAc to Man]β-1→4 N-acetyl-glucosaminyltransferase	2.4.1.-	Fish, birds	[80]
UDP-Galactose:β-N-acetyl glucosamine-β-N-acetyl-galactosamine β-1,3-galactosyltransferase	2.4.1.-	Human	[81]
UDP-GlcNAc:GlcNAcβ1-6 (GlcNAc β1-2)Manα-R (GlcNAc to Man)β 4-GlcNAc-transferase	2.4.1.-	Hen oviduct membranes	[82]
Mucin β 6N-acetylglucosaminyltransferase	2.4.1.-	Cattle	[83]
UDP-N-Acetylglucosamine: Gal β 1-4Glc(NAc)β 1-3 N-acetylglucosaminyltransferase	2.4.1.-	Rat	[69]
UDP-Galactose:2-acetamido-2-deoxy-D-glucose 3 β-galactosyltransferase	2.4.1.-	Pig	[84]
Lactose β-1,3-N-acetylglucosaminyltransferase	2.4.1.-	Human	[61]
UDP-Gal:Gal β (1-4)Glc (or GlcNAc)(α1-3)-galactosyltransferase	2.4.1.-	Bovine colostrum	[85]
UDP-GlcNAc:Gal β 1-4Glc (NAc)β-1,3-N-acetylglucosaminyltransferase	2.4.1.-	Calf	[72]
UDP-GalNAc:GlcNAc β-R β 1-4 N-acetylgalactosaminyltransferase	2.4.1.-	Snail	[86]
UDP-N-Acetylglucosamine polypeptide-N-acetylglucosaminyltransferase	2.4.1.-	*Trypanosoma cruz*	[87]

TABLE 1

Continued

Enzyme	EC number	Source	Ref.
α-Galactosyltransferase	2.4.1.–	*Trypanosoma brucei*	[88]
Lactose β-(1,3)N-acetylglucosaminyltransferase	2.4.1.–	Mammals	[89]
α-1,3-Fucosyltransferase	2.4.1.–	*Schistosoma mansoni*	[90]
UDP-Gal:glucosylceramide β-1,4-galactosyltransferase	2.4.1.–	Rat brain	[91]
N-Acetyllactosamide β1 → 3 and β1 → 6 acetylglycosaminyltransferase	2.4.1.–	Calf thymus	[92]
α-1,3-D-UDP-GlcNAc-GlcNAc-β-1,6(GlcNAc-β-1-2)-Man-α-1-]R-[GlcNAc to Man]β-1 → 4N-acetylglucosaminyltransferase VI	2.4.1.–	Fish, birds	[80]
Hyaluronic acid synthase	2.4.1.–	*Pasteurella multocida*	[93]
UDP-xylose protein xylosetranferase	2.4.2.26	Chicken	[94]
CMP-NeuAc:lactosylceramide (α2-3) sialyltransferase	2.4.99.–	Rat brain	[95]
Cob(I)alamin adenosyltransferase	2.5.1.17	*P. denitrificans*	[96]
Farnesyltranstransferase	2.5.1.29	*Penaeus japonicus*	[97]
β-Adrenergic receptor kinase	2.7.1.126	Bovine brain	[98,99]
ATP sulfurylase	2.7.7.4	*B. stearothermophilus*	[100]

Enzyme	EC number	Source	Ref.
CDP-ethanolamine: diacylglycerol ethanolaminephosphotransferase	2.7.8.1	Bovine liver	[101]
Phosphatidylserine synthase	2.7.8.8	*Bacillus subtilis*	[102]
Phosphatidyl inositol synthase	2.7.8.11	Bacteria, mammals	[103]
UDP-GlcNAc:dolichyl phosphate N-acetylglucosamine-1-phosphotransferase	2.7.8.15	Animals, plants	[104]
UDP-Galactose:N-acetylglucosaminyl(β1→4)-galactosyltransferase	2.7.8.18	Rat	[66,105]
UDP-GlcNAc:serine-protein N-acetylglucosamine-1-phosphotransferase	2.7.8._	*Dictyostelium discoideum*	[106]
GDP-Mannose:serine-protein 1-phosphotransferase	2.7.8._	*Leishmania mexicana*	[107]
Phosphoenolpyruvate synthase	2.7.9.2	*E. coli*	[108]
Histidine kinase	2.7.10._	Plants	[109]
Phenol sulfotransferase	2.8.2.1	Mammals	[110]
Tyrosine sulfotransferase	2.8.2.20	Mammals	[111]
Galactosyl-3-O-sulfotransferase	2.8.2._	Calf thyroid	[112]
IV³ β-Glucuronyl neolactotetraosylceramide sulfotransferase	2.8.2._	Rat brain	[113]
5'-Nucleotidase	3.1.3.5	Rat	[114]
Phosphorylase phosphatase	3.1.3.17	Rat	[115]
UDP-glucose hydrolase	3.1.3._	*Clostridium difficile*	[116]
2',3'-Cyclic nucleotide 2'-phosphodiesterase	3.1.4.16	*Bacillus No A-40-2*	[117]
N-Acetylglucosamine 6-sulfotransferase	3.1.6.14	Mammals	[118]
Bile acid sulfate sulfatase	3.1.6._	*P. testosteroni*	[119]

TABLE 1

Continued

Enzyme	EC number	Source	Ref.
Guanosine-3′,5′-bis(diphosphate) 3′-pyrophosphatase	3.1.7.2	*Streptococcus equisimilis*	[120]
Organophosphate acid anhydrase	3.1.8.1	*Rangia cuneata*	[121]
β-Alanylarginine hydrolase	3.1.13._	Rat brain	[122]
Ribonuclease	3.1._._	*Xenopus laevis (Caff)*	[123]
β-Galactosidase	3.2.1.23	*Tritrichomonas foetus*	[68]
		Saccharopolyspora rectivirgula	[124]
α-Dextrin endo-1,6-α-glucosidase	3.2.1.41	*T. caldophilus*	[125]
Maltose-6′-phosphate glucosidase	3.2.1.122	*Vibrio furnissi*	[126]
6-Phosphoryl-*O*-α-D-glucopyranosyl: phosphoglucohydrolase	3.2.1._	*B. subtilis*	[127]
Carboxymethylcellulase	3.2.1._	*Aspergillus niger,* *Cellulomonas biazotea*	[128]
Dinitrogen reductase–activating glycohydrolase	3.2.1._	*Rhodospirillium rubrum*	[129]
Fructanase	3.2.1._	*Saccarum officanarum*	[130]
Tryptophan aminopeptidase	3.4.11.17	*Trichosporon cutaneum*	[131]

Enzyme	EC number	Source	Reference
Aspartate aminopeptidase	3.4.11.7	Rat brain	[27]
Tripeptidase	3.4.11._	Lactococcus lactis	[132]
X-methyl-his dipeptidase	3.4.13.5	Rat brain	[133]
Dipeptidase	3.4.13.11	Ubiquitous	[134]
Met-X dipeptidase	3.4.13.12	E. coli	[135]
Cytosol-nonspecific dipeptidase	3.4.13.18	Animal	[136]
β-Alanylarginine hydrolase	3.4.13._	Rat brain	[122]
Processing protease	3.4._	Rat liver	[137]
Protein processing peptidase	3.4._	N. crassa	[138]
N-Carbamoyl-L-amino acid amidohydrolase	3.5.1._	Pseudomonas	[139]
β-Citryl-L-glutamate hydrolase	3.5.1._	Rat	[140]
L-Lysinamidase	3.5.1._	Cryptococcus laurenti	[141]
PsbY protein	3.5.1._	Plants	[142]
D-Hydantoinase	3.5._._	Microorganisms	[143]
Allantoate amidohydrolase	3.5.3.9	B. fastidiosus	[144]
Amidinoaspartase	3.5.3.14	P. putida	[145]
3-Guanidoinopropionate amidohydrolase	3.5.3._	P. aeruginosa	[146]
Cyanide-degrading enzyme	3.5._	B. pumilus	[147]
ADP-ribose pyrophosphatase	3.6.1._	Rat liver	[148]
UDP-sugar pyrophosphatase	3.6.1._	Rat retina	[149]
UDP-galactose pyrophosphatase	3.6.1._	Rat retina	[149]
Phosphoadenylsulfatase	3.6.2.2	Mammals	[150]
Oxalacetase	3.7.1.1	Streptomyces cattleya	[151]

TABLE 1

Continued

Enzyme	EC number	Source	Ref.
Oxaloacetate decarboxylase	4.1.1.3	*Corynebacterium glutamicum*	[152]
Imidazole glycerol phenol carboxylase	4.1.1.–	*Pseudomonas*	[153]
Threonine aldolase	4.1.2.5	*Arthrobacter*	[154]
Fructose-1,6-bisphosphate aldolase	4.1.2.13	Plants	[155]
3-Deoxy-D-arabinoheptulosonate-7-phosphate synthase	4.2.1.1	*S. cerevesiae, E. coli*	[156]
D-Threonine aldolase	4.1.2.–	Bacteria	[154]
o-Succinylbenzoic acid synthetase	4.1.99.–	*E. coli*	[157]
Altronic acid hydratase	4.2.1.7	*E. coli*	[158]
Mannonic acid hydratase	4.2.1.8	*E. coli*	[158]
6-Phosphogluconate dehydratase	4.2.1.12	*Zymomas mobilis*	[33]
Imidazoleglycerol phosphate dehydratase	4.2.1.19	*S. cerevisiae*	[159]
D-Glucosaminate dehydratase	4.2.1.26	*P. fluorescens*	[160]
S-Linalool synthase	4.2.1.–	Plants	[161]
2-Hydroxypentadienoic acid hydratase	4.2.1.–	*E. coli*	[162]
Poly(α-L-guluronate) lyase	4.2.2.–	*Corynebacterium*	[163]
Ureidoglycollate lyase	4.3.2.3	Legumes, liver	[164]

Guanylate cyclase	4.6.1.2	Animals	[165,166]
Cytidylate cyclase	4.6.1.6	Animals	[167]
Sabinene hydrate cyclase	4.6.1.9	*Majorana hortensis*	[168]
L-Arabinose isomerase	5.3.1.4	*E. coli*	[169]
D-Mannose isomerase	5.3.1.7	*P. cepacia*	[170]
L-Rhamnose isomerase	5.3.1.14	*Pseudomonas*	[171]
D-Ribose isomerase	5.3.1.20	Bacteria	[172]
Isopentenyldiphosphate δ-isomerase	5.3.3.2	Liver	[173]
Phosphoglycerate phosphomutase	5.4.2.1	*Bacillus* spp.	[174]
Hexosephosphate mutase	5.4.2.–	*Sulfolobus solfataricus*	[175]
Dichloromuconate-lactonizing enzyme	5.5.1.11	*A. eutrophus*	[176]
(4S)-Limonene synthase	5.5.–	*Mentha × piperita*	[177]
Monoterpene cyclase	5.5.–	Plants	[178]
Phytoene synthetase	5.5.–	Plants	[179]
Phenylalanine-tRNA synthetase	6.1.1.20	Ubiquitous	[180]
γ-Glutamylmethylamide synthetase	6.3.4.12	*Methylophaga Sp AA-30*	[181]
Pyruvate carboxylase	6.4.1.1	Chicken liver	[183]
Acetyl-CoA carboxylase	6.4.1.2	Rat liver	[182]
Vitamin K–dependent carboxylase	6.4.–	Calf liver	[184]

structurally characterized. In addition to the copper binding site, the enzyme from pea [193], fenugreek seedlings [194], *Lathyrus odoratus*, *L. sativus* [195], and humans [196] but not from *Hansenula polymorpha* [197] or *Escherichia coli* [198] contains an Mn^{2+} ion. The role of the Mn^{2+} is not known; it is 33 Å from the copper site and so is unlikely to be involved in catalysis [194]. The Mn^{2+} is octahedrally coordinated to three aspartate carboxylates, the amide oxygens of isoleucine and phenylalanine residues, and a water molecule.

2.1.2. Cytochrome c Oxidase

Cytochrome c oxidase (CcO), EC 1.9.3.1, catalyzes the reduction of oxygen to water and pumps protons across the mitochondrial membrane. The number of subunits varies between 3 and 5 in bacteria, and there are up to 13 subunits in mammals. The functional core catalyzes both the oxygen reduction and the proton pumping. Bacterial CcO from *Paracoccus denitrificans* contains a number of redox-active metals, a heme a, a binuclear iron-copper center (heme a_3-Cu$_B$), and two copper ions in a binuclear Cu$_A$ center. Electrons from cytochrome c are transferred to the Cu$_A$ center, then to the heme a, and finally to the heme a_3-Cu$_B$ center where oxygen reduction takes place. In addition to the redox-active metals, CcO contains two non-redox-active divalent metal centers. In mitochondrial CcO these metals are Zn^{2+} and Mg^{2+} but in bacterial CcOs at least 20% of the Mg^{2+} can be replaced by Mn^{2+} and the other metal is Ca^{2+}. The function of these nonredox ions is not known, they may be structurally important but the Mg/Mn site lies directly between the Cu$_A$ and heme a_3 sites [199].

In the enzyme from *Paracoccus denitrificans* the Mn^{2+}/Mg^{2+} ion is bound to Glu-218 in subunit II and Asp-404 and His-403 from subunit I, and at least one and possibly three water molecules [200]. Asp-193 has been shown to have a role in binding Mn^{2+} although in the crystal it is not a ligand [201].

2.2. Dehydrogenases

Dehydrogenases catalyze the reduction of a substrate molecule with NAD^+ as the reducing coenzyme [202]. Most dehydrogenases share common structural features, their NAD binding domains and their folding topology [203], but a family of dehydrogenases has been recognized that does not contain this folding topology. Three members of this family—tartrate dehydrogenase, 3-isopropylmalate dehydrogenase (IPMDH), and isocitrate dehydrogenase (ICDH)—all require a divalent metal ion (Mg^{2+} or Mn^{2+}). Manganese redox chemistry is not involved in the dehydrogenation process, the metal ion probably serves to bind, orient, and activate the substrate. Tartrate dehydrogenase (Table 1) has not been structurally characterized but the other two enzymes are described below.

2.2.1. Isocitrate Dehydrogenase

ICDH catalyzes decarboxylation of isocitrate to α-ketoglutarate and CO_2 via an oxalosuccinate intermediate [204]. Mammalian tissues have two forms of the enzyme. The form found in the mitochondria, EC 1.1.1.41, requires Mn^{2+} or Mg^{2+} and NAD^+ as cofactors; the other form, EC 1.1.1.42, occurs in both the cytosol and the mitochondria, and requires Mg^{2+} and $NADP^+$ as cofactors.

EC 1.1.1.41 is regulated by phosphorylation of a serine residue; phosphorylation blocks entry of isocitrate to the active site [205]. A crystal structure of this enzyme with Mn^{2+} and isocitrate bound has been determined. Isocitrate and Mn^{2+} bind in a pocket between two major domains in which both subunits of the dimer participate. The Mn^{2+} is bound to Asp-283 and Asp-307, two water molecules, and the isocitrate via the carboxylate and an OH group [206].

2.2.2. Isopropylmalate Dehydrogenase

IPMDH, EC 1.1.1.85, catalyzes the third step of the biosynthesis of the amino acid leucine in microrganisms and plants [203]. The reaction involves a dehydrogenation and subsequent decarboxylation of *threo*-D-3-isopropylmalate to 2-oxoisocaproate with the reduction of NAD^+. The monomer of the *E. coli* enzyme requires Mn^{2+} and K^+ for optimum activity. Crystal structures of the enzymes from *Thermus thermophilus* [202], *E. coli* [207], *Thiobacillus ferrooxidans* [208], and *Salmonella typhimurium* [207] have been determined and the enzyme from *Sulfolobus* sp. strain 7 is under investigation [209]. Mn^{2+} ion bound to the *E. coli* enzyme is coordinated to three aspartate residues, two waters, and a sulfate ion. Sulfate is thought to be bound at the position occupied by the substrate, as in the homologous structure of ICDH the C1 carboxylate is bound in the equivalent position [207].

2.3. Peroxidases

2.3.1. Chloroperoxidase

Chloroperoxidase, EC 1.11.1.10, catalyzes the halogenation of the natural product caldariomycin.

$$RH + H_2O_2 + Cl^- \longrightarrow R\text{-}Cl + 2H_2O \tag{1}$$

Although the primary function of chloroperoxidase is chlorination, it also exhibits peroxidase, catalase, and cytochrome P450-like activities. Chloroperoxidase contains a heme group and the iron of the heme is bound to Cys-29. EPR, X-ray fluorescence studies, and the crystal structure of the enzyme from the fungus *Caldariomyces fumago* indicate the presence of Mn^{2+} ions. Mn^{2+} is coordinated by a heme propionate, Glu-104, His-105, Ser-108, and a water molecule. The location of the Mn^{2+} with respect to the heme is similar to that of the Mn^{2+} in manganese-dependent peroxidase (cf. Chap. 17) but the metal coordination sphere is different. The role of the Mn^{2+} in chloroperoxidase is not known, catalytic activity is not altered by the presence or absence of Mn^{2+} [210].

3. TRANSFERASES

Mn^{2+} is involved in many different types of transferase reactions and particularly important reactions involve the transfer of glycosyl groups, the transfer of phosphorus-containing substrates (kinases), DNA and RNA polymerases, and sulfotransferases involved in the biosynthesis of sialic acid groups.

3.1. Kinases

Kinases transfer a phosphate group from a nucleoside triphosphate (ATP or GTP) to a tyrosine, serine, threonine, or histidine residue of proteins or to the OH group of a sugar. The presence of these phosphate groups serves a regulatory function. An Mg^{2+}-nucleotide complex is usually required as the substrate but there are claims in the literature for Mn^{2+}-activated and Mg^{2+}-inactive kinases [211–215] and there are reports of crystal structures with Mn^{2+} bound to a kinase. These structural studies are listed in Table 2 but as most of these kinases are probably activated by Mg^{2+} in vivo they will not be described in detail. Kinases in which it is established that Mn^{2+} participates in vivo are described below.

Reports of Mg^{2+} and Mn^{2+} interacting in a synergistic fashion with kinases have been made with phosphatidylinositol kinase [216], pyruvate kinase (which also requires a monovalent cation) [217], phosphoenolpyruvate kinase [218], and phosphorylase kinase [219]. In the latter case a dinuclear metal binding site has been demonstrated crystallographically.

The basic architecture of the kinase domain and the essential features of substrate recognition have been identified from the studies listed in Table 2 and from other structures of the Mg^{2+}-substituted enzymes. The catalytic core is bilobal; one lobe is a β sheet, the other an

TABLE 2

Structurally Characterized Kinases with Mn^{2+} Bound

Enzyme	EC number	Organism	Ref.
Glycerol kinase	2.7.1.30	*E. coli*	[220]
cAMP-dependent protein kinase	2.7.1.37	Mouse Pig	[221,222] [223]
Phosphorylase kinase	2.7.1.38	Rabbit muscle	[224]
Pyruvate kinase	2.7.1.40	Rabbit muscle	[225]
Acetate kinase	2.7.2.1	*Methanosarcina thermophila*	[226]
Phosphoglycerate kinase	2.7.2.3	Pig muscle Yeast	[227] [228]
Adenylate kinase	2.7.4.3	*B. stearothermophilus*	[229]
Nucleoside diphosphate kinase	2.7.4.6	*Myxococcus xanthus*	[230]

α helix. These are joined by a segment of the polypeptide chain. The substrates bind in a cleft between the two lobes, the nucleotide interacting with the β-sheet lobe and the substrate with the α-helix lobe. The M^{2+} ion is usually coordinated to the β- and γ-phosphoryl groups of the ATP, GTP, or their analogs, but binding to all three phosphates has been observed. Two, three or four water molecules and oxygen atoms from side chains of threonine, serine, aspartic acid, or glutamic acid complete the metal coordination sphere. In some cases no bonds between metal ion and protein are observed [227].

3.1.1. Phosphorylase Kinase

Phosphorylase kinase, EC 2.7.1.38, one of the largest and most complex of the protein kinases, is hexadecameric with a subunit stoichiometry of $(\alpha\beta\gamma\delta)_4$ and an M_r of 1.3×10^6 Da. The γ subunit is the catalytic center. The physiological substrate is glycogen phosphorylase although other substrates have been identified. Phosphorylase kinase has dual specificity; Mg^{2+} causes seryl phosphorylation but Mn^{2+} activates tyrosine phosphorylation. Structural studies of the catalytic core of the γ subunit of rabbit muscle phosphorylase kinase and the binary complex with Mn^{2+}/β,γ-imidoadenosine 5'-triphosphate (AMPPNP) have been reported. Phosphorylase kinase has a dinuclear metal binding site, one Mn^{2+} binds the β- and γ-phosphate oxygens of AMPPNP, two carboxylate oxygens of Asp-167, and two water molecules, and the other Mn^{2+} binds the α- and γ-phosphate oxygens of AMPPNP, the bridging NH between the β- and γ-phosphates of this substrate, the amide oxygen of Asn-154, a carboxylate oxygen of Asp-167, and a water molecule [224]. This AMPPNP binding mode is similar to the carbamoyl phosphate synthesis domain in carbamoyl phosphate synthetase discussed in Sec. 7.2.

3.1.2. Pyruvate Kinase

Pyruvate kinase, EC 2.7.1.40, catalyzes the final step in glycolysis:

Phosphoenolpyruvate + MgADP + H^+ $\longrightarrow$ pyruvate + MgATP (2)

The reaction occurs in two stages, the β-phosphoryl oxygen of MgADP attacks phosphoenolpyruvate forming enolpyruvate and MgATP, and then the enolpyruvate is converted to pyruvate. The enzyme is allosteric and the activity is controlled by a dramatic conformational change in going from the T (inactive) state to the R (active) state [231]. Pyruvate kinase requires a divalent metal ion, a divalent metal nucleotide complex, and K^+ for activity. Mg^{2+} is commonly assumed to be the divalent metal ion used in vivo but pyruvate kinase from *Corynebacterium glutamicum* is activated by Mn^{2+} or Co^{2+} [232], and it has been suggested that intertidal mollusca change the metal cofactor in this enzyme from Mg^{2+} to Mn^{2+} as the mollusc goes from high-tide to low-tide conditions [233]. Crystal structures of the Mn^{2+}-substituted form of the enzyme, in the absence of nucleotide, from rabbit muscle shows that Mn^{2+} is bound to Glu-271 and Asp-295 and the carboxylate oxygen and carbonyl oxygen of the substrate. Mg^{2+} binds to the protein through the same carboxylate side chains. K^+ is located within a well-defined pocket of four oxygen ligands contributed by the carbonyl oxygen of Thr-113, the OH of Ser-76, and O side chain atoms of Asn-74 and Asp-112 [225].

Structures have also been determined with various substrates present. With ATP the γ-phosphate of ATP coordinates to Mg^{2+} and to the K^+ ion. An Mg^{2+}-coordinated oxalate oxygen in an Mg^{2+}oxalate-MgATP complex lies 3.0 Å from γ-phosphate of ATP, and this oxygen is positioned for an attack on the phosphorus [234,235]. In a structure with L-phospholactate present the subunits adopt different conformations within the same crystal. In the open subunits Mg^{2+} is coordinated to Glu-271 and Asp-295 but is not bound to L-phospholactate, which is bound to K^+. When the subunit is in the closed conformation the metal ion is coordinated to Glu-271 and Asp-295 and to the carboxylate oxygen, the bridging ester oxygen, and a nonbridging phosphoryl oxygen of L-phospholactate. L-Phospholactate is still bound to K^+. The Mg^{2+} ion moves about 3.8 Å upon subunit closure [235]. Closure of the active-site cleft involves a rotation of 41° by the one domain relative to the second domain and α carbons of residues in the first domain undergo movements of up to 17.8 Å upon cleft closure.

3.2. DNA and RNA Polymerases

RNA and DNA polymerases are responsible for the transmission of genetic information. These enzymes often contain more than one functional active site. For example, *E. coli* DNA polymerase catalyzes three separate functions, all divalent metal ion-dependent. It has 3',5'-exonuclease, 5',3'-DNA nuclease, and DNA polymerase activity. The 3',5'-exonuclease active site is separated by 33 Å from the polymerase active site and the 5',3'-nuclease active site is separated by some 70 Å from the polymerase active site in the enzyme from *T. aquaticus* [236]. It seems likely that two divalent metal ions are required at each active site. It is not clear as to whether RNA polymerase uses one or two metal ions in catalysis. The structure and function of DNA polymerases have been reviewed recently [237].

3.3. Sugar Transferases

Proteins and lipids are modified by the attachment of carbohydrate groups and further sugar residues can then be added to form complex oligosaccharide structures. These glysolated molecules have a wide range of roles, including determination of membrane and cell wall structure, recognition elements in cell-cell interactions, and the determination of protein structure and folding. Many different enzymes catalyze the glysolation reactions, e.g., 12 different groups and 5 families of galactosyltransferases and twenty-seven families of glycosyltransferases have been recognized on the basis of sequence comparisons [238–240]. In many cases these enzymes catalyze the transfer of a nucleotide sugar residue to an hydroxyl group on the target protein, lipid, or carbohydrate although some use lipid-based dolichol phosphate sugars. Many of these enzymes require divalent metal ions, frequently Mn^{2+}, cf. Table 1, EC 2.4.1._. Little is known about the nature of the metal ion binding site in these enzymes. The concentration of Mn^{2+} required to give maximum activity with these enzymes is usually >1 mM and such a high concentration would normally exclude them from consideration as Mn^{2+}-activated enzymes. However, Mn^{2+} is often the only divalent metal ion tested that shows activity. Mn^{2+} is considered to be the endogenous metal ion in asparagine-linked glycosylation [64], and it has been shown that depletion of Mn^{2+} inhibits both the processing of N-linked oligosaccharides and the addition of oligosaccharides to serine and threonine residues in mammalian cells [241].

Structures of sugar transferases containing Mn^{2+} have been reported, hypoxanthineguanidine phosphoribosyltransferase, EC 2.4.2.8,

from *Trypanosoma cruzi* [242], quinolinic acid phosphoribosyltransferase, EC 2.4.2.19, from *Mycobacterium tuberculosis* [243], and glutamine phosphoribosylpyrophosphate amidotransferase (PRTase), EC
2.4.2.14, from *E. coli* [244]. The Mn^{2+} binding sites (illustrated in Fig. 1)
in the first two of these enzymes are almost identical. One Mn^{2+} is
coordinated by two ribose hydroxyl groups, two pyrophosphate oxygens,
and two water molecules, whereas the other Mn^{2+} is bound to four
water molecules (or three waters and a carboxylate) and α- and β-
pyrophosphate oxygens.

The structure of PRTase contains two domains. One domain has
the phosphoribosylpyrophosphate binding site, the other contains the
active site for glutamine hydrolysis. These active sites are connected by
a solvent inaccessible 20-Å-long channel. Mn^{2+} in the PRTase active
site is octahedrally coordinated to two peptide C=O groups (Pro-302
and Glu-303), to two phosphate oxygens, and to two OH moieties of the
substrate inhibitor 1α-pyrophosphoryl-2α-3α-dihydroxy-4β-cyclopen-
tanemethanol 5-phosphate. This structure also contains an Mn^{2+} located at a lattice contact; this Mn^{2+} is bound to Glu-449 and Asp-471
from a symmetry equivalent molecule, and four water molecules [244].

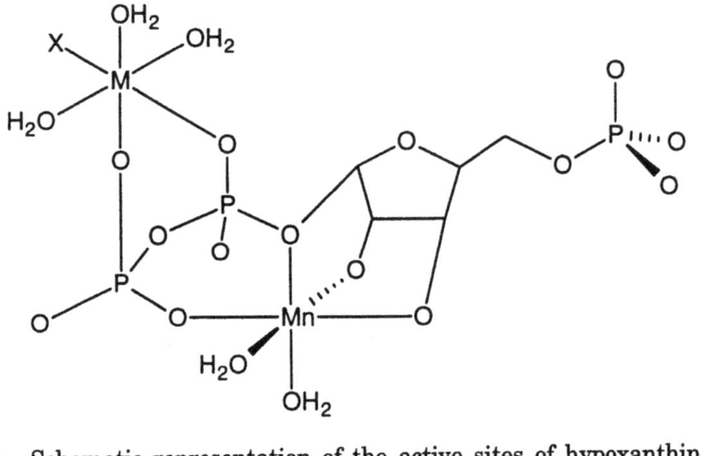

FIG. 1. Schematic representation of the active sites of hypoxanthine guanidine phosphoribosyltransferase from *Trypanosoma cruzi* and quinolinic acid
phosphoribosyltransferase from *Mycobacterium tuberculosis*. In the latter enzyme X is a water molecule and in the former enzyme X is an Asp residue.

3.4. Sulfatases

Cytosolic sulfotransferases of mammalian cells catalyze the transfer of a sulfonate group from 3'-phosphoadenosine 5'-phosphosulfate (PAPS) to a sugar [112], to a lipid [113], to amino acid side chains or an amino group [245]. Human monoamine phenol sulfotransferase is Mn^{2+}-dependent. Sequence comparisons have established that sulfotransferases contain a highly conserved region that is similar to a loop found in many ATP- and GTP-binding proteins and this region is thought to be involved in the binding of PAPS [111]. Crystallographic analysis has revealed considerable structural similarity between arylsulfatases and alkaline phosphatases and alkaline phosphatase has weak sulfatase activity. However, the structurally characterized arylsulfatases [246, 247] have only one metal ion (Mg^{2+} or Ca^{2+}) in the active site, whereas the alkaline phosphatase from *E. coli* has two Zn^{2+} and one Mg^{2+} in close proximity to the phosphoryl group [248,249].

3.5. Adenosyl Transferases

Eukaryotic mRNA is capped at its 5' end by a 7-methyl-GMP moiety, which probably protects the mRNA from digestion. Addition of this 7-methyl-GMP cap is catalyzed by three enzymes; one to remove the 5'-terminal phosphate, the second to form the guanylate derivative, and the third to methylate this derivative. This guanylate derivative is formed from GTP in a reaction that involves an enzyme–GMP adduct. The GMP moiety is then transferred to mRNA. Guanyl transfer reaction requires either Mg^{2+} or Mn^{2+}, which are equally effective. The structure of the capping enzyme, EC 2.7.7.50, from *Chlorella* virus PBCV-1 has been determined [250] and the enzyme has two domains with a cleft between them. There are two conformations of the enzyme in the crystal with GTP bound, one with an open cleft and the other with a closed cleft. Mn^{2+} binds to the closed conformer in the crystal but not to the open form and is bound to the α-phosphate of the nucleotide. The β- and γ-phosphates of GTP were not present in the cleft of the closed form and the α-phosphate was also bound to an active site lysine. These observations are consistent with the formation of a guanylated enzyme intermediate.

3.6. Aryl,Alkyl Transferases

A number of Mn^{2+}- or Mg^{2+}-activated enzymes capable of transferring alkyl and aryl groups are known. The most important of these are the prenyltransferases, reviewed by Ogura and Koyama [251]. Structurally characterized prenyltransferases are Mg^{2+} enzymes that contain three Mg^{2+} ions in the active site [252]. There is one reported structure of an Mn^{2+}-containing enzyme involved in such transferase reactions. Dihydropteroate synthase, EC 2.5.1.15, catalyzes the reaction of p-aminobenzoic acid with 7,8-dihydro-6-hydroxymethylpterin pyrophosphate to give 7,8-dihydropteroate and pyrophosphate. A structure of the enzyme from *Staphylococcus aureus* with hydroxymethylpterin pyrophosphate and Mn^{2+} bound has been determined. Mn^{2+} is bound to the side chain of Asn-11, a β-phosphate oxygen of hydroxymethylpterin pyrophosphate, and two water molecules [253].

The enzyme conferring resistance to the antibiotic fosfomycin, (1R,2S)-1,2-epoxypropylphosphonic acid, is a metalloglutathione transferase, EC 2.5.1.18, which catalyzes the addition of glutathionine to fosfomycin and contains a mononuclear Mn^{2+} center. Sequence alignments and mechanistic considerations suggest that the active site is similar to that in extradiol dioxygenases discussed in Sec. 2.2 [254].

3.6.1. Reverse Transcriptase

Reverse transcriptases, EC 2.7.7.49, are present in all retroviruses and couple DNA-directed and RNA-directed polymerase activities with a ribonuclease H activity to make a double-stranded DNA copy of the single-stranded RNA genome of the retrovirus. This DNA is then integrated into the host genome by the retroviral integrase. Reverse transcriptases usually require metal ions for their activity but only one structure at moderate resolution has been reported containing Mn^{2+}. The structure of the polymerase catalytic fragment (residues 10–278 of the total of 671) of Moloney murine leukemia virus reverse transcriptase has Mn^{2+} ion coordinated to Asp-225 and Asp-224 and possibly two water molecules although the metal site is anisotropically disordered [255].

4. HYDROLASES

Mn^{2+}-activated enzymes are extremely important catalysts of hydrolysis reactions. They are able to hydrolyze esters, glycosidases, peptide and other linear or cyclic $C-N$ bonds, $C-C$ bonds, and acid anhydrides. The best characterized Mn^{2+}-activated hydrolases are the phosphatases, and specific peptidase and protease systems and a number of structurally characterized enzymes are described below.

4.1. Peptide Bonds

4.1.1. Carboxypeptidases

Carboxypeptidases, EC 3.17.4._, which cleave the peptide bond at the carboxylate end of a polypeptide chain are usually Zn^{2+}-containing enzymes but Mn^{2+}-substituted carboxypeptidases are active. Mn^{2+} is bound to procarboxypeptidase B in the rat pancreas [256]. Carboxypeptidase P from pig kidneys [257] and a dipeptidyl carboxypeptidase from the tick *Ixodes scapularis* are activated by Mn^{2+} [258]. Structurally characterized carboxypeptidases have active sites that contain a dinuclear five-coordinate Zn^{2+} center and the Mn-substituted form of carboxypeptidase A also has five-coordinate Mn^{2+} bound to the same ligands as the Zn^{2+} [259,260].

4.1.2. Aminopeptidases

Aminopeptidases catalyze the removal of an amino acid from the N-terminal end of a peptide chain. The best characterized aminopeptidase is the leucine aminopeptidase from bovine lens, which has a dinuclear Zn^{2+} active site. Both binding sites must be occupied for activity to occur; one site must be occupied by Zn^{2+}, but if the other site is occupied by Mn^{2+} there is a significant increase in activity. Leucine aminopeptidases from *E. coli* and *S. typhimurium* have substantial sequence homology with the bovine lens enzyme and the metal-binding residues of the bovine enzyme are conserved. These enzymes are reported to require Mn^{2+} for activity and are inhibited by Zn^{2+} [261]. A number of other aminopeptidases from, for example, *Lactobacillus sake* [262], *Fascolia hepatica* [263], and rat brain [27] are also activated by Mn^{2+}. In addition, di- and tripeptidases from lactobacilli are activated by Mn^{2+} [264,265].

Structurally characterized aminopeptidases have dinuclear metal binding sites. Both bovine lens aminopeptidase, EC 3.4.11.1 [266–268], and the aminopeptidase, EC 3.4.11._, from *Aeromonas proteolytica* [269], have a dinuclear Zn^{2+} active site. Methionine aminopeptidase, EC 3.4.11.18, from *E. coli* [270], and *Pyrococcus furiosus* [271] contains a dinuclear Co^{2+} active site. The proline-specific enzyme, aminopeptidase P, EC 3.4.11.9, from *E. coli* [272,273] has a dinuclear Mn^{2+} active site.

The structure of this tetrameric enzyme from *E. coli* has been determined for a dipeptide-inhibited complex, and for a low-pH, inactive form [272]. Aminopeptidase P has also been investigated using EPR, EXAFS, and XANES [273]. The monomer folds into two domains. The active site, in the C-terminal domain, contains a dinuclear manganese center (the Mn–Mn distance is 3.3 Å). The structure of the active site is shown in Fig. 2. A bridging H_2O or OH^- apparently acts as the

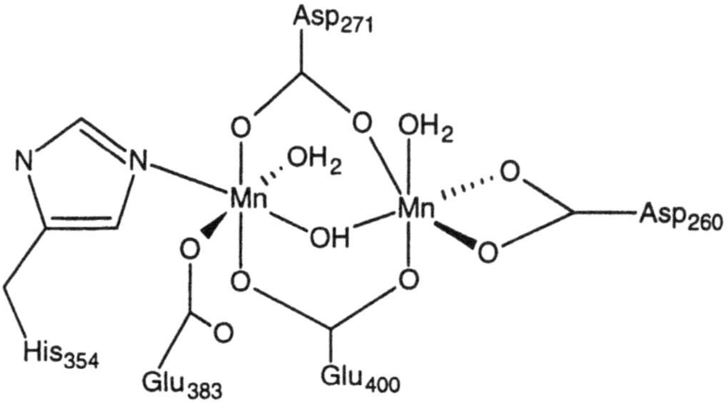

FIG. 2. Schematic representation of the dinuclear active site of aminopeptidase P from *E. coli*.

nucleophile in the attack on the scissile peptide bond of the substrate. In the inactive low-pH form of the enzyme the OH^- group is replaced by a monodentate acetate.

4.1.3. p21ras

p21ras, EC 3.6.1.__, plays a central role in the control of cell proliferation and differentiation. It binds effector molecules such as protein kinase or c-Raf and then a growth signal is transmitted. In the presence of a divalent metal ion Ras proteins have an intrinsic GTPase activity, yielding GDP and PO_4^{3-} which terminates the growth signal. The hydrolysis reaction is thought to involve conversion of a water molecule to an OH^- by the γ-phosphate of the protein-bound GTP. This OH^- subsequently attacks the protonated γ-phosphate resulting in hydrolysis. It has been shown that the GTPase reaction rate is higher in the presence of Mn^{2+} than Mg^{2+}. Mn^{2+} has been extensively used as a probe in EPR and ESEEM experiments to study the metal binding site in p21ras [259,274–276]. Crystal structures of the Mn^{2+}- and Mg^{2+}-substituted forms of a mutant protein show identical metal ion coordination. In the structure with GTP bound M^{2+} is coordinated to Ser-17 and Thr-35, the β- and γ-phosphates of the GTP, and two water molecules, whereas in the GDP form the coordination is to Ser-17, a β-phosphate oxygen, and four water molecules. It is believed that the mechanism of GTP hydrolysis is identical for the two metal forms. Increased rates observed with Mn^{2+} are attributed to Mn^{2+} causing an increase in the pK_a of the γ-phosphate group [20]. This effect would seem to be general for reactions of this type as increased rates with Mn^{2+}-substituted enzymes have been observed with other GTP-binding proteins Ran, Rap1A, and EF-Tu.

4.2. Phosphatases

Phosphatases remove phosphate residues from phosphorylated proteins and sugars. Manganese-activated phosphatases, protein phosphatase, EC 3.1.3.16, alkaline phosphatase, EC 3.1.3.1, purple acid phosphatase, EC 3.1.3.2, inorganic pyrophosphatase, EC 3.6.1.1, phosphodiesterases, EC 3.1.4.16, and phosphotriesterases, EC 3.1.8.1, are considered separately in Chap. 10 [277]. Sugar phosphatases are discussed below.

4.2.1. Inositol Monophosphatase

Inositol monophosphatase, EC 3.1.3.25, an Mg^{2+}-dependent enzyme (Mn^{2+} and Zn^{2+} also support activity), is a crucial enzyme in the recycling of inositol from the inositol pyrophosphate second messengers. A number of crystal structures are available including one containing three Mn^{2+} ions in the active site, illustrated in Fig. 3 [278]. It is believed, however, that one of these Mn^{2+} ions is not involved in the mechanism of enzyme action as it is readily displaced by the addition of PO_4^{3-}. The two functional Mn^{2+} ions are 3.9 Å apart and are bridged by Asp-90; in addition, the five-coordinate Mn^{2+} ion is bound to Glu-70, Thr-95, the backbone oxygen of Ile-92, and a water molecule. The other ion is four-coordinate and is bound to Asp-90, Asp-220, and Asp-93 and a Cl^- or a phosphate oxygen. Both metal ions are believed to bind the sugar phosphate [279].

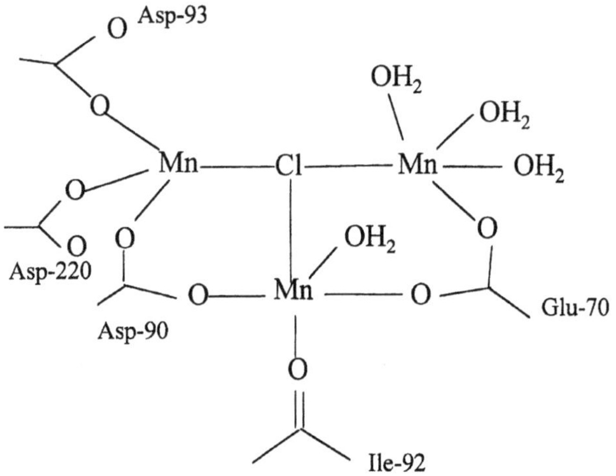

FIG. 3.   Schematic representation of the trinuclear metal binding site in inositol monophosphatase.

4.2.2. *Fructose-1,6-bisphosphatase*

Fructose-1,6-bisphosphatase, EC 3.1.3.11, converts the α form of D-fructose-1,6-bisphosphate to D-fructose-6-phosphate and PO_4^{3-}, is usually tetrameric, and requires two divalent metal ions per subunit. There is evidence that the enzymes from rat and fish brains are Mn^{2+}-activated in vivo [280]. The enzyme is allosterically regulated and occurs in two forms (R and T forms). The structural changes in going from the R form to the T form of the enzyme involve a 16° rotation of the upper dimer with respect to the lower dimer. Crystallographic studies have been performed on Mn^{2+}-containing forms of the enzymes from pig kidney [281,282], mutant forms of the pig kidney enzyme [283,284], and the spinach chloroplast enzyme [285]. In the spinach chloroplast Mn–FBP enzyme complex with the α-analog inhibitor 2,5-anhydro-D-glucitol-1,6-bisphosphate, AhG-1,6-P_2, the two Mn^{2+} are separated by 4.2 Å and are bridged by Glu-97 and Asp-118. Mn1 is also bound to Asp-121, Glu-280, and an O atom of the phosphate of the inhibitor. Mn2 is coordinated to the bridging groups and also bound to Glu-98 and the carbonyl O of Leu-120. Both metals are apparently five-coordinate. In the absence of metal ions the substrate binds in a similar way to the inhibitor AhG-1,6-P_2 so the inhibitor is thought to be a good model for the substrate binding. In the R form, Mn1 is coordinated to the same residues as in the T form but is also bound to a phosphate oxygen of the substrate analog. Mn2 is coordinated to the same groups in both R and T forms. Changes in the coordination of Mn1 causes the metal ion to move about 1.6 Å.

4.3. Esterases

4.3.1. *Nucleases*

Enzymes that participate in the biochemistry of nucleic acids usually require divalent metal ions for activity. The divalent metal ion is most frequently Mg^{2+} and the activation of such enzymes by metal ions has been reviewed [286]. Nucleases are enzymes that catalyze the hydrolysis of polynucleotide chains, endonucleases catalyze the hydrolysis of linkages within the polynucleotide chain, and exonucleases catalyze the hydrolysis from one end of the chain.

4.3.2. Endonucleases

Type II restriction endonucleases require divalent metal ions to cleave both DNA strands in both blunt and sticky end fashion to yield 5'-phosphate and 3'-hydroxyl groups as products. Mg^{2+} is the normal metal ion and cleavage is highly specific with Mg^{2+}. Substitution of Mg^{2+} by Mn^{2+} results in faster rates; however, cleavage can also occur at sites that differ from the native site by one base pair. These enzymes are discussed in more detail in Chap. 11 [287].

4.3.3. Exonucleases

The 5'-exonucleases, EC 3.1.4.1, remove nucleotides from the 5' end of nucleic acid molecules and are essential for DNA replication and repair. A structure of exonuclease III of *E. coli* has been determined in its native form and with Mn^{2+} and dCMP. This enzyme is multifunctional, it also exhibits 3'-repair diesterase, $3' \rightarrow 5'$ exonuclease, 3'-phosphomonoesterase, and ribonuclease activities. The metal nucleotide complex is bound at the bottom of a groove formed by two β sheets and Mn^{2+} is bound to Glu-34 and a nucleotide phosphate oxygen [21]. It is suggested that the role of the metal ion is to polarize the P-O bond, orient the phosphate group for attack, and stabilize the transition state. This active site structure is similar to that of DNase I and RNase H.

The crystal structure of the phage T5 5'-exonuclease that binds both single- and double-stranded linear DNA has also been determined; the active site is in a concave surface at the base of three α helices that form an arch. A mechanism consistent with a mechanism in which single-stranded DNA could slide through the arch has been suggested. The active site contains aspartate residues and two Mn^{2+} binding sites separated by 8.1 Å, but details are currently not available [288].

4.4. Integrases

Retroviral integrases catalyze the insertion of viral DNA into the host DNA. Retroviral integrases contain two metal binding domains. The N-terminal domain includes a zinc finger motif, whereas the central catalytic core domain includes a divalent metal cofactor required for enzymatic activity. The integration reaction occurs in two distinct steps: a specific endonucleolytic cleavage step called "processing," and a polynucleotide transfer or "joining" step [289]. Metal preference for in vitro activity of avian viral S integrase is $Mn^{2+} > Mg^{2+}$ and the coordination sphere of both metals are the same, i.e., two aspartate residues (Asp-64, Asp-121) and four water molecules [290].

4.5. Arginase and Related Enzymes

The enzymes of EC class 3.5.3._ catalyze hydrolysis of guanidinocarboxylic acids to the corresponding ω-amino acid and urea. Arginase, EC 3.5.3.1, a dimanganese enzyme that catalyzes the hydrolysis of L-arginine to urea and L-ornithine, is discussed in detail in Chap. 13 [291]. Enzymes that catalyze similar reactions are dimethylarginase, EC 3.5.3.18, which has been shown to be a Zn^{2+}-dependent enzyme in which the Zn^{2+} plays a structural role [292]; and arginine deiminase, EC 3.5.3.6, which converts L-arginine to L-citrulline and NH_3 which is activated by Mn^{2+} [293]. Some microrganisms do not use the arginase pathway for arginine metabolism but utilize an arginine decarboxylation pathway. Agmatinase, EC 3.5.3.11, which catalyzes the second step in this pathway and formiminoglutamase, EC 3.5.3.8, which hydrolyzes N-formiminoglutamate to glutamate and formamide, have considerable sequence homology with arginase and the metal ligands of arginase are conserved [294]. Other enzymes in this class from *Pseudomonas* species, guanidinoacetase, EC 3.5.3.2 [295], guanidinopropionase, EC 3.5.3.17 [296], guanidinobutyrase, EC 3.5.3.7 [297] and diguanidinobutanase, EC 3.5.3.20 [298], are all activated by Mn^{2+} but structural and sequence data are not available.

5. LYASES

5.1. Carboxykinases and Dehydratases

5.1.1. Phosphoenolpyruvate Carboxykinase

Phosphoenolpyruvate carboxykinases (PCKs) catalyze the reaction:

$$\text{Oxaloacetate} + \text{ATP/GTP} \leftrightarrow \text{phosphoenolpyruvate} + CO_2 + \text{ADP/GDP} \tag{3}$$

This reaction requires either GTP, EC 4.1.1.32, or ATP, EC 4.1.1.49, as the phosphoryl donor and *both* Mn^{2+} and Mg^{2+} cations as cofactors; the Mg^{2+} binds as a nucleoside triphosphate (NTP) complex and Mn^{2+} is bound to the protein. Crystal structures of the *E. coli* PCK enzyme [299], complexed with ATP-Mg^{2+}-oxalate, and with ATP-Mg^{2+}-Mn^{2+}-pyruvate, have been determined [300,301]. When Mg-NTP binds, PCK undergoes domain closure with a 20° rotation of the two domains toward one another, trapping substrates and excluding solvent from the active site. Mg^{2+} and Mn^{2+} are then separated by 5.2 Å. Mg^{2+} is bound by the β- and γ-phosphoryl groups of ATP, three water molecules, and Thr-255. Mn^{2+} is bound to two water molecules, the γ-phosphoryl group of ATP, one oxygen from Asp-269, and two nitrogen donors from Lys-213 and His-232. These Mn^{2+} binding residues are strictly conserved in all ATP- and GTP-dependent PCKs. Pyruvate is bridged to the γ-phosphoryl group of ATP via the Mn^{2+} and two water molecules. No Mg^{2+} binding to the Mn^{2+} binding site is observed in the crystal structure of the ATP-Mg^{2+}-oxalate quaternary complex [302] or in the ATP-Mg^{2+}-pyruvate quaternary complex [301]. The second substrate oxaloacetate is bound in the second coordination sphere of Mn^{2+} hydrogen-bonded to coordinated water molecules.

5.1.2. *Enolase*

Enolase, EC 4.2.1.11, catalyzes the dehydration of 2-phospho-D-glycerate to yield phosphoenolpyruvate and requires a divalent metal ion for activity. Mg^{2+} is regarded as the natural cofactor but a variety of divalent metal ions confer lower activity. There are three metal ion binding sites per subunit. Site 1, the tightest metal ion binding site, is also called the conformational site. Metal binding at this site induces a conformational change that allows the binding of substrate. Following substrate binding a second metal ion binds at site II, the so-called catalytic site. At high metal ion concentrations, site III, an inhibitory site, can be occupied. Crystal structures of enolase in various forms have been reported, i.e., the apoenzyme [303,304], binary complexes of Zn^{2+}- enolase [305], ternary complexes of enolase-Mn^{2+}-phosphoglycolate [304], and quaternary complexes of enolase-2Mn^{2+}-phosphono-hydroxamate (PhAH) [306] and yeast enolase-2Mg^{2+}-PhAH [307,308]; yeast enolase-Mg^{2+}-F-PO_4^{3-} [309], an asymmetric dimer of enolase-2-phospho-D-glycerate/enolase-phosphoenolpyruvate [310,311]. The site I metal has been well characterized in these structural studies, but there is still doubt about the location of the site II metal and the site III binding site has not yet been identified. These difficulties are probably associated with the high (>2 M) concentration of $(NH_4)_2SO_4$ in the usual crystallization medium.

EPR and XAS experiments using Mn^{2+} have been used to characterize the metal binding sites [312,313]. These experiments indicate that two water molecules are bound to Mn^{2+} at site 1 in an enolase–Mn^{2+}–PhAH–Mg^{2+} complex early in the catalytic cycle but that one of the water molecules is lost on conversion to the final enolase–Mn^{2+}–PhAH–Mg^{2+} complex. Mn^{2+} at site II retains two water molecules throughout the cycle. Metal ions at sites I and II are separated by 4.2 Å in the Mg^{2+} structures and 8 Å in the Mn^{2+} structures. Mn^{2+} at site I coordinates to the protein via Asp-246, Asp-320, and Glu-295 (yeast numbering), and also to a water molecule. The carboxylate of the substrate/product is bound in different structures as a bidentate ligand (the metal is octahedral, Mn^{2+}, and Mg^{2+}) or as a monodentate (the metal is five-coordinate, Zn^{2+}, and Mg^{2+}). A carboxylate oxygen and a phosphate oxygen of the substrate/product are bound to the metal at site II; the other four ligands are two water molecules and the carbonyl and OH oxygens of Ser-39.

5.1.3.   D-Glucarate Dehydratase

This enzyme, EC 4.2.1.40, catalyzes the β elimination of water from D-glucarate to yield 5-keto-4-deoxy-D-glucarate. The enzyme from *P. putida* requires Mg^{2+} for activity but both the native enzyme and the Mn^{2+}-substituted enzymes have been structurally characterized [314]. This structure is homologous to both enolase and mandelate racemase and the metal ions are bound to Asp-241, Glu-261, and Asn-295.

5.2. Cyclases

Mn^{2+}-specific cyclases, cf. entries under EC 4.6.1._ in Table 1, have been discovered in specific tissues. One structure is available, that of adenylyl cyclase, EC 4.6.1.1, the enzyme responsible for the conversion of ATP to cAMP. Adenylyl cyclase contains two internally homologous cytoplasmic domains (C1 and C2) which when separated are inactive but catalysis is observed when they are combined. Two metal ions are thought to be required for catalysis; however, the structure contains only one Mg^{2+} ion bound to the C1 domain [315]. A second metal ion binding site (preferring Mn^{2+}) is contained within the C2 domain but its location is not known [316].

6. ISOMERASES

6.1. Keto-aldo Isomerases

Sugar isomerases require a metal ion for activity and use a variety of mechanisms to achieve the isomerization reaction. Xylose isomerase, EC 5.3.1.5, an industrially important enzyme that catalyzes the interconversion of xylose to xylulose via a hydride transfer mechanism, is discussed in detail in Chap. 12 [317].

In addition to xylose isomerase there are a number of Mn^{2+} activated keto-aldo isomerases listed in Table 1 and there are two metal-activated sugar isomerases for which X-ray structural information is available; phosphomannose isomerase (a Zn^{2+}-containing enzyme) [318] and L-fucose isomerase [319].

6.1.1.   L-Fucose Isomerase

L-Fucose isomerase, E.C 5.3.1.3, which catalyzes the isomerization of L-fucose to L-fuculose, Scheme 1 (and also isomerizes D-arabinose to

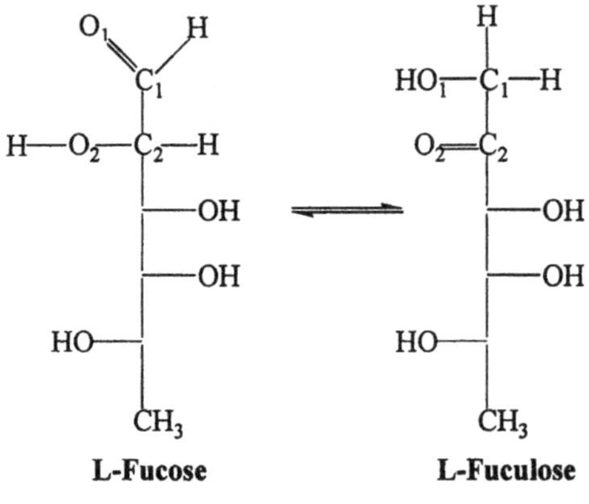

SCHEME 1

D-ribulose), has neither sequence nor structural similarity with other known aldose-ketose isomerases. An X-ray crystal structure of L-fucose isomerase from *E. coli* with an L-fucitol bound to the catalytic center shows that the active site is located between neighboring subunits within each trimer in a 20-Å-deep pocket, terminating at an Mn^{2+} ion. Mn^{2+} is bound to O1 and O2 of L-fucitol, the side chains of Glu-337 and Asp-361 (bidentate with very long bonds to both oxygens), His-528, and a water molecule [319]. It is believed that the fucose is initially bound in its cyclic form but is converted to the open chain conformation before aldose-ketose interconversion occurs. After ring opening, rotation around C2, with concurrent exchange of the O1 and O2 ligand positions at the metal ion, is required. During the isomerization two protons are transferred, one from O1 to O2 and the other from C2 to C1. Asp-361 and Glu-337 are positioned to assist in the transfer of the two protons via an ene-diol intermediate.

6.2. Cycloisomerases

Monoterpene synthases EC 5.5._._ convert allylic pyrophosphates such as farnesyl diphosphate and geranyl diphosphate to mono-, sesqui-, and diterpene natural products. The molecular biology and properties of these enzymes has been reviewed [320]. They require a divalent metal ion as cofactor (usually Mg^{2+} or Mn^{2+}) but with some species, e.g., conifers, Mg^{2+} is not effective [178]. It is of interest that the enzymes responsible for the formation of the allylic pyrophosphates, farnesyl diphosphate synthase, EC 2.5.1.1, 2.5.1.10, and geranyl diphosphate synthase, EC 2.5.1.1, are activated by Mn^{2+} [321,322] and that enzymes responsible for the production of other terpenoids, e.g., (*E*)-β-farnesene, EC 3.6.1._, are also activated by Mn^{2+} [323].

6.2.1. Enolase Superfamily of Enzymes

Members of this family of at least nine different enzymes catalyze very different overall reactions but are structurally similar. Each reaction is initiated by the abstraction of an α proton from a carboxylic acid, and the fate of the intermediate is then determined by the structure of the active site [324]. A number of these enzymes require Mn^{2+} for catalytic activity. The currently accepted mechanism involves the concerted enolization of a carboxylate group using both a general base to abstract the α proton and a general acid to protonate the keto group as it tautomerizes [325–327]. Despite the large difference in the pK_a values of the α protons and the protein bases the reaction rates are rapid, indicating that the enolate intermediate is significantly stabilized relative to the substrate, enabling the activation energy for α-proton abstraction to be lowered [324,325]. Crystal structures of five of these enzymes are now available; the structure of enolase and D-glucarate dehydratase has been described above.

6.2.2. Mandelate Racemase

Mandelate racemase, EC 5.1.2.2, catalyzes the interconversion of R and S enantiomers of mandelic acid [325,328] (Scheme 2). The crystal struc-

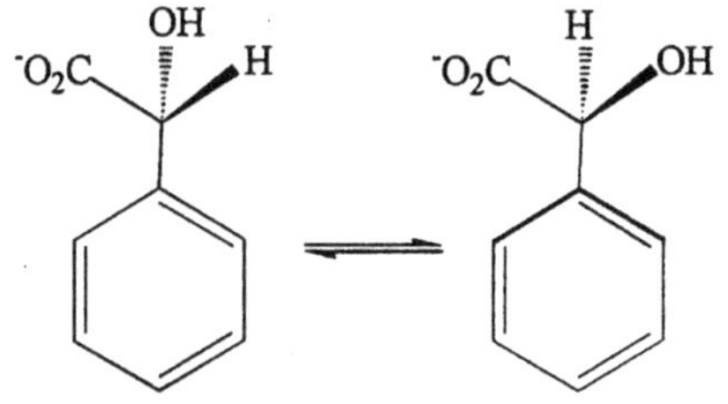

(R) mandelate   (S) mandelate

SCHEME 2

tures of wild-type and mutant forms of mandelate racemase from *P. putida* indicate that the enzyme is octameric, with each monomer composed of an N terminal $\alpha + \beta$ domain, a central α/β-barrel domain, and a C-terminal subdomain [329–333]. The active site is located between the two major domains at the C-terminal end of the β strands. Mandelate racemase requires a divalent metal ion, being most active with Mg^{2+}, but is also activated by Mn^{2+} [334]. The metal ion is ligated by the side chains of Asp-195, Glu-221, and Glu-247 and a sulfate ion which probably occupies the binding site for the carboxylate group of the substrate [329].

6.2.3. Muconate-Lactonizing Enzyme

Muconate-lactonizing enzyme (MLE), EC 5.5.1.1, catalyzes the cyclo-isomerization of *cis,cis*-muconate to muconolactone although the substrate specificity is quite wide [335,336]. Crystal structures of MLE from *P. putida*, mutant forms of this enzyme and of the apo enzyme from *E. coli* have been reported [337–339]. The protein folding is very similar to that of mandelate racemase and the active site, which prefers Mn^{2+} at the same location as in MR, octahedrally coordinated to the protein side chains Asp-198, Glu-224, Asp-249, and three water molecules.

6.2.4. Chloromuconate-Lactonizing Enzyme

Chloromuconate lactonizing enzyme (CMLE), EC 5.5.1.7, catalyzes the cycloisomerization of mono- and disubstituted chloromuconates to chloromuconolactones with concomitant dehalogenation to form diene lactones (Scheme 3) [335,340,341]. The crystal structure of CMLE from

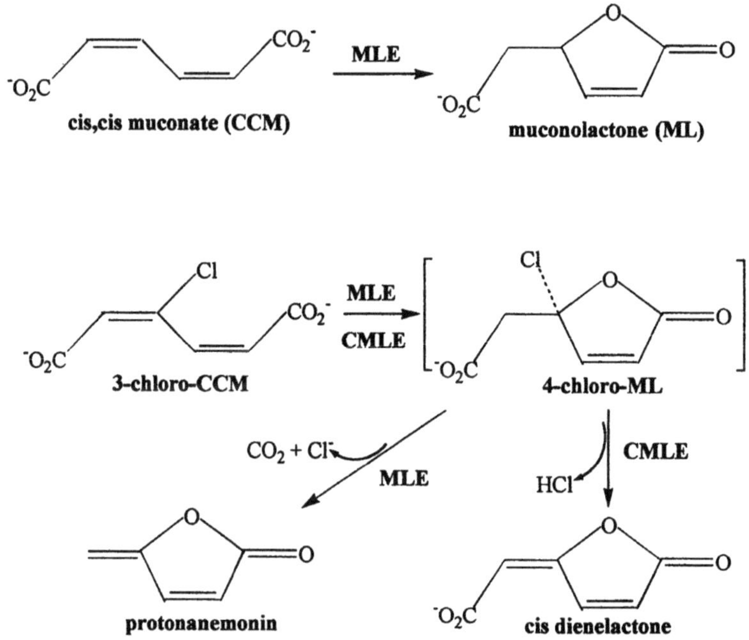

cis,cis muconate (CCM)   muconolactone (ML)

3-chloro-CCM   4-chloro-ML

protonanemonin   cis dienelactone

SCHEME 3

Alcaligenes eutrophus is structurally homologous and has 42% sequence identity with MLE from *P. putida*. The metal ion is coordinated to Asp-194, Glu-220, and Asp-245, and a chloride ion [341,342].

6.2.5. Comparison of MLE, MR, CMLE, D-Glucarate Dehydratase, and Enolase

MR, MLE, CMLE, D-glucarate dehydratase, and enolase are structurally homologous and their active sites are located at the C-terminal end of an α/β barrel. The primary sequences of MR and MLE are approximately 25% identical, whereas the sequences of MLE and yeast enolase are about 15% identical. Both MR and MLE require one divalent metal ion; enolase requires two ions, usually Mg^{2+}, to ensure catalytic activity [337]. The protein-metal ligands of these enzymes are similar, i.e., MR = Asp-195, Glu-221, Glu-247; MLE = Asp-198, Glu-224, Glu-249; enolase (high affinity site) = Asp-246, Glu-295, Asp-320; CMLE = Asp-194, Glu-220, and Asp-245; and D-glucarate dehydratase = Asp-241, Glu-261, and Asn-295. The catalytic bases used by MR are Lys-166 for (S)- and the His-297/Asp-270 dyad for (R)-mandelate racemization [329,333,343]. Enolase uses Lys-345 as its catalytic base [344] and the catalytic base in MLE is Lys-169, and this base apparently performs both the protonation and deprotonation steps [339]. Hence the position of the catalytic bases is conserved although the identities of the residues at those positions differ.

7. LIGASES

Enzymes that catalyze bond-forming reactions often require ATP as an energy source and the ATP is frequently bound to a divalent metal ion, typically Mg^{2+}. However, some of these enzymes are activated by MnATP. Structural determinations of a number of these enzymes reveal a similarity in the secondary structure at the ATP binding site that is also observed in enzymes such as P^{21} ras.

7.1. Glutamine Synthetase

Glutamine synthetase, EC 6.3.1.2, regulates the metabolism of cellular nitrogen and catalyzes the reaction shown in Scheme 4. A divalent metal ion is required for activity and Mn^{2+} or Mg^{2+} is the in vivo activator.

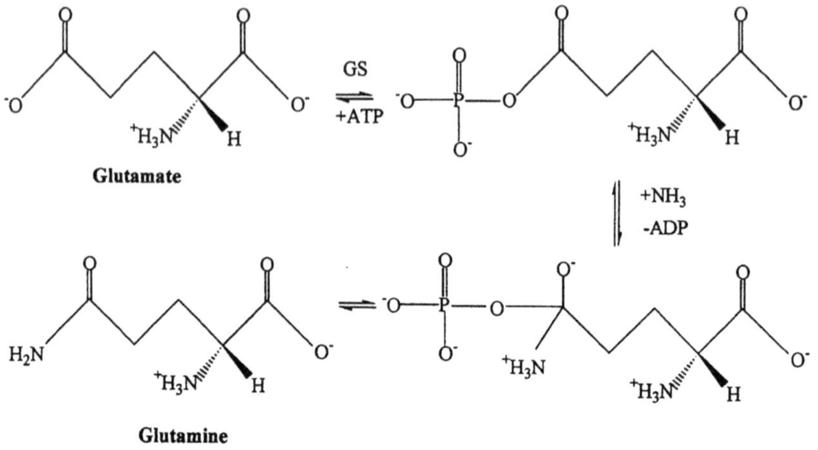

SCHEME 4

X-ray crystal structures of glutamine synthetase from both *S. typhimurium* and *E. coli* are very similar and consist of 12 identical subunits arranged in two face-to-face symmetric hexamers. The active sites are located at the interfaces between adjacent subunits of a hexamer, in funnel-shaped, open-ended cavities. These cavities are approximately 45 Å deep, 30 Å wide at one end, and 10 Å wide at the other. About halfway down this cavity the two catalytically essential divalent metal ions and their ligands form a shelf. Structures of both enzymes were determined with two Mn^{2+} ions bound to the active site, the $Mn^{2+}-Mn^{2+}$ distance is 5.8 Å. One Mn^{2+} is coordinated to side chains of Glu-131, Glu-212, Glu-220, and two water molecules; one water bridges both metal ions. Glu-129, Glu-357, His-269, and two water molecules bind the other Mn^{2+} [345–348].

The proposed mechanism involves the sequential binding of ATP (adjacent to the n_2 Mn^{2+}) and glutamate (adjacent to the n_1 Mn^{2+}), enabling glutamate to attack the γ-phosphorus atom of ATP, forming a γ-glutamyl phosphate intermediate and releasing ADP. Glutamine synthetase then binds ammonia, which attacks the γ-glutamyl phosphate intermediate, forming a tetrahedral intermediate from which inorganic phosphate and glutamine are released [345,349].

7.2. Carbamoyl Phosphate Synthetase

Carbamoyl phosphate is produced by carbamoyl phosphate synthetase (CPS), EC 6.3.4.16, from glutamine, bicarbonate, water, and two ATP molecules via a mechanism that involves a number of consecutive reactions and three unstable intermediates. These intermediates are formed at three separate active sites connected by two molecular tunnels that run through the protein interior. The enzyme is an $(\alpha,\beta)_4$ tetramer and the four small subunits are located at the ends of the molecule. The large subunits have four distinct domains, an oligomerization, an allosteric, a carboxy phosphate, and a carbamoyl phosphate domain. The three active sites contained within the α,β heterodimer are separated by almost 100 Å. Consequently, the catalytic cycles among the three active sites must by coordinated to enable the efficient processing of the highly reactive intermediates—carboxy phosphate, ammonia, and carbamate [350–352]. The active sites for both the carboxy phosphate and carbamoyl phosphate domains contain bound MnADP and monovalent K^+ ions that are octahedrally coordinated by three carbonyl oxygens and three side chain oxygens. The two-nucleotide binding sites of these domains are similar, but they differ with different forms of the enzyme. In the initial structure determination there was an inorganic phosphate and a second manganese ion in the carboxy phosphate domain. The Mn^{2+} ions in this domain are bridged by the Glu-299 carboxylate side chain, inorganic phosphate, and by a phosphate of ADP. Mn1 is also bonded to a water molecule, a second phosphate oxygen of ADP, and the side oxygen of Q-285. Mn2 is bound to Glu-299 (bidentate), the two bridging phosphates, a water molecule, and the backbone carbonyl of Asn-301. The single Mn^{2+} ion in the carbamoyl phosphate domain is also octahedral with two phosphoryl oxygen atoms, a water molecule, and the side chains of Gln-829 and Glu-841. However, in a more recently reported structure with AMPPNP present as a trinucleotide mimic, the carboxy phosphate domain contained only a single Mn^{2+}, bound to Glu-299, Asn-301, two bridging phosphates, and a water, and the carbamoyl phosphate synthetic domain contained two Mn^{2+} ions [353]. These ions are bridged by Glu-841; the Mn^{2+} in the previously identified binding site is also bound to

Glu-829, the α- and γ-phosphate oxygens, and the bridging N of AMP-PNP, and the second Mn^{2+} is bound to the β- and γ-phosphate oxygens of AMPPNP, Asn-843, Glu-841 (bidentate), and a water molecule.

7.3. Aminoacyl-tRNA Synthetases

Aminoacyl-tRNA synthetases link an amino acid to tRNA, which contains the triplet anticodon for that amino acid. Structural and sequence studies have shown that tRNA synthetases can be divided into two different structural frameworks. Members of a subclass of the class II series of enzymes have been structurally characterized with three divalent metal ions (Mg^{2+} or Mn^{2+}) present in the active site. These include glycyl-tRNA synthetase, EC 6.1.1.14 [354], serine-tRNA synthetase (SerRS), EC 6.1.1.11 [355], histidyl-tRNA synthetase, EC 6.1.1.21 [356], and aspartyl-tRNA synthetase, EC 6.1.1.12 [357,358].

Crystal structures of the aspartyl-t-RNA synthetase as the apoenzyme, the ternary complex with ATP and Mn^{2+} or Mg^{2+}, the binary complex with aspartate and with aspartyl adenylate have been determined [359]. The conformation and metal binding properties of the Mn^{2+} and Mg^{2+} forms are identical. There are three metal ions in the active site: Mn1 is bound to β- and γ-phosphate oxygens and four water molecules; Mn2 is bound to α- and β-phosphate oxygens, two water molecules, and Glu-361 and Ser-364; and Mn3 is bound to three water molecules, β- and γ-phosphate oxygens, and Glu-361. Mn2 and Mn3 are bridged by Glu-361, a water molecule, and a β-phosphoryl oxygen.

Structures of three complexes of SerRS with Mn^{2+} and ATP, seryladenylate and Mn^{2+}, and Ap_4A and Mn^{2+} have been determined [355]. The structure of the SerRS-ATP-Mn^{2+} complex revealed a bent conformation of the ATP and three Mn^{2+} ions in the active site [357,358]. One Mn^{2+} ion, Mn1, is octahedrally coordinated to Glu-345, Ser-348, two H_2O molecules, and oxygens from the α- and β-phosphates of ATP. The other two Mn^{2+} ions in this complex both coordinate to the β- and γ-phosphates and are located at either side of the β-O-γ phosphate linkage. One of these Mn^{2+} ions is linked to Mn1 via two bridging ligands, Glu-345, and a water molecule. The other Mn^{2+} forms no bonds to the protein. The SerRS–ATP–Ser–Mn^{2+} complex structure shows only one Mn^{2+} bound at the same position as the principal Mn^{2+} ion of the ATP–Mn^{2+} complex. The structure of the SerRS–Ap$_4$A–Mn^{2+} complex contains one Mn^{2+} ion bound to Glu-345, Ser-348, a water molecule, and the α-, β-, and δ-phosphates of the Ap$_4$A substrate.

8. PROTEINS CONTAINING BOUND MANGANESE

In this section we discuss Mn^{2+}-containing proteins that have no apparent enzymatic function and which have been structurally characterized. Mannose 6-phosphate receptor from mammals is a protein of this type that is structurally uncharacterized [360].

8.1. Lectins

Many virus, plant, and animal species contain carbohydrate-binding proteins, called lectins or agglutinins. Carbohydrate binding activity in legume lectins depends on the presence of two divalent metal ions (Ca^{2+} and Mn^{2+}). Concanavalin A and other lectin proteins are discussed in Chap. 9 [361].

8.2. Integrins

Integrins are plasma membrane proteins that mediate adhesion to other cells and to components of the extracellular matrix. They are implicated in biological functions such as embryogenesis, the immune response, hemostasis, inflammation, and maintenance of tissue integrity [362]. Integrins consist of two subunits: a 120- to 180-kDa α subunit and a 90- to 120-kDa β subunit. There have been 15 α subunits and 8 β subunits identified in humans, and these subunits can combine to form more than 20 different $\alpha\beta$ heterodimers. The integrin subunits consist of a large extracellular domain, a transmembrane domain, and a small cytoplasmic domain that interacts with the actin-containing cytoskeleton [363].

Interaction of integrins with ligands is dependent on the presence of a divalent metal ion, with Mg^{2+} being the most likely under physiological conditions [364]. However, several integrins have a higher affinity for Mn^{2+} ion. The integrins CD11a/CD18 (also known as LFA-1, or $\alpha_L\beta_2$) and CD11b/CD18 (also known as CR3, $\alpha_M\beta_2$, or Mac-1) are expressed in all leukocytes and the CD11a and CD11b domains have been the subject of a number of structural studies with both Mn^{2+} and Mg^{2+} bound to the protein. Two different forms of the domain have been characterized: an "open" form in which two phenylalanines are solvent exposed and a "closed" form in which these phenylalanines are buried in the protein core. The coordination spheres of the metal ions differ in the two forms. These differences do not depend on the nature of the metal ion or on the domain studied. In the open form of CD11b/CD18 Mn^{2+} and Mg^{2+} are located in a shallow crevice at the top of the internal β sheet and are coordinated to two water molecules, four amino acid residues, two serines, a threonine, and an aspartate (or glutamate) side chain from a neighboring domain within the lattice [365]. In the closed form the metal moves about 3 Å, and while the metal–serine and metal–water bonds remain intact the bonds to the threonine and glutamate are broken and replaced by bonds to an aspartate side chain, a water molecule (in CD11b), or a chloride ion (in CD11a), respectively [364,365]. There has been considerable debate as to whether these conformations represent active or inactive structures, which form is active, and whether the open form is a structural artifact [366,367]. Surprisingly, given the similarities in the metal binding sites of CD11a and CD11b, the proteins have significantly different metal ion binding characteristics [368].

8.3.   Diphtheria Toxin Repressor

The diphtheria toxin repressor (DtxR) is a transition metal ion-dependent regulatory element that controls the expression of diphtheria toxin and several genes involved in the synthesis of siderophores in *Corynebacterium diphtheriae*. Crystal structures of DtxR with bound Ni^{2+}, Co^{2+}, Cd^{2+}, and Mn^{2+} have been determined [369–371]. There are three domains in the protein: a DNA binding domain, a metal binding domain, and a flexible domain. There are two metal binding sites in the second domain; site 1 is occupied in all of the structures and Co^{2+} and Mn^{2+} ions are bound tetrahedrally by His-79, Glu-83, His-98, and a sulfate ion. The second metal binding site is only occupied with Mn^{2+}

and Cd^{2+}. In the Mn^{2+} structure the bonding is again tetrahedral and the ligands are Glu-105, His-106, the carbonyl oxygen of Cys-102, and a water molecule. The reasons for differential occupancy of this site in different structures are not understood [371].

8.4. Fur Repressor Protein

Iron uptake and regulation in $E.$ $coli$ have been shown to be mediated by the repressor protein Fur. Mn^{2+} and Cu^{2+} ions have been shown to activate the protein in vitro. Fur binds one Mn^{2+} per monomer, and NMR evidence suggests that His-85, 89, 131, 142, and 144 are possible ligands, along with the oxygen donor residues glutamate and aspartate, which are present at the C terminus [372].

8.5. PsaA

The surface protein PsaA from the bacterium $Streptococcus$ $pneumoniae$ is involved in the uptake of Mn^{2+} and Zn^{2+} by the organism. The crystal structure has been determined and shown to have two $(\beta/\alpha)_4$ domains linked together by a single helix. There is a metal binding site formed in the domain interface by the side chains of His-67, His-139, Glu-205, and Asp-280 but in this structure this site is probably occupied by Zn^{2+} [373].

9. CONCLUSIONS

It is obvious from the results reported above that Mn^{n+} in the active sites of enzymes can catalyze a very wide variety of different reactions. There has been an enormous expansion of our knowledge of Mn-containing enzymes over the last 10 years; however, all of the newly characterized enzymes involve the Mn(II) oxidation state. Whether all the Mn(III)- or Mn(IV)-containing enzymes have already been discovered is for the future to determine. Observed coordination numbers of manganese ion in proteins varies from four to seven. Only nitrogen and oxygen donor atoms are observed; sulfur donors have not yet been observed. Results of the rapidly increasing number of structural studies are beginning to show a number of structural homologies. For example, the binding of the ATP analog AMPPNP to Mn^{2+} in the carboxyphosphate synthetic domain and the carbamoyl phosphate synthetic domain of carbamoyl phosphate synthetase is very similar to the binding of Mn^{2+} and AMPPNP in phosphorylase kinase. One challenge for the future is to understand how the structure of the active site of these enzymes leads to different products.

ACKNOWLEDGMENT

The authors thank Ms. Nicola Morgan for her assistance with literature searching.

ABBREVIATIONS

ADP	adenosine-5'-diphosphate
AhG-1,6-P_2	2,5-anhydro-D-glucitol-1,6-bisphosphate
AMPPNP	β,γ-imidoadenosine-5'-triphosphate
Ap_4A	diadenosine tetraphosphate
ATP	adenosine-5'-triphosphate
cAMP	adenosine 3,5-monophosphate
CcO	cytochrome *c* oxidase
CMLE	chloromuconate-lactonizing enzyme
CMP	cytidine-5'-monophosphate
CPS	carbamoyl phosphate synthetase
DtxR	diphtheria toxin repressor
E.	*Escherichia*
ENDOR	electron nuclear double-resonance spectroscopy
EPR	electron paramagnetic resonance
ESEEM	electron spin-echo envelope modulation
EXAFS	extended X-ray absorption fine structure
FBP	fructose-1,6-biphosphatase
Gal	galactose
GDP	guanosine-5'-diphosphate
Glc	glucosamine

GlcNAc	*N*-acetylglucosamine
GMP	guanosine-5'-monophosphate
GS	glutamine synthase
GTP	guanosine-5'-triphosphate
ICDH	isocitrate dehydrogenase
IPMDH	isopropylmalate dehydrogenase
Man	mannose
MAT	*S*-adenosylmethionine synthetase
MLE	muconate-lactonizing enzyme
MR	mandelate racemase
mRNA	messenger RNA
N.	*Neurospora*
NAD	nicotinamide adenine dinucleotide
NADP	nicotinamide adenine dinucleotide phosphate
NeuAc	*N*-acetylneuraminic acid, i.e., sialic acid
NMP	nucleotide monophosphate
NMR	nuclear magnetic resonance
NTP	nucleotide triphosphate
P.	*Pseudomonas*
PAPS	3'-phosphoadenosine-5'-phosphosulfate
PCK	phosphoenolpyruvate carboxykinase
PhAH	phosphonoacetohydroxamate
PRTase	glutamine phosphoribosylpyrophosphate amido-transferase
T.	*Thermus*
S.	*Saccharomyces*
SerRS	seryl-tRNA synthetase
tRNA	transfer ribonucleic acid
UDP	uridine diphosphate
XAS	X-ray absorption spectroscopy
XANES	X-ray absorption near-edge spectroscopy

REFERENCES

1. F. Archibald, *CRC Crit. Rev. Microbiol.*, *13*, 63–109 (1986).
2. R. L. B. Casareno and J. A. Cowan, *Chem. Commun.*, 1813–1814 (1996).

3. D. W. Christianson, *Prog. Biophys. Mol. Biol.*, *67*, 217–252 (1997).

4. G. C. Dismukes, *Chem. Rev.*, *96*, 2909–2926 (1996).

5. D. J. Klimis-Tavantzis (ed.), *Manganese in Health and Disease*, CRC Press, Boca Raton, FL, 1994.

6. K. H. Nealson and D. Saffarini, *Annu. Rev. Microbiol.*, *48*, 311–343 (1994).

7. V. L. Schramm and F. C. Wedler (eds.), *Manganese in Metabolism and Enzyme Function*, Academic Press, New York, 1986.

8. D. C. Weatherburn, in *Perspectives on Bioinorganic Chemistry*, *Vol. 3* (R. W. Hay, J. R. Dilworth, and K. B. Nolan, eds.), JAI Press, Westport, CT, 1996, pp. 1–113.

9. F. C. Wedler, in *Manganese in Health and Disease* (D. J. Klimis-Tavantzis, ed.), CRC Press, Boca Raton, FL, 1994, pp. 1–37.

10. F. C. Wedler, in *The Role of Glia in Neurotoxicity* (M. Aschner and H. K. Kimbelberg, eds.), CRC Press, Boca Raton, FL, 1996, pp. 155–173.

11. D. T. Richens, in *Perspectives on Bioinorganic Chemistry, Vol. 2* (R. W. Hay, J. R. Dilworth, and K. B. Nolan, eds.), JAI Press, Westport, CT, 1993, pp. 245–292.

12. G. H. Reed and R. R. Poyner, this volume, Chap. 7.

13. C. L. Vermote, I. B. Vipond, and S. E. Halford, *Biochemistry*, *31*, 6089–6097 (1992).

14. M. Andersson, A. Malmendal, S. Linse, I. Ivarsson, S. Forsen, and L. A. Svensson, *Protein Sci.*, *6*, 1139–1147 (1997).

15. D. R. Holland, A. C. Hausrath, D. Juers, and B. W. Matthews, *Protein Sci.*, *4*, 1955–1965 (1995).

16. J. Cha, M. V. Sorensen, Q. Z. Ye, and D. S. Auld, *J. Biol. Inorg. Chem.*, *3*, 353–359 (1998).

17. P. L. Roach, I. J. Clifton, V. Fulop, K. Harlos, G. J. Barton, J. Hajdu, I. Andersson, C. J. Schofield, and J. E. Baldwin, *Nature*, *375*, 700–704 (1995).

18. S. Ragusa, S. Blanquet, and T. Meinnel, *J. Mol. Biol.*, *280*, 515–523 (1998).

19. M. Ghosh, A. M. Grunden, D. M. Dunn, R. Weiss, and M. W. W. Adams, *J. Bacteriol.*, *180*, 4781–4789 (1998).

20. T. Schweins, K. Scheffzek, R. Aßheuer, and A. Wittinghofer, *J. Mol. Biol.*, *266*, 847–856 (1997).

21. C. D. Mol, C. F. Kuo, M. M. Thayer, R. P. Cunningham, and J. A. Tainer, *Nature*, *374*, 381–386 (1995).

22. K. Håkansson, A. Wehnert, and A. Liljas, *Acta Cryst. Sect. D Biol. Cryst.*, *50D*, 93–100 (1993).

23. P. J. Liebowitz, L. S. Schwartzenberg, and A. K. Bruce, *Photochem. Photobiol.*, *23*, 45–50 (1976).

24. S. Mathew, J. Peterson, B. Degaulejac, N. Vicente, M. Denis, J. Bonaventura, and L. L. Pearce, *Comp. Biochem. Physiol. B: Comp. Biochem.*, *113*, 525–532 (1996).

25. C. P. Swann, T. Adewole, and J. H. Waite, *Comp. Biochem. Physiol. B Biochem. Mol. Biol.*, *119*, 755–759 (1998).

26. F. C. Wedler and B. W. Ley, *Neurochem. Res.*, *19*, 139–144 (1994).

27. M. Ramírez, G. Arechaga, S. Garcia, B. Sanchez, P. Lardelli, and J. M. de Gandarias, *Brain Res.*, *522*, 165–167 (1990).

28. J. D. Doherty, N. Salem, Jr., C. J. Lauter, and E. G. Trams, *Neurochem. Res.*, *8*, 493–500 (1983).

29. D. F. Malamud, C. C. DiRusso, and J. R. Aprille, *Biochim. Biophys. Acta*, *485*, 243–247 (1977).

30. M. Sundaramoorthy, K. Kishi, M. H. Gold, and T. L. Poulos, *J. Biol. Chem.*, *272*, 17574–17580 (1997).

31. R. Stein, W. Gross, and C. Schnarrenberger, *Planta*, *202*, 487–493 (1997).

32. W. Y. Chou, S. M. Huang, and G. G. Chang, *Protein Eng.*, *11*, 371–376 (1998).

33. M. Rodriguez, A. G. Wedd, and R. K. Scopes, *Biochem. Mol. Biol. Int.*, *38*, 783–789 (1996).

34. M. Lähdesmäki, and P. Mäntsälä, *Biochim. Biophys. Acta*, *613*, 266–274 (1980).

35. P. Serfozo and P. A. Tipton, *Biochemistry*, *34*, 7517–7524 (1995).

36. A. E. Krafft, J. Winter, V. D. Bokkenheuser, and P. B. Hylemon, *J. Steroid Biochem.*, *28*, 49–54 (1987).

37. V. Ansanay, S. Dequin, B. Blondin, and P. Barre, *FEBS Lett.*, *332*, 74–80 (1993).

38. S. G. Bhat and C. S. Vaidyanathan, *Eur. J. Biochem.*, *68*, 323–331 (1976).

39. J. Markiewicz and S. Strumilo, *Biochem. Arch.*, *13*, 127–129 (1997).

40. J. C. Schabort and D. J. J. Potgieter, *Biochim. Biophys. Acta*, *151*, 47–54 (1968).

41. R. Cammack, A. Chapman, W.-P. Lu, A. Karagouni, and D. P. Kelly, *FEBS Lett.*, *253*, 239–243 (1989).

42. D. P. Kelly, J. K. Shergill, W. P. Lu, and A. P. Wood, *Antonie van Leeuwenhoek*, *71*, 95–107 (1997).

43. P. M. Nair and L. C. Vining, *Biochim. Biophys. Acta*, *96*, 318–327 (1965).

44. Y. M. Jiang, G. Zauberman, and Y. Fuchs, *Postharvest Biol. Technol.*, *10*, 221–228 (1997).

45. M. J. Rodríguez Maranón, A. R. Hoy, and R. B. van Huystee, *Cell. Mol. Biol.*, *40*, 871–879 (1994).

46. M. Hamberg, C. Su, and E. Oliw, *J. Biol. Chem.*, *273*, 13080–13088 (1998).

47. C. Su and E. H. Oliw, *J. Biol. Chem.*, *273*, 13072–13079 (1998).

48. O. V. Maltseva, I. P. Solyanikova, and L. A. Golovleva, *Eur. J. Biochem.*, *226*, 1053–1061 (1994).

49. S. Fujita, N. Binsaari, M. Maegawa, N. Samura, N. Hayashi, and T. Tono, *J. Agric. Food Chem.*, *45*, 59–63 (1997).

50. A. Kelm, L. Shaw, R. Schauer, and G. Reuter, *Eur. J. Biochem.*, *251*, 874–884 (1998).

51. R. Mineyama, K. Mikami, and K. Saito, *Microbios*, *82*, 7–19 (1995).

52. S. Das and F. D. Gillin, *Biochem. J.*, *280*, 641–647 (1991).

53. H. Kitagawa, M. Ujikawa, K. Tsutsumi, J. Tamura, K. W. Neumann, T. Ogawa, and K. Sugahara, *Glycobiology*, *7*, 905–911 (1997).

54. K. Ng, E. Handman, and A. Bacic, *Biochem. J.*, *317*, 247–255 (1996).

55. M. Malissard, L. Borsig, S. Dimarco, M. G. Grutter, U. Kragl, C. Wandrey, and E. G. Berger, *Eur. J. Biochem.*, *239*, 340–348 (1996).

56. J. Mendicino and S. Sangadala, *Mol. Cell. Biochem.*, *185*, 135–145 (1998).

57. S. Ghosh, J. W. Kyle, S. Dastgheib, F. Daussin, Z. X. Li, and S. Basu, *Glycoconjugate J.*, *12*, 838–847 (1995).

58. M. Bortolato, J. Radisson, G. Azzar, and R. Got, *Int. J. Biochem.*, *24*, 243–248 (1992).

59. H. Coste, M. B. Martel, G. Azzar, and R. Got, *Biochim. Biophys. Acta*, *814*, 1–7 (1985).

60. N. Taniguchi, N. Yokosawa, S. Gasa, and A. Makita, *J. Biol. Chem.*, *257*, 10631–10637 (1982).

61. A. Takeya, O. Hosomi, and T. Kogure, *Jpn. J. Med. Sci.*, *38*, 1–8 (1985).

62. T. Szumilo, G. P. Kaushal, and A. D. Elbein, *Biochemistry*, *26*, 5498–5505 (1987).

63. S. N. Bocca, A. Rothschild, and J. S. Tandecarz, *Plant Physiol. Biochem.*, *35*, 205–212 (1997).

64. T. L. Hendrickson, and B. Imperiali, *Biochemistry*, *34*, 9444–9450 (1995).

65. J. J. J. Liu, W. Odegard, and B. O. Delumen, *Plant Physiol.*, *109*, 505–511 (1995).

66. M. J. Elices and I. J. Goldstein, *J. Biol. Chem.*, *263*, 3354–3362 (1988).

67. M. J. Elices, D. A. Blake, and I. J. Goldstein, *J. Biol. Chem.*, *261*, 6064–6072 (1986).

68. M. Vella and P. Greenwell, *Glycoconj. J.*, *14*, 883–887 (1997).

69. Y. Tsuji, T. Urashima, and T. Matsuzawa, *Biochim. Biophys. Acta*, *1289*, 115–121 (1996).

70. S. Oguri, M. T. Minowa, Y. Ihara, N. Taniguchi, H. Ikenaga, and M. Takeuchi, *J. Biol. Chem.*, *272*, 22721–22727 (1997).

71. I. Brockhausen, K. L. Matta, J. Orr, and H. Schachter, *Biochemistry*, *24*, 1866–1874 (1985).

72. H. Kawashima, K. Yamamoto, T. Osawa, and T. Irimura, *J. Biol. Chem.*, *268*, 27118–27126 (1993).

73. N. Malagolini, F. Dall'Olio, and F. Serafini-Cessi, *Biochem. Biophys. Res. Commun.*, *180*, 681–686 (1991).

74. D. K. Chou and F. B. Jungalwala, *J. Biol. Chem.*, *268*, 21727–21733 (1993).

75. F. Piller and J. P. Cartron, *J. Biol. Chem.*, *258*, 12293–12299 (1983).

76. N. Malagolini, F. Dall'Olio, S. Guerrini, and F. Serafini-Cessi, *Glycoconj. J.*, *11*, 89–95 (1994).

77. A. Suzuki, N. Shibata, M. Suzuki, F. Saitoh, H. Oyamada, H. Kobayashi, S. Suzuki, and Y. Okawa, *J. Biol. Chem.*, *272*, 16822–16828 (1997).

78. C. A. R. Wiggins and S. Munro, *Proc. Natl. Acad. Sci. USA*, *95*, 7945–7950 (1998).

79. A. Suzuki, N. Shibata, M. Suzuki, F. Saitoh, Y. Takata, A. Oshie, H. Oyamada, H. Kobayashi, S. Suzuki, and Y. Okawa, *Eur. J. Biochem.*, *240*, 37–44 (1996).

80. T. Taguchi, K. Kitajima, S. Inoue, Y. Inoue, J. M. Yang, H. Schachter, and I. Brockhausen, *Biochem. Biophys. Res. Commun.*, *230*, 533–536 (1997).

81. M. Amado, R. Almeida, F. Carneiro, S. B. Levery, E. H. Holmes, M. Nomoto, M. A. Hollingsworth, H. Hassan, T. Schwientek, P. A. Nielsen, E. P. Bennett, and H. Clausen, *J. Biol. Chem.*, *273*, 12770-12778 (1998).

82. I. Brockhausen, E. Hull, O. Hindsgaul, H. Schachter, R. N. Shah, S. W. Michnick, and J. P. Carver, *J. Biol. Chem.*, *264*, 11211–11221 (1989).

83. P. A. Ropp, M. R. Little, and P. W. Cheng, *J. Biol. Chem.*, *266*, 23863–23871 (1991).

84. B. T. Sheares and D. M. Carlson, *J. Biol. Chem.*, *258*, 9893–9898 (1983).

85. O. Hosomi and A. Takeya, *Nippon Juigaku Zasshi*, *51*, 961–968 (1989).

86. H. Mulder, B. A. Spronk, H. Schachter, A. P. Neeleman, D. H. van den Eijnden, M. De Jong-Brink, J. P. Kamerling, and J. F. Vliegenthart, *Eur. J. Biochem.*, *227*, 175–185 (1995).

87. J. O. Previato, M. Sola-penna, O. A. Agrellos, C. Jones, T. Oeltmann, L. R. Travassos, and L. Mendonca-Previato, *J. Biol. Chem.*, *273*, 14982–14988 (1998).

88. S. Pingel, U. Rheinweiler, V. Kolb, and M. Duszenko, *Biochem. J.*, *338*, 545–551 (1999).

89. E. H. Holmes, *Arch. Biochem. Biophys.*, *260*, 461–468 (1988).

90. K. Shinoda, Y. Morishita, K. Sasaki, Y. Matsuda, I. Takahashi, and T. Nishi, *J. Biol. Chem.*, *272*, 31992–31997 (1997).

91. T. Nomura, M. Takizawa, J. Aoki, H. Arai, K. Inoue, E. Wakisaka, N. Yoshizuka, G. Imokawa, N. Dohmae, K. Takio, M. Hattori, and N. Matsuo, *J. Biol. Chem.*, *273*, 13570–13577 (1998).

92. D. H. van den Eijnden, W. M. Blanken, H. Winterwerp, and W. E. Schiphorst, *Eur. J. Biochem.*, *134*, 523–530 (1983).

93. P. L. DeAngelis, *Biochemistry*, *35*, 9768–9771 (1996).

94. M. L. McNatt, F. M. Fiser, M. J. Elders, B. S. Kilgore, W. G. Smith, and E. R. Hughes, *Biochem. J.*, *160*, 211–216 (1976).

95. U. Preuss, X. B. Gu, T. J. Gu, and R. K. Yu, *J. Biol. Chem.*, *268*, 26273–26278 (1993).

96. L. Debussche, M. Couder, D. Thibaut, B. Cameron, J. Crouzet, and F. Blanche, *J. Bacteriol.*, *173*, 6300–6302 (1991).

97. C. S. Wu and N. N. Chuang, *J. Exp. Zool.*, *275*, 346–354 (1996).

98. J. L. Benovic, F. Mayor, Jr., C. Staniszewski, and R. J. Lefkowitz, *J. Biol. Chem.*, *262*, 9026–9032 (1987).

99. J. L. Benovic, *Meth. Enzymol.*, *200*, 351–362 (1991).

100. M. Onda, A. Morimoto, A. Simoide, K. Iwata, and H. Nakajima, *Biosci. Biotechnol. Biochem.*, *60*, 1740–1742 (1996).

101. A. Mancini, F. Del Rosso, R. Roberti, P. Orvietani, L. Coletti, and L. Binaglia, *Biochim. Biophys. Acta*, *1437*, 80–92 (1999).

102. S. K. Saha, Y. Furukawa, H. Matsuzaki, I. Shibuya, and K. Matsumoto, *Biosci. Biotech. Biochem.*, *60*, 630–633 (1996).

103. M. E. Monaco, M. Feldman, and D. L. Kleinberg, *Biochem. J.*, *304*, 301–305 (1994).

104. G. P. Kaushal, and A. D. Elbein, *J. Biol. Chem.*, *260*, 16303–16309 (1985).

105. J. R. Wilson, J. A. Deinhart, and M. M. Weiser, *Biochim. Biophys. Acta*, *924*, 323–331 (1987).

106. S. Merello, A. J. Parodi, and R. Couso, *J. Biol. Chem.*, *270*, 7281–7287 (1995).

107. J. M. Moss, G. E. Reid, K. A. Mullin, J. L. Zawadzki, R. J. Simpson, and M. J. McConville, *J. Biol. Chem.*, *274*, 6678–6688 (1999).

108. G. Harauz and W. Li, *Biochem. Biophys. Res. Commun.*, *241*, 599–605 (1997).

109. R. L. Gamble, M. L. Coonfield, and G. E. Schaller, *Proc. Natl. Acad. Sci. USA*, *95*, 7825–7829 (1998).

110. S. William, P. Ramaprasad, and C. Kasinathan, *Arch. Biochem. Biophys.*, *338*, 90–96 (1997).

111. Y. Sakakibara, Y. Takami, T. Nakayama, M. Suiko, and M. C. Liu, *J. Biol. Chem.*, *273*, 6242–6247 (1998).

112. Y. Kato and R. G. Spiro, *J. Biol. Chem.*, *264*, 3364–3371 (1989).

113. D. K. H. Chou and F. B. Jungalwala, *J. Biol. Chem.*, *268*, 330–336 (1993).

114. M. J. Irons and P. J. O'Brien, *Exp. Eye Res.*, *45*, 813–821 (1987).

115. Z. Zhang, G. Bai, S. Deans-Zirattu, M. F. Browner, and E. Y. C. Lee, *J. Biol. Chem.*, *267*, 1484–1490 (1992).

116. W. P. Ciesla, Jr. and D. A. Bobak, *J. Biol. Chem.*, *273*, 16021–16026 (1998).

117. Y. Ikura and K. Horikoshi, *Agric. Biol. Chem.*, *54*, 3205–3509 (1990).

118. R. G. Spiro and V. D. Bhoyroo, *Biochem. J.*, *331*, 265–271 (1998).

119. Y. Tazuke and K. Matsuda, *Biosci. Biotech. Biochem.*, *56*, 1584–1588 (1992).

120. U. Mechold, M. Cashel, K. Steiner, D. Gentry, and H. Malke, *J. Bacteriol.*, *178*, 1401–1411 (1996).

121. R. Ray, L. J. Boucher, C. A. Broomfield, and D. E. Lenz, *Biochim. Biophys. Acta*, *967*, 373–381 (1988).

122. N. Kunze, H. Kleinkauf, and K. Bauer, *Eur. J. Biochem.*, *160*, 605–613 (1986).

123. E. Caffarelli, L. Maggi, A. Fatica, J. Jiricny, and I. Bozzoni, *Biochem. Biophys. Res. Commun.*, *233*, 514–517 (1997).

124. M. Harada, M. Inohara, M. Nakao, T. Nakayama, A. Kakudo, Y. Shibano, and T. Amachi, *J. Biol. Chem.*, *269*, 22021–22026 (1994).

125. C. H. Kim, O. Nashiru, and J. H. Ko, *FEMS Microbiol. Lett.*, *138*, 147–152 (1996).

126. C. L. Bouma, J. Reizer, A. Reizer, S. A. Robrish, and J. Thompson, *J. Bacteriol.*, *179*, 4129–4137 (1997).

127. J. Thompson, A. Pikis, S. B. Ruvinov, B. Henrissat, H. Yamamoto, and J. Sekiguchi, *J. Biol. Chem.*, *273*, 27347–27356 (1998).

128. K. S. Siddiqui, M. J. Azhar, M. H. Rashid, T. M. Ghuri, and M. I. Rajoka, *Folia Microbiol.*, *42*, 303–311 (1997).

129. B. S. Antharavally, R. P. Poyner, and P. W. Ludden, *J. Am. Chem. Soc.*, *120*, 8897–8898 (1998).

130. M. E. Legaz, R. De Armas, M. Martínez, M. Medina, and C. Vincente, *Plant Physiol. Biochem. (Paris)*, *29*, 601–605 (1991).

131. A. Iwayama, T. Kimura, O. Adachi, and M. Ameyama, *Agric. Biol. Chem.*, *47*, 2483–2493 (1983).

132. Y. Sanz, F. Mulholland, and F. Toldra, *J. Agric. Food Chem.*, *46*, 349–353 (1998).

133. L. R. Hegstrand and T. H. Kalinke, *J. Neurochem.*, *45*, 300–307 (1985).

134. F. Aranishi, T. Watanabe, K. Osatomi, M. Cao, K. Hara, and T. Ishihara, *J. Marine Biotechnol.*, *6*, 157–162 (1998).

135. J. L. Brown and J. F. Krall, *Biochem. Biophys. Res. Commun.*, *42*, 390–397 (1971).

136. K. S. Hui, M. P. Hui, and A. Lajtha, *J. Neurosci. Res.*, *20*, 231–240 (1988).

137. W.-J. Ou, A. Ito, H. Okazaki, and T. Omura, *EMBO J.*, *8*, 2605–2612 (1989).

138. B. Schmidt, E. Wachter, W. Sebald, and W. Neupert, *Eur. J. Biochem.*, *144*, 581–588 (1984).

139. T. Ishikawa, K. Watabe, Y. Mukohara, and H. Nakamura, *Biosci. Biotechnol. Biochem.*, *60*, 612–615 (1996).

140. M. Asakura, Y. Nagahashi, M. Hamada, M. Kawai, K. Kadobayashi, M. Narahara, S. Nakagawa, Y. Kawai, T. Hama, and M. Miyake, *Biochim. Biophys. Acta*, *1250*, 35–42 (1995).

141. B. Ceskis, H. Sekeka, K. Janulaitiene, A. Pauliukonis, and D. Kazlauskas, *Int. J. Biochem.*, *19*, 973–980 (1987).

142. A. E. Gau, H. H. Thole, A. Sokolenko, L. Altschmied, R. G. Hermann, and E. K. Pistorius, *Mol. Gen. Genet.*, *260*, 56–68 (1998).

143. G. J. Kim and H. S. Kim, *Biochem. J.*, *330*, 295–302 (1998).

144. Z. W. Xu, F. E. De Windt, and C. van der Drift, *Arch. Biochem. Biophys.*, *324*, 99–104 (1995).

145. T. Yorifuji and S. Furuyoshi, *Agric. Biol. Chem.*, *50*, 1327–1328 (1986).

146. T. Yorifuji, K. Sawada, and C. Tokuda, *Agric. Biol. Chem.*, *50*, 3077–3082 (1986).

147. P. R. Meyers, P. Gokool, D. E. Rawlings, and D. R. Woods, *J. Gen. Microb.*, *137*, 1397–1400 (1991).

148. J. Canales, R. M. Pinto, M. J. Costas, M. T. Hernandez, A. Miro, D. Bernet, A. Fernandez, and J. C. Cameselle, *Biochim. Biophys. Acta*, *1246*, 167–177 (1995).

149. J. A. Martina, J. L. Daniotti, and H. J. F. Maccioni, *J. Neurochem.*, *64*, 1274–1280 (1995).

150. A. Farooqui, *Int. J. Biochem.*, *12*, 529–536 (1980).

151. D. R. Houck and E. Inamine, *Arch. Biochem. Biophys.*, *259*, 58–65 (1987).

152. M. S. M. Jetten and A. J. Sinskey, *Antonie Van Leeuwenhoek Int. J. Gen. Mol. Microbiol.*, *67*, 221–227 (1995).

153. A. Lack and G. Fuchs, *J. Bacteriol.*, *174*, 3629–3636 (1992).

154. J. Q. Liu, T. Dairi, N. Itoh, M. Kataoka, S. Shimizu, and H. Yamada, *J. Biol. Chem.*, *273*, 16678–16685 (1998).

155. B. Pelzer-Reith, A. Penger, and C. Schnarrenberger, *Plant Mol. Biol.*, *21*, 331–140 (1993).

156. J. P. Akowski and R. Bauerle, *Biochemistry*, *36*, 15817–15822 (1997).

157. A. Weische, W. Garvert, and E. Leistner, *Arch. Biochem. Biophys.*, *256*, 223–231 (1987).

158. J.-L. Dreyer, *Eur. J. Biochem.*, *166*, 623–630 (1987).

159. T. R. Hawkes, P. G. Thomas, L. S. Edwards, S. J. Rayner, K. W. Wilkinson, and D. W. Rice, *Biochem. J.*, *306*, 385–397 (1995).

160. R. Iwamoto, H. Taniki, J. Koishi, and S. Nakura, *Biosci. Biotechnol. Biochem.*, *59*, 408–411 (1995).

161. E. Pichersky, E. Lewinsohn, and R. Croteau, *Arch. Biochem. Biophys.*, *316*, 803–807 (1995).

162. J. R. Pollard and T. D. H. Bugg, *Eur. J. Biochem.*, *251*, 98–106 (1998).

163. Y. Matsubara, R. Kawada, K. Iwasaki, T. Oda, and T. Muramatsu, *J. Protein Chem.*, *17*, 29–36 (1998).

164. Y. Takada and T. Noguchi, *Biochem. J.*, *235*, 391–397 (1986).

165. T. Tomita, S. Tsuyama, Y. Imai, and T. Kitagawa, *J. Biochem.*, *122*, 531–536 (1997).

166. L. R. Potter, *Biochemistry*, *37*, 2422–2429 (1998).

167. R. P. Newton, B. J. Salvage, and N. A. Hakeem, *Biochem. J.*, *265*, 581–586 (1990).

168. T. W. Hallahan and R. Croteau, *Arch. Biochem. Biophys.*, *264*, 618–631 (1988).

169. S. Banerjee, F. Anderson, and G. K. Farber, *Protein Eng.*, *8*, 1189–1195 (1995).

170. P. Allenza, M. J. Morrell, and R. W. Detroy, *Appl. Biochem. Biotechnol.*, *24/25*, 171–182 (1990).

171. S. H. Bhuiyan, Y. Itami, and K. Izumori, *J. Ferment. Bioeng.*, *84*, 319–323 (1997).

172. A. D. Elbein and K. Izumori, *Meth. Enzymol.*, *89*, 547–550 (1982).

173. H. Sagami and K. Ogura, *J. Biochem. (Tokyo)*, *94*, 975–979 (1983).

174. M. Chander, B. Setlow, and P. Setlow, *Can. J. Microbiol.*, *44*, 759–767 (1998).

175. B. Solow, K. M. Bischoff, M. J. Zylka, and P. J. Kennelly, *Protein Sci.*, *7*, 105–111 (1998).

176. A. E. Kuhm, M. Schlömann, H.-J. Knackmuss, and D. H. Pieper, *Biochem. J.*, *266*, 877–883 (1990).

177. J. I. Rajaonarivony, J. Gershenzon, J. Miyazaki, and R. Croteau, *Arch. Biochem. Biophys.*, *299*, 77–82 (1992).

178. T. J. Savage, M. W. Hatch, and R. Croteau, *J. Biol. Chem.*, *269*, 4012–4020 (1994).

179. U. Neudert, I. M. Martinez-Ferez, P. D. Fraser, and G. Sandmann, *Biochim. Biophys. Acta*, *1392*, 51–58 (1998).

180. A. Jack, J. E. Ladner, D. Rhodes, R. S. Brown, and A. Klug, *J. Mol. Biol.*, *111*, 315–328 (1977).

181. T. Kimura, I. Sugahara, K. Hanai, and Y. Tonomura, *Biosci. Biotechnol. Biochem.*, *56*, 708–711 (1992)

182. K. G. Thampy, and S. J. Wakil, *J. Biol. Chem.*, *260*, 6318–6323 (1985).

183. B. G. Werneburg and D. E. Ash, *Biochemistry*, *36*, 14392–14402 (1997).

184. L. Uotila, *Arch. Biochem. Biophys.*, *264*, 135–143 (1988).

185. L. Que, Jr., this volume, Chap. 15.

186. U. Griepenburg, K. Blasczyk, R. Kappl, J. Hüttermann, and G. Auling, *Biochemistry*, *37*, 7992–7996 (1998).

187. G. Auling and H. Follmann, in *Metalloenzymes Involving Amino Acid-Residue and Related Radicals* (H. Sigel and A. Sigel, eds.), Vol. 30 of *Metal Ions in Biological Systems*, Marcel Dekker, New York, 1994, pp. 131–161.

188. J. W. Whittaker, this volume, Chap. 18.

189. D. W. Yoder, J. Hwang, and J. E. Penner-Hahn, this volume, Chap. 16.

190. M. H. Gold, H. L. Youngs, and M. D. Sollewijn Gelpke, this volume, Chap. 17.

191. G. T. Babcock and C. W. Hoganson, this volume, Chap. 19.

192. R. J. Debus, this volume, Chap. 20.

193. V. Kumar, D. M. Dooley, H. C. Freeman, J. M. Guss, I. Harvey, M. A. McGuirl, M. C. J. Wilce, and V. M. Zubak, *Structure*, *4*, 943–955 (1996).

194. M. Sebela, L. Luhová, I. Frébort, S. Hirota, H. G. Faulhammer, V. Stuzka, and P. Pec, *J. Exp. Bot.*, *48*, 1897–1907 (1997).

195. M. Sebela, L. Luhová, I. Frébort, H. G. Faulhammer, S. Hirota, L. Zajoncova, V. Stuzka, and P. Pec, *Phytochem. Anal.*, *9*, 211–222 (1998).

196. M. J. Crabbe, R. D. Waight, W. G. Bardsley, R. W. Barker, I. D. Kelly, and P. F. Knowles, *Biochem. J.*, *155*, 679–687 (1976).

197. R. B. Li, J. P. Klinman, and F. S. Mathews, *Structure*, *6*, 293–307 (1998).

198. M. R. Parsons, M. A. Convery, C. M. Wilmot, K. D. S. Yadav, V. Blakely, A. S. Corner, S. E. V. Phillips, M. J. McPherson, and P. F. Knowles, *Structure*, *3*, 1171–1184 (1995).

199. H. Michel, J. Behr, A. Harrenga, and A. Kannt, *Annu. Rev. Biophys. Biomol. Struct.*, *27*, 329–356 (1998).

200. C. Ostermeier, A. Harrenga, U. Ermler, and H. Michel, *Proc. Natl. Acad. Sci. USA*, *94*, 10547–10553 (1997).

201. H. Witt, A. Wittershagen, E. Bill, B. O. Kolbesen, and B. Ludwig, *FEBS Lett.*, *409*, 128–130 (1997).

202. K. Imada, M. Sato, N. Tanaka, Y. Katsube, Y. Matsuura, and T. Oshima, *J. Mol. Biol.*, *222*, 725–738 (1991).

203. G. Wallon, K. Yamamoto, H. Kirino, A. Yamagishi, S. T. Lovett, G. A. Petsko, and T. Oshima, *Biochim. Biophys. Acta*, *1337*, 105–112 (1997).

204. B. L. Stoddard, A. Dean, and D. E. Koshland, Jr., *Biochemistry*, *32*, 9310–9316 (1993).

205. R. D. Chen, J. A. Grobler, J. H. Hurley, and A. M. Dean, *Protein Sci.*, *5*, 287–295 (1996).

206. J. H. Hurley, A. M. Dean, J. L. Sohl, D. E. Koshland, Jr., and R. M. Stroud, *Science*, *249*, 1012–1016 (1990).

207. G. Wallon, G. Kryger, S. T. Lovett, T. Oshima, D. Ringe, and G. A. Petsko, *J. Mol. Biol.*, *266*, 1016–1031 (1997).

208. K. Imada, K. Inagaki, H. Matsunami, H. Kawaguchi, H. Tanaka, N. Tanaka, and K. Namba, *Structure*, 6, 971–982 (1998).

209. T. Suzuki, H. Moriyama, R. Hirose, M. Sakurai, N. Tanaka, and T. Oshima, *Acta Cryst. Sect. D. Biol. Cryst.*, 54, 444–445 (1998).

210. M. Sundaramoorthy, J. Terner, and T. L. Poulos, *Structure*, 3, 1367–1377 (1995).

211. J. R. Goldenring, M. Oddsdottir, and I. M. Modlin, *Biochem. Biophys. Res. Commun.*, 142, 559–566 (1987).

212. A.-P. Ernould, G. Ferry, J.-M. Barret, A. Genton, and J. A. Boutin, *Eur. J. Biochem.*, 214, 503–514 (1993).

213. T. Peng, J. R. C. Hunter, and J. W. Nelson, *Virology*, 216, 184–196 (1996).

214. S. Stocchetto, O. Marin, G. Carignani, and L. A. Pinna, *FEBS Lett.*, 414, 171–175 (1997).

215. K.-T. Yu, Y. N. Khalaf, and M. P. Czech, *J. Biol. Chem.*, 262, 16677–16685 (1987).

216. P. Steinert, J. B. Wissing, and K. G. Wagner, *Plant Sci.*, 101, 105–114 (1994).

217. Y. H. Baek and T. Nowak, *Arch. Biochem. Biophys.*, 217, 491–497 (1982).

218. M. H. Lee, C. A. Hebda, and T. Nowak, *J. Biol. Chem.*, 256, 12793–12801 (1981).

219. D. J. Owen, M. E. Noble, E. F. Garman, A. C. Papageorgiou, and L. N. Johnson, *Structure*, 3, 467–482 (1995).

220. J. H. Hurley, H. R. Faber, D. Worthylake, N. D. Meadow, S. Roseman, D. W. Pettigrew, and S. J. Remington, *Science*, 259, 673–677 (1993).

221. J. H. Zheng, E. A. Trafny, D. R. Knighton, N.-H. Xuong, S. S. Taylor, L. F. Ten Eyck, and J. M. Sowadski, *Acta Cryst. Sect. D Biol. Cryst.*, 49, 362–365 (1993).

222. R. A. Engh, A. Girod, V. Kinzel, R. Huber, and D. Bossemeyer, *J. Biol. Chem.*, 271, 26157–26164 (1996).

223. D. Bossemeyer, R. A. Engh, V. Kinzel, H. Ponstingl, and R. Huber, *EMBO J.*, 12, 849–859 (1993).

224. E. D. Lowe, M. E. M. Noble, V. T. Skamnaki, N. G. Oikonomakos, D. J. Owen, and L. N. Johnson, *EMBO J.*, 16, 6646–6658 (1997).

225. T. M. Larsen, L. T. Laughlin, H. M. Holden, I. Rayment, and G. H. Reed, *Biochemistry*, 33, 6301–6309 (1994).

226. K. A. Buss, C. Ingram-Smith, J. G. Ferry, D. A. Sanders, and M. S. Hasson, *Protein Sci.*, *6*, 2659–2662 (1997).

227. A. May, M. Vas, K. Harlos, and C. Blake, *Proteins*, *24*, 292–303 (1996).

228. H. C. Watson, N. P. Walker, P. J. Shaw, T. N. Bryant, P. L. Wendell, L. A. Fothergill, R. E. Perkins, S. C. Conroy, M. J. Dobson, M. F. Tuite, A. J. Kingsman, and S. M. Kingsman, *EMBO J.*, *1*, 1635–1640 (1982).

229. M. B. Berry and G. N. Phillips, Jr., *Proteins Struct. Funct. Genet.*, *32*, 276–288 (1998).

230. R. L. Williams, D. A. Oren, J. Muñoz-Dorado, S. Inouye, M. Inouye, and E. Arnold, *J. Mol. Biol.*, *234*, 1230–1247 (1993).

231. A. Mattevi, M. Bolognesi, and G. Valentini, *FEBS Lett.*, *389*, 15–19 (1996).

232. M. S. M. Jetten, M. E. Gubler, S. H. Lee, and A. J. Sinskey, *Appl. Environ. Microbiol.*, *60*, 2501–2507 (1994).

233. A. de Zwaan, D. A. Holwerda, and A. D. Addink, *Comp. Biochem. Physiol. [B]*, *52*, 469–472 (1975).

234. T. M. Larsen, M. M. Benning, I. Rayment, and G. H. Reed, *Biochemistry*, *37*, 6247–6255 (1998).

235. T. M. Larsen, M. M. Benning, G. E. Wesenberg, I. Rayment, and G. H. Reed, *Arch. Biochem. Biophys.*, *345*, 199–206 (1997).

236. Y. Kim, S. H. Eom, J. M. Wang, D. S. Lee, S. W. Suh, and T. A. Steitz, *Nature*, *376*, 612–616 (1995).

237. (a) C. A. Brautigam and T. A. Steitz, *Curr. Opin. Struct. Biol.*, *8*, 54–63 (1998).
    (b) C. M. Joyce and T. A. Steitz, *Annu. Rev. Biochem.*, *63*, 777–822 (1994).

238. C. Breton, E. Bettler, D. H. Joziasse, R. A. Geremia, and A. Imberty, *J. Biochem.*, *123*, 1000–1009 (1998).

239. J. A. Campbell, G. J. Davies, V. Bulone, and B. Henrissat, *Biochem. J.*, *326*, 929–939 (1997).

240. J. A. Campbell, G. J. Davies, V. Bulone, and B. Henrissat, *Biochem. J.*, *329*, 719 (1998).

241. R. J. Kaufman, M. Swaroop, and P. Murtha-Riel, *Biochemistry*, *33*, 9813–9819 (1994).

242. P. J. Focia, S. P. Craig III, and A. E. Eakin, *Biochemistry*, *37*, 17120–17127 (1998).

243. V. Sharma, C. Grubmeyer, and J. C. Sacchettini, *Structure*, *6*, 1587–1599 (1998).

244. J. M. Krahn, J. H. Kim, M. R. Burns, R. J. Parry, H. Zalkin, and J. L. Smith, *Biochemistry*, *36*, 11061–11068 (1997).

245. R. G. Spiro, Y. Yasumoto, and V. Bhoyroo, *Biochem. J.*, *319*, 209–216 (1996).

246. G. Lukatela, N. Krauss, K. Theis, T. Selmer, V. Gieselmann, K. von Figura, W. Saenger, *Biochemistry*, *37*, 3654–3664 (1998).

247. C. S. Bond, P. R. Clements, S. J. Ashby, C. A. Collyer, S. J. Harrop, J. J. Hopwood, and J. M. Guss, *Structure*, *5*, 277–289 (1997).

248. P. J. O'Brien and D. Herschlag, *J. Am. Chem. Soc.*, *120*, 12369–12370 (1998).

249. J. E. Murphy, B. Stec, L. Ma, and E. R. Kantrowitz, *Nature Struct. Biol.*, *4*, 618–622 (1997).

250. K. Håkansson, A. J. Doherty, S. Shuman, and D. B. Wigley, *Cell*, *89*, 545–553 (1997).

251. K. Ogura and T. Koyama, *Chem. Rev.*, *98*, 1263–1276 (1998).

252. K. U. Wendt and G. E. Schulz, *Structure*, *6*, 127–133 (1998).

253. I. C. Hampele, A. D'Arcy, G. E. Dale, D. Kostrewa, J. Nielsen, C. Oefner, M. G. Page, H. J. Schönfeld, D. Stüber, and R. L. Then, *J. Mol. Biol.*, *268*, 21–30 (1997).

254. B. A. Bernat, L. T. Laughlin, and R. N. Armstrong, *Biochemistry*, *36*, 3050–3055 (1997).

255. M. M. Georgiadis, S. M. Jessen, C. M. Ogata, A. Telesnitsky, S. P. Goff, and W. A. Hendrickson, *Structure*, *3*, 879–892 (1995).

256. H. Kodama, N. Shimojo, and K. T. Suzuki, *Biochem. J.*, *278*, 857–862 (1991).

257. S. Hedeager-Sorenson and A. J. Kenny, *Biochem. J.*, *229*, 251–257 (1985).

258. J. M. C. Ribeiro and T. N. Mather, *Exp. Parasitol.*, *89*, 213–221 (1998).

259. S. Rowsell, R. A. Pauptit, A. D. Tucker, R. G. Melton, D. M. Blow, and P. Brick, *Structure*, *5*, 337–347 (1997).

260. H. M. Greenblatt, H. Feinberg, P. A. Tucker, and G. Scoham, *Acta Cryst. Sect. D Biol. Cryst.*, *54D*, 289–305 (1998).

261. C. J. Stirling, S. D. Colloms, J. F. Collins, G. Szatmari, and D. J. Sherratt, *EMBO J.*, *8*, 1623–1627 (1989).

262. Y. Sanz and F. Toldra, *J. Agric. Food Chem.*, *45*, 1552–1558 (1997).

263. D. Acosta, F. Goni, and C. Carmona, *J. Parasitol.*, *84*, 1–7 (1998).

264. M. D. Fernandez-Espla and M. C. Martin-Hernandez, *J. Dairy Sci.*, *80*, 1497–1504 (1997).

265. M. Simitsopoulou, A. Vafopoulou, T. Cholipapadopoulou, and E. Alichanidis, *Appl. Environ. Microbiol.*, *63*, 4872–4876 (1997).

266. H. Kim and W. N. Lipscomb, in *Advances in Enzymology, Vol. 68* (A. Meister, ed.), John Wiley and Sons, New York, 1994, pp. 153–213.

267. N. Sträter and W. N. Lipscomb, *Biochemistry*, *34*, 14792–14800 (1995).

268. N. Sträter and W. N. Lipscomb, *Biochemistry*, *34*, 9200–9210 (1995).

269. B. Chevrier, H. Dorchymont, C. Schalk, C. Tarnus, and D. Moras, *Eur. J. Biochem.*, *237*, 393–398 (1996).

270. S. L. Roderick and B. W. Matthews, *Biochemistry*, *32*, 3907–3912 (1993).

271. T. H. Tahirov, H. Oki, T. Tsukihara, K. Ogasahara, K. Yutani, K. Ogata, Y. Izu, S. Tsunasawa, I. Kato, *J. Mol. Biol.*, *284*, 101–124 (1998).

272. M. C. J. Wilce, C. S. Bond, N. E. Dixon, H. C. Freeman, J. M. Guss, P. E. Lilley, and J. A. Wilce, *Proc. Natl. Acad. Sci. USA*, *95*, 3472–3477 (1998).

273. L. B. Zhang, M. J. Crossley, N. E. Dixon, P. J. Ellis, M. L. Fisher, G. F. King, P. E. Lilley, D. MacLachlan, R. J. Pace, and H. C. Freeman, *J. Biol. Inorg. Chem.*, *3*, 470–483 (1998).

274. B. F. Bellew, C. J. Halkides, G. J. Gerfen, R. G. Griffin, and D. J. Singel, *Biochemistry*, *35*, 12186–12193 (1996).

275. C. J. Halkides, B. F. Bellew, G. J. Gerfen, C. T. Farrar, P. H. Carter, B. Ruo, D. A. Evans, R. G. Griffin, and D. J. Singel, *Biochemistry*, *35*, 12194–12200 (1996).

276. D. G. Latwesen, M. Poe, I. G. Leigh, and G. A. Reed, *Biochemistry*, *31*, 4946–4950 (1992).

277. F. Rusnak, this volume, Chap. 10.

278. R. Bone, L. Frank, J. P. Springer, and J. R. Atack, *Biochemistry*, *33*, 9468–9476 (1994).

279. J. R. Atack, H. B. Broughton, and S. J. Pollack, *FEBS Lett.*, *361*, 1–7 (1995).

280. S. Chattoraj-Bhattacharyya and A. L. Majumder, *Arch. Biochem. Biophys.*, *316*, 63–69 (1995).

281. Y. Zhang, J.-Y. Liang, S. Huang, H. Ke, and W. N. Lipscomb, *Biochemistry*, *32*, 1844–1857 (1993).

282. V. Villeret, S. Huang, Y. Zhang, and W. N. Lipscomb, *Biochemistry*, *34*, 4307–4315 (1995).

283. G. Q. Lu, B. Stec, E. L. Giroux, and E. R. Kantrowitz, *Protein Sci.*, *5*, 2333–2342 (1996).

284. B. Stec, R. Abraham, E. Giroux, and E. R. Kantrowitz, *Protein Sci.*, *5*, 1541–1553 (1996).

285. V. Villeret, S. H. Huang, Y. P. Zhang, Y. F. Xue, and W. N. Lipscomb, *Biochemistry*, *34*, 4299–4306 (1995).

286. J. A. Cowan, *Chem. Rev.*, *98*, 1067–1087 (1998).

287. G. S. Baldwin, N. A. Gormley, and S. E. Halford, this volume, Chap. 11.

288. T. A. Ceska, J. R. Sayers, G. Stier, and D. Suck, *Nature*, *382*, 90–93 (1996).

289. G. Bujacz, J. Alexandratos, and A. Wlodawer, *J. Biol. Chem.*, *272*, 18161–18168 (1997).

290. G. Bujacz, M. Jaskólski, J. Alexandratos, A. Wlodawer, G. Merkel, R. A. Katz, and A. M. Skalka, *Structure*, *4*, 89–96 (1996).

291. D. E. Ash, J. D. Cox, and D. W. Christianson, this volume, Chap. 13.

292. R. Bogumil, M. Knipp, S. M. Fundel, and M. Vasak, *Biochemistry*, *37*, 4791–4798 (1998).

293. H. Baur, E. Luethi, V. Stalon, A. Mercenier, and D. Haas, *Eur. J. Biochem.*, *179*, 53–60 (1989).

294. J. Perozich, J. Hempel, and S. M. Morris, *Biochim. Biophys. Acta*, *1382*, 23–37 (1998).

295. Y. Shirokane, M. Utsushikawa, and M. Nakajima, *Clin. Chem.*, *33*, 394–397 (1987).

296. T. Yorifuji, I. Sugai, H. Matsumoto, and A. Tabuchi, *Agric. Biol. Chem.*, *16*, 1362–1367 (1982).

297. T. Yorifuji, M. Kato, T. Kobayashi, S. Ozaki, and S. Ueno, *Agric. Biol. Chem.*, *44*, 1127–1134 (1980).

298. S. M. Shoeb, M. Kaneoke, E. Shimizu, and T. Yorifuji, *Appl. Microbiol. Biotechnol.*, *44*, 94–99 (1995).

299. A. Matte, H. Goldie, R. M. Sweet, and L. T. J. Delbaere, *J. Mol. Biol.*, *256*, 126–143 (1996).

300. L. W. Tari, A. Matte, U. Pugazhenthi, H. Goldie, and L. T. J. Delbaere, *Nature Struct. Biol.*, *3*, 355–363 (1996).

301. L. W. Tari, A. Matte, H. Goldie, and L. T. J. Delbaere, *Nature Struct. Biol.*, *4*, 990–994 (1997).

302. A. Matte, L. W. Tari, H. Goldie, and L. T. J. Delbaere, *J. Biol. Chem.*, *272*, 8105–8108 (1997).

303. B. Stec and L. Lebioda, *J. Mol. Biol.*, *211*, 235–248 (1990).

304. S. Duquerroy, C. Camus, and J. Janin, *Biochemistry*, *34*, 12513–12523 (1995).

305. L. Lebioda, B. Stec, and J. M. Brewer, *J. Biol. Chem.*, *264*, 3685–3693 (1989).

306. E. L. Zhang, M. Hatada, J. M. Brewer, and L. Lebioda, *Biochemistry*, *33*, 6295–6300 (1994).

307. J. E. Wedekind, R. R. Poyner, G. H. Reed, and I. Rayment, *Biochemistry*, *33*, 9333–9342 (1994).

308. J. E. Wedekind, G. H. Reed, and I. Rayment, *Biochemistry*, *34*, 4325–4330 (1995).

309. L. Lebioda, E. Zhang, K. Lewinski, and J. M. Brewer, *Proteins Struct. Funct. Genet.*, *16*, 219–225 (1993).

310. E. Zhang, J. M. Brewer, W. Minor, L. A. Carreira, and L. Lebioda, *Biochemistry*, *36*, 12526–12534 (1997).

311. T. M. Larsen, J. E. Wedekind, I. Rayment, and G. H. Reed, *Biochemistry*, *35*, 4349–4358 (1996).

312. R. R. Poyner and G. H. Reed, *Biochemistry*, *31*, 7166–7173 (1992).

313. S. K. Wang, R. A. Scott, L. Lebioda, Z. H. Zhou, and J. M. Brewer, *J. Inorg. Biochem.*, *58*, 209–221 (1995).

314. A. M. Gulick, D. R. J. Palmer, P. C. Babbitt, J. A. Gerlt, and I. Rayment, *Biochemistry*, *37*, 14358–14368 (1998).

315. J. J. G. Tesmer, R. K. Sunahara, A. G. Gilman, and S. R. Sprang, *Science*, *278*, 1907–1916 (1997).

316. T. Mitterauer, M. Hohenegger, W. J. Tang, C. Nanoff, and M. Freissmuth, *Biochemistry*, *37*, 16183–16191 (1998).

317. R. Bogumil, R. Kappl, and J. Hütterman, this volume, Chap. 12.

318. A. Cleasby, A. Wonacott, T. Skarzynski, R. E. Hubbard, G. J. Davies, A. E. Proudfoot, A. R. Bernard, M. A. Payton, and T. N. Wells, *Nature Struct. Biol.*, *3*, 470–479 (1996).

319. J. E. Seemann and G. E. Schulz, *J. Mol. Biol.*, *273*, 256–268 (1997).

320. J. Bohlmann, G. Meyergauen, and R. Croteau, *Proc. Natl. Acad. Sci. USA*, *95*, 4126–4133 (1998).

321. M. Clastre, B. Bantignies, G. Feron, E. Soler, and C. Ambid, *Plant Physiol.*, *102*, 205–211 (1993).

322. A. J. Chen and C. D. Poulter, *J. Biol. Chem.*, *268*, 11002–11007 (1993).

323. J. Crock, M. Wildung, and R. Croteau, *Proc. Natl. Acad. Sci. USA*, *94*, 12833–12838 (1997).

324. P. C. Babbitt and J. A. Gerlt, *J. Biol. Chem.*, *272*, 30591–30594 (1997).

325. S. L. Bearne and R. Wolfenden, *Biochemistry*, *36*, 1646–1656 (1997).

326. J. A. Gerlt and P. G. Gassman, *Biochemistry*, *32*, 11943–11952 (1993).

327. J. A. Gerlt and P. G. Gassman, *J. Am. Chem. Soc.*, *115*, 11552–11568 (1993).

328. G. L. Kenyon, J. A. Gerlt, G. A. Petsko, and J. W. Kozarich, *Acc. Chem. Res.*, *28*, 178–188 (1995).

329. D. J. Neidhart, P. L. Howell, G. A. Petsko, V. M. Powers, R. Li, G. L. Kenyon, and J. A. Gerlt, *Biochemistry*, *30*, 9264–9273 (1991).

330. J. A. Landro, J. A. Gerlt, J. W. Kozarich, C. W. Koo, V. J. Shah, G. L. Kenyon, and D. J. Neidhart, *Biochemistry*, *33*, 635–643 (1994).

331. A. T. Kallarakal, B. Mitra, J. W. Kozarich, J. A. Gerlt, J. G. Clifton, G. A. Petsko, and G. L. Kenyon, *Biochemistry*, *34*, 2788–2797 (1995).

332. B. Mitra, A. T. Kallarakal, J. W. Kozarich, J. A. Gerlt, J. G. Clifton, G. A. Petsko, and G. L. Kenyon, *Biochemistry*, *34*, 2777–2787 (1995).

333. S. L. Schafer, W. C. Barrett, A. T. Kallarakal, B. Mitra, J. W. Kozarich, J. A. Gerlt, J. G. Clifton, G. A. Petsko, and G. L. Kenyon, *Biochemistry*, *35*, 5662– 5669 (1996).

334. J. A. Fee, G. D. Hegeman, and G. L. Kenyon, *Biochemistry*, *13*, 2528–2532 (1974).

335. R. Blasco, R. M. Wittich, M. Mallavarapu, K. N. Timmis, and D. H. Pieper, *J. Biol. Chem.*, *270*, 29229–29235 (1995).

336. M. D. Vollmer, H. Hoier, H.-J. Hecht, U. Schell, J. Gröning, A. Goldman, and M. Schlömann, *Appl. Environ. Microbiol.*, *64*, 3290–3299 (1998).

337. M. S. Hasson, I. Schlichting, J. Moulai, K. Taylor, W. Barrett, G. L. Kenyon, P. C. Babbitt, J. A. Gerlt, G. A. Petsko, and D. Ringe, *Proc. Natl. Acad. Sci. USA*, *95*, 10396–10401 (1998).

338. S. Helin, P. C. Kahn, B. L. Guha, D. G. Mallows, and A. Goldman, *J. Mol. Biol.*, *254*, 918–941 (1995).

339. U. Schell, S. Helin, T. Kajander, M. Schlömann, and A. Goldman, *Proteins*, *34*, 125–136 (1999).

340. M. D. Vollmer and M. Schlömann, *J. Bacteriol.*, *177*, 2938–2941 (1995).

341. H. Hoier, M. Schlömann, A. Hammer, J. P. Glusker, H. L. Carrell, A. Goldman, J. J. Stezowski, and U. H. Heinemann, *Acta Cryst. Sect. D Biol. Cryst.*, *50*, 75–84 (1994).

342. G. J. Kleywegt, H. Hoier, and T. A. Jones, *Acta Cryst. Sect. D Biol. Cryst.*, *52*, 858–863 (1996).

343. J. A. Landro, A. T. Kallarakal, S. C. Ransom, J. A. Gerlt, J. W. Kozarich, D. J. Niedhart, and G. L. Kenyon, *Biochemistry*, *30*, 9274–9281 (1991).

344. R. R. Poyner, L. T. Laughlin, G. A. Sowa, and G. H. Reed, *Biochemistry*, *35*, 1692–1699 (1996).

345. S.-H. Liaw and D. Eisenberg, *Biochemistry*, *33*, 675–681 (1994).

346. M. R. Witmer, D. Palmieri-Young, and J. J. Villafranca, *Protein Sci.*, *3*, 1746–1759 (1994).

347. M. R. Witmer, D. Palmieri-Young, J. J. Villafranca, in *Techniques*

in Protein Chemistry (J. W. Crabb, ed.), Academic Press, San Diego, 1994, pp. 321–329.

348. M. M. Yamashita, R. J. Almassy, C. A. Janson, D. Cascio, and D. Eisenberg, *J. Biol. Chem.*, *264*, 17681–17690 (1989).

349. L. P. Reynaldo, J. J. Villafranca, and W. D. Horrocks, *Protein Sci.*, 5, 2532–2544 (1996).

350. J. B. Thoden, S. G. Miran, J. C. Phillips, A. J. Howard, F. M. Raushel, and H. M. Holden, *Biochemistry*, *37*, 8825–8831 (1998).

351. F. M. Raushel, J. B. Thoden, G. D. Reinhart, and H. M. Holden, *Curr. Opin. Chem. Biol.*, *2*, 624–632 (1998).

352. J. B. Thoden, F. M. Raushel, M. M. Benning, I. Rayment, and H. M. Holden, *Acta Cryst. Sect. D. Biol. Cryst.*, *55*, 8–24 (1999).

353. J. B. Thoden, G. Wesenberg, F. M. Raushel, and H. M. Holden, *Biochemistry*, *38*, 2347–2357 (1999).

354. J. G. Arnez, A.-C. Dock-Bregeon, and J. M. P. Moras, *J. Mol. Biol.*, *286*, 1449–1459 (1999).

355. H. Belrhali, A. Yaremchuk, M. Tukalo, C. Berthet-Colominas, B. Rasmussen, P. Bösecke, O. Diat, and S. Cusack, *Structure*, *3*, 341–352 (1995).

356. J. G. Arnez, J. G. Augustine, D. Moras, and C. S. Francklyn, *Proc. Natl. Acad. Sci. USA*, *94*, 7144–7149 (1997).

357. S. Cusack, *Curr. Opin. Struct. Biol.*, *7*, 881–889 (1997).

358. C. Berthet-Colominas, L. Seignovert, M. Hartlein, M. Grotli, S. Cusack, and R. Leberman, *EMBO J.*, *17*, 2947–2960 (1998).

359. E. Schmidt, L. Moulinier, S. Fujiwara, T. Imanaka, J.-C. Thierry, and D. Moras, *EMBO J.*, *17*, 5227–5237 (1998).

360. Z. Ma, J. H. Grubb, and W. S. Sly, *J. Biol. Chem.*, *266*, 10589–10595 (1991).

361. A. J. Kalb(Gilboa), J. Habash, N. S. Hunter, H. J. Price, J. Raftery, and J. R. Helliwell, this volume, Chap. 9.

362. C. Chothia and E. Y. Jones, *Annu. Rev. Biochem.*, *66*, 823–862 (1997).

363. J. Joseph-Silverstein and R. L. Silverstein, *Cancer Invest.*, *16*, 176–182 (1998).

364. A. D. Qu and D. J. Leahy, *Proc. Natl. Acad. Sci. USA*, *92*, 10277–10281 (1995).

365. J. O. Lee, P. Rieu, M. A. Arnaout, and R. Liddington, *Cell*, *80*, 631–638 (1995).

366. R. Li, P. Rieu, D. L. Griffith, D. Scott, and M. Amin Arnaout, *J. Cell. Biol.*, *143*, 1523–1534 (1998).

367. E. T. Baldwin, R. W. Sarver, G. L. Bryant, Jr., K. A. Curry, M. B. Fairbanks, B. C. Finzel, R. L. Garlick, R. L. Heinrikson, N. C. Horton, L. L. Kelley, A. M. Mildner, J. B. Moon, J. E. Mott, V. T. Mutchler, C. S. Tomich, K. D. Watenpaugh, and V. H. Wiley, *Structure*, *6*, 923–935 (1998).

368. D. W. Griggs, C. M. Schmidt, and C. P. Carron, *J. Biol. Chem.*, *273*, 22113–22119 (1998).

369. N. Schiering, X. Tao, H. Y. Zeng, J. R. Murphy, G. A. Petsko, and D. Ringe, *Proc. Natl. Acad. Sci. USA*, *92*, 9843–9850 (1995).

370. X. Ding, H. Zeng, N. Schiering, D. Ringe, and J. R. Murphy, *Nature Struct. Biol.*, *3*, 382–387 (1996).

371. X. Y. Qiu, E. Pohl, R. K. Holmes, and W. G. J. Hol, *Biochemistry*, *35*, 12292–12302 (1996).

372. M. Y. Hamed and J. B. Neilands, *J. Inorg. Biochem.*, *53*, 235–248 (1994).

373. M. C. Lawrence, P. A. Pilling, V. C. Epa, A. M. Berry, A. D. Ogunniyi, and J. C. Paton, *Structure*, *6*, 1553–1561 (1998).

9

Manganese(II) in Concanavalin A and Other Lectin Proteins

A. Joseph Kalb(Gilboa),[1]* Jarjis Habash,[2] Nicola S. Hunter,[2] Helen J. Price,[2] James Raftery,[2] and John R. Helliwell[2]*

[1]Department of Structural Biology, The Weizmann Institute of Science, Rehovot, Israel

[2]Section of Structural Chemistry, Department of Chemistry, University of Manchester, Manchester M13 9PL, UK

*Corresponding authors.

1. INTRODUCTION: THE BIOLOGY AND MOLECULAR BIOLOGY OF CONCANAVALIN A

Concanavalin A is a member of a family of widely distributed plant proteins originally known as hemagglutinins and currently known also as plant lectins. The specificity and reversibility of carbohydrate recognition by lectins has made them useful for identification and characterization of carbohydrate structures during cell growth, differentiation, malignancies, and metastases [1]. No specific biological function has been unequivocally attributed to the plant lectins; however, their saccharide binding property may be important in cell-to-cell crosslinking and in cell attachment by viral proteins [2]. Most important is the usefulness of the lectins in providing quantitative structural and thermodynamic data leading to a basic understanding of protein-carbohydrate recognition. Concanavalin A is the most extensively studied plant lectin ever since its isolation as bisphenoid crystals in 1919 by the Nobel Laureate, James B. Sumner [3]. The protein is found in large quantities in the Jack bean *Canavalia ensiformis* (Fig. 1) and comprises more than 5% of the dry weight of the bean. It has been suggested that such large

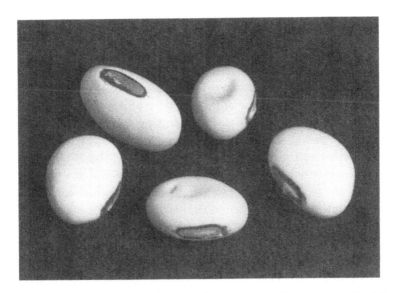

FIG. 1.   Jack beans, maximum length ≈2 cm, from which concanavalin A is extracted and purified.

amounts of the lectin are needed by the plant in order to form an impervious crosslinked matrix as a defense mechanism. Such plant defense could be a valuable tool and is one of the approaches that has been considered for genetic modification of crops to confer pest resistance (e.g., involving snowdrop lectin to deal with aphids [4]).

   At the molecular level, structural details of concanavalin A have been revealed by X-ray crystallography; it is the first lectin whose saccharide binding site was characterized in molecular detail [5]. The saccharide binding site geometry relies in part on an unusal nonproline cis-peptide, stabilized by a calcium ion, which in turn is stabilized by a transition metal ion, usually manganese. Thus, very specific molecular recognition for the protein's cognate sugars (glucoside and mannoside) is achieved. This chapter reviews the structural work on concanavalin A, with special emphasis on recent advances in ultrahigh-resolution and multiwavelength anomalous dispersion (MAD) X-ray crystallography using synchrotron radiation, and also neutron crystallography using the recently developed neutron Laue technique, as well as details of the isolation and purification and related spectrocopic and calorimetric results. The precise structural description of the Mn site is emphasized.

2.   ISOLATION AND CHARACTERIZATION

Concanavalin A was first isolated by Sumner by fractional crystallization from an aqueous extract of Jack bean meal [3]. The final step involved selective dissolution of the concanavalin A crystals by treatment
with saturated NaCl at 40°C. The resulting solution had the ability to
agglutinate red blood cells or glycogen at extremely high dilution and
the protein was therefore identified as the Jack bean hemagglutinin.
Surprisingly, when the same crystals were dissolved in a warm sucrose
solution, the protein was found to have lost its agglutinating power [6].
This led to the novel conclusion that concanavalin A binds simple sugars as well as naturally occurring polysaccharides. Sumner and co-
workers used Svedberg's newly developed technique of sedimentation-
diffusion in the ultracentrifuge to determine the molecular weight of
concanavalin A [7]. They also characterized concanavalin A as a metalloprotein on the basis of the observation that acidification destroyed the
ability to agglutinate red cells but that this property was recovered
when certain essential metal ions were supplied [8,9]. One of the essential metals identified in the acidic dialyzate was manganese. The
stoichiometry of saccharide and metal binding was, however, not studied until many years after Sumner's pioneering work [10,11].
    Several alternative methods of isolation, based on the saccharide
binding property of concanavalin A, have been devised in the last few
decades and are in widespread use today. Sephadex, a synthetically
crosslinked form of dextran, adsorbs concanavalin A selectively from an
aqueous Jack bean extract [12,13]. The pure protein can be recovered
by elution with simple sugars such as glucose or by acidification. A synthetic affinity medium designed to have a high density of glucoside moieties has been used to produce what appears to be an extremely pure
preparation of concanavalin A [14]. One clear advantage of Sumner's
crystallization method over the more fashionable affinity methods is
that it avoids exposing the protein to sugars.

2.1.   Molecular Weight

Determination of the molecular weight of concanavalin A is complicated
by the tendency of the molecule to aggregate in solution [15]. Below pH

5.8, the molecular weight is approximately 50 kDa; around neutrality it is a mixture of two species of 50 and 100 kDa; and above pH 7 larger aggregates of ill-defined molecular weight appear. The behavior of concanavalin A under denaturing conditions is also complex: it is a mixture of intact subunits of 25 kDa; and two fragments of 12 and 13 kDa, respectively, which together make up a complete subunit of 25 kDa [16]. Sequence analysis confirms that the intact subunit of concanavalin A has a molecular weight of 25 600 consisting of 237 amino acid residues and that the two fragments comprise residues 1–119 and 120–237. In the native protein, the intact and nicked subunits coexist, the two fragments folding exactly as the corresponding parts of the intact subunit. Various methods for purification of intact subunits have been reported [17,18].

2.2. Stoichiometry

Direct binding studies by the method of equilibrium dialysis established the equivalent binding weight for the simple saccharide, methyl α-D-glucopyranoside, to be approximately 30 kDa, corresponding to one subunit of concanavalin A [10]. Similar values were determined for equivalent binding weights for several metal ions [11,19]. Taken together, this suggests that the operational unit in concanavalin A is the 25-kDa monomer. The simple form of the binding curves also suggests that there is no intersubunit cooperativity. On the other hand, there is a unique form of site–site interaction *within* the individual subunit: metal-free (also known as "demetallized") concanavalin A binds one of the following divalent metal ions—Zn, Co, Ni, Mn, or Cd—with a stoichiometry of one metal ion per subunit but does not bind Ca or saccharide; saturated with any one of the above five metals (we will call such one-metal species M-concanavalin A) the protein binds one equivalent of Ca per subunit but does not bind saccharide; only the two-metal species, M,Ca-concanavalin A, can bind one equivalent of saccharide per subunit. These findings indicate that there are two distinct metal binding sites, a transition metal binding site and a calcium binding site, and that both must be occupied for saccharide to be bound [11]. X-ray crystallographic studies, described in Sec. 8, have revealed the structural links among the three sites (two metal binding sites and one saccharide binding site) as well as the mechanism of interaction among them [5,20–23].

It is appropriate in a review such as this to point out an intriguing problem concerning stoichiometry of concanavalin A: as isolated from the Jack bean, concanavalin A contains *sub*stoichiometric quantities of manganese—from 20% to 40% of one equivalent [24,25]. Considering the ability of concanavalin A to accommodate five different metal ions in the transition metal binding site, one might imagine that the naturally occurring protein contains a mixture of these, whose distribution reflects the environmental abundance and the relative affinity of each of them. There is, however, no experimental evidence concerning the metal ion population in naturally occurring concanavalin A. In Sec. 6 we describe an experiment designed to determine the fraction of transition-metal binding sites occupied by Mn in a concanavalin A crystal. However, several observations suggest that the transition metal binding site might be enriched in Mn during crystallization due to the protein then being in the presence of excess Mn^{2+} (unlike in the Jack bean itself).

2.3.   Thermodynamics of Metal Binding

Association constants and the corresponding values of free energy of binding have been determined for the binding of the five metals mentioned in the previous section to the transition metal binding site and for calcium and cadmium to the calcium binding site [19]. The metals that bind to the transition metal binding site vary widely in ionic radius (0.7–1 Å) and have in common that they are divalent ions with affinity for nitrogen ligands as well as oxygen ligands. Their affinity for concanavalin A correlates well with their affinity for ammonia or imidazole. The two metals that bind to the calcium binding site, on the other hand, have nearly the same ionic radius. The possibility of binding a heavy metal such as cadmium to both sites has proven to be very useful in X-ray crystallographic research [26].

2.4.   Thermodynamics of Saccharide Binding

A systematic study of binding of simple sugars to concanavalin A has been carried out by direct binding measurements based on equilibrium dialysis [27]; thermodynamics of binding of several oligosaccharides has been studied by means of microcalorimetry [28]. An unexpected result, supported by both studies, is that the energetic cost of replacing one hydroxyl group with a hydrogen atom is approximately the same for each of the three hydroxyl groups involved in direct interaction with the saccharide binding site and is approximately 2 kcal/mol (Table 1) [29]. The same energetic cost is associated with removal of the exocyclic $-CH_2$ of carbon-6.

An interesting observation, first described in Ref. 30 and recently confirmed [27], is that the effectiveness of a saccharide in dissolving crystals of saccharide-free concanavalin A is highly correlated with its binding constant. This can afford a simple method for estimation of binding constants and is especially useful for weakly interacting saccharides.

TABLE 1

Free Energy of Association of Simple and Complex
Saccharides with Concanavalin A[a]

Saccharide	Free energy of association, G (kcal/mol)	Reduction in complex stability, ΔG (kcal/mol)	Ref.
MMP	−5.3	—	27
3-Deoxy-MMP	−2.7	2.6	27
6-Deoxy-MMP	−3.0	2.3	27
MGP	−4.6	—	27
2-Deoxy-MGP	−4.9	−0.3	27
4-Deoxy-MGP	−2.0	2.6	27
Trimannoside	−7.8	—	28
2-Deoxytrimannoside	−7.8	0.0	28
3-Deoxytrimannoside	−6.3	1.5	28
4-Deoxytrimannoside	−6.0	1.8	28
6-Deoxytrimannoside	−6.1	1.7	28

[a]Effect on complex stability of removal of OH-2, OH-3, OH-4, and OH-6 from the interacting sugar. MMP, methyl α-D-mannopyranoside; MGP, methyl α-D-glucopyranoside; "trimannoside," methyl-3,6-di-O-(α-D-mannopyranosyl)-α-D-mannopyranoside. The deoxy analogs of the trimannoside refer to the mannoside moiety that binds to the saccharide binding site, namely the α(1-6) arm.

3. SPECTROSCOPIC STUDIES

The possibility of preparing concanavalin A with any one of several metal ions in the transition metal binding site makes a variety of spectroscopic methods available for study of this site. This has also served as an impetus for determination of exact crystal structures for the various single-metal species.

3.1. Magnetic Resonance Spectroscopy

Manganese is particularly useful in this respect because it is the key to several varieties of magnetic resonance spectroscopy. Electron paramagnetic resonance (EPR) spectra of single crystals as well as of solutions of concanavalin A have been measured at Q-band frequency leading to a detailed description of the magnetic parameters of the transition metal binding site [31,32]. Recently, the pulsed EPR technique has been applied to single crystals, crystalline powders, and frozen solutions of Mn,Ca-concanavalin A in order to study the superhyperfine interactions between the Mn ion and hydrogen or nitrogen atoms in the transition metal binding site [33]. A classic study of Mn-mediated nuclear magnetic resonance (NMR) relaxation kinetics was used to deduce the mode of binding of ^{13}C-labeled methyl α-D-glucopyranoside bound to the saccharide binding site [34]. Many years later, these results were shown to be essentially correct by X-ray crystallographic structure determination of the corresponding crystalline complex [5]. NMR relaxation dispersion studies were used to investigate the kinetics of the interaction of concanavalin A with Mn, Ca, and saccharides [35]. Cobalt has been used as a chemical shifting nucleus in a study of the role of histidine in Co,Ca-concanavalin A [36]. ^{113}Cd NMR spectroscopy was used to deduce the existence of an additional site for cadmium in Cd,Cd-concanavalin A whose location and chemical nature were later determined by X-ray crystallography [37,38].

3.2. Circular Dichroism Spectroscopy

Far UV circular dichroism (CD) spectroscopy was used to estimate the secondary structure of concanavalin A [39]. The high content of β structure and the absence of helical structure deduced from this study is consistent with the β-barrel fold assigned to concanavalin A on the basis of X-ray crystallography [40,41]. Visible CD spectroscopy of the Co absorption bands of Co-concanavalin A provided the first evidence that the transition metal binding site must be geometrically asymmetric [42], a result that has recently been confirmed in fine detail by ultrahigh-resolution X-ray crystallography (see [43] and Sec. 5).

3.3. X-ray Absorption Fine-Structure Spectroscopy (XAFS)

First shell distances and coordination numbers in the transition metal binding site of Zn-concanavalin A and Zn,Ca-concanavalin A have been measured for the protein in microcrystalline suspensions [44]. These studies suggest that coordination in the transition metal binding site changes from hexa- to pentacoordinate on binding of calcium at the calcium binding site. A recent X-ray crystallographic study of Zn-concanavalin A and Zn,Ca-concanavalin A, however, shows the Zn ion to be hexacoordinate in both states [45].

4. CRYSTALS OF CONCANAVALIN A: INTRODUCTION AND EARLY HISTORY

Sumner originally isolated concanavalin A by fractional crystallization from aqueous extracts of the Jack bean [3]. Many years later, crystals suitable for X-ray studies, belonging to the orthorhombic space group I222, were obtained by gradually lowering the salt concentration of high-salt solutions of the purified protein by means of dialysis [46]. The crystals, though odd-shaped, have unusually excellent crystallographic properties, diffracting to 1.2 Å at room temperature [47] and to 0.85 Å at 100 K [43], and displaying low crystal mosaicity (approximately 0.2°).

4.1. Crystals of Saccharide-Free Concanavalin A

Crystal morphology can be controlled by suitable adjustment of initial supersaturation [48–50]. Lowering supersaturation by decreasing protein concentration, by increasing temperature, or by adjustment of pH below or above the pH of minimum solubility results in crystals of a very regular morphology with no change in the diffraction limit or crystal mosaicity. This can be important in certain experiments, such as single-crystal EPR spectroscopy, where it is essential to have crystals of regular morphology to facilitate orientation of the crystallographic axes relative to the magnetic field [51]. Crystal size is very difficult to control; however, very large crystals (3 mm in the largest dimension) suitable for neutron diffraction experiments are occasionally formed (see Sec. 7). A highly pure commercial preparation of lyophilized, salt-free concanavalin A produces small crystals (maximum dimension 0.2 mm) under standard crystallization conditions [50]. There is good evidence that this behavior is the result of stock solutions of this preparation containing a large endogenous population of stable crystal nuclei small enough to pass through the microfilter (0.2 µm) normally used before setting up crystallization trials. The population of these nuclei can be substantially reduced by incubation of the concentrated stock solution of concanavalin A in saturated NaCl at 40°C for 2 h, producing a stock solution that crystallizes slowly and gives a normal size distribution of crystals, including very large ones.

Crystals of concanavalin A of the same space group and similar cell dimensions as described above can be produced by salting out at high concentration of phosphate salts [41].

4.2.   Crystals of Demetallized, M- and M,Ca-Concanavalin A

As isolated from the Jack bean, concanavalin A contains less than stoichiometric amounts of manganese [14]. This can be removed by acidification and the resulting demetallized concanavalin A can be titrated at neutral pH with one of the metal ions Ni, Co, Zn, Mn, or Cd to produce stoichiometric one-metal species: M-concanavalin A, and, on addition of calcium, the corresponding M,Ca-concanavalin A where M stands for one of the five metals listed above [19]. Suitable crystallization conditions have been described for de-metallized, M- (M = Zn) and M,Ca- (M = Ni, Co, Zn, Mn, or Cd) concanavalin A and the structure of each of these species has been determined by X-ray crystallography [20,22, 23,38,52–54].

4.3. Crystals of Saccharide Complexes of Concanavalin A

The problem of crystallization of saccharide complexes of concanavalin A proved to be a serious barrier to progress in investigation of the atomic details of the protein–saccharide interaction. Once the anomalous solubility of these complexes was understood, however, it became feasible to crystallize several such complexes [5,55,56]. Whereas saccharide-free concanavalin A is virtually insoluble in water or dilute salts, the saccharide complexes can be dissolved in dilute salt solutions at extraordinarily high concentration (120–200 mg/mL). Preparation of suitable stock solutions of the saccharide complexes therefore involves dissolution of crystals of saccharide-free concanavalin A in a minimal volume of the saccharide. Recently, a general method has been proposed for crystallization of carbohydrate complexes of concanavalin A [57]. A recent review [58] summarizes essential data for 19 crystal forms of concanavalin A and its complexes. Photographs of a representative group of these are shown in Fig. 2.

5. ULTRAHIGH-RESOLUTION X-RAY PROTEIN CRYSTALLOGRAPHY

The purpose of investigating the protein at ultrahigh resolution was to realize sufficient X-ray data that the protein model could be refined with small molecule accuracy, i.e., where the X-ray data to parameter ratio is approaching an order of magnitude. This occurs at 1 Å or better diffraction resolution. Atoms become resolved in electron density maps at around 1.2 Å resolution. Our objectives were then more ambitious and would allow the determination of protonation states of side chain carboxyl groups and, in the current context, the accurate definition of the Mn metal binding site. The first study we conducted was at 0.94 Å resolution [43] and was of native concanavalin A, i.e., protein as isolated from the Jack bean. Here we describe the 0.92-Å study of the protein where the demetallized protein has been reconstituted in vitro with Mn and then Ca ions. The apparently very slight improvement in resolution from 0.94 Å to 0.92 Å conceals an increase of the number of unique

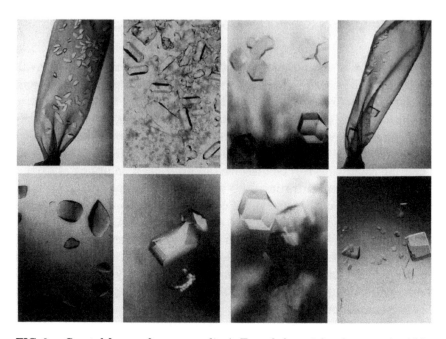

FIG. 2.   Crystal forms of concanavalin A. From left to right, they are: (*top*) Native saccharide-free concanavalin A crystals growing in a dialysis bag. (*bottom*) Close-up showing this "seed-like" crystal shape. Orthorhombic crystals (space group I222). (*top*) Native saccharide-free concanavalin A crystals showing a faceted morphology, grown at a temperature of 30°C. (*bottom*) One such large crystal showing details of the facets. These are also space group I222 and with the same unit cell parameters as the "seed-like" crystals. (*top*) α-Methylglucoside-bound concanavalin A (cubic crystals) in a dialysis bag showing several views (space group I2$_1$3). (*bottom*) Close-up of a large cubic crystal. (*top*) Demetallized concanavalin A crystals growing in a dialysis bag (space group P2$_1$22$_1$). (*bottom*) α-Methylmannoside-bound concanavalin A complex crystals (orthorhombic, space group P2$_1$2$_1$2$_1$).

X-ray diffraction data from 117 000 to 138 000 reflections (anomalous pairs merged). Inversion of the crystallographic full-matrix refinement elements in both studies yielded explicit standard uncertainties of atomic positions and thereby of bond and ligand distances and angles. Comparison of these two structures [43,59], similar in many respects, allows another way to evaluate the structural accuracies achieved. To realize these X-ray diffraction resolutions has required improvements in technology (synchrotrons and charge coupled device X-ray electronic area detectors) and of technique (cryo-freezing of the protein crystal sample and small-molecule style protein model refinement) [60–62]. The geometry around the metal is seen in Fig. 3a and b. Table 2 gives the metal–ligand distances. There are two, clearly distinguished, longer axial ligands (the His 24 imidazole nitrogen atom and a bound water oxygen) and four shorter ligand distances in the square plane. The interbond angles are, within 5°, close to 90°. The geometry thus corresponds to a distorted octahedron in agreement with evidence from single-crystal and solution EPR spectroscopy results described in Sec. 3.2.

6. MANGANESE MULTIWAVELENGTH ANOMALOUS DISPERSION (MAD) PROTEIN CRYSTALLOGRAPHY

An experiment has been conducted to evaluate the occupancy of manganese at the transition metal binding site in concanavalin A crystallized from naturally occurring ("native") concanavalin A in the presence of an excess of Mn^{2+}. Native concanavalin A crystal diffraction data were collected using synchrotron radiation at the "XRD" multipole wiggler beam line of ELETTRA in Trieste tuned to the manganese K absorption edge (1.896 Å) and data at three X-ray wavelengths were measured. Firstly, to guide the selection of these wavelengths, a number of crystals were packed into a thin-walled glass capillary and the Mn fluorescence spectrum was measured at the Mn K edge. The fluorescence scan showed the Mn signal clearly. Full X-ray diffraction datasets were then collected at the inflection point of the absorption edge, at the peak absorption point, and at a remote wavelength. The crystallographic Patterson vector maps derived from these three datasets, in various combinations, show clear peaks (not shown here) and therefore confirm that the Mn occupancy in native concanavalin A at the transition metal binding site is high rather than low [63]. This is consistent with the ultrahigh resolution 0.94-Å protein model refinement of native concanavalin A [43], which put the value of the Mn ion occupancy at about 85% [64]. Obviously the remaining 15% may be trace impurities in the protein as isolated from the Jack bean, and indeed the repopulation of other pure transition metal ions is possible.

(a)

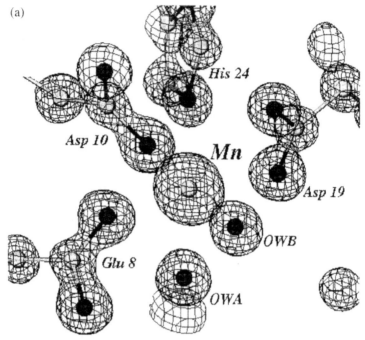

FIG. 3.   Synchrotron X-ray crystallography, ultra-high-resolution (0.92 Å) study. (a) Electron density image of the manganese and its binding environment. (b) Atomic displacement parameters (ADPs) for the direct manganese ligand atoms derived from the protein model refinement; for the nitrogen the whole histidine-24 side-chain ring is shown, residues 10 and 19 are both aspartic acids, residue 8 is a glutamic acid, OWA and OWB are bound water molecule oxygens. See Sec. 8 for details of shared ligands, involving residues Asp10 and Asp19, with the neighboring Ca ion.

7.   NEUTRON LAUE DIFFRACTION

Structural studies by neutron diffraction permit elucidation of hydrogen/deuterium (H/D) exchange. This approach exploits the difference in neutron scattering lengths between hydrogen and deuterium, which is not present in X-ray diffraction. The neutron scattering length is -0.374 for hydrogen but 0.667 for deuterium. Moreover, the positioning of water hydrogens is possible by using heavy water; for ordinary water the two hydrogens almost exactly cancel out the oxygen neutron-scattering cross-section (the neutron-scattering cross-section for oxygen is 0.5805).

(b)

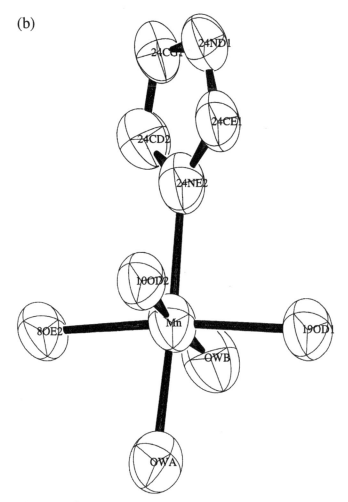

FIG. 3.   Continued

Ultrahigh-resolution X-ray protein crystallography can yield water hydrogens as well but requires them to be very well ordered. Neutron diffraction of a deuterated protein crystal, although always constrained to be at only medium high resolution, has the advantage that the deuterium atoms, which scatter strongly, need not be so well ordered to be orientated. Obviously, disordered and completely mobile deuteriums on waters cannot be resolved by either X-ray or neutron diffraction. In this chapter reasonably ordered deuteriums on two waters liganded via

TABLE 2

Bond Lengths and Bond Angles from the Synchrotron X-ray
0.92-Å-Resolution Concanavalin A Model Refinement
for Manganese in the Transition Metal Binding Site[a]

Ligand	24NE2	OWA	19OD1	OWB	8OE2	10OD2
24NE2	2.222 (6)		90.6	90.5	93.2	86.4
OWA		2.269 (6)	91.5	94.0	85.4	89.3
19OD1			2.178 (5)	82.1		95.0
OWB				2.166 (6)	88.5	
8OE2					2.170 (5)	94.6
10OD2						2.146 (5)

[a]Ligand atoms labeled as in Fig. 3b. The diagonal terms are manganese–ligand bond distances with standard uncertainties in brackets for the last digit. Off-diagonal terms are ligand–manganese–ligand bond angles in degrees (standard uncertainties for the angles are 0.2°).

Note: The corresponding values for this site in native concanavalin A can be found in [43]; these two sets of distances agree within a range of 0.004–0.016 Å, i.e., average deviation 0.012 Å, and the bond angle differences lie in the range 0.0–0.5° with an average deviation of 0.24°.

their oxygen atoms to the manganese are described below. On a very practical note, normally it requires months to record measurements from a protein crystal in a neutron monochromatic beam, but this can be cut to a matter of days using the neutron Laue diffraction technique [65,66].

In this study deuterated concanavalin A protein crystals were prepared using successive transfers between deuterated artificial mother liquors over a 4-month period. First of all, an X-ray refinement to 1.8 Å resolution of a deuterated crystal, prepared under identical conditions to the one used in the neutron experiment, was used as the starting model for the neutron refinement. The X-ray structure comprised 3564 protein atoms, the two metals (Mn and Ca), and 148 oxygen atoms of the bound waters [67].

The neutron study [67] has revealed directly that the deuterium atoms of the two bound waters are pointing away from the Mn atom (Fig. 4), in correspondence with the chemistry of the metal–ligand

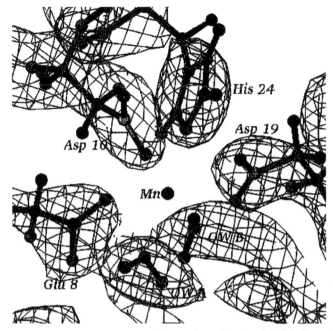

FIG. 4.   Neutron Laue crystallography nuclear density Mn binding site at 2.4 Å resolution. The pairs of deuterium atoms for each of the two water molecules OWA and OWB are thereby determined and are pointing away from the Mn, as expected.

charge interaction. The His24 imidazole nitrogen shows no deuterium at that position. The carboxyl side chains show no nuclear density either for H or D, which is consistent with the absence of protonation, i.e., the single negative charge on the two carboxyl side chains balancing the divalent positive charge on the Mn ion.

8.   ROLE OF MANGANESE IN SACCHARIDE BINDING IN CONCANAVALIN A AND OTHER LEGUME LECTINS

Manganese, as well as the other divalent metal ions that can occupy the transition metal binding site, plays an indirect but crucial role in creating the saccharide binding site in concanavalin A [11]. Although the Mn ion is located approximately 13 Å from the saccharide binding site, its presence (or that of one of the other four metals) is absolutely essential for saccharide binding to occur, as outlined in Sec. 2.2.

The process whereby binding of Mn leads to creation of the saccharide binding site was first proposed on the basis of comparison between the crystal structure of native concanavalin A and a relatively low-resolution structure of the demetallized protein [20]. This initial hypothesis, substantially modified on the basis of recent medium- and high-resolution X-ray crystallographic studies of demetallized concanavalin A [22], Zn-concanavalin A, Zn,Ca-concanavalin A [23], and several saccharide complexes of concanavalin A [5,21,26,68], is based on the observation that the amino acid residues that constitute the transition metal binding site, the calcium binding site, and the saccharide binding site are located in a crevice near the surface of the protein created by the conjunction of several loops (Fig. 5). In the demetallized protein, these loops are disordered. Nonetheless, three out of four of the transition metal-binding ligands—Glu8, Asp10, and His24—are close enough to their positions in the native structure to enable Mn to bind, albeit weakly, at this *"proto*-transition metal binding site." Binding of the divalent Mn ion causes several readjustments of the metal binding region, partially neutralizing the negative charge, optimizing the orientation of Asp10 for binding of calcium, and stabilizing the position of Asp19 in the vicinity of the nascent calcium binding site, without actually creating the calcium binding site as it exists in the native protein. The structural changes leading to the tightly knit bimetallic site as it exists in Mn,Ca-concanavalin A and, simultaneously, to the creation of the saccharide binding site are the consequence of calcium binding. Asp19 moves into the ligation sphere of the metal ions, bridging between Mn and Ca; Asp10 reorients to provide a second bridge between the two metals; Asn14 is drawn into the ligation sphere of calcium as is Tyr12; and two water ligands bridge between calcium and two saccharide-binding ligands, Arg228 and Asp208, also facilitating the trans-to-cis isomerization of the Ala207–Asp208 peptide bond. Simultaneously, a distant saccharide-binding loop (Thr97–Glu102) undergoes a large readjustment, bringing the peptide nitrogen atoms of Leu99 and Tyr100 into the correct positions for saccharide binding.

Since the isolation of concanavalin A, many other legume lectins have been isolated and characterized [58]. Eighteen of these from 17 different legumes have been studied by X-ray crystallography and are heavily represented by more than 70 crystal structures (25 of which are

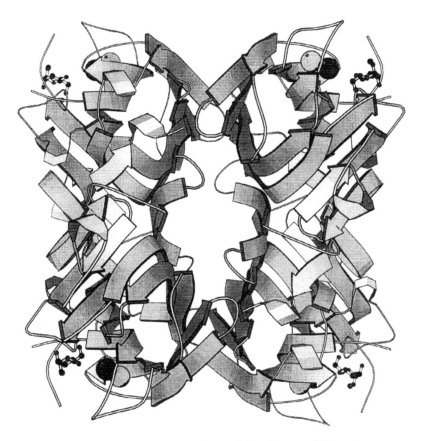

FIG. 5.   A tetramer of concanavalin A in "ribbon diagram" format; arrows represent β-sheet strands, the predominant secondary structure in this protein. Spheres represent the metal ions with the manganese ions in light shading and the calcium ions in dark shading. Saccharide in "ball-and-stick" form and all atoms shown. Each monomer of concanavalin A (molecular weight 25 kDa) binds one Mn^{2+}, one Ca^{2+}, and one such saccharide. Based on Refs. 8, 21, and 68; prepared using MOLSCRIPT [70].

structures of concanavalin A and its metal and saccharide complexes) in the Protein Data Bank. The members of this large family of proteins have much in common at the level of primary, secondary, and tertiary structure. However, they contain saccharide binding sites with widely varying sugar specificity. Nevertheless, they all possess an Mn,Ca bimetallic site that must be occupied by both metals for saccharide binding to be possible. It is thus likely that they have a common mechanism of site–site interaction involving Mn and Ca as demonstrated for concanavalin A. The possibility of preparing demetallized crystals and one-metal crystals is, so far, unique to concanavalin A and has been the key to elucidation of this detailed mechanism.

Involvement of transition metal ions in saccharide binding is a unique feature of the legume lectin family [58]. With one exception, all other known classes of lectins of plant, animal, bacterial, and viral origin (represented by crystal structures of 42 proteins of these classes) bind their conjugate saccharide without the involvement of metal ions [69]. In the case of C-lectins, a calcium ion in the saccharide binding site is directly coordinated to two ring oxygens of the bound sugar.

The biological role of concanavalin A and of the other members of the legume lectin family is still a subject for speculation. On the basis of structural analysis, we may conclude that, whatever the biological activity of the lectin, the concentration of free metal ions can provide a subtle, indirect control mechanism of its activity.

9. CONCLUDING REMARKS

The detailed definition of the Mn,Ca-saccharide-binding protein concanavalin A has been achieved via a variety of crystal structures, the most detailed of which is a 0.92-Å resolution structure for the saccharide-free crystal form based on advanced synchrotron radiation techniques. Moreover, for this crystal form the hydrogen atom positions of bound water have now been positioned definitively on the basis of 2.4-Å resolution data from the newly developed technique of neutron Laue protein crystallography. Thus an accurate description of the structure and nature of the environment of the Mn transition metal atom has been achieved as a principal benefit of these structural studies.

These structures are also serving as a test bed for the development and application of advanced spectroscopic techniques such as single-crystal pulsed EPR to concanavalin A (via the Mn(II) d^5 high-spin probe) and to proteins in general. In another methods development application, these structures, particularly those of the saccharide complexes of concanavalin A, serve as a test bed for the direct calculation of the energetics of protein–ligand interaction [68], experimental values for which have been determined by microcalorimetry.

The intricate role played by manganese, and therefrom calcium, in saccharide binding has also been revealed by careful structural analysis of crystals of several intermediate forms of the protein and of its saccharide complexes. Evolution of this particular molecular architecture, highly conserved across the family of legume lectins, may be favored because it results in a good match between the binding affinities of the saccharides and their levels in the living organisms and because it may allow indirect control via free metal ion levels in the medium. In other classes of saccharide-binding proteins such as animal lectins and sugar-binding enzymes a transition metal atom is not utilized. In some animal lectins (C-lectins) calcium is utilized but as a direct ligand to the sugar.

Intensive study of concanavalin A and its Mn binding site continues to constitute a powerful link between development of new scientific methods in basic protein research and practical applications in various fields of applied research.

ACKNOWLEDGMENTS

J.R.H. thanks the Wellcome Trust for research grant support (salary of Dr. J. Habash). The British Council UK/Israel Fund is thanked for a joint collaboration grant to A.J.K.G. and J.R.H. (which supported the Ph.D. stipend of Ms. H. Price). The BBSRC provided financial support for SG computer molecular graphics workstations and the SG Challenge (on which the 0.92-Å protein model refinements were run), partial salary support of Dr. J. Raftery and a Ph.D. research studentship to Ms. N. Hunter. Beam time was awarded to J.R.H. at the synchrotron sources at Daresbury (UK), CHESS Cornell (USA), and ELETTRA (Trieste) and, more recently, at the Institut Laue Langevin neutron source at Grenoble, France for the X-ray and neutron protein crystallography data collection, respectively, on which this structural studies program was conducted. J.R.H. warmly thanks Dr. A. Karplus, then of Cornell University's Section of Biochemistry, for the gift of five beans from Prof. J. B. Sumner's original jar of beans.

REFERENCES

1. (a) H. Bittiger and H. P. Schnebli, *Concanavalin A as a Tool*, John Wiley and Sons, New York (1976). (b) H. Ben-Bassat and N. Goldblum, *Proc. Natl. Acad. Sci. USA*, *72*, 1046–1049 (1975). (c) J. C. Brown and R. C. Hunt, *Int. Rev. Cytol.*, *52*, 277–349 (1978).

2. J. Balzarini, J. Neyts, D. Schols, M. Hosaya, E. van Damme, W. Peumans, and E. de Clerq, *Antiviral Res.*, *18*, 191–207 (1992).

3. J. B. Sumner, *J. Biol. Chem.*, *37*, 137–142 (1919).

4. V. A. Hilder, K. S. Powell, A. M. R. Gatehouse, J. A. Gatehouse, L. N. Gatehouse, Y. Shi, W. D. O. Hamilton, A. Merryweather, C. A. Newell, J. C. Timans, W. J. Peumans, E. van Damme, and D. Boulter, *Transgenic Res.*, *4*, 18–25 (1995).

5. Z. Derewenda, J. Yariv, J. R. Helliwell, A. J. Kalb(Gilboa), E. J. Dodson, M. Z. Papiz, T. Wan, and J. Campbell, *EMBO J.*, *8*, 2189–2193 (1989).

6. J. B. Sumner and S. F. Howell, *J. Bacteriol.*, *32*, 227–237 (1936).

7. J. B. Sumner, N. Gralen, and I. B. Eriksson-Quensel, *J. Biol. Chem.*, *125*, 45–48 (1938).

8. As in many key experiments, serendipity and clear thinking played important roles in this discovery. Acidification was actually the control for a peptic digestion experiment designed to test the hypothesis that agglutination was a protein-mediated property. Failure of the pepsin-free control to cause agglutination suggested that essential metals were split off at low pH.

9. J. B. Sumner and S. F. Howell, *J. Biol. Chem.*, *115*, 583–588 (1936).

10. J. Yariv, A. J. Kalb, and A. Levitzki, *Biochim. Biophys. Acta*, *165*, 303–305 (1968).

11. A. J. Kalb and A. Levitzki, *Biochem. J.*, *109*, 669–672 (1968).

12. B. B. L. Agrawal and I. J. Goldstein, *Biochim. Biophys. Acta*, *147*, 262–271 (1967).

13. M. O. J. Olson and I. E. Liener, *Biochemistry*, *6*, 105–111 (1967).

14. I. Matsumoto, H. Kitagaki, Y. Akai, Y. Ito, and N. Seno, *Anal. Biochem.*, *116*, 103–110 (1981).

15. A. J. Kalb and A. Lustig, *Biochim. Biophys. Acta*, *168*, 366–367 (1968).

16. J. L. Wang, B. A. Cunningham, and G. M. Edelman, *Proc. Natl. Acad. Sci. USA*, *68*, 1130–1134 (1971).

17. B. A. Cunningham, J. L. Wang, M. N. Pflumm, and G. M. Edelman, *Biochemistry*, *11*, 3233–3239 (1972).

18. G. H. McKenzie and W. H. Sawyer, *J. Biol. Chem.*, *248*, 549–556 (1973).

19. M. Shoham, A. J. Kalb, and I. Pecht, *Biochemistry*, *12*, 1914–1917 (1973).

20. M. Shoham, A. Yonath, J. L. Sussman, J. Moult, W. Traub, and A. J. Kalb(Gilboa), *J. Mol. Biol.*, *131*, 137–155 (1979).

21. J. H. Naismith, C. Emmerich, J. Habash, S. J. Harrop, J. R. Helliwell, W. N. Hunter, J. Raftery, A. J. Kalb (Gilboa), and J. Yariv, *Acta Crystallogr.*, *D50*, 847–858 (1994).

22. J. Bouckaert, R. Loris, F. Poortmans, and L. Wyns, *Prot. Struct. Funct. Gen.*, *23*, 510–524 (1995).

23. J. Bouckaert, F. Poortmans, L. Wyns, and R. Loris, *J. Biol. Chem.*, *271*, 16144–16150 (1996).

24. T. Uchida and T. Matsumoto, *Biochim. Biophys. Acta*, *257*, 230–234 (1972).

25. This has proven useful in preparing single crystals of concanavalin A for pulsed EPR studies where dilution of Mn with Cd is needed to minimize spin–spin relaxation enhancement.

26. S. J. Harrop, J. R. Helliwell, T. C. M. Wan, A. J. Kalb(Gilboa), L. Tong, and J. Yariv, *Acta Crystallogr.*, *D52*, 143–155 (1996).

27. A. Evdokimov, M.Sc. thesis, The Weizmann Institute of Science, Rehovot, Israel (1996).

28. D. Gupta, T. K. Dam, S. Oscarson, and C. F. Brewer, *J. Biol. Chem.*, *272*, 6388–6392 (1997).

29. Clearly, stability of the complex is not proportional to the number of hydrogen bonds formed between the bound saccharide and the protein. If this were the case, the free energy increment would be greatest for OH-6, which participates in three hydrogen bonds, and least for OH-3, which participates in only one. (See H bonding scheme in Ref. 5.)

30. A. J. Kalb(Gilboa), F. Frolow, J. Yariv, and M. Eisenstein, *Acta Crystallogr.*, *D51*, 1077–1079 (1995).

31. E. Meirovitch, Z. Luz, and A. J. Kalb(Gilboa), *J. Am. Chem. Soc.*, *96*, 7538–7542 (1974).

32. E. Meirovitch, Z. Luz, and A. J. Kalb(Gilboa), *J. Am. Chem. Soc.*, *96*, 7542–7546 (1974).

33. P. Manikandan, R. Carmieli, T. Shane, A. J. Kalb(Gilboa), and D. Goldfarb, in preparation (1999).

34. C. F. Brewer, H. Sternlicht, D. M. Marcus, and A. P. Grollman, *Biochemistry*, *12*, 4448–4457 (1973).

35. R. D. Brown, C. F. Brewer, and S. H. Koenig, *Biochemistry*, *16*, 3883–3896 (1977).

36. J. P. Carver, B. H. Barber, and B. J. Fuhr, *J. Biol. Chem.*, 3141–3146 (1977).

37. A. R. Palmer, D. B. Bailey, W. D. Behnke, A. D. Cardin, P. P. Yang, and P. D. Ellis, *Biochemistry*, *19*, 5063–5070 (1980).

38. J. H. Naismith, J. Habash, S. Harrop, J. R. Helliwell, W. N. Hunter, T. C. M. Wan, S. Weisgerber, A. J. Kalb(Gilboa), and J. Yariv, *Acta Crystallogr.*, *D49*, 561–571 (1993).

39. W. D. McCubbin, K. Oikawa, and C. M. Kay, *Biochim. Biophys. Res. Commun.*, *43*, 666–674 (1971).

40. G. M. Edelman, B. A. Cunningham, G. N. Reeke, Jr., J. W. Becker, M. J. Waxdal, and J. L. Wang, *Proc. Natl. Acad. Sci. USA*, *69*, 2580–2584 (1972).

41. K. D. Hardman and C. F. Ainsworth, *Biochemistry*, *11*, 4910–4919 (1972).

42. A. J. Kalb and I. Pecht, *Biochim. Biophys. Acta*, *303*, 264–268 (1973).

43. A. Deacon, T. Gleichmann, A. J. Kalb(Gilboa), H. Price, J. Raftery, G. Bradbrook, J. Yariv, and J. R. Helliwell, *J. Chem. Soc. Faraday Trans.*, *93*, 4305–4312 (1997).

44. A. J. Kalb, E. A. Stern, and S. M. Heald, *J. Mol. Biol.*, *135*, 501–506 (1979).

45. J. Bouckaert, F. Poortmans, L. Wyns, and R. Loris, *J. Biol. Chem.*, *271*, 16144–16150 (1996).

46. J. Greer, H. W. Kaufman, and A. J. Kalb, *J. Mol. Biol.*, *48*, 365–366 (1970).

47. A. J. Kalb(Gilboa), J. Yariv, J. R. Helliwell, and M. Z. Papiz, *J. Cryst. Growth*, *88*, 537–540 (1988).

48. S. More and W. Saenger, *J. Cryst. Growth*, *153*, 35–42 (1995).

49. E. Kashimoto, G. Sazaki, K. Hasegawa, T. Nakada, S. Miyashita, H. Komatsu, K. Sato, Y. Matsuura, and H. Tanaka, *J. Cryst. Growth*, *186*, 461–470 (1998).

50. Y. Elan and A. J. Kalb(Gilboa), unpublished results. Unfortunately, this behavior is not observed in every lot of the commercial preparation and some lots crystallize only after several weeks or not at all.

51. D. Goldfarb, T. Shane, and A. J. Kalb(Gilboa), in preparation (1999).

52. A. Jack, J. Weinzierl, and A. J. Kalb, *J. Mol. Biol.*, *58*, 389–395 (1971).

53. K. D. Hardman, R. C. Agarwal, and M. J. Freiser, *J. Mol. Biol.*, *157*, 69–86 (1982).

54. C. Emmerich, J. R. Helliwell, M. Redshaw, J. H. Naismith, S. J. Harrop, J. Raftery, A. J. Kalb(Gilboa), and J. Yariv, *Acta Crystallogr.*, *D50*, 749–756 (1994).

55. J. Yariv, A. J. Kalb(Gilboa), M. Z. Papiz, J. R. Helliwell, S. J. Andrews, and J. Habash, *J. Mol. Biol.*, *195*, 759–760 (1987).

56. A. J. Kalb(Gilboa), F. Frolow, J. Yariv, and M. Eisenstein, *Acta Crystallogr.*, *D51*, 1077–1079 (1995).

57. D. N. Moothoo and J. H. Naismith, *Acta Crystallogr.*, *D55*, 353–355 (1999).

58. R. Loris, T. Hamelryck, J. Bouckaert, and L. Wyns, *Biochim. Biophys. Acta*, *1383*, 9–36 (1998).

59. H. J. Price, Ph.D. thesis, University of Manchester, in preparation (1999).

60. J. R. Helliwell, *Macromolecular Crystallography with Synchrotron Radiation*, Cambridge University Press, 1992.

61. J. R. Helliwell and M. Helliwell, *Chem. Commun.*, 1598–1602 (1996).

62. G. M. Sheldrick, *SHELXL96*, University of Göttingen (1996).

63. N. S. Hunter, Ph.D. thesis, University of Manchester, in preparation (1999).

64. A. M. Deacon, Ph.D. thesis, University of Manchester (1997).

65. J. R. Helliwell, *Nature Struct. Biol.*, *4*, 874–876 (1997).

66. J. Habash, J. Raftery, S. Weisgerber, A. Cassetta, M. S. Lehmann, P. Hoghoj, C. Wilkinson, J. W. Campbell, and J. R. Helliwell, *J. Chem. Soc. Faraday Trans.*, *93*(24), 4313–4317 (1997).

67. J. Habash, J. Raftery, R. B. Nuttall, C. Wilkinson, M. S. Lehmann, A. J. Kalb(Gilboa), and J. R. Helliwell, in preparation.

68. G. M. Bradbrook, T. Gleichmann, S. J. Harrop, J. Habash, J. Raftery, A. J. Kalb(Gilboa), J. Yariv, I. H. Hillier, and J. R. Helliwell, *J. Chem. Soc. Faraday Trans.*, *94*(11), 1603–1611 (1998).

69. E. Bettler, R. Loris, and A. Imberty, 3D Lectin Database, *http://www.cermav.cnrs.fr/databank/lectine/* (1999).

70. P. J. Kraulis, *J. Appl. Crystallogr.*, *24*, 946–950 (1991).

10

Manganese-Activated Phosphatases

Frank Rusnak

Department of Biochemistry & Molecular Biology
and the Section of Hematology Research,
Mayo Clinic, Rochester, MN 55905, USA

1. INTRODUCTION: PHOSPHATE ESTERS IN BIOLOGICAL SYSTEMS

Phosphorus is an essential biological element that can be found in numerous structures. The principal biochemical forms are phosphoanhydrides and phosphate mono- and diesters of alcohols, although a few phosphoramidates such as phosphocreatine and phosphoarginine are known (Fig. 1). In addition, sulfur-containing analogs of phosphate esters, e.g., phosphorothioates, are becoming widely used as biochemical reagents [1,2]. Of particular relevance for this chapter are phosphate monoesters of serine, threonine, and tyrosine side chain -OH groups in polypeptides. Phosphorylation of these amino acid sides by protein kinases and dephosphorylation by protein phosphatases represents a universal mechanism for biological regulation. The family of protein phosphatases that includes protein phosphatases 1 (PP1), 2A (PP2A), and 2B (PP2B or calcineurin) are metalloenzymes that can be activated by Mn^{2+}. Protein phosphatase 2C (PP2C), although evolutionarily unrelated to the above phosphatases, is also activated by Mn^{2+}. Despite the

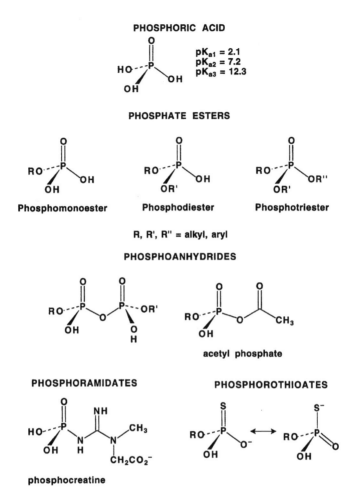

PHOSPHORIC ACID

pK$_{a1}$ = 2.1
pK$_{a2}$ = 7.2
pK$_{a3}$ = 12.3

PHOSPHATE ESTERS

Phosphomonoester   Phosphodiester   Phosphotriester

R, R', R'' = alkyl, aryl

PHOSPHOANHYDRIDES

acetyl phosphate

PHOSPHORAMIDATES   **PHOSPHOROTHIOATES**

phosphocreatine

FIG. 1. Phosphate esters are one of the predominant forms of phosphorus in biological systems. Values for phosphoric acid acidity constants are from Smith and Martell [95].

lack of sequence homologies, these and other enzymes involved in phosphate ester hydrolysis reactions share a common active site architecture accommodating metal cofactors. These and other phosphatases—their structure and mechanism, and what is known about their interaction with Mn^{2+}—will be discussed below.

Phosphate esters can exist in numerous chemical structures and various degrees of protonation. The parent compound is phosphoric acid, which can exist in four ionization states $(0, 1-, 2-, 3-)$ given three ionizable protons with pK_a values of 2.1, 7.2, and 12.3 [95] (Fig. 1). Phosphate monoesters are more acidic with pK_a values over 1 pH unit lower than phosphoric acid (Table 1). At physiological pH (about 7.0–7.4), most biological phosphate monoesters exist as the dianion ($\approx$5% as the monoanion). Phosphomonoesterases that operate at physiological pH have active sites tailored for these highly charged substrates. In certain biological environments, the pH is significantly higher or lower, and in fact, classes of alkaline and acid phosphatases have evolved that function efficiently at nonphysiological pH. Phosphate diesters have one ionizable proton with a pK_a near unity [3] and carry a net charge of 1– at nearly all values of pH. Phosphotriesters are neutral in solution.

TABLE 1
pK_a Values for Selected Phosphomonoesters[a]

Compound	pK_{a1}	pK_{a2}
NH$_2$ | H$_2$O$_3$POCH$_2$CHCO$_2$H L-Phosphoserine	0.7	5.67 $\pm$ 0.03
CH$_3$ (ring) OPO$_3$H$_2$ 4-Methylphenylphosphate	0.56	5.80
NO$_2$ (ring) OPO$_3$H$_2$ p-Nitrophenylphosphate	0.30 $\pm$ 0.02	4.96 $\pm$ 0.02

[a]The pK_a values for L-phosphoserine were obtained from Smith and Martell [106], while these values for phenylphosphate and p-nitrophenylphosphate are from Bourne and Williams [107].

2. CLASSIFICATION OF METAL-ACTIVATED PHOSPHATASES

Enzymes that hydrolyze phosphate esters are classified according to the *Enzyme Commission of the International Union of Biochemistry and Molecular Biology* designation [4]. These enzymes fall under the division and subclass of hydrolases acting on ester bonds. These enzymes catalyze the cleavage of P-O bonds of phosphate esters and anhydrides, and subsequent transfer of the phosphoryl group to water according to the reaction in Scheme 1. Numerous subsubclasses are identified in the 1992 edition of *Enzyme Nomenclature*, distinguished by their substrate specificity and position of bond cleavage [4].

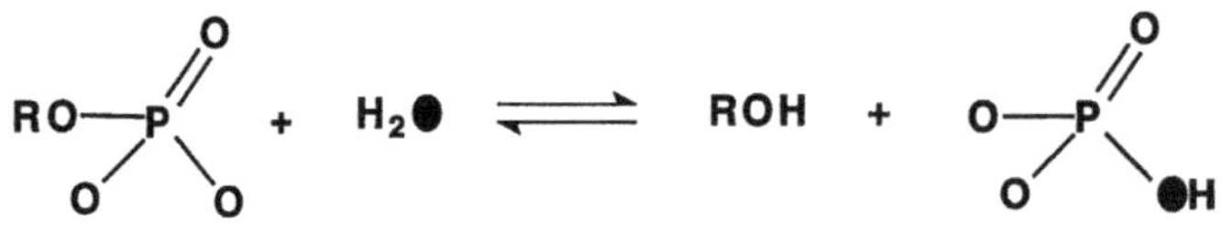

SCHEME 1

The vast majority of enzymes that hydrolyze phosphate esters and anhydrides are metalloenzymes or metal-activated enzymes. One of the fundamental issues that arises with regard to metal-activated enzymes is the identity of the metal ion used by the enzyme in vivo. For enzymes with tightly bound metal ions that survive chromatographic purification, the identity can be determined by analytical and/or spectroscopic methods. For example, purified *Escherichia coli* [5] and calf intestine [6] alkaline phosphatases contain stoichiometric quantities of Zn^{2+} and Mg^{2+}. The native metals in phosphotriesterase from *Pseudomonas diminuta* are thought to be a pair of Zn^{2+} ions [7]. Of the protein phosphatases, calcineurin from bovine brain has been shown to contain iron and zinc in near-stoichiometric quantities [8,9]. Although none of these enzymes appear to utilize Mn^{2+} as a native metal cofactor, most can be activated to some extent by Mn^{2+} ions.

2.1. Phosphomonoesterases

The phosphoric monoester hydrolases ("phosphatases") represent one of the largest subsubclasses of enzymes. These enzymes hydrolyze pri-

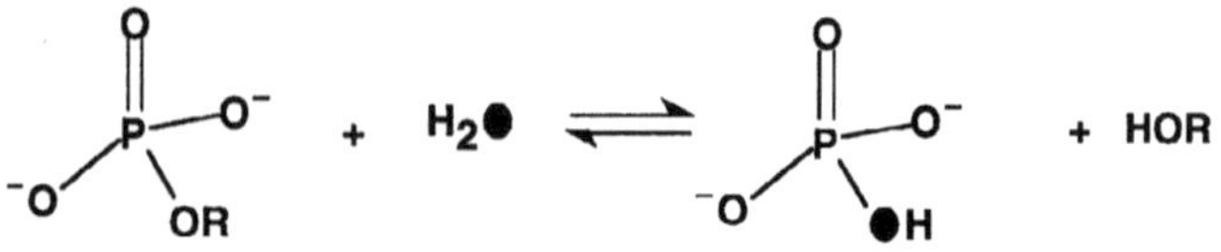

SCHEME 2

marily phosphate monoesters as substrates, producing an alcohol and orthophosphate as products (Scheme 2). These can be further distinguished by their physiological substrate specificity.

2.1.1.   Nonspecific Phosphatases

Alkaline phosphatase (EC 3.1.3.1) was one of the first phosphatases to be characterized both structurally and mechanistically [10]. Alkaline phosphatases are found in both prokaryotic and eukaryotic species with the enzyme from *E. coli* encoded for by the *phoA* gene being the best characterized member of this family in terms of structural and mechanistic information. Alkaline phosphatases have been isolated from a variety of other eukaryotic and prokaryotic sources [11]. The enzymes from *E. coli* and mammals have related amino acid sequences and are both Zn/Mg metalloenzymes [10]. Alkaline phosphatase is considered a nonspecific phosphatase since it can hydrolyze a number of phosphate monoesters with comparable catalytic efficiency regardless of the chemical nature of the R group [11]. In addition, alkaline phosphatase can hydrolyze *O-* and *S*-phosphorothioates and phosphoramidates [10].

The reason for similar catalytic rates for different substrates is due to a rate-determining step for hydrolysis involving breakdown of a common phosphoenzyme intermediate (Scheme 3). The phosphoenzyme intermediate is formed upon transfer of the phosphoryl group from substrate to an active site serine residue as will be discussed in more de-

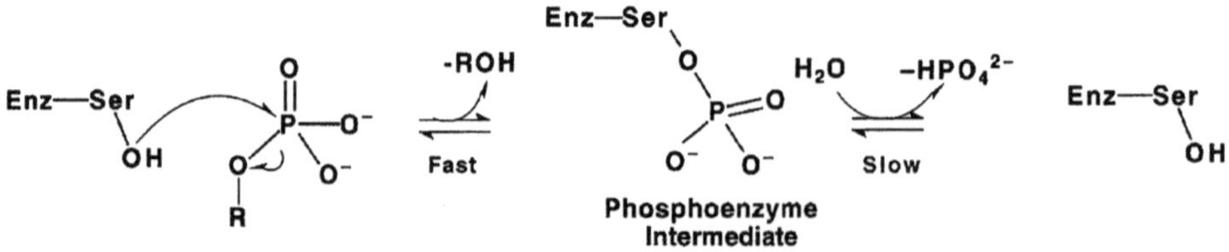

SCHEME 3

tail below. The rate-determining step occurs when the phosphoryl group is transferred to water for pH <7 and release of product phosphate for pH >7. Since the R group of the product alcohol has departed by this time, the measured kinetic constants are largely invariant for substrates with different R groups [12,13]. The existence of a phosphoenzyme intermediate is consistent with stereochemical studies of the enzyme-catalyzed reaction, which shows that the stereochemistry about the phosphorus atom undergoes net retention of stereochemical configuration resulting from successive nucleophilic displacement reactions [14]. Indeed, a phosphoenzyme intermediate has been observed by ^{31}P-NMR methods [15] and X-ray crystallography of the Cd-substituted enzymes [16] (reviewed in [10,11]).

2.1.2. Protein Phosphatases

Serine/threonine protein phosphatases represent yet another class of metal-dependent phosphatases. PP1, PP2A, calcineurin, and PP2C represent the major eukaryotic protein phosphatases in signal transduction pathways [17]. Recent work has identified homologs of the PP1/PP2A/calcineurin family of enzymes in cyanobacteria [18] and the archea [19–21]. The members of this family contain a conserved amino acid sequence called the phosphoesterase motif, $\mathbf{DXH(X)}_n\mathbf{GDXXD(X)}_m$ GNHD/E [22–24]. This motif is manifested as a $\beta\alpha\beta\alpha\beta$ secondary structure element that positions two active site metal ions with ligands provided by four conserved residues noted above in bold. Besides the protein phosphatases, additional enzymes in this family that have been identified by sequence analysis include a protein phosphatase from bacteriophage λ, diadenosine tetraphosphatase, 2′,3′-cyclic nucleotide phosphodiesterase, 5′-nucleotidase, exonucleases from E. coli and Bacillus subtilis, acid sphingomyelin phosphodiesterase, a UDP-sugar pyrophosphatase, and an RNA intron lariat-debranching enzyme [22,24].

PP2C is a member of an unrelated superfamily of metal-containing phosphatases. Members of this family include eukaryotic PP2C homologs; a PP2C domain in fungal adenylate cyclases; a phosphatase in plants designated KAPP (kinase-associated protein phosphatase) that is composed of an amino terminal signal anchor, a kinase interaction domain, and a type 2C protein phosphatase catalytic region; and prokaryotic homologs from B. subtilis (SpoIIE protein), Mycobacterium genitalium, and Synechocystis species [25]. The conserved features of the PP2C family include a number of invariant residues in the active site that coordinate two Mg^{2+} or two Mn^{2+} ions [26].

The substrates for the protein phosphatases are phosphoserine, phosphothreonine, and phosphotyrosine residues of proteins that have been phosphorylated by protein kinases [17]. In vivo, the serine/threonine protein phosphatases hydrolyze serine/threonine phosphate monoesters while tyrosine phosphatases are deemed responsible for the hydrolysis of phosphotyrosine residues. However, the serine/threonine phosphatases have broad substrate specificity in vitro, e.g., protein phosphotyrosine residues can also be hydrolyzed [27]. Besides protein and peptide substrates, small nonphysiological phosphate monoesters such as p-nitrophenylphosphate (pNPP), naphthylphosphate, and phosphoenolpyruvate can be efficiently dephosphorylated [28,29].

Although not originally classified as a protein phosphatase but rather a nonspecific phosphomonoesterase, purple acid phosphatases can dephosphorylate bone matrix phosphoproteins [30,31]. This and the fact that purple acid phosphatase shares a similar active site architecture to PP1, PP2A, and calcineurin suggests that it is a member of the same superfamily and it may serve similar roles in vivo.

2.2. Phosphodiesterases

Phosphodiesterases catalyze the hydrolysis of phosphate diesters, yielding an alcohol and a phosphomonoester as products. These enzymes are specific for phosphodiesters and do not further hydrolyze the product phosphomonoester (Scheme 4). A number of enzymes in this class can

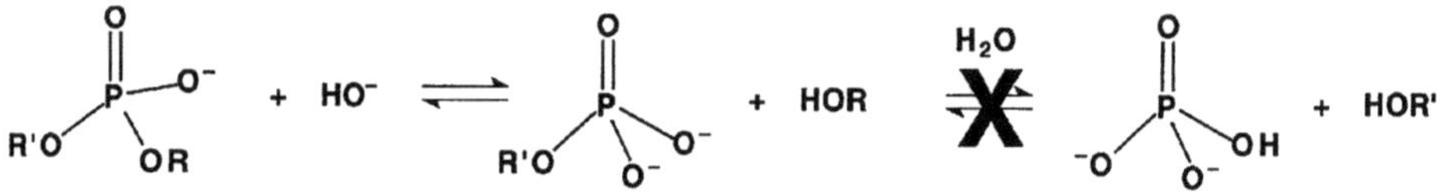

SCHEME 4

act on polynucleotides (e.g., exo- and endonucleases) and utilize divalent metal ions such as Mn^{2+} as activators. The substrates of these enzymes are $3',5'$-phosphodiesters of ribo- or deoxyribonucleic acids. These enzymes and the role of metal activation has been reviewed recently [32]. Furthermore, the following chapter in this volume by Baldwin, Gormley, and Halford focuses on Mn^{2+} as a probe for endonucleases. Therefore, metal-dependent phosphodiesterases will not be further discussed here.

2.3. Phosphotriesterases

Phosphotriesterases are unique enzymes which, unlike phosphomono- and diesterases, act on substrates that bear no negative charge. Nevertheless, there are similarities in the active site and proposed mechanism for hydrolysis between phosphotriesterases and other phosphoesterases. The phosphotriesterase from *P. diminuta* has been studied extensively by Raushel and co-workers. The enzyme catalyzes the hydrolysis of a variety of organophosphorus triester insecticides such as paraoxon as well as phosphorothioate triesters dursban, parathion, and diazinon [33]. The native enzyme contains Zn^{2+} but a wide variety of divalent metal ions can be substituted with only slight decreases of activity [7]. Phosphotriesterases are members of a large superfamily that includes enzymes involved in the hydrolysis of amide bonds, indicating a distant but common evolutionary relationship [34].

2.4. Inorganic Pyrophosphatases

Inorganic pyrophosphatases catalyze the hydrolysis of pyrophosphate to two molecules of orthophosphate (Scheme 5). A structure-based se-

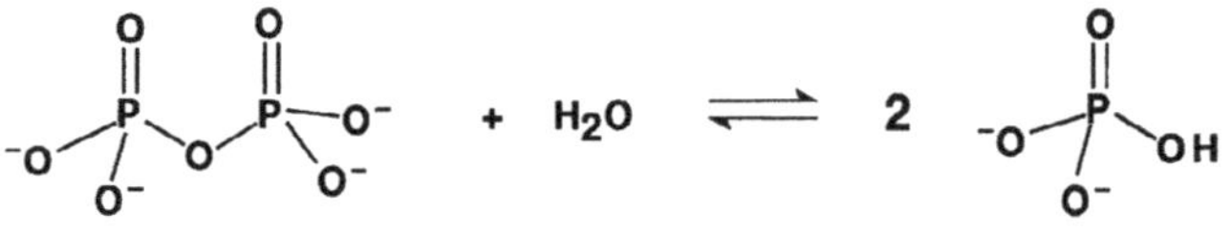

SCHEME 5

quence alignment of inorganic pyrophosphatases revealed 14 charged and polar conserved residues as participating in the catalytic mechanism [35]. Six of these form a group at the bottom of the active site and bind two of the four essential metal ions. In the presence of orthophosphate, the yeast enzyme binds four metal ions and two phosphate molecules [36]. The native metal is most likely Mg^{2+}, but both Mg^{2+} [35,37] and Mn^{2+} [36,38] have been used in crystallography and X-ray diffraction experiments.

3. PHOSPHATASE STRUCTURE AND ACTIVE SITE METAL ION GEOMETRY

3.1. Alkaline Phosphatase

Alkaline phosphatase is a dimeric enzyme containing one active site per subunit. Each active site consists of two Zn^{2+} ions, an Mg^{2+} ion, a nucleophilic serine residue (Ser102) that participates in the formation of the phosphoenzyme intermediate noted in Scheme 3, and an arginine residue (Arg166) involved in holding the substrate in place (Fig. 2) [16]. The two zinc ions participate directly in catalysis while the magnesium ion is thought to play a structural role. One zinc ion (Zn_1) is coordinated by two nitrogen atoms from His331 and His412 and both oxygen atoms from Asp327. The second zinc ion, Zn_2, is 4.06 Å from Zn_1 and has a single nitrogen ligand from His370 and two oxygen ligands, one from the side chain carboxylate of Asp51 whose other carboxylate oxygen atom bridges to the Mg^{2+} ion, and a second oxygen from the carboxylate of Asp369 [39]. The X-ray structure of the phosphate-inhibited enzyme

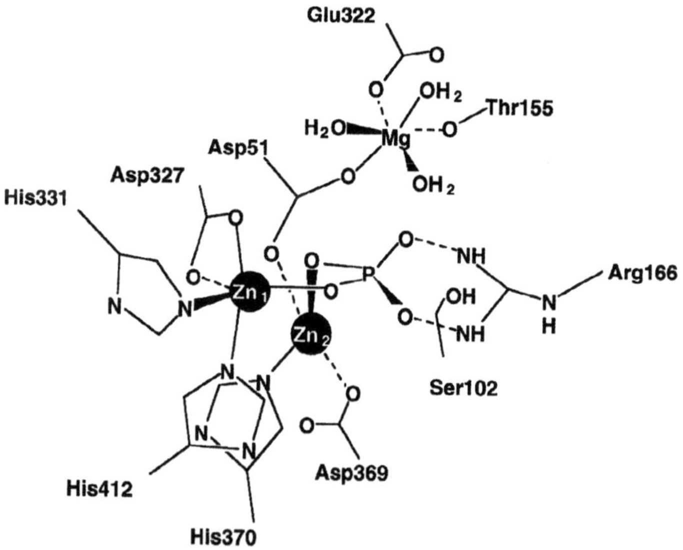

FIG. 2.   Active site of *E. coli* alkaline phosphatase. Figure adapted from the 2.0-Å resolution X-ray structure of the product-inhibited complex, Protein Data Bank entry 1ALK [16].

shows two oxygen atoms of phosphate coordinating to each Zn^{2+} ion, resulting in a phosphate bridge between these two metals. Two of the phosphate oxygens are also hydrogen-bonded to Arg166, presumably to help position the substrate during catalysis. The Mg^{2+} ion coordination is octahedral with oxygen ligands donated from the side chain carboxyls of Glu322 and Asp51, the side chain -OH of Thr155, and three water molecules.

In the phosphate complex, the -OH group of the catalytic serine, Ser102, is 4.6–4.9 Å from Zn_1, 2.1–2.2 Å from Zn_2, and 2.6–2.8 Å from the phosphorus atom of bound phosphate (Fig. 2). In the phosphate-free enzyme, the hydroxyl group of Ser102 is coordinated to Zn_2, an interaction that stabilizes the deprotonated form necessary for nucleophilic attack on the phosphate ester [16,39]. The role of the other zinc ion, Zn_1, is to stabilize developing charge on the leaving group in the first half of the reaction leading up to the formation of the phosphoenzyme intermediate. Interestingly, the roles of Zn_1 and Zn_2 are reversed in the second half of the reaction in which the phosphoenzyme intermediate is hydrolyzed and the enzyme regenerated for another round of substrate turnover. In the second step, Zn_1 lowers the pK_a of the nucleophile, a coordinated water molecule, while Zn_2 stabilizes the developing negative charge on the leaving group, which in this step is the serine alkoxide. This two-step mechanism, summarized in Fig. 3, shows the transition states in both the first and second steps of the reaction as a pentacoordinated intermediate characteristic of an associative mechanism (see Sec. 4.1 below). There is still some debate as to whether alkaline phosphatase proceeds by an associative or dissociative transition state. The experimental evidence regarding this issue has been reviewed thoroughly in [40]. Nevertheless, the transition state of a dissociative mechanism is expected to have a trigonal bipyramidal geometry not unlike that of the pentacoordinated intermediate shown in Fig. 3.

Mn^{2+} can substitute for the native Zn^{2+} ions but yields an enzyme with lower activity, $\approx 7\%$, compared to 100% for the native Zn_2/Mg enzyme [41]. The interaction of alkaline phosphatase with Mn^{2+} has been studied by electron paramagnetic resonance (EPR) spectroscopy and nuclear magnetic relaxation dispersion by Coleman and colleagues [42–44]. The addition of up to two equivalents of Mn^{2+} to the dimer yielded an X-band EPR spectrum characteristic of a mononuclear Mn^{2+} site in a ligand field with a large rhombic distortion, representing the

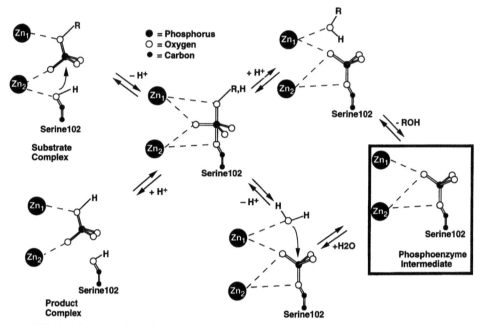

FIG. 3.   Proposed mechanism for *E. coli* alkaline phosphatase. The figure is adapted from the mechanism proposed by Kim and Wyckoff [16]. Phosphate ester cleavage proceeds along the top while hydrolysis of the phosphoenzyme intermediate is shown at the bottom.

binding of one Mn^{2+} ion to a site in each subunit normally occupied by a Zn^{2+} ion. Phosphate addition to this form produces changes in the EPR spectrum of bound Mn^{2+} and broadening of the ^{31}P-NMR spectrum of phosphate is observed, indicating that the phosphorus atom is in close proximity to the paramagnetic Mn^{2+} ion. The addition of two additional equivalents of Mn^{2+} yielded EPR spectra typical of Mn^{2+} in a symmetric environment. No evidence could be found for the formation of an exchange-coupled dinuclear $(Mn^{2+})_2$ cluster, although the presence of adjacent metal sites normally occupied by Zn^{2+} (metal–metal distance ≈ 4 Å) suggests that the formation of such a cluster should be observable by EPR measurements [45]. The absence of EPR spectra characteristic of an exchange-coupled $(Mn^{2+})_2$ cluster was taken to infer the absence of a bridging ligand, which is the case for the X-ray structures of the Zn^{2+} and Cd^{2+} enzymes but not for the Cu^{2+}-substituted enzyme [46].

3.2. Inorganic Pyrophosphatase

Inorganic pyrophosphatases from *E. coli*, *Thermus thermophilus*, and *Saccharomyces cerevisiae* have been purified and their structures solved by X-ray methods [35–38,47]. The enzymes from *E. coli* and *S. cerevisiae* are dimers and have absolute requirements for divalent metal ions, with Mg^{2+} the likely physiological metal ion. The reaction mechanism is thought to proceed by the binding of two metal ions in the absence of substrate, with two additional metal ions binding as a complex with pyrophosphate according to Scheme 6 [48].

$$Mg_2E + Mg_2PP_i \rightleftharpoons Mg_2E\cdot Mg_2PP_i \rightleftharpoons Mg_2E\cdot(MgP_i)_2 \rightleftharpoons Mg_2E + 2MgP_i$$

SCHEME 6

Catalysis is thought to proceed by the direct transfer of the phosphoryl group to water without the formation of a phosphoenzyme intermediate as observed in *E. coli* alkaline phosphatase. In the *E. coli* enzyme containing 1.5 Mg^{2+} ions per monomer, one Mg^{2+} ion is bound in the active site coordinated to Asp65, Asp70, and Asp102, while the second Mg^{2+} ion is shared by the two subunits and stabilizes the dimer interface [37]. In the X-ray structure of the yeast enzyme complexed without and with phosphate, Mn^{2+} was used in place of Mg^{2+} [38]. In the absence of phosphate, two Mn^{2+} ions bind and one of the Mn^{2+} ions is in an identical environment as that seen in the *E. coli* enzyme and is coordinated by three water molecules and Asp115, Asp120, and Asp152, which align with Asp65, Asp70, and Asp102 in the *E. coli* enzyme. A second Mn^{2+} ion is present and directly coordinated to five water molecules and only one protein residue, Asp120. In the presence of product phosphate, each subunit of the yeast enzyme binds four Mn^{2+} ions and two molecules of phosphate [36]. The structure of this complex allowed the authors to propose a hypothetical transition state (Fig. 4) which posits a metal-coordinated hydroxide serving as the nucleophile (hydroxide coordinated to Mn_2), while the other Mn^{2+} ions tether the substrate and stabilize the developing negative charge on the leaving group. Of significance is the finding that the basic group on the enzyme responsible for protonation of the leaving group appears to be a metal-coordinated hydroxide ion, which is shown coordinated to Mn_3 in Fig. 4 [49,50].

The binding of Mn^{2+} to yeast inorganic pyrophosphatase has also been studied by NMR and EPR techniques [51] and agree with the X-

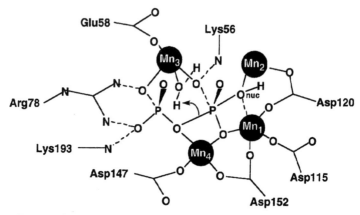

FIG. 4. Proposed transition state of yeast inorganic pyrophosphatase. The figure is adapted based on the structure of the enzyme complexed with two molecules of phosphate and four Mn^{2+} ions, Protein Data Bank entry 1WGJ [36,38]. Mn_2 is postulated to be the metal ion that coordinates the nucleophilic hydroxide, identified as O_{nuc} in the figure, while a second Mn^{2+}-coordinated water molecule is the general acid which donates a proton to the leaving group.

ray data indicating that two Mn^{2+} ions bind to the enzyme in the absence of substrate. A third Mn^{2+} was also shown to bind in the presence of phosphate, a result consistent with equilibrium dialysis experiments which found that catalysis proceeds when either three or four (and possibly five) Mg^{2+} ions bind per active site [48]. Also in agreement with the X-ray data, the distance between metal ions was shown to decrease upon binding of phosphate although the metal–metal distances measured by dipolar relaxation techniques were significantly longer than what has been determined by X-ray diffraction methods.

3.3. Phosphotriesterase

The active site of phosphotriesterase from *P. diminuta* has been solved reconstituted with Cd^{2+} [52] and Zn^{2+} [53]. The active site consists of a dinuclear metal center of two divalent cations (Fig. 5). In the $(Cd^{2+})_2$ enzyme, the metal ions are separated by 3.8 Å and are coordinated by four histidines, an aspartyl carboxylate group, and up to three solvent mol-

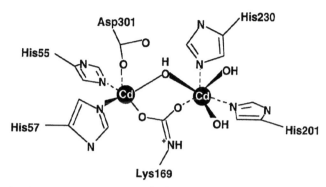

FIG. 5. Active site architecture of phosphotriesterase from *Pseudomonas diminuta*. The schematic is based on the active site of the cadmium-reconstituted enzyme at 2.0 Å, Protein Data Bank entry 1PSC [52].

ecules, one of which forms a μ-hydroxo bridge between the two Cd^{2+} ions. Of interest was the finding that a carbamylated lysine residue provided a second bridging ligand between metal ions. A carbamylated lysine residue is also a bridging ligand to the active site $(Ni^{2+})_2$ cluster of urease from *Klebsiella aerogenes* [54]. In fact, the dinuclear metal center and overall tertiary fold of urease and phosphotriesterase are quite similar [34]. The structure of the $(Zn^{2+})_2$ enzyme superimposes on the structure of the $(Cd^{2+})_2$ enzyme with root mean square deviation (rmsd) of 0.20 Å for the polypeptide chain backbone atoms and just 0.4 Å rmsd for all protein atoms [53]. However, the metal–metal distance in the $(Zn^{2+})_2$ enzyme is shorter at 3.3 Å and there are also slight decreases in metal–ligand distances, presumably reflecting the smaller ionic radius of zinc compared to cadmium.

The mechanism of phosphotriestease was studied by following the hydrolysis of paraoxon (diethyl 4-nitrophenylphosphate) in ^{18}O-H_2O. Hydrolysis yielded *p*-nitrophenol, and diethylphosphate containing the ^{18}O label. These results demonstrate nucleophilic attack by water/hydroxide at the phosphorus atom concomitant with P-O bond scission. Hydrolysis of the chiral substrate *O*-ethyl-*O*-(4-nitrophenyl)phenyl-phosphonothioate resulted in inversion of stereochemistry about the phosphorus atom, indicating a direct, in-line displacement reaction of an activated water molecule at the phosphorus atom of the phosphotriester substrate [55] (Scheme 7).

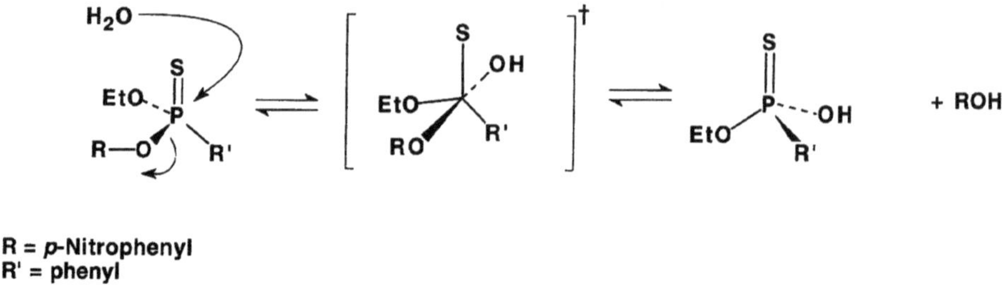

R = p-Nitrophenyl
R' = phenyl

SCHEME 7

Recently, the three-dimensional structure of a gene product in the *E. coli* genome homologous to phosphotriesterase has also been solved [56]. The *E. coli* enzyme does not catalyze the hydrolysis of nonspecific phosphotriesters and the identity of the physiological substrate remains elusive. One significant difference in the active site of this enzyme is the substitution of the carbamylated lysine residue with a carboxylate group from a glutamic acid side chain. In addition to the *E. coli* enzyme, phosphotriesterase homologs have been found in other species including mammals [34].

EPR investigation of Mn^{2+}-substituted phosphotriesterase revealed formation of a antiferromagnetically coupled dinuclear $(Mn^{2+})_2$ cluster [57]. The spectrum was characterized by a multiline spectrum displaying 26 hyperfine lines from ^{55}Mn near $g = 2.0$ separated by ≈ 45 G rather than the more typical ≈ 90 G splitting of a mononuclear Mn^{2+} ion. An estimation of the magnitude of the exchange interaction based on the temperature dependence of the EPR spectra yielded a value of $J = 5 \pm 1$ cm^{-1} and an estimate of Mn^{2+}–Mn^{2+} distances of 3.6–4.3 Å. The presence of a bridging ligand was inferred and candidates included an aquo ligand, an imidazole from histidine, or a carboxylate from aspartate or glutamate.

3.4. Purple Acid Phosphatase

X-ray structures of kidney bean purple acid phosphatase have been obtained for the iron-zinc form of the enzyme initially at 2.9 Å resolution [58] and further refined to 2.65 Å resolution [59]. Additional structures of the enzyme complexed with phosphate and tungstate at 2.7 and 3.0 Å resolution, respectively, have also been obtained [59]. The active site consists of a dinuclear Fe^{3+}-Zn^{2+} cluster with a metal–metal distance of 3.26 Å. The structure of the kidney bean enzyme complexed with phosphate is shown in Fig. 6.

As with PP1 and calcineurin, a phosphoesterase motif that forms a metal-binding $\beta\alpha\beta\alpha\beta$ secondary structure is present in purple acid phosphatase. The phosphoesterase motif in purple acid phosphatases, $D(X)_n GDXXY(X)_m GNHD/E$, is similar to that in protein phosphatases but differs by the absence of a histidine residue in the loop between the first β sheet/α helix and the presence of a tyrosine residue in the loop between the second β sheet/α helix. These substitutions and the presence of an additional histidine ligand outside this motif bring about a

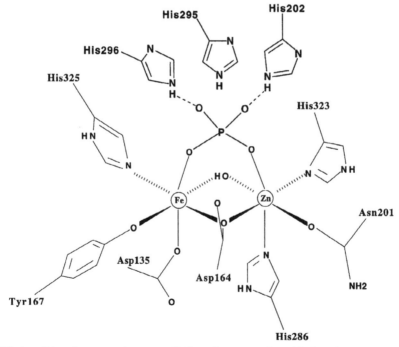

FIG. 6. Dinuclear metal center of kidney bean purple acid phosphatase in complex with product phosphate. The active site dinuclear Fe^{3+}-Zn^{2+} center, its ligands, and surrounding active site residues is depicted and based on the 2.7-Å resolution X-ray structure, Protein Data Bank entry 4KBP [59].

net replacement of a putative water/hydroxide ligand with a tyrosine residue in the coordination sphere of the Fe^{3+} ion of purple acid phosphatase.

In addition to nitrogen and oxygen ligands from amino acid side chains, three solvent molecules were modeled into the coordination sphere of the unliganded enzyme: one bridging hydroxide, a terminal hydroxide on the Fe^{3+} ion, and a terminal aqua ligand on the Zn^{2+} ion. At the resolution obtained, these could not be unambiguously observed in the electron density maps but were modeled based on preferred geometries and spectroscopic evidence [59]. The presence of at least one metal- coordinated solvent molecule is likely, however, as a mechanism involving a hydroxide coordinated to the Fe^{3+} ion that participates in a single-step nucleophilic displacement reaction has been proposed [60,61]. This mechanism is based on stereochemical analysis indicating that the phosphate ester undergoes *inversion* of stereochemistry upon hydrolysis [62]. A single displacement mechanism is in contrast to the mechanism of alkaline phosphatase, which shows *retention* of stereochemistry and is taken to indicate that a phosphoenzyme intermediate is not formed in the purple acid phosphatase reaction. Additional support for this mechanism comes from data which indicate that phosphate binding to the mammalian enzyme involves initial coordination to the divalent ion (Fe^{2+}, Zn^{2+}) with displacement of an aquo ligand followed by a slower isomerization that leads to phosphate bridging the two metal ions [60]. Nucleophilic attack on the substrate by a hydroxide coordinated to Fe^{3+} would result in a product complex with phosphate coordinating to both metal ions. In fact, this structure is observed in the product/product analog complexes with phosphate and tungstate, which shows these anion inhibitors bound in place of the two terminal water molecules via two oxygen atoms, resulting in a nearly symmetric bridge between the two metal ions (Fig. 6).

In addition to the metal ions and their accompanying ligands, three histidine residues are also part of the active site of purple acid phosphatase. In the phosphate- and tungstate-inhibited enzymes, the N_ε atoms of His202 and His296 interact with the oxygen atoms of the anion inhibitor (Fig. 6). His202 is homologous to His151 in calcineurin and His76 in bacteriophage λ protein phosphatase, residues that have been proposed to participate in the enzyme reaction as active site general acids and/or bases (Fig. 7) [63]. Notably absent in the active site of

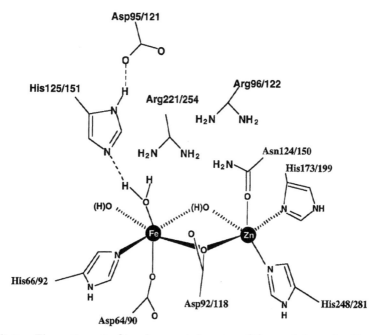

FIG. 7. The active site dinuclear metal center of the protein serine/threonine phosphatases. The drawing is based on the 2.1-Å resolution structure of human calcineurin, Protein Data Bank entry 1AUI [76]. The ligand numbering provides the residue number of rabbit muscle PP1 (first number) and calcineurin (second number). One or more of the metal ions in the X-ray structures of PP1 was likely to be Mn^{2+} due to its presence in the purification and/or crystallization buffers [73,74]. In PP1, the site occupied by iron was modeled as pentacoordinate in a square-pyramidal or trigonal pyramidal geometry. The higher resolution X-ray structure of calcineurin identified an additional solvent molecule and octahedral coordination for the iron atom.

purple acid phosphatase is an arginine present in alkaline phosphatase (Fig. 2), calcineurin/PP1 (see Fig. 7), and inorganic pyrophosphatases (Fig. 4). The presence of a histidine residue in purple acid phosphatase rather than an arginine was used to hypothesize the shift in the pH optimum of purple acid phosphatases (≈6) [61,64,65] compared to the analogous protein phosphatases (≈7–8) [66,67].

Derivatives of kidney bean purple acid phosphatase containing Mn^{2+} have been prepared [68]. In that study, the apoenzyme was prepared and the activity of the enzyme assessed after adding back various metal ions. Essentially full activity was obtained when the apo-enzyme was incubated with Fe^{3+} and either Fe^{2+}, Zn^{2+}, or Co^{2+}. Tenfold lower but measurable activity was obtained when Fe^{3+} and Mn^{2+} were added, allowing the authors to conclude that separate binding sites exist for the Fe^{3+} and divalent metal ions. This result implies the formation of an Fe^{3+}-Mn^{2+} dinuclear metal center but thus far no spectroscopic proof for this has been forwarded. There have also been earlier reports of a Mn^{3+}-dependent acid phosphatase from sweet potato [69–71]. Subsequent studies by Hefler and Averill, however, have found that this enzyme contains 2 mol of iron and insignificant amounts of manganese [72].

3.5.   Protein Phosphatases 1 and 2B (Calcineurin)

The protein serine/threonine phosphatases also accommodate dinuclear metal centers. In the X-ray structure of PP1, Mn^{2+} was included in purification and/or crystallization buffers and evidence for both manganese and iron were obtained by X-ray emission spectroscopy of crystals used for X-ray diffraction [73,74]. In X-ray structures of calcineurin, iron and zinc were modeled into the active site based on previous metal analyses [8] and homology to the structure of purple acid phosphatase [75,76]. The presence of iron and zinc in the bovine enzyme was confirmed by metal analyses and EPR spectrometry, which hypothesized the presence of a dinuclear Fe^{3+}- Zn^{2+} cluster (Fig. 7) [9].

A comparison of the metal coordination of PP1, calcineurin, and purple acid phosphatase indicates many similarities (compare Figs. 6 and 7). Thus, in the absence of phosphate, the Zn^{2+} sites are identical with the only difference being an additional solvent molecule as an axial ligand in purple acid phosphatase that is situated in place of the phosphate oxygen atom at that site in Fig. 6. As noted above, electron density for this solvent molecule in the purple acid phosphatase structure could not be unambiguously assigned but was modeled in place to preserve octahedral geometry [58,59]. With a few exceptions, the geometry at the Fe^{3+} site is also highly conserved. The most notable difference is the presence of a tyrosine and a histidine coordinated to the Fe^{3+} site in purple acid phosphatase, substituted by a histidine and water molecule in calcineurin and PP1. The absence of a tyrosine ligand in PP1 and calcineurin explains the lack of detectable absorbance in the UV/Vis spectra of these enzymes for $\lambda \geq 300$ nm [9]. Although few mechanistic or structural data have been obtained on PP2A, this enzyme is highly homologous to calcineurin and PP1 and can be activated by divalent metal ions [77]. As such PP2A is expected to contain a dinuclear metal center analogous to that shown in Fig. 7.

Mn^{2+}, although not a native metal ion, is a potent activator of PP1 [78–83], PP2A [77], and calcineurin [8,28,84–88]. As noted above in the X-ray studies, Mn^{2+} appears to be incorporated into PP1 following purification and/or crystallization in buffers containing Mn^{2+} although it was not ascertained whether Mn^{2+} occupied one or both metal sites. In the case of the phosphatase from bacteriophage λ, Mn^{2+} is also an excellent activator. Room temperature and low-temperature EPR spectrometry has been used to investigate Mn^{2+} binding to λ protein phosphatase [89]. Titration of the enzyme with Mn^{2+} indicated one binding site with micromolar affinity and a second site with about 100-fold lower affinity. The high-affinity binding site is characterized by a rhombic mononuclear Mn^{2+} EPR signal. The binding of the second Mn^{2+} results in a multiline EPR spectrum with narrow hyperfine splitting (≈ 39 G) indicative of a spin-coupled $(Mn^{2+})_2$ cluster similar to that observed for Mn^{2+}-substituted phosphotriesterase, discussed above in Sec. 3.3. An estimate of the exchange interaction found a J value of 1–3 cm^{-1}, possibly indicating a weak aquo ligand bridging the two Mn^{2+} ions. Further studies will clarify whether Mn^{2+} activation of PP1, PP2A, and calcineurin results from Mn^{2+} binding in one or both metal sites.

3.6. Protein Phosphatase 2C

It is intriguing to note that in spite of the absence of sequence homology to PP1, calcineurin, or purple acid phosphatase, PP2C also contains a dinuclear metal center [26]. In the case of the recombinant PP2C, crystals were obtained in the presence of $MnCl_2$, thus placing two Mn ions 4.0 Å apart in the active site (Fig. 8). The metal coordination of PP2C differs considerably with one metal coordinated by an oxygen atom from the backbone carbonyl of Gly61, one oxygen from the side chain carboxylate of Asp60, and four solvent molecules, one bridging to the second metal. Two terminal solvent molecules and three oxygen atoms from

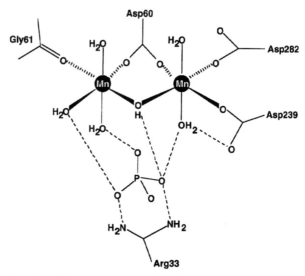

FIG. 8.   Active site of human protein phosphatase 2C. (Adapted from Figure 6 in [26].)

Asp239, Asp282, and the second carboxylate oxygen from Asp60 complete the coordination of the second metal ion. Another major difference was the manner in which phosphate binds to the enzyme. Cocrystallization localized the phosphate molecule in the active site but without direct coordination to either metal. Rather, the coordination between the phosphate molecule and the metal ions was via a second-sphere interaction with four metal-coordinated solvent molecules involved in hydrogen bonding to the phosphate oxygen atoms (Fig. 8).

The catalytic mechanism of PP2C has not been investigated in detail although metal-coordinated water molecules have been proposed as both the attacking nucleophile and the general acid responsible for protonation of the leaving group [26]. In that regard, the mechanism resembles that worked out in detail for inorganic pyrophosphatase. Nevertheless, the uniqueness of the active site structure of PP2C compared to the other phosphatases, in particular the mode of interaction with phosphate, suggests that an alternative mechanism is possible. One possibility would be an outer sphere mechanism in which substrate and/or product do not interact directly with the metal ions but indirectly through metal-coordinated solvent molecules. Further experimentation may reveal whether this is the case.

4.   MECHANISMS OF HYDROLYSIS

4.1.   Chemical Aspects

Chemical (non-enzymatic) hydrolysis of phosphate esters has been studied in detail and different mechanisms have been found for phosphate mono-, di-, and triesters. The mechanisms differ in the degree of bond formation between the phosphorus atom and the incoming nucleophile and the extent of bond cleavage to the leaving group. In one extreme, termed the dissociative mechanism, the transition state involves substantial bond cleavage to the leaving group but little bond formation to the nucleophile (Fig. 9). In the transition state of this mechanism, the phosphoryl group resembles the metaphosphate anion, PO_3^-. In the other extreme, the associative mechanism, bond formation to the nucleophile, precedes dissociation of the leaving group and the transition state resembles a pentacoordinated phosphorane. The concerted mechanism has substantial bond formation to the nucleophile and bond cleavage to the leaving group, with both occurring to varying degrees in the transition state.

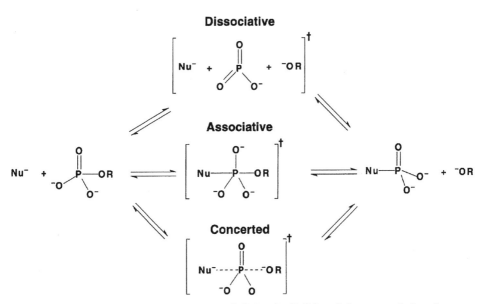

FIG. 9.   Limiting mechanistic possibilities for P-O bond cleavage of phosphate esters.

Mechanistic studies have been used to study the transition state of phosphate esters in solution [40]. Experimental data including Brønsted analyses and isotope effect studies indicate that both the monoanion and dianion forms of phosphate monoesters undergo solution state reactions characterized by the dissociative mechanism with extensive P-O bond cleavage and only a small degree of bond formation to the nucleophile. In the transition state of phosphate monoester at low pH where the monoanion predominates, substantial charge neutralization of the leaving group occurs by an intramolecular proton transfer reaction. In the case of phosphate di- and triesters, the transition state is usually more associative and is characterized by greater bond formation to the nucleophile and less P-O bond cleavage.

4.2. Active Site Metal Ions: Functional Roles

4.2.1. Metal–Phosphoryl Group Interactions

In enzyme reactions, transition state stabilization plays a key role in catalysis and is likely to be one mechanism for catalysis of the metal-dependent phosphatases. In most of the phosphatases noted above, structural studies indicate that product phosphate and/or product analogs (e.g., tungstate) coordinate directly to the metal ions. This implies that the substrate phosphoryl group also coordinates to one or more metal ions during catalysis. For phosphate mono- and diesters, the substrate carries a significant negative charge that would effectively shield the phosphorus atom and hinder nucleophilic attack. Metal coordination would effectively neutralize this charge, making the phosphorus atom more electrophilic and prone to nucleophilic attack by a hydroxide ion or active site nucleophile. This interaction has been used to argue that the normally dissociative transition state of phosphate monoesters in solution may become more associative in the presence of metal ions [90]. Hengge has eloquently discussed this hypothesis and argued that it is not likely that coordination of the phosphoryl group oxygen atoms to the metal ion(s) can bring about a change in the enzyme-catalyzed reaction from a dissociative one, as observed in solution hydrolysis, to a purely associative transition state [40]. In the case of phosphotriesterase, the substrate is uncharged and this type of stabilization by the dinuclear metal center is unnecessary, suggesting that the multinuclear metal center in this enzyme and possibly other phosphatases may have other roles.

Isotope effect studies have been performed on phosphotriesterase [91], alkaline phosphatase [92], calcineurin [93], and, recently, the protein phosphatase from bacteriophage λ that is homologous to calcineurin and PP1 [67]. Primary and secondary isotope effects for the phosphotriesterase reaction have been studied using the substrate [^{18}O]-O,O-diethyl-O-(4-carbamoylphenyl)phosphate. The isotope effects were comparable in magnitude to the isotope effects for alkaline hydrolysis of this substrate and indicative of an associative transition state but without the formation of a stable phosphorane intermediate. In the case of alkaline phosphatase, a step other than the chemical step involving bond formation to the nucleophile and P-O bond cleavage was rate limiting and the isotope effects were suppressed and near unity. This was also the case for calcineurin at pH 7.0 but increasing the pH to 8.5 resulted in isotope effects indicative of substantial P-O bond cleavage in the transition state and a small but measurable negative charge on the leaving group. Similar results were obtained for bacteriophage λ protein phosphatase where the chemical step was rate limiting and the isotope effects fully expressed [67]. These results were taken to indicate that the transition state in the enzyme-catalyzed hydrolysis of phosphate monoesters resembles the dissociative transition state of phosphate monoesters in solution. Thus the change to an associative mechanism anticipated by the presence of metal ions in the enzyme active site does not appear to occur.

4.2.2. General Acid Catalysis: Charge Neutralization on the Leaving Group

For all phosphate esters, if P-O bond scission occurs in the transition state, this would result in significant buildup of negative charge on the leaving group. For most biological substrates, the leaving group is an alcohol. For the protein serine/threonine phosphatases, the leaving group is the alkoxide of a serine or threonine residue, the conjugate acid of which will have a $pK_a \geq 14$. Thus neutralization of the charge by protonation (general acid catalysis) or metal coordination would lower the energy of the transition state and increase the rate of the reaction. As noted above, isotope effect studies of calcineurin and bacteriophage λ protein phosphatase are consistent with charge neutralization of the leaving group. In the λ phosphatase, additional isotope effect studies were performed with a mutant form of the enzyme in which an active site histidine residue, proposed to be the general acid that protonates the leaving group, was mutated to asparagine (H76N). The H76N mutant enzyme exhibited increased isotope effects consistent with additional negative charge buildup on the leaving group, as might be expected for deleting an active site general acid. However, the isotope effects were smaller than expected for a full negative charge and therefore an additional possibility involving charge neutralization by one or more of the metal ions was considered [67].

The analogous histidine residue in PP1/calcineurin is His125/151 (Fig. 7) and His202 in purple acid phosphatase (Fig. 6). In the crystal structure of phosphate-inhibited calcineurin, His151 is within H bonding distance of the most solvent-exposed oxygen atom of phosphate and is close enough to donate a proton to the leaving group [75]. Similar orientations are observed in PP1 with bound anion inhibitors modeled in the active site [73,74] and in purple acid phosphatase with phosphate and tungstate bound at the active site [59]. Mertz et al. addressed the possibility that this histidine is involved in proton donation to the leaving group by comparing relative k_{cat} values for substrates that have different pK_a values of the respective leaving group [63]. "Activated" phosphate esters such as pNPP have good leaving groups by virtue of their low pK_a (p-nitrophenol $pK_a = 7.2$) compared to substrates such as phenyl phosphate (pK_a of phenol = 10) or a phosphoseryl peptide (pK_a serine side chain -OH $\approx$ 14). Thus, hydrolysis of pNPP requires less catalytic assistance than either phenyl phosphate or a phosphoseryl peptide substrate since the developing negative charge on the leaving group can be effectively delocalized by the electron-withdrawing nitro substituent of p-nitrophenol. As such, if His151 is serving as a proton donor to the leaving group, one would expect larger effects on relative k_{cat} values (wild-type vs. mutant) for substrates with poorer leaving groups. Although mutagenesis of H151 to glutamine (H151Q) resulted in a 460- to 1300-fold decrease in k_{cat} compared to wild-type enzyme, less than a 3-fold difference in relative k_{cat} was found for calcineurin using pNPP vs. a phosphopeptide substrate despite a difference in basicity of the leaving group of $>10^6$. With bacteriophage λ protein phosphatase, mutagenesis of His76 to Asn resulted in the same 500- to 600-fold decrease in k_{cat} using either pNPP or phenyl phosphate, i.e., essentially no difference in relative k_{cat} values for these two substrates ($\Delta pK_a = 2.75$). These results suggest that removal of this histidine by mutagenesis did not affect the ability to protonate the leaving group.

4.2.3. General Base Catalysis

We have postulated that His151 in calcineurin (and His76 in bacterio-phage λ protein phosphatase) acts in concert with the dinuclear metal center by interacting with the nucleophilic solvent molecule [63]. Thus, H151 could either serve as a general base to remove the proton from the metal-coordinated water molecule, or it may position the oxygen atom of this solvent molecule for an optimum in-line attack on the phosphate ester. In the X-ray structure of calcineurin, the N_ε atom of His151 is H-bonded to one of two terminal solvent molecules on the Fe^{3+} site (Fig. 7) [76]. Interestingly, Asp121 is within H-bonding distance of His151. Indeed, mutagenesis of the residues analogous to Asp121 in PP1 (Asp95) or λ protein phosphatase (Asp52) resulted in an $\approx 10^2$-fold decrease in k_{cat}. Thus, the interaction of this conserved histidine/aspartate pair with a terminal aqua/hydroxo ligand on the Fe^{3+} is analogous to the Asp-His-Ser catalytic triad of serine proteases. The "Asp-His-HO-metal" motif can be thought of as a catalytic tetrad, with the metal ion serving to lower the pK_a of the nucleophilic water molecule while the Asp-His functions as a catalytic base to assist in hydroxide formation.

4.2.4. Lewis Acid Catalysis: Lowering the pK_a of the Nucleophile

Metal-coordinated solvent molecules have been implicated in many of the above phosphatase reactions. In many of these reactions, the metal ion is functioning as a Lewis acid, effectively lowering the pK_a of a co-ordinated nucleophile or water molecule. In the first step in the reaction catalyzed by alkaline phosphatase, Zn_2 is coordinated to the active site nucleophile, Ser102, while in the second step, coordination of a water molecule by Zn_1 occurs, thereby lowering the pK_a of these and increasing their nucleophilicity. Similar mechanisms have been discussed above for purple acid phosphatase, inorganic pyrophosphatase, and phosphotriesterase. In the case of the protein serine/threonine phosphatase, Yu et al. have studied the effect of redox state of the iron ion in the active site of calcineurin [9,94]. In the native iron-zinc enzyme, treatment of the Fe^{3+}-Zn^{2+} form of bovine calcineurin with sodium dithionite ($Na_2S_2O_4$) reduced the iron to the ferrous oxidation state and led to a loss of activity toward pNPP. In the di-iron form of the enzyme, a similar inactivation occurred upon reduction of the mixed-valence

Fe^{3+}-Fe^{2+} state to the Fe^{2+}-Fe^{2+} state. These results were taken to indicate a requirement for an Fe^{3+} ion in the active site. Considering the possibility that the Fe^{3+} ion activates the nucleophilic water in the reaction, the loss of activity upon reduction to Fe^{2+} is consistent with a decreased Lewis acidity associated with a Fe^{2+} ion compared to an Fe^{3+} ion. The pK_a of water coordinated to aqueous Fe^{3+} is 2.13 compared to 8.44 for Fe^{2+}, a more than 10^6-fold difference in acidity [95].

Besides the requirement for a Fe^{3+} ion, additional studies utilizing the di-iron form of calcineurin indicated a requirement for a divalent metal ion in the other metal site ($M^{2+} = Zn^{2+}$, Fe^{2+}). In the case of the native iron-zinc bovine enzyme, higher oxidation states of Zn^{2+} are not biologically relevant. However, replacement of the Zn^{2+} ion with Fe^{2+} afforded the chance to explore the activity of an additional redox state, the Fe^{3+}-Fe^{3+} state. Calcineurin in the mixed-valence Fe^{3+}-Fe^{2+} state could be oxidized by H_2O_2 to the diferric state, a process that could be quantitatively followed by EPR spectrometry [94]. Oxidation to the diferric state resulted in loss of activity as judged using pNPP as substrate. This also occurs with mammalian purple acid phosphatase which, when isolated under aerobic conditions, is obtained in the inactive Fe^{3+}-Fe^{3+} oxidation state [61,96–99]. Treatment of oxidized purple acid phosphatase with mild reductants such as ascorbate or β-mercaptoethanol yields the active Fe^{3+}-Fe^{2+} enzyme. The requirement for a divalent metal ion in this site may indicate that this metal ion interacts with the substrate and/or product through one or more of the phosphate oxygen atoms. If this site is occupied by a solvent molecule that is displaced by incoming substrate, the presence of Fe^{3+} in this site will result in a stronger bond to the solvent compared to Fe^{2+} and make it more difficult for substrate to displace the solvent molecule. Alternatively, the presence of a trivalent metal ion in this position may result in product inhibition. Crystallographic data indicate that the product of the reaction, phosphate, coordinates to both metal ions and must be displaced to prepare the enzyme for another round of catalysis. Association constants of Fe^{3+} with HPO_4^{2-} ($\log K = 8.30$, 25°C, $I = 0.5$ M) are nearly 10^5-fold larger than for Fe^{2+} ($\log K = 3.5$, 25°C, $I = 0$ M) [95]. Yet another possibility for the requirement for a divalent metal ion in this site would be to coordinate a solvent molecule that serves as a general acid in the reaction. This type of role was discussed above in the reaction catalyzed by inorganic pyrophosphatase. In that enzyme, a water molecule coordinated to one of the Mn^{2+} ions was proposed to be the general acid that donates a proton to the leaving group (cf. Fig. 4).

4.3. Conserved Nonligand Active Site Residues

Besides the commonality of multinuclear metal ion cofactors, the active sites of these phosphatases consist of other nonligand residues that are essential for catalysis. The presence of a conserved histidine-aspartate pair in the protein serine/threonine phosphatases was discussed above in Secs. 4.2.2 and 4.2.3. In addition, most of the enzymes discussed above have one or more basic residues present in the active site. Together with the metal ions, these basic residues generate a region of positive electrostatic potential. Thus, in alkaline phosphatase, PP1/calcineurin, inorganic pyrophosphatase, and PP2C, arginine residues are present in the active site and either hydrogen-bond to the negatively charged phosphate oxygen atoms or are close enough that such an interaction in the substrate complex could occur. In purple acid phosphatase, an arginine is absent but an imidazole group from one or more histidine residues is thought to be a functional substitute. Depending on the enzyme/substrate, mutagenesis usually results in decreases in k_{cat}, increases in substrate K_m, or increases in the K_I for product phosphate (Table 2) [49,100–105]. These results are consistent with roles for these basic residues in substrate binding and/or transition state stabilization.

5. CONCLUSIONS

It is intriguing that these active sites can accommodate a wide variety of metal ions. In many instances the native metal ion is spectroscopically silent (e.g., Zn^{2+}, Mg^{2+}), making it difficult to study. Mg^{2+} also suffers from the fact that it diffracts X-rays poorly due to low electron density. These features have resulted in the use of transition metals as probes of the active site. In the phosphatases discussed here, Mn^{2+} has proven to be a useful surrogate. Mn^{2+} was useful in X-ray diffraction studies of inorganic pyrophosphatase due to its more favorable diffraction characteristics compared to Mg^{2+}. Furthermore, Mn^{2+} is paramagnetic and amenable to EPR and NMR studies. As such, the use of metal

TABLE 2

Effect of Site-Directed Mutagenesis of Conserved Active Site Basic Residues on the Kinetic Parameters for Wild-Type and Mutant Phosphatases

Enzyme	Mutation	k_{cat} (s^{-1})	K_M (M)	k_{cat}/K_m (M^{-1} s^{-1})	K_I (HPO$_4^{2-}$) (μM)	Ref.
Alkaline phosphatase	Wild type	19.0[a]	5.5 × 10^{-6}	3.5 × 10^6	—	[104]
	R166K	4.4[a]	5.2 × 10^{-6}	8.4 × 10^5	—	
	R166Q	1.4[a]	65.9 × 10^{-6}	2.1 × 10^4	—	
	Wild type	13.6[a]	7.4 × 10^{-6}	1.8 × 10^6	14.3[c]	[105]
	R166S	0.44[a]	7.6 × 10^{-6}	5.8 × 10^4	417[c]	
	R166A	0.33[a]	13.8 × 10^{-6}	2.4 × 10^4	665[c]	
Inorganic pyrophosphatase						
E. coli pyrophosphatase	Wild type	200	4.3 × 10^{-6}	4.7 × 10^7		[49]
	K29R	14	82 × 10^{-6}	1.7 × 10^5		
	R43K	100	21 × 10^{-6}	4.8 × 10^6		
	K142R	283	83 × 10^{-6}	3.4 × 10^6		

Protein serine/threonine phosphatases

Calcineurin					
	Wild type	14.1^a	37×10^{-3}	3.8×10^2	—	[103]
	R122A	$<0.0026^a$	ND	—	—
	R254A	0.077^a	90×10^{-3}	0.86	—
Protein phosphatase 1					
	Wild type	14.3^b	3.5×10^{-6}	4.1×10^6	—	[101]
	R96E	0.054^b	8.9×10^{-6}	6.1×10^3	—
	Wild type	39^b	10.6×10^{-6}	3.7×10^6	—	[102]
	R96A	0.09^b	6.9×10^{-6}	1.3×10^4	—
	R221S	0.2^b	105×10^{-6}	1.9×10^3	—
	Wild type	9.0^b	2.8×10^{-6}	3.2×10^6	—	[108]
	R221Q	0.44^b	11×10^{-6}	4.0×10^4	—
λ Protein phosphatase					
	Wild type	$2000^{a,d}$	10.3×10^{-3}	1.9×10^5	710	[100]
	R53A	$0.70^{b,d}$	10.1×10^{-3}	6.9×10^1	>2000
	R73A	$88^{b,d}$	6.3×10^{-3}	1.4×10^4	>2000

[a] pNPP as substrate.
[b] Phosphorylase a as substrate.
[c] K_I for orthophosphate.
[d] Reaction in the presence of 1 mM $MnCl_2$.
ND, not determined.

analogs such as Mn^{2+} has provided insight into structural and mechanistic details. Nevertheless, one has to be cautious that the use of a different metal ion may lead to an altered structure and/or change in the mechanism of an enzyme. We have noted that Mn^{2+} substitution in purple acid phosphatase and alkaline phosphatase resulted in lower activity compared with Zn^{2+}. In other instances, Mn^{2+} results in higher activities (e.g., protein serine/threonine phosphatases) and examples of altered substrate specificity have been documented [32]. These facts should be considered in all studies that utilize a nonnative metal ion as a structural and mechanistic probe.

A comparison of the active sites of six different classes of enzymes involved in phosphate ester hydrolysis reveals numerous similarities in the active sites of these enzymes. Despite the fact that substrates range from highly negatively charged phosphate monoesters and pyrophosphate to neutral triester substrates, these enzymes have two or more metal ions present as dinuclear or multinuclear centers. In all cases, the metal ions are proposed to interact with the substrate, either directly via coordination of the phosphate ester oxygen atoms, or through a second-sphere mechanism (e.g., PP2C). Such interactions can reduce the charge on the phosphoryl group, making it easier to undergo nucleophilic attack. Metal-coordinated amino acid side chains (e.g., Ser 102 in alkaline phosphatase) and ligated solvent molecules play key roles as nucleophiles that attack the phosphate ester substrate in an S_N^2 type mechanism. In these interactions, the metal serves to lower the pK_a of the conjugate acid, facilitating its deprotonation to form the more nucleophilic anionic species. Additional active site residues may participate in general base catalysis in concert with the metal ion to deprotonate the nucleophile. Water molecules bound to the metal ions have also been proposed as general acids that donate protons to the leaving group, with the metal ions functioning to lower the pK_a of the donated proton. In some cases, the developing negative charge on the leaving group is stabilized by a direct metal interaction or possibly by protonation via an active site residue.

These common structural features are remarkable given the fact that these enzymes do not appear to be homologous and thus derived from a common ancestor. It is intriguing to speculate that these common features represent an optimal active site architecture based on convergent evolution. At present, the structures of only a handful of these enzymes have been determined and their mechanisms rigorously characterized. It is anticipated that future studies may reveal whether there are unifying chemical principles regarding the mechanism for phosphate ester hydrolysis by these and other phosphatases.

ACKNOWLEDGMENTS

The author gratefully acknowledges support from the National Institutes of Health (GM46865) and the Mayo Foundation. The author also thanks Nancy Wengenack for critical reading of the manuscript.

ABBREVIATIONS

EPR   electron paramagnetic resonance
NMR   nuclear magnetic resonance
pNPP   *para*-nitrophenyl phosphate
PP1   protein phosphatase 1
PP2A   protein phosphatase 2A
PP2B   protein phosphatase 2B or calcineurin
PP2C   protein phosphatase 2C
PP_i inorganic diphosphate
rmsd   root mean square deviation

REFERENCES

1. P. A. Frey and R. D. Sammons, *Science, 228*, 541–545 (1985).

2. C. A. Stein, J. L. Tonkinson, and L. Yakubov, *Pharmacol. Ther., 52*, 365–384 (1991).

3. C. R. Cantor and P. R. Schimmel, *Biophysical Chemistry*, W. H. Freeman and Company, New York, 1980.

4. E. C. Webb, *Enzyme Nomenclature 1992: Recommendations of the Nomenclature Committee of the International Union of Biochemistry and Molecular Biology on the Nomenclature and Classification of Enzymes*, Academic Press, San Diego, 1992, p. 320.

5. W. F. Bosron, F. S. Kennedy, and B. L. Vallee, *Biochemistry*, *14*, 2275–2282 (1975).

6. M. Fosset, D. Chappelet-Tordo, and M. Lazdunski, *Biochemistry*, *13*, 1783–1788 (1974).

7. G. A. Omburo, J. M. Kuo, L. S. Mullins, and F. M. Raushel, *J. Biol. Chem.*, *267*, 13278–13283 (1992).

8. M. M. King and C. Y. Huang, *J. Biol. Chem.*, *259*, 8847–8856 (1984).

9. L. Yu, A. Haddy, and F. Rusnak, *J. Am. Chem. Soc.*, *117*, 10147–10148 (1995).

10. J. E. Coleman, *Annu. Rev. Biophys. Biomol. Struct.*, *21*, 441–483 (1992).

11. J. E. Coleman and P. Gettins, *Adv. Enzymol.*, *55*, 381–452 (1983).

12. R. Han and J. E. Coleman, *Biochemistry*, *34*, 4238–4245 (1995).

13. A. D. Hall and A. Williams, *Biochemistry*, *25*, 4784–4790 (1986).

14. J. A. Gerlt, J. A. Coderre, and S. Mehdi, *Adv. Enzymol.*, *55*, 291–380 (1983).

15. P. Gettins and J. E. Coleman, *J. Biol. Chem.*, *258*, 408–416 (1983).

16. E. E. Kim and H. W. Wyckoff, *J. Mol. Biol.*, *218*, 449–464 (1991).

17. S. Shenolikar and A. C. Nairn, *Adv. Second Messenger Phosphoprot. Res.*, *23*, 3–121 (1991).

18. C.-C. Zhang, A. Friry, and L. Peng, *J. Bacteriol.*, *180*, 2616–2622 (1998).

19. J. Leng, A. J. M. Cameron, S. Buckel, and P. J. Kennelly, *J. Bacteriol.*, *177*, 6510–6517 (1995).

20. B. Solow, J. C. Young, and P. J. Kennelly, *J. Bacteriol.*, *179*, 5072–5075 (1997).

21. B. Mai, G. Frey, R. V. Swanson, E. J. Mathur, and K. O. Stetter, *J. Bacteriol.*, *180*, 4030–4035 (1998).

22. E. V. Koonin, *Prot. Sci.*, *3*, 356–358 (1994).

23. G. J. Barton, P. T. W. Cohen, and D. Barford, *Eur. J. Biochem.*, *220*, 225–237 (1994).

24. D. L. Lohse, J. M. Denu, and J. E. Dixon, *Structure*, *3*, 987–990 (1995).

25. P. Bork, N. P. Brown, H. Hegyi, and J. Schultz, *Prot. Sci.*, *5*, 1421–1425 (1996).

26. A. K. Das, N. R. Helps, P. T. W. Cohen, and D. Barford, *EMBO J.*, 15, 6798–6809 (1996).

27. A. Donella-Deana, M. H. Krinks, M. Ruzzene, C. Klee, and L. A. Pinna, *Eur. J. Biochem.*, 219, 109–117 (1994).

28. C. J. Pallen and J. H. Wang, *J. Biol. Chem.*, 258, 8550–8553 (1983).

29. C. J. Pallen, M. L. Brown, H. Matsui, K. J. Mitchell, and J. H. Wang, *Biochem. Biophys. Res. Commun.*, 131, 1256–1261 (1985).

30. B. Ek-Rylander, M. Flores, M. Wendel, D. Heinegård, and G. Andersson, *J. Biol. Chem.*, 269, 14853–14856 (1994).

31. B. Ek-Rylander, T. Barkhem, J. Ljusberg, L. Ohman, K. K. Andersson, and G. Andersson, *Biochem. J.*, 321, 305–311 (1997).

32. J. A. Cowan, *Chem. Rev.*, 98, 1067–1087 (1998).

33. D. P. Dumas, S. R. Caldwell, J. R. Wild, and F. M. Raushel, *J. Biol. Chem.*, 264, 19659–19665 (1989).

34. L. Holm and C. Sander, *Proteins*, 28, 72–82 (1997).

35. J. Kankare, G. S. Neal, T. Salminen, T. Glumhoff, B. S. Cooperman, R. Lahti, and A. Goldman, *Prot. Eng.*, 7, 823–830 (1994).

36. E. H. Harutyunyan, I. P. Kuranova, B. K. Vainshtein, W. E. Höhne, V. S. Lamzin, Z. Dauter, A. V. Teplyakov, and K. S. Wilson, *Eur. J. Biochem.*, 239, 220–228 (1996).

37. J. Kankare, T. Salminen, R. Lahti, B. S. Cooperman, A. A. Baykov, and A. Goldman, *Biochemistry*, 35, 4670–4677 (1996).

38. P. Heikinheimo, J. Lehtonen, A. Baykov, R. Lahti, B. S. Cooperman, and A. Goldman, *Structure*, 4, 1491–1508 (1996).

39. B. Stec, M. J. Hehir, C. Brennan, M. Nolte, and E. R. Kantrowitz, *J. Mol. Biol.*, 277, 647–662 (1998).

40. A. C. Hengge, in *Comprehensive Biological Catalysis: A Mechanistic Reference, Vol. 1, Reactions of Electrophilic Carbon, Phosphorus and Sulfur* (M. Sinnott, ed.), Academic Press, San Diego, 1998, pp. 517–542.

41. M. L. Applebury, B. P. Johnson, and J. E. Coleman, *J. Biol. Chem.*, 245, 4968–4976 (1970).

42. P. H. Haffner, F. Goodsaid-Zalduondo, and J. E. Coleman, *J. Biol. Chem.*, 249, 6693–6695 (1974).

43. R. E. Weiner, J. F. Chlebowski, P. H. Haffner, and J. E. Coleman, *J. Biol. Chem.*, 254, 9739–9746 (1979).

44. C. Schulz, I. Bertini, M. S. Viezzoli, R. D. Brown, III, S. H. Koenig, and J. E. Coleman, *Inorg. Chem.*, *28*, 1490–1496 (1989).

45. G. H. Reed and G. D. Markham, *Biol. Magn. Res.*, *6*, 73–142 (1984).

46. I. Bertini, C. Luchinat, M. S. Viezzoli, L. Banel, S. H. Koenig, M. Leung, and J. E. Coleman, *Inorg. Chem.*, *28*, 352–358 (1989).

47. A. Teplyakov, G. Obmolova, K. S. Wilson, K. Ishii, H. Kaji, T. Samejima, and I. Kuranova, *Prot. Sci.*, *3*, 1098–1107 (1994).

48. A. A. Baykov, T. Hyytia, S. E. Volk, V. N. Kasho, A. V. Vener, A. Goldman, R. Lahti, and B. S. Cooperman, *Biochemistry*, *35*, 4655–4661 (1996).

49. T. Salminen, J. Käpylä, P. Heikinheimo, J. Kankare, A. Goldman, J. Heinonen, A. A. Baykov, B. S. Cooperman, and R. Lahti, *Biochemistry*, *34*, 782–791 (1995).

50. P. Heikinheimo, P. Pohjanjoki, A. Helminen, M. Tasanen, B. S. Cooperman, A. Goldman, A. Baykov, and R. Lahti, *Eur. J. Biochem.*, *239*, 138–143 (1996).

51. W. B. Knight, D. Dunaway-Mariano, S. C. Ransom, and J. J. Villafranca, *J. Biol. Chem.*, *259*, 2886–2895 (1984).

52. M. M. Benning, J. M. Kuo, F. M. Raushel, and H. M. Holden, *Biochemistry*, *34*, 7973–7978 (1995).

53. J. L. Vanhooke, M. M. Benning, F. M. Raushel, and H. M. Holden, *Biochemistry*, *35*, 6020–6025 (1996).

54. E. Jabri, M. B. Carr, R. P. Hausinger, and P. A. Karplus, *Science*, *268*, 998–1004 (1995).

55. V. E. Lewis, W. J. Donarski, J. R. Wild, and F. M. Raushel, *Biochemistry*, *27*, 1591–1597 (1988).

56. J. L. Buchbinder, R. C. Stephenson, M. J. Dresser, J. W. Pitera, T. S. Scanlan, and R. J. Fletterick, *Biochemistry*, *37*, 5096–5106 (1998).

57. M. Y. Chae, G. A. Omburo, P. A. Lindahl, and F. M. Raushel, *J. Am. Chem. Soc.*, *115*, 12173–12174 (1993).

58. N. Sträter, T. Klabunde, P. Tucker, H. Witzel, and B. Krebs, *Science*, *268*, 1489–1492 (1995).

59. T. Klabunde, N. Sträter, R. Frölich, H. Witzel, and B. Krebs, *J. Mol. Biol.*, *259*, 737–748 (1996).

60. M. A. S. Aquino, J.-S. Lim, and A. G. Sykes, *J. Chem. Soc. Dalton Trans.*, 429–436 (1994).

61. M. Dietrich, D. Münstermann, H. Suerbaum, and H. Witzel, *Eur. J. Biochem.*, *199*, 105–113 (1991).

62. E. G. Mueller, M. W. Crowder, B. A. Averill, and J. R. Knowles, *J. Am. Chem. Soc.*, *115*, 2974–2975 (1993).

63. P. Mertz, L. Yu, R. Sikkink, and F. Rusnak, *J. Biol. Chem.*, *272*, 21296–21302 (1997).

64. M. Merkx and B. A. Averill, *Biochemistry*, *37*, 8490–8497 (1998).

65. M. Merkx and B. A. Averill, *Biochemistry*, *37*, 11223–11231 (1998).

66. B. L. Martin and D. J. Graves, *J. Biol. Chem.*, *261*, 14545–14550 (1986).

67. R. H. Hoff, P. Mertz, F. Rusnak, and A. C. Hengge, (1999), *J. Am. Chem. Soc. 121*, 6382–6390.

68. J. L. Beck, M. J. McArthur, J. de Jersey, and B. Zerner, *Inorg. Chim. Acta*, *153*, 39–44 (1988).

69. Y. Sugiura, H. Kawabe, and H. Tanaka, *J. Am. Chem. Soc.*, *102*, 6582–6584 (1980).

70. Y. Sugiura, H. Kawabe, H. Tanaka, S. Fujimoto, and A. Ohara, *J. Biol. Chem.*, *256*, 10664–10670 (1981).

71. Y. Sugiura, H. Kawabe, H. Tanaka, S. Fujimoto, and A. Ohara, *J. Am. Chem. Soc.*, *103*, 963–964 (1981).

72. S. K. Hefler and B. A. Averill, *Biochem. Biophys. Res. Commun.*, *146*, 1173–1177 (1987).

73. J. Goldberg, H.-B. Huang, Y.-G. Kwon, P. Greengard, A. C. Nairn, and J. Kuriyan, *Nature*, *376*, 745–753 (1995).

74. M.-P. Egloff, P. T. W. Cohen, P. Reinemer, and D. Barford, *J. Mol. Biol.*, *254*, 942–959 (1995).

75. J. P. Griffith, J. L. Kim, E. E. Kim, M. D. Sintchak, J. A. Thomson, M. J. Fitzgibbon, M. A. Fleming, P. R. Caron, K. Hsiao, and M. A. Navia, *Cell*, *82*, 507–522 (1995).

76. C. R. Kissinger, H. E. Parge, D. R. Knighton, C. T. Lewis, L. A. Pelletier, A. Tempczyk, V. J. Kalish, K. D. Tucker, R. E. Showalter, E. W. Moomaw, L. N. Gastinel, N. Habuka, X. Chen, F. Maldonado, J. E. Barker, R. Bacquet, and J. E. Villafranca, *Nature*, *378*, 641–644 (1995).

77. L. Cai, Y. Chu, S. E. Wilson, and K. K. Schlender, *Biochem. Biophys. Res. Commun.*, *208*, 274–279 (1995).

78. N. Berndt and P. T. W. Cohen, *Eur. J. Biochem.*, *190*, 291–297 (1990).

79. Z. Zhang, G. Bai, S. Deans-Zirattu, M. F. Browner, and E. Y. C. Lee, *J. Biol. Chem.*, *267*, 1484–1490 (1992).

80. D. R. Alessi, A. J. Street, P. Cohen, and P. T. W. Cohen, *Eur. J. Biochem.*, *213*, 1055–1066 (1993).

81. Y. Chu, S. E. Wilson, and K. K. Schlender, *Biochem. Biophys. Acta*, *1208*, 45–54 (1994).

82. Y. Chu, E. Y. C. Lee, and K. K. Schlender, *J. Biol. Chem.*, *271*, 2574–2577 (1996).

83. S. Endo, J. H. Connor, B. Forney, L. Zhang, T. S. Ingebritsen, E. Y. C. Lee, and S. Shenolikar, *Biochemistry*, *36*, 6986–6992 (1997).

84. M. M. King and C. Y. Huang, *Biochem. Biophys. Res. Commun.*, *114*, 955–961 (1983).

85. C. J. Pallen and J. H. Wang, *J. Biol. Chem.*, *259*, 6134–6141 (1984).

86. R. C. Gupta, R. L. Khandelwal, and P. V. Sulakhe, *FEBS Lett.*, *169*, 251–255 (1984).

87. H.-C. Li, *J. Biol. Chem.*, *259*, 8801–8807 (1984).

88. D. J. Wolff and D. W. Sved, *J. Biol. Chem.*, *260*, 4195–4202 (1985).

89. F. Rusnak, L. Yu, S. Todorovic, and P. Mertz (1999), *Biochemistry* *38*, 6943–6952.

90. A. Hassett, W. Blättler, and J. R. Knowles, *Biochemistry*, *21*, 6335–6340 (1982).

91. S. R. Caldwell, F. M. Raushel, P. M. Weiss, and W. W. Cleland, *Biochemistry*, *30*, 7444–7450 (1991).

92. A. C. Hengge, W. A. Edens, and H. Elsing, *J. Am. Chem. Soc.*, *116*, 5045–5049 (1994).

93. A. C. Hengge and B. L. Martin, *Biochemistry*, *36*, 10185–10191 (1997).

94. L. Yu, J. Golbeck, J. Yao, and F. Rusnak, *Biochemistry*, *36*, 10727–10734 (1997).

95. R. M. Smith and A. E. Martell, *Critical Stability Constants*, Vol. 4, Plenum Press, New York, 1976.

96. J. C. Davis, S. S. Lin, and B. A. Averill, *Biochemistry*, *20*, 4062–4067 (1981).

97. J. C. Davis and B. A. Averill, *Proc. Natl. Acad. Sci. USA*, *79*, 4623–4627 (1982).

98. B. C. Antanaitis and P. Aisen, *J. Biol. Chem.*, *260*, 751–756 (1985).

99. B. A. Averill, J. C. Davis, S. Burman, T. Zirino, J. Sanders-Loehr, T. M. Loehr, J. T. Sage, and P. G. Debrunner, *J. Am. Chem. Soc.*, *109*, 3760–3767 (1987).

100. S. Zhuo, J. C. Clemens, R. L. Stone, and J. E. Dixon, *J. Biol. Chem.*, *269*, 26234–26238 (1994).

101. J. Zhang, Z. Zhang, K. Brew, and E. Y. C. Lee, *Biochemistry*, *35*, 6276–6282 (1996).

102. H.-B. Huang, A. Horiuchi, J. Goldberg, P. Greengard, and A. C. Nairn, *Proc. Natl. Acad. Sci. USA*, *94*, 3530–3535 (1997).

103. A. Mondragon, E. C. Griffith, L. Sun, F. Xiong, C. Armstrong, and J. O. Liu, *Biochemistry*, *36*, 4934–4942 (1997).

104. J. E. Butler-Ransohoff, D. A. Kendall, and E. T. Kaiser, *Proc. Natl. Acad. Sci. USA*, *85*, 4276–4278 (1988).

105. A. Chaidaroglou, D. J. Brezinski, S. A. Middleton, and E. R. Kantrowitz, *Biochemistry*, *27*, 8338–8343 (1988).

106. R. M. Smith and A. E. Martell, *Critical Stability Constants*, Vol. 6, Plenum Press, New York, 1989.

107. N. Bourne and A. Williams, *J. Org. Chem.*, *49*, 1200–1204 (1984).

108. L. Zhang and E. Y. C. Lee, *Biochemistry*, *36*, 8209–8214 (1997).

11

Manganese(II) as a Probe for the Mechanism and Specificity of Restriction Endonucleases

Geoffrey S. Baldwin, Niall A. Gormley, and Stephen E. Halford

Department of Biochemistry, School of Medical Sciences,
University of Bristol, University Walk,
Bristol, BS8 1TD, UK

1. INTRODUCTION

1.1. Restriction and Modification of DNA

To date, 3015 restriction-modification (R/M) systems have been identified from many different species of bacteria, across virtually all bacterial genera [1]. R/M systems consist of two enzymic activities, which act to defend bacterial cells against foreign DNA entering the cell [2]. One is a modification methyltransferase that methylates a particular base within a specific DNA sequence, the recognition site for that particular R/M system. The other is a restriction endonuclease that recognizes the same DNA sequence as the methyltransferase and cleaves DNA in response to this sequence [3]. However, the restriction enzyme cannot cleave DNA previously modified by the methyltransferase. Thus, neither the genomic DNA of the cell nor invading DNA with methylated sites is cleaved, but invading DNA that carries unmethylated sites is destroyed by the restriction enzyme unless the methyltransferase modifies every site before the endonuclease has cleaved any one site [4].

R/M systems are classified by their protein compositions and cofactor requirements into three main types [4]. In the type I and type III systems, both restriction and modification activities are executed by a multimeric protein with different subunits for each activity [5]. Their modification activities require S-adenosylmethionine (AdoMet) as the methyl donor while their nuclease activities need both Mg^{2+} and ATP, and also AdoMet as an allosteric activator. Type I and type III endonucleases can only cleave DNA that has the requisite recognition site(s), yet the cleavage occurs not at the recognition site but elsewhere along the same DNA molecule [6,7]. These enzymes bind to DNA at their recognition sites but then translocate the adjacent nonspecific DNA past themselves in an ATP-dependent process prior to cleaving the DNA [5]. The roles of Mg^{2+} in these reactions have still to be elucidated. Given the common roles of divalent metal ions in phosphodiester chemistry [8], Mg^{2+} is likely to participate in the hydrolysis of both the DNA and ATP. It is not yet known whether other metal ions, such as Mn^{2+}, can also support the activities of type I or type III restriction enzymes.

1.2. Type II Restriction Endonucleases

Type II R/M systems, on the other hand, employ two separate enzymes for modification and restriction. The former requires only AdoMet as a cofactor for DNA methylation and the latter only Mg^{2+} for DNA cleavage [3,9]. The recognition sites for the majority of type II R/M systems are continuous sequences of palindromic DNA, 4, 6, or 8 bp long, though the palindrome is interrupted in some cases by a spacer containing a fixed number of base pairs of undefined sequence [1]. The type II restriction enzymes cut both strands of the DNA at fixed positions, either in or adjacent to the recognition site. The precision with which the type II restriction enzymes cleave DNA at specific loci has resulted in multitudinous applications of these enzymes in the analysis and reconstruction of DNA [3]. Consequently, more information is currently available about type II enzymes than either type I or type III systems. This chapter therefore focuses on the type II endonucleases with particular reference to *Eco*RV, the restriction enzyme that has perhaps been studied in most detail [10,11, and references therein]. *Eco*RV cleaves DNA at the sequence GAT↓ATC, at the position marked [12].

Type II restriction enzymes have dissimilar amino acid sequences, apart from a small cluster of carboxylic acid residues that bind the Mg^{2+} ions needed for DNA cleavage [9], yet they can have similar tertiary structures [13]. For example, the *Eco*RV, *Bgl*I, and *Pvu*II proteins all have similar structures [14–17], as do *Eco*RI and *Bam*HI [18,19], though there is little similarity between *Eco*RV and *Eco*RI. The enzymes in both the *Eco*RV and *Eco*RI families are dimers of identical subunits. They interact symmetrically with their palindromic recognition sites, so that essentially all of the contacts from one subunit of the protein to one half of the DNA are duplicated by the second subunit with the other half of the DNA. One active site in the dimer is positioned to cleave one strand of the DNA while the other active site attacks the second strand. The endonuclease can then cleave both strands at a single site before dissociating from the DNA [20]. However, some restriction enzymes are active only after interacting with two sites at separate locations on the DNA. For example, the *Sfi*I endonuclease is a tetrameric protein that can cut DNA only after binding two copies of its recognition site, either looping out the intervening DNA on a molecule with two sites or holding together two DNA molecules with one *Sfi*I site on each [21]. Once bound to two sites, *Sfi*I can cut both strands at both sites before leaving the DNA [22]. Conversely, the *Fok*I endonuclease is a monomeric protein that has the catalytic functions for cutting just one DNA strand [23]. Two monomers of *Fok*I bound to separate sites may need to interact with each other before being able to make a double-strand break [24,25].

Type II endonucleases often retain some DNA cleavage activity with Mn^{2+} or Co^{2+} in place of Mg^{2+} but most other divalent metal ions, such as Ca^{2+}, Ni^{2+}, or Zn^{2+}, give zero or near-zero levels of activity [26]. However, the substitution of Mg^{2+} by Mn^{2+} perturbs both the specificity and the kinetics of these enzymes [27–30]. Nevertheless, the perturbations caused by Mn^{2+} shed considerable light onto their mechanisms for DNA recognition and cleavage.

2.   DNA RECOGNITION AND CLEAVAGE

2.1.   DNA Sequence Recognition: Roles of Metal Ions

The central property of restriction endonucleases, with regard to both biological function and biotechnological applications, is their discrimination between different DNA sequences, so that they virtually never cleave DNA other than at their unmodified recognition sites [31]. For enzymes like *Sfi*I, the requirement for two recognition sites provides a safety check against DNA cleavages at incorrect sequences, since both sites have to possess the correct sequence before the reaction can start. But apart from these special enzymes, the discrimination is achieved by individual proteins acting at individual sites. Even so, *Eco*RV, for instance, cleaves DNA with an extraordinarily high specificity for its recognition site under its optimal reaction conditions in the presence of Mg^{2+} [32,33]. The only other sites where cleavages are detectable have sequences that differ from the cognate site by 1 bp yet these noncognate sites are cleaved between 10^6 and 10^9 times more slowly than the cognate site, depending on which particular bp was changed and on the sequence flanking the site [34]. Other dimeric restriction enzymes, such as *Eco*RI and *Taq*I, show similar efficiencies to *Eco*RV in discriminating between alternative sequences in their DNA cleavage reactions [35,36].

In all known crystal structures of a restriction enzyme bound to its recognition sequence, an extensive network of hydrogen bonds exists between the nucleotide bases in the recognition sequence and the relevant amino acids in the protein [13–19,23]. For *Eco*RV, a crystal structure of the enzyme bound to nonspecific DNA is also available and this shows none of the hydrogen-bonding network to the nucleotide bases seen in the specific complex [14]. Hence, it might have been thought that a significant fraction of the specificity for DNA cleavage would have arisen from binding to the recognition site in preference to other sequences.

In contrast to this expectation, equilibrium binding studies on *Eco*RV with a 381-bp DNA fragment containing one *Eco*RV site, in the absence of divalent metal ions, revealed a series of DNA–protein complexes with 1, 2, 3, ..., n molecules of protein per molecule of DNA [37]. The same series of complexes were found with DNA lacking an *Eco*RV site and an analysis of the binding equilibria, by methods from statistical mechanics, gave the same equilibrium constant for each successive association, even when the DNA had an *Eco*RV site [37]. Numerous studies on the binding of *Eco*RV to duplex oligonucleotides 12–30 bp long that either have or lack its recognition sequence have also shown that *Eco*RV has the same affinity for different DNA sequences under its optimal reaction conditions except for the absence of Mg^{2+} [33,38,39]. DNA binding by an active restriction enzyme cannot be studied in the presence of Mg^{2+} because the DNA would be cleaved. Nonetheless, two approaches have been used to study the effect of divalent metal ions on DNA binding: either an active site mutant of *Eco*RV in the presence of Mg^{2+} or the wild-type enzyme in the presence of an inactive cofactor, Ca^{2+} [40,41]. In both cases, the divalent metal ion caused *Eco*RV to bind to DNA specifically at its recognition sequence.

Many other restriction enzymes bind to DNA in the absence of divalent metal ions without any preference for their recognition sites [36] while binding specifically to their recognition sites in the presence of Ca^{2+} [42]. These include *Bgl*I [66], an enzyme with a similar structure to *Eco*RV. In contrast, *Eco*RI and *Bam*HI, enzymes with structures unlike *Eco*RV, show some specificity for their recognition sites in binding to DNA without metal ions [43] yet Ca^{2+} can still enhance the affinity of such enzymes for their recognition sites [44]. These differences corroborate the distinction between the *Eco*RV-like and the *Eco*RI-like restriction enzymes noted previously [13,36]. Nevertheless, in both families, DNA sequence recognition is a function, either exclusively (in the case of *Eco*RV) or extensively (in the case of *Eco*RI), of an enzyme–DNA–

metal ion ternary complex rather than the enzyme–DNA binary complex [10].

2.2. Mechanism of DNA Cleavage: Roles of Metal Ions

For all restriction enzymes where the stereochemical path of phosphodiester hydrolysis is known, the reaction proceeds with inversion of configuration at the phosphorus [45–47]. This indicates the direct hydrolysis of the phosphodiester bond by water as opposed to a two-step reaction involving a covalent enzyme–DNA intermediate. The role(s) of divalent metal ions in such reactions can be any one of, or any combination of, the following [48]: positioning the substrate and/or the hydrolytic water; enhancing the nucleophilicity of the phosphorus; activating the attacking water; neutralizing the negative charge in the transition states; facilitating the departure of the leaving group. A single metal ion at the active site of an enzyme cannot fulfill all of these functions. Even so, many nucleases have just one divalent metal ion at their active sites, whose function may be to enhance the susceptibility of the phosphodiester to nucleophilic attack, by coordination to one of the nonbridging oxygens [49]. However, many other nucleases contain two metal ions at their active sites [8] and a general mechanism has been proposed for how two metal ions might fulfill all of the functions noted above [50].

Attempts have been made to account for phosphodiester hydrolysis by different restriction enzymes with a uniform one-metal-ion mechanism [9], but it now appears that these enzymes differ among themselves with respect to the number of metal ions per active site. X-ray crystallography on EcoRI revealed just one Mg^{2+} ion at the active site [18] and the biochemical data on EcoRI also support a one-metal-ion mechanism [26]. But with EcoRV, $BglI$, and BamHI, the addition of Mg^{2+} or Ca^{2+} to crystals of the protein bound to its recognition sequence can lead to two metal ions per active site [15,16,51]. In both BamHI and $BglI$, the metal ions are positioned at either side of the scissile phosphate, in accordance with the general two-metal-ion mechanism [50]. In contrast, only one of the ions in EcoRV is positioned to interact with the scissile phosphate [15,52]. However, the structure of EcoRV is of an inactive conformation: Mg^{2+} fails to promote DNA cleavage in the cocrystals. Molecular dynamics on the EcoRV–DNA complex suggest that the generation of the catalytically competent state involves a flip in the pucker of the deoxyribose 3' to the scissile bond, which moves the target phosphate to a position where it can interact with both metal ions [11].

A substantial volume of biochemical data indicate that phosphodiester hydrolysis by EcoRV requires at least two metal ions [26,53]. In particular, stopped-flow studies identified a rapid process early in the reaction pathway that involved the binding of Mg^{2+} to a high-affinity site and a slower process, concomitant with phosphodiester hydrolysis, that involved the binding of Mg^{2+} to a low-affinity site [53]. Though the biochemical data can be related to a mechanism in which only one metal ion plays a direct role in catalysis, with the other ion fulfilling a structural role elsewhere in the protein [52], two metal ions playing direct roles at the active site provides the simplest interdigitation of the biochemical and the crystallographic data on EcoRV [11,15].

3.   RESTRICTION ENDONUCLEASES WITH MANGANESE

3.1.   Perturbations to DNA Recognition

The plasmid pAT153, a 3658-bp circle of supercoiled DNA with one recognition site for EcoRV, has been widely used as a substrate for the EcoRV endonuclease [10,20]. EcoRV reactions on this DNA are monitored by using agarose gel electrophoresis to separate the intact substrate from open-circle DNA, cleaved in one strand, and from full-length linear DNA, cleaved at the EcoRV site in both strands. If cleavage of the recognition site is followed by cleavages at other sites, the full-length linear DNA is cut into several fragments. Figure 1 shows an experiment in which pAT153 was incubated for a fixed time span with increasing concentrations of EcoRV in the presence of either $MgCl_2$ or $MnCl_2$. With Mg^{2+} as cofactor, the supercoiled DNA was converted solely to the full-length linear product: no other cleavages occurred even at the highest enzyme concentration tested. In contrast, the reactions with Mn^{2+} yielded the full-length linear DNA at low enzyme concentrations but just a 10-fold increase in the concentration of EcoRV caused DNA cleavages at many additional sites. The additional sites are located on pAT153 at positions where the sequence differs from the EcoRV recognition site by 1 bp [28]. Cleavage of these noncognate sites in the pres-

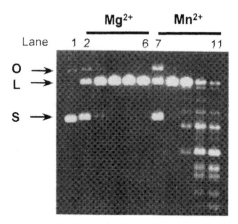

FIG. 1.   Specificity of DNA cleavage by $EcoRV$ with Mg^{2+} or Mn^{2+}. Various concentrations of $EcoRV$ endonuclease were added to reactions containing pAT153 (1 μg) in 50 mM Hepes (pH 7.5) and 100 mM NaCl, with either $MgCl_2$ or $MnCl_2$ (each at 10 mM). Lane 1 had no $EcoRV$ enzyme. The concentrations of $EcoRV$ in lanes 2–6 were 0.1 nM, 1 nM, 10 nM, 100 nM, and 1 μM, respectively: likewise in lanes 7–11. Lanes 2–6 contained $MgCl_2$ and lanes 7–11 $MnCl_2$, as indicated above the gel. After 1 h at 25°C, the DNA was extracted with phenol/chloroform and subjected to agarose gel electrophoresis. The mobilities of the supercoiled (S), open-circle (O), and linear (L) forms of the plasmid are marked on the left of the gel.

ence of Mg^{2+} is only detected after reactions at higher $EcoRV$ levels and/or longer time spans than those used in Fig. 1 [34].

     With Mg^{2+}, $EcoRV$ cleaves its cognate recognition site about 10^6 times faster than the "best" of the noncognate sites on pAT153 but the ratio falls to about 6 with Mn^{2+} as the cofactor [28]. Mn^{2+} thus virtually eliminates the ability of this enzyme to discriminate between cognate and noncognate sites. This effect is particular to Mn^{2+}. The only other metal ion known to support significant activity by $EcoRV$ is Co^{2+} but Co^{2+} acts like Mg^{2+} in focusing DNA cleavage to the recognition site [11]. However, this effect is not particular to $EcoRV$. Many other restriction enzymes cleave DNA at sites other than their recognition sites more readily with Mn^{2+} as the cofactor than with Mg^{2+} [27,29]. For example, $BglI$ cleaves DNA specifically at its recognition site in the presence of either Mg^{2+} or Co^{2+}, but Mn^{2+} again leads to DNA cleavages at many noncognate sites, even at low enzyme concentrations [66].

The data from experiments on restriction enzymes with Mn^{2+} in place of Mg^{2+} thus validate the notion [10] that the specificity of these enzymes for DNA cleavages at their target sequences is determined principally by the metal ion cofactor. In the case of $EcoRV$, the protein binds equally well to cognate and noncognate sites on DNA in the absence of divalent metal ions [37], but Ca^{2+} promotes binding to the recognition sequence without permitting DNA cleavage [41]. The $EcoRV$–DNA complex at the recognition site therefore has a higher affinity for divalent metal ions than the complexes at other DNA sequences. In effect, the metal ion guides the protein to its recognition site [40]. Consequently, Mg^{2+} or Co^{2+} cause cleavages almost exclusively at the cognate site [11,32]. However, the complexes formed between $EcoRV$ and noncognate DNA have a higher affinity for Mn^{2+} than Mg^{2+} [28]. Catalytically active $EcoRV$–DNA–metal ion complexes are thus formed at noncognate DNA sites more readily with Mn^{2+} than with Mg^{2+}.

3.2. Perturbations to Catalytic Mechanisms

Under steady-state conditions with the DNA in molar excess of the enzyme, the turnover rate (k_{cat}) for $EcoRV$ at its recognition site on pAT153 is lower with Mn^{2+} as the cofactor than with Mg^{2+} (Table 1). Nonetheless, the low activity with Mn^{2+} yielded an indication that two metal ions were involved in phosphodiester hydrolysis by $EcoRV$. $EcoRV$ has no activity at all with Ca^{2+} and its Mg^{2+}-dependent activity is inhibited by Ca^{2+} [26]. In contrast, Ca^{2+} enhances the Mn^{2+}-dependent activity of $EcoRV$ (Fig. 2). Mn^{2+} and Ca^{2+} thus act synergistically to give a higher activity than either metal ion alone. Similar experiments with combinations of metal ions have since been used to validate two-metal-ion mechanisms for various ribozymes [54,55].

The steady-state k_{cat} cannot by itself reveal the role of Mn^{2+} since the complete turnover of $EcoRV$ involves many steps: the initial binding of the protein to anywhere on the DNA; the transfer to the recognition site; incorporation of metal ions; two hydrolytic reactions, one on each strand of the DNA; the release of the product(s) cleaved in either one or both strands [53]. The question then arises as to which step, or which combination of steps, is the rate-limiting event that determines k_{cat}. To answer this question, single-turnover reactions with excess

TABLE 1

DNA Cleavage Kinetics by *Eco*RV with Mg^{2+} or Mn^{2+} Cofactors[a]

Metal ion	Conc. (mM)	pAT153		Oligonucleotide		
		k_{cat} (s^{-1})	k_h (s^{-1})	k_{cat} (s^{-1})	k_h (s^{-1})	k_r (s^{-1})
Mg^{2+}	1	0.012	0.30	0.13	0.28	0.38
	10	0.015	3.4	0.66	2.7	n.d.
Mn^{2+}	1	n.d.	n.d.	0.078	4.9	0.036
	10	0.00067	26	0.072	14.6	n.d.

[a]Reactions on the plasmid pAT153 were carried out at 25°C in RV buffer with either $MgCl_2$ or $MnCl_2$ at the indicated concentrations. RV buffer is 50 mM Tris-HCl (pH 7.5), 100 mM NaCl, 10 mM β-mercaptoethanol, and 100 μg/mL serum albumin. Reactions on the oligonucleotide (the duplex form of GACGATATCGTC) were carried out at 25°C in 50 mM Hepes (pH 7.5), with either $MgCl_2$ or $MnCl_2$ at the indicated concentrations and with an NaCl concentration adjusted to give an ionic strength of 0.1 M. Values for k_{cat} are from fitting steady-state velocities at varied substrate concentrations to the Michaelis-Menten equation. Values for k_h and k_r refer, respectively, to the DNA cleavage step and the product-release step in single-turnover reactions. n.d., not determined.

*Eco*RV over pAT153 were studied by the quench-flow method [20]. The quench-flow analysis yielded rate constants for the DNA cleavage steps in the reaction pathway (k_h values, one for each strand) that were very similar to each other and were much faster than the steady-state k_{cat} (Table 1). The step that limits the turnover rate must therefore be located in the reaction pathway after the cleavage of both strands. The effect of Mn^{2+} on k_{cat} is thus probably due to a reduced rate for product dissociation. Surprisingly, Mn^{2+} gave a much faster rate for the DNA cleavage step (k_h) in the reaction pathway on pAT153 than the natural cofactor Mg^{2+} (Table 1).

The dissection of the reaction pathway of a restriction enzyme into its individual steps is facilitated by using as the substrate a DNA duplex made from synthetic oligonucleotides instead of a large plasmid: for example, the self-complementary sequence, GAC<u>GATATC</u>GTC, where the underlined bases denote the *Eco*RV recognition site [53, 56,57]. As with pAT153, steady-state reactions of *Eco*RV on the 12-bp

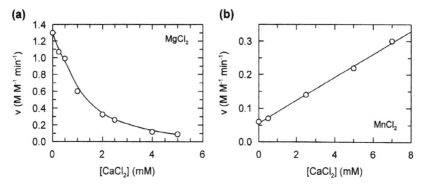

FIG. 2.   Effect of Ca^{2+} on *Eco*RV with Mg^{2+} or Mn^{2+}. The reactions contained 0.5 nM *Eco*RV endonuclease and 10 nM pAT153 in RV buffer (for a definition, see Table 1) at 25°C, with either 5 mM $MgCl_2$ (panel a) or 0.5 mM $MnCl_2$ (panel b), and the concentration of $CaCl_2$ indicated on the x axis. Samples were removed from each reaction at timed intervals and mixed immediately with EDTA prior to analysis of the DNA by electrophoresis through agarose. Reaction velocities were calculated from the initial zero-order decline in the concentration of the DNA substrate and are given on the y axes. (Data from [26], with permission. Copyright © American Chemical Society [1995].)

substrate in the presence of Mn^{2+} gave lower k_{cat} values than those with Mg^{2+} (Table 1). (It is impossible to cite ratios of rates with Mn^{2+} or Mg^{2+}, or between oligonucleotide or plasmid substrates, because the actual rates vary with the concentration of each metal ion [11].) Yet the rate constants for phosphodiester hydrolysis (k_h) on the 12-bp substrate, determined by quench-flow analysis of single turnovers (Fig. 3a and b), were again faster with Mn^{2+} as the cofactor in place of Mg^{2+} (Table 1). With both metal ions, phosphodiester hydrolysis occurred on the oligonucleotide at virtually the same rate as on pAT153 but the steady-state k_{cat} values with the 12-bp DNA were considerably faster than those with the plasmid (Table 1).

An advantage of oligonucleotide substrates for restriction enzymes is that the reaction can be monitored continuously by spectrophotometric methods, instead of stopping the reaction at timed intervals and then separating intact substrate from cleaved product [56]. If the products from cleaving a duplex oligonucleotide are too short to remain double-stranded at the relevant temperature, the reaction causes an in-

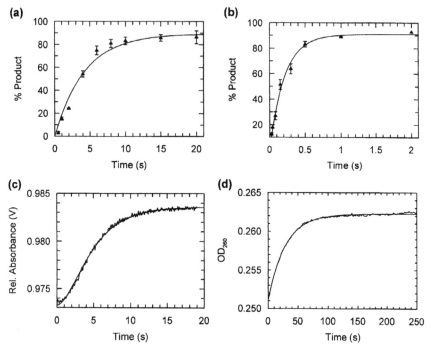

FIG. 3.   Formation and release of cleaved DNA during *Eco*RV reactions with
Mg^{2+} or Mn^{2+}. The reactions at 25°C contained 2 µM *Eco*RV endonuclease and
1 µM DNA (the duplex form of GACGATATCGTC) in 50 mM Hepes (pH 7.5)
and 97 mM NaCl, with either 1 mM $MgCl_2$ (panels a and c) or 1 mM $MnCl_2$ (panels b and d). The reactions in a and b were carried out by mixing in the quench-
flow apparatus a solution of enzyme and divalent metal ion chloride with a solution of DNA and divalent metal ion chloride and then, after the time delay
indicated on the *x* axis, quenching the reaction in NaOH. The 6-bp products were
separated from the 12-bp substrate by HPLC and the percentage of the total
DNA present as 6-bp products (▲, error bars denote standard deviations from
repeats) is shown on the *y* axis. The solid lines denote the exponential curves
that optimally fit the data, to give $k_h = 0.24$ s^{-1} for the reaction with Mg^{2+} (panel
a) and $k_h = 4.9$ s^{-1} for the reaction with Mn^{2+} (panel b). The reactions in c and d
were carried out by using the same mixing procedure as above in either a
stopped-flow (panel c) or a bench-top spectrophotometer (panel d), the increase
in A_{260} was monitored during the course of the reaction. The solid line in c is
the optimal fit of the data to the equation for [C] in a two-step A → B → C pathway, to give rate constants (k_h or k_r) of 0.39 s^{-1} and 0.38 s^{-1} for the *Eco*RV reaction with Mg^{2+}. The solid line in d is the optimal fit to a single exponential, to
give $k_r = 0.036$ s^{-1} for the *Eco*RV reaction with Mn^{2+}. (Data from [11] and [53],
with permission. Copyrights © American Chemical Society [1995] and Acade-
mic Press [1999].)

crease in A_{260}, due to the hyperchromic shift as the products melt to single strands. However, in single-turnover reactions on the 12-bp substrate, the 6-bp products melt to single strands only after dissociating from the enzyme and the hyperchromic shift then chronicles product release [53]. In the presence of Mg^{2+}, the stopped-flow record of A_{260} displayed an initial lag phase prior to a subsequent increase over the same scale as that for phosphodiester hydrolysis (Fig. 3c). The lag phase denotes a sequential reaction pathway for the conversion of the enzyme–substrate complex (ES) to free enzyme and product (E + P): where k_h is the rate constant for the hydrolysis of the enzyme-bound DNA and k_r that for the release of the cleaved DNA from the enzyme–product complex (EP). This analysis yielded values for k_h and k_r that were similar to each other and to the value for k_h from quench-flow measurements (Fig. 3a). The k_{cat} calculated from these values for k_h and k_r matched the k_{cat} from steady-state experiments [53]. The k_{cat} from the Mg^{2+}-dependent reactions of *Eco*RV on the 12-bp substrate is larger

$$ES \xrightarrow{k_h} EP \xrightarrow{k_r} E + P$$

than that from pAT153, not because of any difference in the rate of phosphodiester hydrolysis but rather because of faster product release.

In marked contrast to the behavior with Mg^{2+}, the increase in A_{260} during single turnovers of *Eco*RV on the 12-bp substrate in the presence of Mn^{2+} occurred over a very much longer time scale than that for phosphodiester hydrolysis (Fig. 3d) and followed a single exponential. It yielded a value for k_r that was similar to that for the steady-state k_{cat} (Table 1). This demonstrates directly that Mn^{2+} results in a much slower release of the cleaved products than Mg^{2+}, so that even the release of the 6-bp products from the 12-bp substrate, which is relatively rapid with Mg^{2+}, is much slower than the DNA cleavage step. Other experiments have also shown that the *Eco*RV–DNA–Mn^{2+} complexes are substantially more stable than *Eco*RV–DNA–Mg^{2+} complexes [11,30].

3.3.   Rescue of Mutant Enzymes

Mn^{2+} has proved to be a useful tool for studying mutationally altered forms of the *Eco*RV endonuclease. In contrast to wild-type *Eco*RV, which has a faster turnover with Mg^{2+} than Mn^{2+}, many mutants are more active with Mn^{2+} as the cofactor than with Mg^{2+} and are effectively rescued by Mn^{2+} [58–60]. In many instances, the Mg^{2+}- dependent activity of the mutant protein is far below that of the wild-type enzyme with Mg^{2+} but the Mn^{2+}-dependent activity of the mutant approaches that of the wild-type with Mn^{2+}. This behavior has been observed with mutants carrying alterations to either DNA recognition or catalytic functions.

The fact that mutants with altered catalytic functions can have similar turnover rates to the wild-type enzyme in Mn^{2+}, but much lower turnover rates in Mg^{2+}, can be accounted for readily by the effect of Mn^{2+} on the individual steps of the EcoRV reaction. The DNA cleavage step (k_{h}) in the reaction pathway on pAT153 is about 200 times faster than the steady-state k_{cat} in 10 mM $MgCl_2$, but it is about 40 000 times faster than the k_{cat} in 10 mM $MnCl_2$ (Table 1). Consequently, a mutation that causes a 10 000-fold reduction in the rate constant for phosphodiester hydrolysis may result in a 50-fold lower k_{cat} than the wild-type enzyme in the presence of Mg^{2+} but the same k_{cat} as the wild-type in the presence of Mn^{2+}. To affect the k_{cat} with Mn^{2+}, the mutation needs to cause a >40 000-fold reduction in the rate constant for the hydrolytic step. On the other hand, the ability of mutants with altered DNA recognition functions to cleave DNA more readily with Mn^{2+} than with Mg^{2+} may be the mirror image of the ability of wild-type EcoRV to cleave noncognate DNA more readily with Mn^{2+} than with Mg^{2+} (Fig. 1). In both cases, a mismatch between the protein and the DNA, which prohibits DNA cleavage with Mg^{2+}, is circumvented by Mn^{2+}.

Random mutagenesis of EcoRV followed by a genetic selection in E. coli for the null phenotype yielded one mutant of EcoRV, I91L, in which an isoleucine near the active site was replaced by leucine [60]. Like many other mutants of EcoRV, I91L had a very low activity in vitro with Mg^{2+} and was more active with Mn^{2+} but it differed from the usual pattern in that its Mn^{2+}-dependent activity was actually higher than that of the wild-type enzyme [61]. Indeed, the Mn^{2+}-dependent activity of I91L was similar to that of the wild-type enzyme with Mg^{2+}. Moreover, in contrast to wild-type EcoRV, which readily cleaves DNA at noncognate sequences in the presence of Mn^{2+} (Fig. 1), I91L cleaved DNA specifically at the recognition site in the presence of Mn^{2+}. Thus, the conservative substitution of an isoleucine by leucine converted

*Eco*RV from being an Mg^{2+}-dependent restriction enzyme to a sequence-specific endonuclease dependent on Mn^{2+}. However, since I91L had been identified by a genetic selection for zero activity, this mutant cannot have shown its high Mn^{2+}-dependent activity in vivo. Instead, *Eco*RV must be utilizing only Mg^{2+} in vivo.

4. CONCLUSIONS

4.1. Loss of Specificity by Restriction Endonucleases and Other Enzymes

Many restriction enzymes behave like *Eco*RV in losing their ability to discriminate between cognate and noncognate DNA sequences on replacing Mg^{2+} as the cofactor with Mn^{2+} [27,29]. However, restriction enzymes are not the only enzymes that act on DNA whose activities in vitro are profoundly altered by substituting Mg^{2+} with Mn^{2+}. Many other enzymes carry out aberrant reactions on DNA in the presence of Mn^{2+} even though these are barely detectable in the presence of Mg^{2+}. For instance, DNA polymerases incorporate incorrect nucleotides at much higher frequencies with Mn^{2+} as the cofactor compared to Mg^{2+} [62]. Similarly, the transposition of phage Mu DNA can be duplicated in vitro, in the presence of Mg^{2+}, by the MuA and the MuB proteins acting in concert, but in the presence of Mn^{2+}, the reaction no longer requires MuB and can be completed by MuA alone [63].

In order to cleave DNA at a particular site, a restriction enzyme needs to bind to both that site and to a metal ion, and to hydrolyze two phosphodiester bonds within the lifetime of the protein–DNA–metal complex. Mn^{2+} facilitates DNA cleavages by *Eco*RV at noncognate sites through both of these factors. *Eco*RV–DNA–Mn^{2+} complexes are more stable than *Eco*RV–DNA–Mg^{2+} complexes [11], and the rate constants for phosphodiester hydrolysis with Mn^{2+} are faster than those with Mg^{2+} (Fig. 3). The same combination of enhancements to both complex stability and chemical reactivity occurs upon switching the metal ion cofactor for the *Taq*I restriction enzyme from Mg^{2+} to Mn^{2+} [29]. These two factors may account for why many other enzymes acting on nucleic acids also catalyze aberrant reactions in the presence of Mn^{2+}.

4.2.   Roles of Metal Ions in Phosphodiester Hydrolysis

Metal ions at the active sites of nucleases are often coordinated to a non-bridging oxygen on the phosphorus at the scissile bond [8] and the metal is then thought to act by withdrawing electrons from the phosphorus so as to enhance its susceptibility to nucleophilic attack, increasing the associative nature of the transition state [64]. If so, the rate enhancement should correlate to the electronegativity of the metal ion. This model might seem to be supported by Mn^{2+} giving faster rate constants for phosphodiester hydrolysis by EcoRV than Mg^{2+}, since Mn^{2+} is more electronegative than Mg^{2+}. Co^{2+} is even more electronegative than Mn^{2+} yet it supports DNA cleavage by EcoRV at almost the same rate as Mg^{2+} [11]. Moreover, if the rate enhancement was solely a function of the electronegativity of the metal ion, then the substitution of Mg^{2+} with Ca^{2+} should cause only a modest reduction in the rate constant for the DNA cleavage step, perhaps 30-fold, yet EcoRV has no detectable activity with Ca^{2+} [26]. The principal role of either metal ion at the active site of EcoRV is thus unlikely to be the withdrawal of electrons from the phosphorus so as to enhance its susceptibility to nucleophilic attack.

The inability of Ca^{2+} to support DNA cleavage by EcoRV may be due to its ionic radius being about 0.3 Å larger than that of Mg^{2+}, while Mn^{2+} and Co^{2+} have radii that are within 0.1 Å of that for Mg^{2+}. This in turn suggests that the metal ions play crucial roles in the positioning of the reacting groups at the active site of the enzyme [11]. The precise positioning of the catalytic functions can be a major factor in enzymatic rate enhancements [65]. However, the molecule of water that carries out the hydrolytic reaction must not only be positioned precisely but must also be activated. Both of these requirements can be met by generating the attacking nucleophile by the deprotonation of a water bound to one of the metal ions, as indicated by the pH dependence of phosphodiester hydrolysis by EcoRV [30]. The hydroxide ion that acts as the nucleophile will be present at a much higher concentration at neutral pH if it originates from a metal-bound water rather than bulk water, since the first pK_a of $Mg(H_2O)_6^{2+}$ is about 5 log units lower than the pK_a of bulk water [55]. The positioning and the activation of the water is probably the principal function of one of the metal ions at the active site of EcoRV [11]. Even though the pK_a of the metal-bound water will be lowered still further by replacing Mg^{2+} with a more electronegative metal such as Mn^{2+} or Co^{2+}, the enhanced concentration of hydroxide on a strongly electronegative metal may then be counterbalanced by that hydroxide ion having a reduced nucleophilicity [55].

ACKNOWLEDGMENTS

We thank Bernard Connolly, Alfred Pingoud, and Fritz Winkler for extensive discussions over many years and for supplying data ahead of publication. The work in Bristol was funded by the Biotechnology and Biological Sciences Research Council and by the Wellcome Trust.

ABBREVIATIONS AND DEFINITIONS

AdoMet	S-adenosylmethionine
ATP	adenosine 5'-triphosphate
bp	base pair(s)
Hepes	N-[2-hydroxyethyl]piperazine-N'-[2-ethanesulfonic acid]
HPLC	high-pressure liquid chromatography
R/M	restriction-modification
Tris	Tris(2-aminoethyl)amine

REFERENCES

1. R. J. Roberts and D. Macelis, *Nucl. Acids Res.*, *26*, 312–313 (1999).

2. W. Arber, *Science*, *205*, 361–365 (1979).

3. R. J. Roberts and S. E. Halford, in *Nucleases* (S. M. Linn, R. S. Lloyd, and R. J. Roberts, eds.), Cold Spring Harbor Laboratory Press, New York, 1993, pp. 35–88.

4. G. G. Wilson and N. E. Murray, *Annu. Rev. Genet.*, *19*, 585–627 (1991).

5. T. A. Bickle, in *Nucleases* (S. M. Linn, R. S. Lloyd, and R. J. Roberts, eds.), Cold Spring Harbor Laboratory Press, New York, 1993, pp. 89–109.

6. A. Meisel, P. Mackeldanz, T. A. Bickle, D. H. Krüger, and C. Schroeder, *EMBO J.*, *14*, 2958–2966 (1995).

7. M. D. Szczelkun, M. S. Dillingham, P. Janscak, K. Firman, and S. E. Halford, *EMBO J.*, *15*, 6335–6347 (1996).

8. D. E. Wilcox, *Chem. Rev.*, *96*, 2435–2458 (1996).

9. A. Pingoud and A. Jeltsch, *Eur. J. Biochem.*, *246*, 1–22 (1997).

10. S. E. Halford, J. D. Taylor, C. L. M. Vermote, and I. B. Vipond, in *Nucleic Acids and Molecular Biology*, Vol. 7 (F. Eckstein and D. M. J. Lilley, eds.), Springer-Verlag, Berlin, 1993, pp. 47–69.

11. G. S. Baldwin, R. B. Sessions, S. G. Erskine, and S. E. Halford, *J. Mol. Biol.*, *288*, 785–797 (1999).

12. I. Schildkraut, C. D. B. Banner, C. C. Rhodes, and S. Parekh, *Gene*, *27*, 327–329 (1984).

13. A. K. Aggarwal, *Curr. Opin. Struct. Biol.*, *5*, 11–19 (1995).

14. F. K. Winkler, D. W. Banner, C. Oefner, D. Tsernoglou, R. S. Brown, S. P. Heathman, R. K. Bryan, P. D. Martin, K. Petratos, and K. S. Wilson, *EMBO J.*, *12*, 1781–1795 (1993).

15. D. Kostrewa and F. K. Winkler, *Biochemistry*, *34*, 683–696 (1995).

16. M. Newman, K. Lunnen, G. Wilson, J. Greci, I. Schildkraut, and S. E. V. Phillips, *EMBO J.*, *17*, 5466–5476 (1998).

17. X. Cheng, K. Balendiran, I. Schildkraut, and J. Anderson, *EMBO J.*, *13*, 3927–3935 (1994).

18. J. R. Rosenberg, *Curr. Opin. Struct. Biol.*, *1*, 104–113 (1991).

19. M. Newman, T. Strzelecka, L. F. Dorner, J. Greci, I. Schildkraut, and A. K. Aggarwal, *Science*, *269*, 656–663 (1995).

20. S. G. Erskine, G. S. Baldwin, and S. E. Halford, *Biochemistry*, *36*, 7567–7576 (1997).

21. L. M. Wentzell and S. E. Halford, *J. Mol. Biol.*, *281*, 433–444 (1998).

22. T. J. Nobbs, M. D. Szczelkun, L. M. Wentzell, and S. E. Halford, *J. Mol. Biol.*, *281*, 419–432 (1998).

23. D. A. Wah, J. A. Hirsch, L. F. Dorner, I. Schildkraut, and A. K. Aggarwal, *Nature*, *388*, 97–100 (1997).

24. D. A. Wah, J. Bitinaite, I. Schildkraut, and A. K. Aggarwal, *Proc. Natl. Acad, Sci. USA*, *95*, 10564–10569 (1998).

25. J. Bitinaite, D. A. Wah, A. K. Aggarwal, and I. Schildkraut, *Proc. Natl. Acad, Sci. USA*, *95*, 10570–10575 (1998).

26. I. B. Vipond, G. S. Baldwin, and S. E. Halford, *Biochemistry*, *34*, 697–704 (1995).

27. M.-T. Hsu and P. Berg, *Biochemistry*, *17*, 131–138 (1978).

28. C. L. M. Vermote and S. E. Halford, *Biochemistry*, *31*, 6082–6089 (1992).

29. W. Cao, A. N. Mayer, and F. Barany, *Biochemistry*, *34*, 2276–2283 (1995).

30. N. P. Stanford, S. E. Halford, and G. S. Baldwin, *J. Mol. Biol.*, *288*, 105–116 (1999).

31. J. D. Taylor, A. J. Goodall, C. L. M. Vermote, and S. E. Halford, *Biochemistry*, *29*, 10727–10733 (1990).

32. J. D. Taylor and S. E. Halford, *Biochemistry*, *28*, 6198–6207 (1989).

33. J. Alves, U. Selent, and H. Wolfes, *Biochemistry*, *34*, 11191–11197 (1995).

34. J. D. Taylor and S. E. Halford, *Biochemistry*, *31*, 90–97 (1992).

35. V. Thielking, J. Alves, A. Fliess, G. Maass, and A. Pingoud, *Biochemistry*, *29*, 4681–4692 (1990).

36. J. A. Zebala, J. Choi, and F. Barany, *J. Biol. Chem.*, *267*, 8097–8105 (1992).

37. J. D. Taylor, I. G. Badcoe, A. R. Clarke, and S. E. Halford, *Biochemistry*, *30*, 8743–8753 (1991).

38. M. D. Szczelkun and B. A. Connolly, *Biochemistry*, *34*, 10724–10733 (1995).

39. S. G. Erskine and S. E. Halford, *J. Mol. Biol.*, *275*, 759–772 (1998).

40. V. Thielking, U. Selent, E. Köhler, A. Landraf, H. Wolfes, J. Alves, and A. Pingoud, *Biochemistry*, *31*, 3727–3732 (1992).

41. I. B. Vipond and S. E. Halford, *Biochemistry*, *34*, 1113–1119 (1995).

42. R. Skirgaila and V. Siksyns, *Biol. Chem.*, *379*, 595–598 (1988).

43. S. E. Halford and N. P. Johnson, *Biochem. J.*, *149*, 411–422 (1980).

44. R. D. Whitaker, L. F. Dorner, and I. Schildkraut, *J. Mol. Biol.*, *285*, 1525–1536 (1999).

45. B. A. Connolly, F. Eckstein, and A. Pingoud, *J. Biol. Chem.*, *259*, 10760–10764 (1984).

46. J. A. Grasby and B. A. Connolly, *Biochemistry*, *31*, 7855–7861 (1992).

47. K. Mizuuchi, T. Nobbs, S. E. Halford, K. Adzuma, and J. Qin, *Biochemistry*, *38*, 4640–4648 (1999).

48. W. P. Jencks, *Catalysis in Chemistry and Enzymology*, McGraw-Hill, New York, 1969.

49. D. Suck, *Curr. Opin. Struct. Biol.*, *2*, 84–92 (1992).

50. T. A. Steitz, *Curr. Opin. Struct. Biol.*, *3*, 31–38 (1993).

51. H. Viadiu and A. K. Aggarwal, *Nature Struct. Biol.*, *5*, 910–916 (1998).

52. D. Groll, A. Jeltsch, U. Selent, and A. Pingoud, *Biochemistry*, *36*, 11389–11401 (1997).

53. G. S. Baldwin, I. B. Vipond, and S. E. Halford, *Biochemistry*, *34*, 705–714 (1995).

54. T. Ohmichi and N. Sugimoto, *Biochemistry*, *36*, 3514–3521 (1997).

55. W. B. Lott, B. W. Pontius, and P. H. von Hippel, *Proc. Natl. Acad. Sci. USA*, *95*, 542–547 (1998).

56. T. R. Waters and B. A. Connolly, *Anal. Biochem.*, *204*, 204–209 (1992).

57. T. R. Waters and B. A. Connolly, *Biochemistry*, *33*, 1812–1819 (1994).

58. C. L. M. Vermote, I. B. Vipond, and S. E. Halford, *Biochemistry*, *31*, 6089–6097 (1992).

59. U. Selent, T. Rüter, E. Köhler, M. Liedtke, V. Thielking, J. Alves, T. Oelgeschläger, H. Wolfes, F. Peters, and A. Pingoud, *Biochemistry*, *31*, 4808–4815 (1992).

60. I. B. Vipond and S. E. Halford, *Biochemistry*, *35*, 1701–1711 (1996).

61. I. B. Vipond, B.-J. Moon, and S. E. Halford, *Biochemistry*, *35*, 1712–1721 (1996).

62. W. S. El-Deiry, A. G. So, and K. M. Downey, *Biochemistry*, *27*, 546–553 (1988).

63. T. A. Baker, M. Mizuuchi, and K. Mizuuchi, *Cell*, *65*, 1003–1013 (1991).

64. S. J. Benkovic and K. J. Schray, in *The Enzymes*, Vol. 8 (P. D. Boyer, ed.), Academic Press, New York, 1973, pp. 201–238.

65. W. R. Cannon, S. F. Singleton, and S. J. Benkovic, *Nature Struct. Biol.*, *3*, 821–833 (1996).

66. N. A. Gormley and S. E. Halford, in preparation.

12

Role of the Binuclear Manganese(II) Site in Xylose Isomerase

Ralf Bogumil,[1] Reinhard Kappl,[2] and Jürgen Hüttermann[2]

[1]Fakultät für Biologie, Universität Konstanz, Fach X
910-Sonnenbühl, D-78457 Konstanz, Germany

[2]Fachrichtung Biophysik und Physikalische Grundlagen der Medizin,
Universität des Saarlandes, Klinikum, Bau 76,
D-66421 Homburg (Saar), Germany

1.   INTRODUCTION

D-Xylose isomerase (XylI) (EC 5.3.1.5), an intracellular bacterial enzyme, is one of the most widely used industrial enzymes [1]. The physiological reaction catalyzed by the enzyme is the reversible isomerization of the five-carbon aldose D-xylose to D-xylulose as part of the xylose metabolic pathway in microorganisms. It also converts D-glucose, a six-carbon analog of D-xylose, to D-fructose in a reaction that is industrially applied to the production of high-fructose corn syrup [1,2]. Xylose isomerases are homotetrameric enzymes and have an absolute requirement for divalent metal cations (Mg^{2+}, Mn^{2+}, or Co^{2+}) for activity. The structures of XylI from different bacterial species—*Streptomyces rubiginosus* [3–7], *Streptomyces olivochromogenes* [8,9], *Arthrobacter* [10,11], and *Actinoplanes missouriensis* [12,13]—have been solved by X-ray crystallography and were found to be very similar. Each subunit folds into a main domain that has a typical "triose phosphate isomerase barrel" motif [14] comprising an eight-stranded parallel β sheet surrounded by eight α helices and a C-terminal helical domain that forms a large loop embracing a neighboring subunit. The active site containing a binuclear metal center is located near the center of the barrel as it is in other enzymes that contain a parallel β barrel. The residues, which ligate to the metal ions and other important residues, are conserved in all species studied so far. The two metal binding sites are bridged by Glu217 (symmetric μ-1,3 carboxylate bridge) and are separated by 490 pm in the substrate-free form [7]. Thus, XylI belongs to the growing family of enzymes with binuclear metal centers in the active site. In particular, the manganese enzymes with binuclear active sites have been reviewed previously [15] and are also discussed in various chapters of this book.

In the last 10 years extensive work by a variety of groups was undertaken to elucidate the structural and mechanistic aspects of the isomerization reaction and to understand the role and the spectroscopic properties of the metal binding sites. Mainly on the basis of X-ray crystallographic work, a metal-mediated 1,2-hydride shift mechanism was postulated, which is now the generally accepted scheme for the mechanism (Fig. 1). This is in contrast to the well-studied proton transfer mechanism, which involves the formation of an ene-diol or diolate intermediate, and is utilized by the metal ion–independent phosphosugar isomerases such as triose-phosphate isomerase [16,17].

In this chapter we will focus on the spectroscopic characterization of the binuclear metal site. Since the interpretation of the data is in part based on the structural work we will first briefly summarize the results from the various X-ray crystal structures in Sec. 2. Thereafter, in Sec. 3 kinetic data, metal ion dissociation constants, and the spectroscopic work excluding the manganese(II)-substituted enzyme will be covered. In Sec. 4 the X- and Q-band EPR studies of the manganese(II)-substituted XylI and the interactions with substrates and inhibitors are presented. Finally, in Sec. 5 the catalytic mechanism and the role of the binuclear manganese site is discussed, which reveals that there are still some incongruous results by comparing the spectroscopic and the structural work.

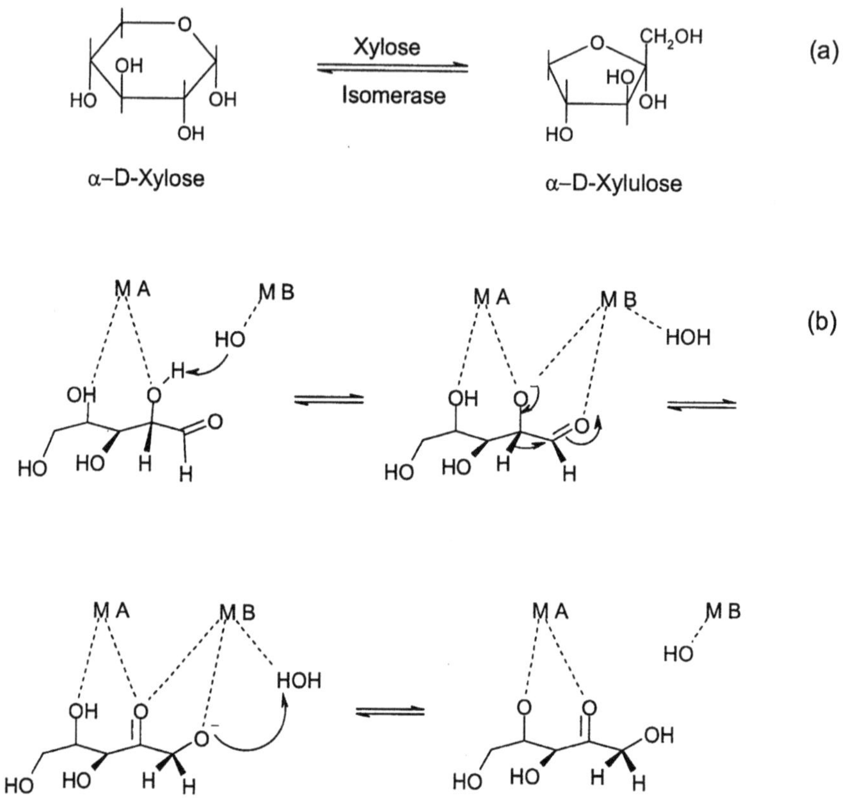

FIG. 1. (a) The reaction catalyzed by xylose isomerase (XylI). (b) Scheme of the hydrid shift mechanism for the isomerization reaction. A detailed description is given in Sec. 5.1.

2. X-RAY CRYSTAL STRUCTURES OF XYLOSE ISOMERASES

A detailed discussion of the various crystallographic studies on XylI is beyond the scope of this chapter and the reader is referred to the original work. Here, we rather restrict ourselves to questions concerning the active site. The so-far-determined X-ray structures of the XylI from the different bacterial sources are very similar to each other with a highly conserved active site. Therefore, we do not have to discuss the X-ray structures from the different organisms separately. The first crystallographic study, which revealed the coordination sphere of both metal sites, was published in 1989 by Carrell et al. [4]. The arrangement of ligands for the manganese-substituted enzyme of *Streptomyces rubiginosus* [7] and the nomenclature of both metal sites is presented in Fig. 2. In Mn^{2+}-XylI the coordination geometry of both binding sites is octahedral; metal binding site 1 (or A-site) is constituted by four carboxylate groups and two water ligands and in site 2 (or B-site) the metal is coordinated to one histidine, three carboxylate groups (one of them bidentate) and one water or OH^- ligand.

Within a short time several crystal structures of the enzyme with various substrates and inhibitors bound and with different cations became available. Based on these structures and in accordance with most biochemical and kinetic studies, a detailed mechanism for the isomerization was proposed [7,11,18,19]. This mechanism involves several steps: (1) binding of the cyclic α anomer of the substrate, (2) enzyme-catalyzed ring opening followed by a rearrangement during which the substrate adopts an extended conformation, (3) isomerization is facili-

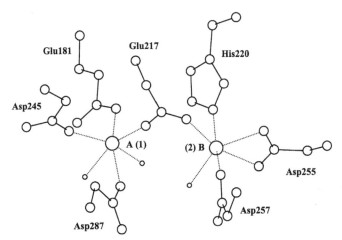

FIG. 2.   Structure of the binuclear manganese(II) site in xylose isomerase (XylI). The Mn^{2+} ions (large spheres) are octahedrally coordinated; the bonds of the metal ions are indicated by the dashed lines. Three of the ligands are water molecules represented by the small spheres. The assignment of the two metal sites is given. For all following presentations of structures the given numbering of amino acid residues is adopted and the A site is always located on the left side. The structure was extracted from the pdb structure file 1xis [7].

tated through a metal-ion mediated 1,2-hydride shift (cf. Fig. 1b), and
(4) ring closure as a reverse of the ring opening step [11]. This mechanism accounts for the majority of the biochemical properties of XylI including the following: (1) XylI specifically reacts with the α anomers of
its substrates and the initial product also maintains the α configuration [20,21]; (2) the hydrogen transfer is stereospecific, consistent with
a planar intermediate in which the O-1 and O-2 oxygens are in a cis position and the hydrogen transfer occurs at one site of the plane and the
transferred proton does not exchange with solvent protons [20,22]; (3)
the requirement of two divalent metal ions for substrate binding and
catalysis. Below we will discuss some X-ray structures with substrates
and inhibitors in more detail with a focus on the substrates/inhibitors
that have also been used in the EPR spectroscopic studies.

2.1.   X-Ray Crystal Structures with the Acyclic Inhibitor Xylitol

The acyclic polyols xylitol and sorbitol closely resemble the open-chain
configurations of the substrates D-xylose and D-glucose. They are competitive inhibitors of the isomerization and the K_i value for xylitol (K_i =
0.89 mM) is about 10 times lower than the K_m value for D-xylose (K_m =
7.3 mM [23], K_m and K_i values are given for the Mn^{2+}-activated enzyme).
Several crystal structures with xylitol and sorbitol have been reported
and in all of these structures the inhibitor has been found in a very similar linear orientation [5,7,10–12]. Figure 3 shows the active sites with
the bound inhibitor (derived from pdb-structure file 1xig), which is
bound in a linear fashion and strongly interacts with the metal in the
A site by coordinating with the O-2 and O-4 oxygens of the hydroxyl
groups, which replace two metal-bound water molecules. This results in
a similar octahedral geometry for this binding site as in the structure
without inhibitor. The B-site metal retains its octahedral ligation. In
one structure with xylitol a ligation of the O-1 hydroxyl of the xylitol to
the B-site metal was also discussed resulting in a monodentate binding
of Asp255 to the B-site metal [12]. The two hydrogen bonds between
Lys183 and the O-1 hydroxyl and between His54 and the O-5 hydroxyl
are also important as demonstrated by site-directed mutagenesis studies in which these important residues have been replaced (see below).
In contrast to the crystal structures in the presence of substrates only

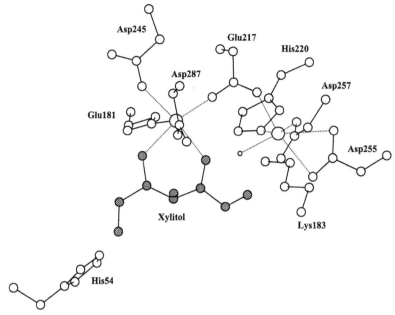

FIG. 3. X-ray structure of the active site of XylI with the inhibitor xylitol-bound (obtained from the pdb-structure file 1xig). The inhibitor is shaded in gray and is bound to the A-site Mn²⁺. In addition to the metal-bound residues both amino acid side chains of Lys183 and His54 in hydrogen bond distance to the inhibitor are given.

one position is found for the metal ion in the B site for the inhibitor xylitol.

2.2. X-Ray Crystal Structures with Substrates and a Transition State Analog

The binding of the substrates D-xylose and D-glucose to the active site of XylI has been intensively studied by several groups using X-ray crystallography [4,5,7,8,11,12,18]. However, the interpretation of the substrate electron density is not straightforward. Since the crystals are catalytically active, the substrate electron density represents a mixture of substrate and product present at equilibrium. Moreover, as a result of the relative low affinity of the substrate for the enzyme, the observed electron density also represents an average of bound and unbound active sites. A further complication is that electron density maps of several crystal structures in the presence of substrate are consistent with two alternate positions of the metal ion in the B site, indicating a movement of this metal ion upon substrate binding or catalysis.

The most striking feature of the crystal structures with D-xylose was that the sugar was generally found in an extended open-chain conformation rather than the cyclic hemiacetal conformation normally found in the free sugars. However, in some crystal structures electron density indicative for the cyclic form has also been observed [7,19]. The binding conformation of the extended form of the sugar was very similar to the binding of the inhibitor xylitol, but as a major difference to the structure with xylitol the metal ion in the B site was observed in two alternate positions [7,8,13]. One position of the metal ion is almost identical to the position of the metal ion in the substrate free form (see Table 1). In this form the two Mn^{2+} are 4.9 Å apart. In the second alternate position (B* or 2* position with a rather low occupancy of only 0.17) the Mn^{2+} is about 1.8 Å away from the first position and is directed toward the substrate. The Mn^{2+} in the B* site is now coordinated to both the O-1 and O-2 oxygens of the substrate and in this form the metal–metal distance is significantly shortened to about 3.5 Å. In addition to the bridging carboxylate Glu217 the metal ions are now also bridged by the O-2 of the substrate. Recently, a similar arrangement of the two metal ions could be stabilized and characterized by X-ray crystallography using a potent inhibitor of the enzyme [9]. The inhibitor D-threonohydroxamic acid (THA) was designed to mimic the putative transition state assuming a hydride shift mechanism. The structure of the postulated transition state for the hydride transfer step in such a mechanism for the substrate xylose should have partial negative charges in the O-1 carbonyl oxygen and the O-2 oxygen and partial double-bond character between C-1 and C-2. THA was chosen to best mimic these desired steric and electronic features (see Fig. 4) and a very high affinity was observed for this inhibitor (K_i <100 nM) [9]. In the X-ray crystal structure with THA [9], the inhibitor is bound in analogous fashion to the extended form of the substrate. However, in this structure the metal ion in the B site is only observed in one position, which is similar to the B* position found with the substrate. Figure 4 shows the structure of the active site with the bound inhibitor THA. The metal–metal

TABLE 1

Metal Coordination and Distances in Mn^{2+} Xylose Isomerase

			Structure with D-xylose		
	Native structure			Distance	
Site	Ligand	Distance[a]	Ligand	B site	B* site
B	OE1 Glu217	2.11		2.12	2.71
	OE2 Glu217				2.51
	NE2 His220	2.32		2.43	2.09
	OD1 Asp255	2.34		2.28	
	OD2 Asp255	2.29		2.29	
	OD2 Asp257	2.24		2.30	
	H_2O	2.23		2.23	1.92
			O1-xylose		2.61
			O2-xylose		2.35
A	OE1 Glu181	2.09		2.14	
	OE2 Glu217	2.12		2.17	
	OD1 Asp245	2.18		2.18	
	OD2 Asp287	2.15		2.19	
	H_2O	2.42			
	H_2O	2.62			
			O2-xylose	2.31	
			O4-xylose	2.34	
Metal-metal distance		4.9		4.9	3.5

[a]Distances are given in Ångstrom and were taken from [7].

distance in this structure, which should resemble the transition state of the reaction, is 4.1 Å.

2.3. X-Ray Crystal Structure of the Cyclic Substrate Analog 5-Thio-α-D-glucose

The anomeric specificity of XylI predicts binding of the cyclic α-anomeric form of the sugar. The binding of cyclic-α-substrate analogs should

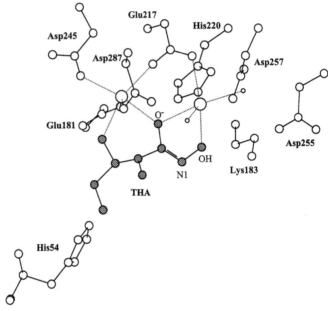

FIG. 4.   Structure of the active site of XylI with the inhibitor THA bound (pdb-structure file 2gyi [9]). The magnesium ions at a distance of 4.1 Å are represented by the large spheres, the water molecules bound to the B-site metal as small spheres replacing the ligands Asp255 and Asp257. THA is shaded in gray and adopts a similar arrangement as xylitol or the linear substrate. Lys183 and His54 are within hydrogen bond distance to THA. The double-bond character between N1 and C2 is indicated as well as the negative charge of the C-2 oxygen.

therefore represent the first step in the catalysis. In the cyclic substrate analog 5-thio-α-D-glucose the cyclic hemiacetal conformation is stabilized by the sulfur and no enzymatic ketose formation has been found for this sugar [22]. Instead, a competitive inhibition is observed with a K_i value of 22.5 mM [24]. Two similar X-ray crystal structures with this cyclic substrate analog have been reported for *Streptomyces rubiginosus* and for the *Arthrobacter* enzyme [5,11]. Figure 5 depicts the mode of binding of 5-thio-α-D-glucose to the Mn^{2+}- substituted *Arthrobacter* enzyme. The α anomer of the sugar is directly ligated to the Mn^{2+} in the A site, creating an octahedral geometry for this metal ion. Note that in contrast to the inhibitor xylitol and the open-chain form of the substrates, which ligate with the O-2 and O-4 oxygens to the A sites, the

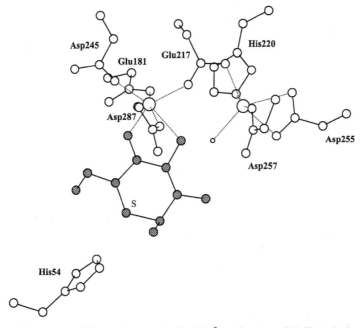

FIG. 5. Structure of the active site in the Mn^{2+}-substituted XylI with the cyclic substrate analog 5-thio-α-D-glucose (from pdb-structure file 1xli [11]),which is shown in gray. The oxygens O3 and O4 are ligands to the A-site Mn^{2+}. No metal movement was observed for this complex. His54 is in hydrogen bond distance to the sulfur atom of the cyclic sugar.

cyclic form binds via the O-3 and O-4 hydroxyl groups. Furthermore, there is no direct interaction of the cyclic substrate analog with the Mn^{2+} in the B site. Due to the position of His54 in hydrogen bonding distance to the ring sulfur a base-catalyzed ring opening by this residue was initially proposed as the first step in catalysis and it was speculated that this is the rate-determining step in catalysis [7,11]. However, additional work by various groups has challenged both assumptions. Deuterium isotope effects on the rate of glucose isomerization and other kinetic work indicated that the hydrogen transfer reaction and not the ring opening is the rate-limiting step in the catalytic process [24–26]. Site-directed mutagenesis has been used to prove the function of specific active site residues in XylI and His54 was one of the first targets. The replacement of His54 with other amino acids revealed that this residue is not essential for catalysis since the catalytic activity in the variant proteins was not abolished, although a reduced activity was found [5,12,26]. However, these studies indicate that His54 is important in governing the anomeric specificity.

3.   THE TWO METAL BINDING SITES

3.1.   Affinities and Activation by Different Metal Ions

The activation of XylI by the divalent cations Mg^{2+}, Mn^{2+}, and Co^{2+} has been known for a long time [2,27] and under most conditions Mg^{2+} appears to be the physiological cofactor [28]. Based on the kinetic parameters two distinct groups of XylI can be differentiated. The XylI from group I (Actinomycetaceae) such as *Streptomyces, Arthrobacter, Ampullariella,* and *Actinoplanes* are best activated by Mg^{2+} followed by Co^{2+} and Mn^{2+}. For XylI from more divergent strains such as *Escherichia, Bacillus,* and *Lactobacillus,* Mn^{2+} is superior to Mg^{2+} and Co^{2+} with the physiological pentose substrates, whereas Co^{2+} is the preferred metal ion for the interconversion of D-glucose to D-fructose [23,29]. In addition to their catalytic role, stabilization of XylI by metal ions has been recognized for many years [2] and Co^{2+} was found to be superior to Mg^{2+} as protector against thermal denaturation [30]. A variety of other divalent (Ca^{2+}, Pb^{2+}, Cd^{2+}, Zn^{2+}, VO^{2+}) and trivalent (Eu^{3+}, Al^{3+}, Sm^{3+}) cations can also bind to the enzyme but are inhibitory [31–33,35].

The first clear evidence that there are two different metal binding sites per monomer was presented in 1988 by Callens et al. [33]. These authors revealed by equilibrium dialysis and spectrometric studies that the XylI from *Streptomyces violaceoruber* binds 2 mol Co^{2+}/mol of monomer. From conformational changes shown by UV difference absorption spectrometry on M(II) binding the following dissociation constants were estimated for the tight binding site: $K_{Co} \leq 3 \cdot 10^{-7}$ M and $K_{Mg} = 1 \cdot 10^{-5}$ M. For the second binding site the $K_{Co} = 2.5 \cdot 10^{-5}$ M was obtained by equilibrium dialysis and visible difference spectra. Recently, the dissociation constants for Mn^{2+}, Co^{2+}, and Mg^{2+} for XylI from five different species have been determined by titrating the metal ion-free enzymes with the respective metal ions using the enzyme activity as indicator of the formation of the active complex [29]. It was found that the metal ion binding is stronger in the order $Mn^{2+} > Co^{2+} \gg Mg^{2+}$ with dissociation constants for the enzymes from *Streptomyces sp.* and *Streptomyces violaceoruber* in the range of $4-8 \cdot 10^{-8}$ M (Mn^{2+}), $4-6 \cdot 10^{-7}$ M (Co^{2+}), and $10^{-5}-10^{-6}$ M (Mg^{2+}). A high- and low-affinity site for the binding of Mn^{2+} and Co^{2+} was not observed. These results seem to be in contrast with the spectroscopic metal binding studies for the enzyme from *Streptomyces rubiginosus* summarized below (Sec. 3.2), which clearly show that a high- and low-affinity metal binding site for these cations exists. Note, however, that in the spectroscopic titration experiment no substrate was present, whereas for the determination of the dissociation constants the enzyme activity using D-xylose as substrate was monitored. Thus, a possible explanation for the discrepancies could be that the affinities of the two metal sites are influenced by the presence of the substrate D-xylose due to the direct interaction of the substrate with the metal ions. The substrate-free forms then should contain two binding sites with different affinities, whereas these differences are less significant upon substrate binding. Furthermore, as expected for a binuclear metal site with a bridging carboxylate group, and as shown by Mn^{2+}-EPR spectroscopy, there is a significant change in the ligand field of the B site upon occupation of the A site even without addition of substrate. These interactions between the two metal sites should complicate the determination of the binding constants. Thus, the model used for the determination of the dissociation constants assuming random and independent metal sites [29] probably has some limitations in such a case.

3.2. Spectroscopic Characterization of the Two Metal Binding Sites

Xylose isomerases can be isolated from various D-xylose-producing organisms in high yields using conventional protein isolation strategies. Since XylI is one of the major industrial enzymes, many groups have also obtained the enzyme through collaboration with industrial partners. For our spectroscopic work the protein from *Streptomyces rubigi-*

nosus was used (Kali Chemie AG, Hannover, Germany). In the last years several XylI have been cloned and expressed in *E. coli* for protein engineering studies [5,13,26]. The metal-free XylI is stable and can be prepared by incubation of XylI with excess of EDTA followed by gel filtration [31]. Using the metal-free XylI several metal-substituted forms can easily be prepared by incubation with stoichiometric amounts of the respective metal ions. The metal concentration in the figures and descriptions below is generally given in mol/mol tetramer. In the case where more than one metal was used (mixed-metal samples) they are denoted in such a way that the occupation of the B site is indicated first (e.g., $4Cd^{2+}/4Mn^{2+}$-enzyme means Cd^{2+} in the B site).

3.2.1. Co^{2+}-Substituted Xylose Isomerase

The Co^{2+}-substituted form of the enzyme has been studied with electronic absorption, circular dichroism (CD), and magnetic CD (MCD) spectroscopy [31,33]. Figure 6 shows the electronic absorption spectra of metal-free XylI titrated with Co(II). After the addition of Co^{2+} time-dependent changes in the visible spectra are observed. Incubation with up to 4 Co^{2+}/tetramer immediately generates a relatively intense spectrum with two maxima at 505 nm ($\varepsilon = 170$ M^{-1} cm^{-1}) and 586 nm ($\varepsilon = 240$ M^{-1} cm^{-1}), which changes with time (2 h) to an absorption spectrum with only one not-well-resolved maximum at 545 nm ($\varepsilon = 20$ M^{-1} cm^{-1}) and a much lower extinction coefficient characteristic for an octahedral metal coordination [31] (spectrum with 4 Co^{2+} in Fig. 6). Therefore, after equilibrium is reached the high affinity Co^{2+} binding site has an octahedral or distorted octahedral symmetry. This binding site corresponds to the B site in Fig. 2. After addition of further 4 Co^{2+}, the second binding site (A site) is occupied with the maxima at 505 and 586 nm. The spectral characteristics in the electronic absorption and in the MCD spectra are consistent with a distorted tetrahedral or pentacoordinated complex structure for this binding site [31]. In the X-ray structure of XylI from *Actinoplanes missouriensis* a tetrahedral coordination with four carboxylate ligands has been found for the A site in the Co^{2+}- or Mg^{2+}-substituted enzyme [13]. In contrast, in the Mn^{2+}-substituted XylI two additional water ligands are bound creating an octahedral geometry for the A site as shown by both EPR [32] and X-ray crystallo-

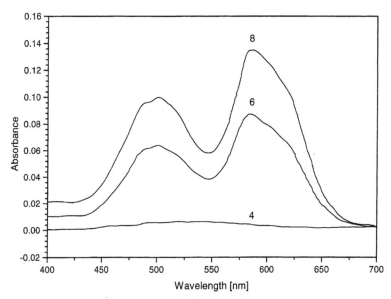

FIG. 6.   Electronic absorption spectra of Co^{2+}-substituted XylI from *Strepto-myces rubiginosus*. The metal-free apoenzyme (0.16 mM) in 0.01 M Hepes buffer, pH 7.4 was titrated with increasing molar excesses of Co^{2+} and the spectra with 4, 6, and 8 Co^{2+} are shown. The spectra were recorded after a 2-h incubation and have been corrected by subtracting the contribution of the apoenzyme [31].

graphic work [4,7]. The complex geometry in the B site is octahedral for all three cations as shown by both spectroscopic and X-ray structural work. Upon incubation with substrates or inhibitors the A site is also octahedral with Mg^{2+} and Co^{2+} due to additional binding to the two hydroxyl groups of the substrates/inhibitors. Since octahedral Co^{2+} complexes have a low molar absorption coefficient the binding of substrates/inhibitors can be studied by Co^{2+} visible spectroscopy monitoring the decrease in the intense absorption bands of the A site [31]. Using the characteristic absorption bands of the Co^{2+}-substituted enzyme the competition between Co^{2+} and other metal ions for both binding sites can be studied and the visible spectroscopy of these "mixed-metal" derivatives provides information about the distribution of the metal ions among both sites. These studies have demonstrated that the B site is the high-affinity metal binding site for the divalent Co^{2+}, Mn^{2+}, VO^{2+}, Cd^{2+}, and Pb^{2+} cations, while trivalent ions like Eu^{3+}, Sm^{3+}, and Al^{3+} have higher affinity for the A site [31,32,34,35]. Mg^{2+} is an exception since it is a divalent ion, which seems to have higher affinity for the A site. This was indicated by some X-ray structures in which Mg^{2+} was only found in the A site and this would also correlate with the prefer- ence of Mg^{2+} for oxygen ligands [10,11].

3.2.2. VO^{2+}-Substituted Xylose Isomerase

The VO^{2+}-substituted XylI and mixed-metal derivatives with Co^{2+} and VO^{2+} and with Cd^{2+} and VO^{2+} have been studied with electronic absorp- tion, electron paramagnetic resonance (EPR), electron nuclear double res- onance (ENDOR), and electron spin-echo envelope modulation [35,36]. Since only the B site of XylI contains a nitrogen ligand (His220), the two binding sites could be clearly differentiated using ^{14}N-ENDOR spec- troscopy. Thus, ^{14}N-ENDOR spectra of the $4VO^{2+}$-XylI gave for the first time direct evidence that the binding site with the histidine ligand is the high-affinity site for most divalent cations and permitted correla- tion of the spectroscopically defined A and B sites with the two metal sites 1 and 2 found in the X-ray crystallographic work. This information was used in Fig. 2.

3.3. Catalytic Activity of Mixed-Metal Derivatives of Xylose Isomerase

Especially the large diamagnetic heavy metal ions Cd^{2+} and Pb^{2+} ex- hibit a high affinity for the B site and can therefore block this site se- lectively in order to study the spectroscopic characteristics of the A site. Kinetic measurements on different mixed-metal derivatives have shown that both binding sites must be occupied with Mg^{2+}, Co^{2+}, or Mn^{2+} cations to obtain catalytically active species indicating that both metal sites are involved in the catalytic process. The catalytic activity of XylI with only the B site occupied ($4Mn^{2+}$-XylI or $4Co^{2+}$-XylI) is very low and increases with the occupation of the A site. The $4Co^{2+}/4Mn^{2+}$-XylI has a catalytic activity comparable with $4Co^{2+}/4Co^{2+}$-XylI. In contrast, in mixed-metal derivatives in which the B site is occupied with Cd^{2+} or

Pb^{2+} and the A site with Mn^{2+} or Co^{2+}, the catalytic activity is almost completely lost, although spectroscopic studies reveal that the substrate can still bind to the A site [31,32,34].

4. EPR STUDIES OF MANGANESE-SUBSTITUTED XYLOSE ISOMERASE

4.1. Characterization of Mn^{2+}-EPR Spectra

Some preliminary remarks on the interpretation of continuous wave EPR spectra of Mn^{2+} in enzymes and proteins seem appropriate to facilitate the comprehension of the spectral characteristics of Mn^{2+}-substituted XylI presented in this paragraph. A thorough discussion of the theoretical background is presented, for example, in [37] and in Chap. 7 of this book. The divalent manganese ion with a $3d^5$ electron configuration has an electron spin of $S = 5/2$ and a nuclear spin of $I = 5/2$. A negligible spin-orbit coupling (i.e., the g factor is close to the free electron value of 2.0023) is responsible for relatively long relaxation times of the complexed ion, which result in rather narrow EPR linewidths even for solutions at room temperature. Typically, the Mn^{2+}-hexaaquacomplex shows six hyperfine lines at $g \cong 2$ due to the nuclear spin manifold $(2I + 1)$. The magnitude of the hyperfine splitting depends on the symmetry of the complex, an octahedrally coordinated Mn^{2+} shows values of approximately 9.5 mT, a tetrahedral complex of about 6–7 mT for the hyperfine coupling [38]. In some cases a superhyperfine interaction of ligands with a nuclear spin (e.g. ^{14}N: $I = 1$) in the first coordination sphere can be resolved.

The sixfold degeneracy of the $S = 5/2$ high-spin state of the Mn^{2+} ion is lifted by the asymmetry of the ligand field often present in proteins. In such a noncubic environment the $\pm 1/2$, $\pm 3/2$, and $\pm 5/2$ Kramer doublets adopt different energies in the absence of an external magnetic field that is called *zero field splitting* (zfs). These Kramer doublets are further split in an external magnetic field and the electronic transitions between the various energy levels $(-5/2 \leftrightarrow -3/2, -3/2 \leftrightarrow -1/2, -1/2 \leftrightarrow +1/2, +1/2 \leftrightarrow +3/2, +3/2 \leftrightarrow +5/2)$ obeying the selection rule $\Delta M_s = \pm 1$ are the origin of five possible fine-structure resonances. In addition, each of these may show six hyperfine lines arising from the nuclear spin manifold

$I = 5/2$ with $\Delta M_I = \pm 0$. Hence up to 30 EPR lines can be present in an EPR spectrum of an Mn^{2+} complex. The zfs interaction is correlated to the molecular frame and is orientation-dependent, reflecting the properties of the ligand environment of the Mn^{2+} ion. For small molecules in solution with a sufficiently high tumbling rate the anisotropic zfs contributions are averaged to zero because the zfs tensor D is traceless. Larger molecules, like proteins in solution, frozen solution, or powders of Mn^{2+} complexes with a "static" but random orientation of molecules, are yielding anisotropic EPR line patterns (powder spectra), which can span several hundred mT in field depending on the magnitude of the zfs.

Because the ligand field is always somewhat variable within an ensemble of protein molecules, the zfs parameters are quite variable too. As a consequence the four outer fine-structure transitions, $\pm 5/2 \leftrightarrow \pm 3/2$ and $\pm 3/2 \leftrightarrow \pm 1/2$ are often found to be extremely broadened even beyond detection because their resonance positions are explicitly dependent on the orientation-sensitive D tensor. In contrast, the central transition $-1/2 \leftrightarrow +1/2$ is influenced by the zfs in second and third order only, so that broadening effects are less pronounced. This usually gives rise to the buildup of flanks around the signal, which is always found at $g \approx 2$, and to a distortion and broadening of the six hyperfine lines. The largest intensity of all fine-structure transitions is observed for the central transition and by analysis of the spectral features of this transition, all information on the zfs can be extracted. An analytical expression for the simulation of the spectral properties of the central transition has been developed for Mn^{2+} systems, in which the zfs parameter is clearly smaller than the electronic Zeeman interaction ($D \ll g\beta H$) [39] and was successfully applied to several manganese-containing enzymes [37]. However, in cases where the zfs is in the order of or larger than the electronic Zeeman interaction ($D \gtrsim g\beta H$) a treatment of the complete Hamiltonian is required.

We have adopted the program based on the analytical formalism for simulation of the central transition in the EPR spectra of Mn^{2+}-substituted xylose isomerase. It also takes into account the above-mentioned distribution in zfs parameters, which is essential for improvement of the quality of fit to the experimental spectra. For the majority of Mn^{2+}-substituted XylI samples the condition $D \ll g\beta H$ was fulfilled.

Within a molecule-fixed axis system the zfs can be expressed by two parameters: D, the axial zfs term, and E, the rhombic zfs term. These two parameters, together with their corresponding variabilities, are obtained from simulations of the perturbation of the six Mn^{2+} hyperfine lines induced by the zfs. Each hyperfine line may split into a doublet or a rhombic pattern depending on the values of D and E. The larger D becomes the more the individual components of each hyperfine line are separated until they eventually overlap and, in particular, increase the overall width of the EPR pattern. On the other hand, the variation in these parameters contributes to an intrinsic linewidth and broadens the resonances.

It is of advantage to apply higher field and frequency to EPR spectroscopy of Mn^{2+} proteins because resolution is enhanced by the reduction of the effects of the zfs and of the superposition of the outer fine-structure resonances with the central transition. In addition, contributions of "forbidden" transitions within the hyperfine manifold (with $\Delta M_I = 1$) are largely suppressed [40]. Due to these extra lines the complexity of an EPR spectrum at X-band frequencies (9.5 GHz) impedes a straightforward interpretation. Hence, experiments were mostly performed at Q-band frequencies (34.5 GHz) to gain better resolution necessary for a detailed simulation.

4.2. EPR of Different Metal-Substituted Xylose Isomerase Samples

It has been pointed out in Sec. 3.2 that the divalent cations Co^{2+}, Mn^{2+}, Cd^{2+}, and Pb^{2+} preferably bind to the high-affinity B site. Careful displacement studies [31,32] have demonstrated that Mn^{2+} is nearly exclusively incorporated into the A site whenever the B site has been blocked by a prior incubation of the metal-free apoenzyme with stoichiometric amounts (i.e., 4 mol of metal ion/mol of tetramer) of one of the other cations. In such a way the Mn^{2+} ion was used to monitor the effects that a metal ion in the B site is exerting on the A site. The corresponding enzyme preparations are designated as $4M^{2+}/3.5Mn^{2+}$ to indicate that M^{2+} is in the B site and Mn^{2+} is occupying the A site (only 3.5 mol Mn^{2+} were added to the samples to avoid an excess and contributions of unbound Mn^{2+}). Due to the time dependence in the occupation of the metal sites, the apoenzyme was incubated with the first metal for 2 h before the second metal was added (see Sec. 3.2). To exclude the presence of unbound Mn^{2+} the samples were tested by liquid phase EPR at room temperature.

When metal-free apoenzyme is titrated with up to 4 mol Mn^{2+}/mol tetramer, the X-band EPR spectrum in Fig. 7a is recorded, which shows a poorly resolved Mn^{2+} hyperfine structure for the central transition around $g \approx 2$ together with very broad features arising from other fine structure transitions, which are indicative for a considerable zfs with a

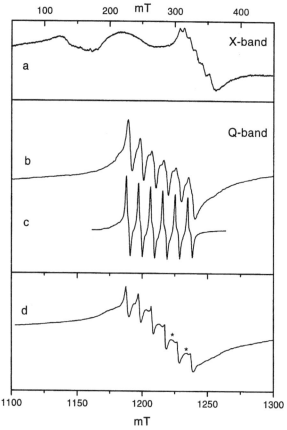

FIG. 7. EPR spectra of XylI titrated with up to 4 mol per mol tetramer in X band (a) (77 K, 9.5 GHz) and in Q band (b) (110 K, 34.5 GHz) showing the gain in resolution for the spectrum at higher frequency. A simulation of the zfs-broadened spectrum is shown in trace c. Trace d is obtained for the 8Mn^{2+} XylI which has a reduced linewidth of the hyperfine resonances. The weak features marked by asterisks are due to small amounts of 4Mn^{2+} species.

wide distribution in D and E. Comparable X-band spectra have been published for various enzymes, e.g., phosphoglucomutase [41], pyruvate kinase [42,43], and isocitrate dehydrogenase [44], for which the authors estimated magnitudes of the zfs parameter D between 45 and 60 mT. For comparison the Q-band spectrum (Fig. 7b) is much better resolved for which a width of the low-field hyperfine line of approximately 2.9 mT is measured. The hyperfine lines toward higher magnetic field are broader and eventually a poorly resolved doublet subsplitting is detected (yielding a width of 4.8 mT for the high-field hyperfine line). Broad flanks are framing the hyperfine pattern. Apart from the intense central transition no clearly visible additional fine-structure resonances were detected.

Systematic simulations for the central transition resulted in a satisfying concurrence in overall spectral and linewidth, hyperfine and subsplitting only for values of D between 45 and 48 mT, and allowing for a Gaussian distribution in D of about 9 mT. The corresponding rhombicity parameter E/D was adjusted between 0.2 and 0.3. The simulated pattern is presented in Fig. 7c for which a hyperfine value of 9.4 mT and an intrinsic linewidth of 0.7 mT were used. The variation in D causes the poorly resolved subsplitting of hyperfine lines as well as the broad low-field shoulder. Similar distributions in zfs parameters were necessary to simulate the spectra of lyophilized powders of Mn^{2+}-Ca^{2+} concanavalin A [45]. The relatively large variation (9 mT) in D values for simulation also explains the absence of outer fine-structure transitions (e.g., at lower fields), since these are, in first order, explicitly dependent on D and E. Therefore in the Q-band spectrum they are smeared out over a wide range in magnetic field beyond detection. The effect of a variation in zfs parameters is less pronounced for the central transition, leading mainly to a buildup of the outer flanks and a drastic broadening of the zf-split hyperfine lines. Since the displacement and titration studies indicate a higher affinity of Mn^{2+} for the B site, the A site should not be occupied in the $3Mn^{2+}$ XylI sample. A magnetic interaction of partially Mn^{2+}/Mn^{2+} occupied metal sites is therefore excluded, so that the appearance of the broad shoulders and the large linewidth are solely due to a distribution in the zfs parameter D. The spread of 9 mT in D may result from a disordered and disturbed environment of the Mn^{2+} ion in the B site that obviously gains structural flexibility due to the absence of restraints from the unoccupied A site. This interpretation is supported by experiments on XylI samples, for which up to 8 mol

Mn^{2+}/mol tetramer were titrated so that all metal sites are occupied. In this sample (Fig. 7d) a hyperfine sextet with reduced linewidth (1.5 mT) is apparent. In between the high-field hyperfine lines broad weak shoulders can be distinguished (marked with asterisks). By comparison they are identical to the zf-split left doublet line of the $3Mn^{2+}$ + XylI pattern and arise from a small proportion of the enzyme in which only the B site is occupied. The other doublet line is superimposed onto the narrower resonance of $8Mn^{2+}$ XylI. Together with the X-band titration studies [32] it appears that in $8Mn^{2+}$ XylI both sites acquire a more symmetric ligation environment resulting in reduced effects of the zfs on the spectra. This observation is in line with the interpretation of effects of the second metal ion on the zfs in EPR spectra of binuclear model complexes. It was found that the second metal ion attenuates the bridging ligand field potential (see Ref [15] and references therein).

For the mixed-metal sample $4Co^{2+}$/$3.5Mn^{2+}$ a very symmetric spectrum with a splitting of 9.1 mT between the first two hyperfine lines and a linewidth of 1.2 mT was obtained (Fig. 8a). The pattern closely resembles that of the narrow major component in $8Mn^{2+}$ XylI, indicating a comparable symmetry of the ligand environment. By comparison with X-band EPR and UV/Vis spectra it was shown that more than 90% of Mn^{2+} occupy the A site, while Co^{2+} is in the B site. No EPR signal of the paramagnetic Co^{2+} is observed at a temperature of 110 K because of the fast relaxation of the high-spin state (S = 3/2). The simulation of the pattern yielded values of D = 12 mT with nearly axial symmetry (E/D = 1:8) [32] (see Table 2).

Significantly different spectra were obtained when Cd^{2+} or Pb^{2+} are located in the B site. For $4Cd^{2+}$/$3.5Mn^{2+}$ XylI a splitting of the hyperfine line was observed (for comparison, see Fig. 10a below), which could be simulated with a value D = 39 mT and maximal rhombicity applying a variation in D of about 1.5 mT (Table 1) [32]. An even more pronounced anisotropy of the central transition was detected in $4Pb^{2+}$/$3.5Mn^{2+}$ XylI, from which a larger D value of about 54 mT and a rhombicity $E/D \approx$ 1:4 was derived by spectra simulation. The variation in D had to be increased to 4 mT, which, however, was still considerably smaller than for the $3Mn^{2+}$ sample. The simulation data for the three mixed-metal samples are compiled in Table 2. A corresponding change to larger effects of the zfs term was also found in the X-band spectra [32].

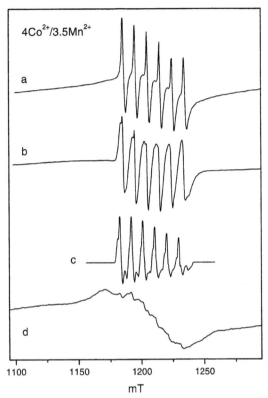

FIG. 8.   Q-band EPR spectra of $4Co^{2+}/3.5Mn^{2+}$ XylI at 110 K without any additive (a) and with the inhibitor xylitol (b) indicating an increase in zfs parameters. Trace c is a simulation of spectrum b. After addition of an excess of the substrate xylose the extremely broadened spectrum d is recorded.

The drastic increase in zfs parameters when Co^{2+} (or Mn^{2+}) are substituted with Cd^{2+} or Pb^{2+} in the B site reflects the enhanced distortion of the immediate environment of Mn^{2+} in the A site, which, on the other hand, might be responsible for the loss of activity for the latter cations. The disorder or tension within the A site may be mediated by the carboxylate group of the amino acid Glu217 (see Fig. 2), which bridges both metal binding sites. The extent of the disturbance seems to be directly connected to the ionic radii of the ions bound to the B site, which are definitely larger for Cd^{2+} (109 pm) and Pb^{2+} (133 pm) compared to Co^{2+} (88 pm) or Mn^{2+} (97 pm) [46]. Hence the larger ions in the

TABLE 2

zfs Parameters of Mixed-Metal Samples
of Mn^{2+}-Substituted Xylose Isomerase and After
Addition of Inhibitor, Substrate, or Substrate Analogs

| Sample | Simulation of central transition[a] | | Estimates[b] |
	D (mT)	E/D	D (mT)
$3Mn^{2+}$	45–48	0.2–0.3	
$8Mn^{2+}$	≈12	<0.15	
+ xylitol	34	1/4	
+ D-xylose			50–60
$4Co^{2+}/3.5Mn^{2+}$	12	<1/8	
+ xylitol	34	1/4	
+ D-xylose[c]			50–60
+ substrate analogs[c]			50–60
$4Cd^{2+}/3.5Mn^{2+}$	39	1/3	
+ xylitol	≈50	≈1/4	
+ D-xylose			75–85
+ substrate analogs			65–85
$4Pb^{2+}/3.5Mn^{2+}$	≈54	1/4	
+ xylitol			60
+ D-xylose			75–85

[a]Simulations were performed for the $-1/2 \leftrightarrow 1/2$ transition with a modified version of the program of [37].
[b]According to [41].
[c]The spectra are extremely broadened.

B site render the crystal field around Mn^{2+} in the A site more anisotropic. The effect is maximal for Pb^{2+} with the largest D value and an increased distribution of the parameters. In a similar way, the absence of a metal ion in the A site with Mn^{2+} bound to the B site as in the $3Mn^{2+}$ enzyme is supposed to allow more disorder by the carboxylate group of Glu217, which in turn lowers the symmetry around Mn^{2+} and gives rise to the large zf splitting and the distinct distribution of zfs parameters for the $3Mn^{2+}$ species. It is remarkable that the division into enzymes governed by small zfs (Co^{2+} or Mn^{2+} in the B site) and large zfs

$(Cd^{2+}$ and Pb^{2+} in the B site) is correlated to the catalytic activity of these metal-substituted enzymes. Probably Co^{2+} or Mn^{2+} in the B site are rendering a complex geometry in the A site that is comparable to that of the natural cofactor Mg^{2+} which, with respect to ionic radii (86 pm), is similar to these two metal cations.

4.3.   Interactions with Inhibitors, Substrates, and Substrate Analogs

The EPR properties of the Mn^{2+} cation in the A site of XylI were used to monitor the influence of the binding of inhibitors, substrates, or substrate analogs to the binuclear active site in XylI. When the inhibitor xylitol, which is a linear chain molecule, is added to $4Co^{2+}/3.5Mn^{2+}$ XylI some additional powder-type features besides the hyperfine lines become apparent in the Q-band spectrum (Fig. 8b). They are indicative for an increased zfs parameter D and a rhombic component E/D. Systematic simulations for the $-1/2 \leftrightarrow 1/2$ transition resulted in a good agreement to the experimental spectrum concerning total spectral width and the zf-split line pattern for a value of D of 34 mT and a rhombicity of about 1:4 (Fig. 8c), applying a small variation in D values of 4 mT to adjust to the observed linewidth [34]. The D value increased considerably in comparison with the $4Co^{2+}/3.5Mn^{2+}$ without the inhibitor (12 mT, E/D = 1:8), but is still smaller than the D value of the more distorted $4Cd^{2+}/3.5Mn^{2+}$ species without inhibitor (39 mT, E/D = 1:3) [32] (see also Table 2).

Drastic changes of the EPR spectrum of $4Co^{2+}/3.5Mn^{2+}$ XylI were observed upon addition of the substrate D-xylose (Fig. 8d). The overall spectral width increased from approximately 65 mT to 111 mT and the pattern is broadened without resolved hyperfine interaction for the central transition. There are very broad shoulders visible around field positions 1125 and 1275 mT, which are related to other fine-structure transitions. The EPR feature is indicative of a large zf-splitting for which, in the absence of simulation parameters, only a rough estimate of D between 50 and 60 mT (Table 2) can be inferred from the field positions of the outer transitions according to the scheme suggested for axial symmetry [41]. From the variation of substrate concentration (up to 250 mol D-xylose/mol monomer) and reaction time (up to 24 h), the amount of enzyme without bound substrate was estimated to be smaller than 5% and the presence of nonequilibrium states was excluded [34]. For a quantitative binding higher amounts of the substrate D-xylose are needed than in the case of the inhibitor xylitol. This is in agreement with the higher affinity of the competitive inhibitor xylitol compared to D-xylose (see Sec. 2).

A very similar behavior upon incubation with either the inhibitor xylitol or with an excess of D-xylose is observed for the $8Mn^{2+}$-XylI specimen (in which both binding sites are occupied by Mn^{2+}). The spectrum with bound xylitol (Fig. 9a) is closely related to that of $4Co^{2+}/3.5Mn^{2+}$ with inhibitor (Fig. 8b), showing approximately the same zfs parameters. Since both binding sites are now contributing to the spectrum of $8Mn^{2+}$ XylI with inhibitor, it becomes obvious that both the A and the B sites are not very different with respect to their ligand environment (zfs parameters) and that they are very similar to that of Mn^{2+} in the A site of $4Co^{2+}/3.5Mn^{2+}$. The comparability to the $4Co^{2+}/3.5Mn^{2+}$ XylI specimen also applies to the interaction with D-xylose, which again yields an extremely broadened spectrum with barely resolvable hyperfine structure (Fig. 9b). In analogy, from the positions of outer fine-struc-

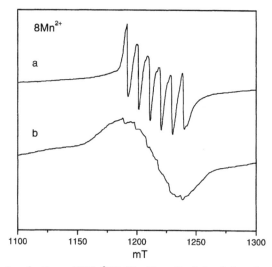

FIG. 9.   After incubation of $8Mn^{2+}$XylI with xylitol the Q-band spectrum shows an increase in zfs (trace a) and an extreme broadening after addition of the substrate xylose (b).

ture transitions comparable D values of 50–60 mT are estimated. Control measurements at X-band frequencies, besides the central transition, also exhibit very broad zfs resonances extending from 200 mT to more than 450 mT (not shown), corroborating the predominance of such large zfs.

The picture that emerges from studying the interactions of xylitol and D-xylose with inactive $4Cd^{2+}/3.5Mn^{2+}$ XylI (and also with $4Pb^{2+}/3.5Mn^{2+}$ XylI) is in contrast to the findings for both catalytically active XylI samples. It is noted that the Q-band spectrum of $4Cd^{2+}/3.5Mn^{2+}$ XylI without any additive (Fig. 10a) shows zfs parameters slightly larger than in $4Co^{2+}/3.5Mn^{2+}$ with xylitol (see Table 2). Addition of xylitol to this sample induces an additional increase of zfs parameters, producing a well-separated low-field line and an increased overall spectral width (75 vs. 84 mT) (Fig. 10b). Simulation of the $-1/2 \leftrightarrow 1/2$ transition with a D value around 50 mT reproduced the position of the low-field line (6.1 mT downfield of the first hyperfine resonance) and the spectral width reasonably well. However, finer details like the pattern of forbidden transitions between the manganese hyperfine lines and line intensities could not be obtained (Fig. 10c).

The addition of xylose to $4Cd^{2+}/3.5Mn^{2+}$ XylI samples (25 mol/mol monomer) brings about drastic spectral changes. The overall spectral width of the $-1/2 \leftrightarrow 1/2$ transition increases to about 92 mT and additional zf split resonances are flanking the original hyperfine sextet (Fig. 10d). The biphasic line shape of the low-field resonance is indicative for intermediate rhombic distortion, since in case of complete rhombicity ($E/D = 1:3$) typically absorptive line shapes are expected [37]. In contrast to the $4Co^{2+}/3.5Mn^{2+}$ XylI sample with xylose the line pattern is well resolved and does not show a pronounced broadening. Attempts to simulate the spectral pattern of the $-1/2 \leftrightarrow 1/2$ transition gave no satisfying results, which seems to be due to the involved large D values at or above the limits of the applicability of the used simulation routine. From an analysis of the outer zf transitions, clearly discernible in the Q-band spectrum of Fig. 10e recorded with an enhanced field scan (500 vs. 200 mT for traces a–d), a D value of approximately 75–85 mT is estimated (Table 2) according to the scheme suggested in [41]. The other catalytically inactive XylI species, $4Pb^{2+}/3.5Mn^{2+}$, behaves in an identical manner as $4Cd^{2+}/3.5Mn^{2+}$ upon addition of xylitol and D-xylose showing an increasing zfs. In the case of D-xylose also a well-resolved

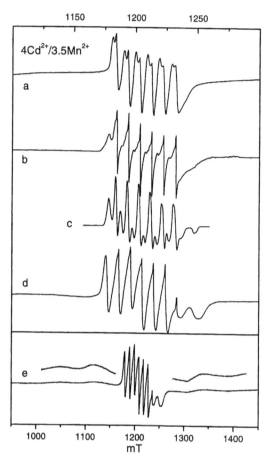

FIG. 10.   The Q-band spectrum (110 K) of catalytically inactive 4Cd^{2+}/3.5Mn^{2+} XylI in the absence of any additive is characterized by considerable zfs splitting (a), which increases further upon addition of xylitol (b). Trace c is the corresponding simulation. Spectrum d is obtained after addition of xylose exhibiting a large zfs contribution, but maintaining a well-resolved line pattern. Broad lines of outer fine structure transitions are visible in spectrum e.

line pattern is obtained. Because D is already too large for a simulation of the central transition, only estimates of this value could be given [34] (see Table 2).

To gain more detailed insight into the binding mode of the substrate to the binuclear active site and, in particular, to address the questions regarding the binding of the extended and cyclic forms of the substrate, which creates multiple binding possibilities [4,7,8,11,13,19], cyclic substrate analogs were incubated with metal-substituted XylI. 5-Thio-α-D-glucose is an analog of the reactive substrate anomer with the ring oxygen replaced by a sulfur and no enzymatic ketose formation is observed for this sugar. In the X-ray structure of Collyer et al., 5-thio-α-D-glucose is found in a cyclic form with C-3 and C-4 OH ligated to the A-site metal [11] (see Fig. 5). The compound 2-deoxy-D-glucose was used to test the importance of the C-2 hydroxyl group for the binding of the substrates. For comparison the spectra in the presence of the substrates D-glucose, D-fructose, and D-xylulose were also collected. D-Glucose and D-xylose have identical atomic conformations except for the presence of an additional CH_2OH group at the C-6 position in D-glucose.

Addition of the three D-glucose derivatives to $4Co^{2+}/3.5Mn^{2+}$ XylI yielded the spectra in Fig. 11a–c. They closely resemble those after addition of D-xylose to the mixed metal sample or to $8Mn^{2+}$ (Figs. 8d and 9b). They are also characterized by an extreme broadening of the overall spectral width amounting up to 120 mT. On the low-field side of the $-1/2 \leftrightarrow 1/2$ transition broad features around 1130 mT are discernible, e.g., for $4Co^{2+}/3.5Mn^{2+}$ XylI with 5-thio-α-D-glucose, which may arise from other electronic transitions. The hyperfine sextet pattern on top of the poorly resolved central transition presumably arises from metal sites with no glucose derivatives bound in a similar intensity as for $4Co^{2+}/3.5Mn^{2+}$ XylI with D-xylose in lower concentration as in Fig. 8d [34]. It should be noted that the same behavior of spectral broadening is also found in the measurements with D-fructose and D-xylulose.

In contrast to the active XylI sample the incubation of $4Cd^{2+}/3.5Mn^{2+}$ XylI with the D-glucose derivatives results in all cases in well-resolved line patterns, which extend over a field range of approximately 100–120 mT and are indicative for a large zero field splitting. The spectra all show roughly the same overall spectral width but differ considerably in their individual line pattern. These distinct spectral features are probably resulting from a variation of the ratio E/D rather than of the magnitude of the zero field splitting D. They demonstrate the high sensitivity of Mn^{2+} EPR spectroscopy to the different modes of binding of the glucose derivatives. Attempts to simulate the complex line patterns failed because of the large zfs parameters involved. From the very broad resonances barely visible in larger field scans in Q-band as well as from X-band spectra a rough estimate of D in the range from 65 to 85 mT could be obtained [34].

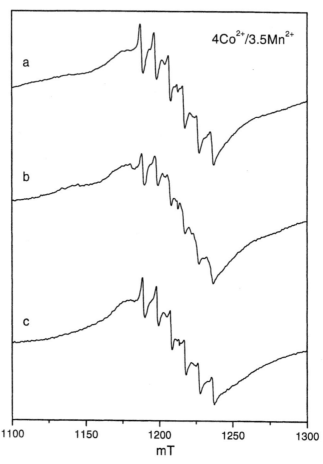

FIG. 11. The Q-band spectra of $4Co^{2+}/3.5Mn^{2+}$XylI show an extreme line broadening after addition of the substrate D-glucose (a), and the substrate analogs 5-thio-D-glucose (b) and 2-deoxy-D-glucose (c). The sharp lines on top of the broad feature originate from metal sites without bound glucose derivative.

4.4. Summary of EPR Results

The EPR data of the mixed-metal and $8Mn^{2+}$ XylI provide evidence for an octahedral coordination of Mn^{2+} in the A site. The ^{55}Mn-hyperfine coupling in all samples studied is in the range of 9.1–9.5 mT, a charac-teristic value for octahedral Mn^{2+} complexes (e.g., $Mn(H_2O)_6^{2+}$, $A = 9.5$ mT), whereas in tetrahedral complexes the hyperfine coupling is usually smaller (6–7 mT). In contrast, electronic absorption and MCD spectroscopic studies indicate a tetrahedral or pentacoordinated Co^{2+} in the A site [31], and X-ray crystallographic analysis revealed a tetrahedral arrangement of four carboxylate groups for Co^{2+} or Mg^{2+} in this site [13]. These differences between Mn^{2+} and Co^{2+} can be explained with the different properties of complex formation. The d^5 ion Mn^{2+} strongly favors an octahedral coordination sphere in aqueous solution, whereas Co^{2+} with a d^7 configuration can form relatively stable tetrahedral complexes. In the X-ray structures of the Mn^{2+}-substituted enzyme an octahedral coordination sphere is also found with two water molecules bound in addition to the four carboxylate groups (see Fig. 2).

The EPR analysis suggests a direct interaction of xylitol with Mn^{2+} in the A site because significant changes are observed in the EPR spectra of all xylitol complexes ($4Co^{2+}/3.5Mn^{2+}$, $4Cd^{2+}/3.5Mn^{2+}$, $4Pb^{2+}/3.5Mn^{2+}$). In all cases an increase in the zf-splitting D was seen in comparison to the spectra without xylitol. This finding can be attributed to a more distorted ligand arrangement of the Mn^{2+}, although the zf splitting is still relatively small compared to the EPR spectra with substrates. The replacement of the two water ligands with hydroxyl groups from the xylitol could explain these changes (see Fig. 3). Slight distortions of the ligand sphere of the Mn^{2+} might be expected, since the two hydroxyl groups are not as flexible as the water ligands. At present no X-ray data are available for the Cd^{2+}- and Pb^{2+}-substituted enzyme, but the same trend (increase in zf splitting) observed in the EPR spectra indicates a similar binding of the acyclic inhibitor xylitol to these samples.

The predominant feature obtained from binding of the substrate D-xylose to the catalytically active XylI-samples ($8Mn^{2+}$, $4Co^{2+}/3.5Mn^{2+}$) is an extreme spectral broadening without any resolved hyperfine interactions. Nearly identical spectral patterns are evident in the EPR spectra with other substrates (D-xylulose, D-glucose, D-fructose) and also in the EPR spectra with the two cyclic substrate analogs 5-thio-α-D-glucose and 2-deoxy-D-glucose. This spectral effect was attributed to the induction of a dipolar interaction between Mn^{2+} in the A site and the paramagnetic Co^{2+} or Mn^{2+} (in the case of the $8Mn^{2+}$ enzyme) in the B site upon binding substrate or cyclic substrate analogs [34]. This assignment is strongly supported by the results obtained with the catalytically inactive samples, in which the B site is loaded with diamagnetic Cd^{2+} or Pb^{2+} ions. In these samples incubation with substrates gives rise to significant changes in the EPR spectra, but despite these large changes in zf splitting, well-resolved resonances are detected.

In the substrate-free form the two metal binding sites in XylI were found to be 4.9 Å apart and to be bridged by a common ligand (Glu217). The respective EPR spectra of $4Co^{2+}/3.5Mn^{2+}$ and $8Mn^{2+}$ XylI did not reveal any significant contributions of dipolar or exchange interactions between the metals in the two binding sites [32]. However, in the X-ray structure of Mn^{2+}-substituted XylI with xylose two different positions for the metal in the B site were resolved, one of which had a rather low occupancy (site B*). The distance of this site to site A was found to be reduced to about 3.5 Å (see Table 1 [7]). Such a reduced distance between the two paramagnetic metals in sites A and B* could give rise to a drastically enlarged magnetic dipolar interaction, which is sensitively depending on the distance r between the dipoles ($\sim 1/r^3$) and the relative orientation of their magnetic moments [37,38]. The appearance of a very similar, extremely broadened spectrum in $8Mn^{2+}$ XylI with xylose is indicative for a dominant role of the $1/r^3$ dependence in line broadening, since for Mn^{2+} the g tensor is assumed to be nearly isotropic and close to the free electron value (see Sec. 4.1). An estimate with the simple point dipole model yields a threefold increase in magnetic interaction for the observed shift of the metal into the B* site. Because the distance-dependent dipolar contribution is very sensitive to spatial disorder of the metal sites in the protein molecules, it is potentially responsible for a wide distribution of interaction values, which in turn are reducing the spectral resolution. Attributing the spectral pattern of the complexes with substrates to dipolar interactions, it is postulated that the distances between the two metal ions are decreased compared to the substrate free form.

The dipolar interactions in XylI are not induced by binding of the acyclic inhibitor xylitol but are clearly evident in the spectra with the cyclic inhibitor 5-thio-α-D-glucose. Because its spectra are very similar to those of the substrates, it is suggested that the substrates bind in the cyclic form to both the catalytic active and the inactive mixed-metal samples. Further support comes from the measurements with 2-deoxy-D-glucose. According to the different X-ray structures, the extended form of the substrates binds with O-2 and O-4 to the metal in the A site, while in the cyclic form O-3 and O-4 ligate to the metal ion. The similarity of the EPR spectra of 2-deoxy-D-glucose to the spectra with substrates makes O-3 and O-4 the most likely candidates for metal ion binding [34].

A metal ion movement upon substrate binding was postulated on the basis of several X-ray structures of XylI in the presence of substrate

[7,8,11,13]. The EPR data, particularly the dipolar interaction between the sites occupied with paramagnetic metal ions, give direct spectroscopic evidence for such a movement. However, the results indicate some discrepancies with the crystallographic analysis concerning the origin of this dynamic behavior (see Sec. 5.1).

5. THE CATALYTIC MECHANISM AND THE ROLE OF THE BINUCLEAR CENTER

5.1. Implications from EPR Studies

On the whole the spectroscopic work is in good agreement with the proposed metal-mediated hydride shift mechanism for this enzyme, which was mainly derived from X-ray crystallographic work (cf. Fig. 1b). However, from the spectroscopic findings several implications concerning particularly the first step in the catalytic cycle, the binding of the cyclic α anomer of the sugar, have to be discussed in some detail. It was evidenced above that the largely symmetric coordination environment in the $8Mn^{2+}$ and the $4Co^{2+}/3.5Mn^{2+}$ XylI is consistent with the EPR spectra with small zfs contributions. The corresponding scheme of the complex is shown in Fig. 12 (Scheme I) with a roughly octahedral ligand arrangement in sites A and B. Site A is coordinated with two additional water ligands while in site B probably an OH^- ion is a ligand. The inhibitor xylitol is binding via the O-2 and O-4 hydroxyl groups to the Mn^{2+} in site A replacing the water ligands (Fig. 12, II). This rearrangement (with these less flexible groups) seems to be responsible for the increased zfs of the EPR spectra.

When xylose or cyclic substrate analogs are added, there is always a drastic spectral broadening observed in EPR, which is correlated to a metal movement from site B to B*. The distance found in X-ray structures for the low-occupancy B* site is reduced to from 4.9 to 3.5 Å. This is indicated in Fig. 12 (III), where both B sites in the presence of the cyclic substrate are shown. Since the spectral broadening is also found for α-D-thioglucose, for which a ring opening is not possible, it is concluded that the metal movement is induced directly by binding of the cyclic form of the substrate. It seems plausible that the structural rearrangement occurring upon binding of the rather bulky ring via the O-3 and O-4 hydroxyls to the A site is mediated via the bridging Glu217 to site B, so that the metal is moving to its new position. It is noted that

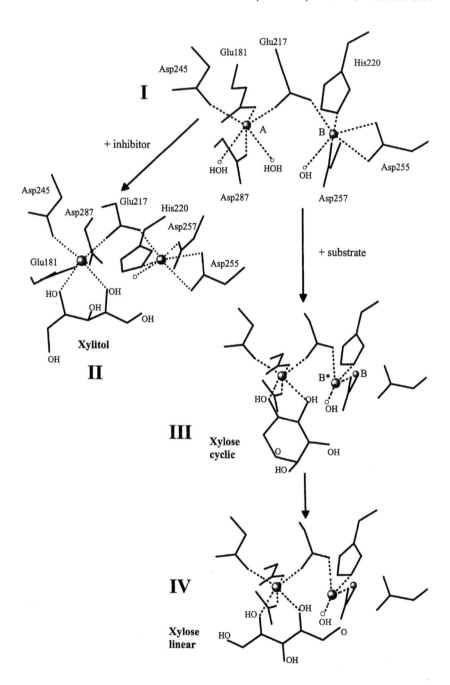

the distance between O-3 and O-4 is only 2.5 Å compared to the distance of 2.95 Å between O-2 and O-4 in the inhibitor xylitol. This correlated disturbance of the ligand environment in site A could possibly represent, together with other steric or electronic changes, the trigger for the metal movement. This is in contrast to the interpretation from X-ray crystallography, where it was postulated that the metal movement is following the ring opening step and occurs when the linear extended form is bound [7,8,11]. It was suggested that the C-2 hydroxyl group is deprotonated by an OH$^-$ ion bound to the B site and that this negative charge is the driving force that induces the shift of the metal ion to the B* position. Within such a picture the EPR results on the enzyme–xylitol complex appear contradictory because one would also expect that a deprotonation of the O-2 hydroxyl of the xylitol might be possible. This should induce a metal shift which in turn should yield a drastic broadening of the EPR spectrum. However, such effects are not observed for this complex (see Sec. 4.3) and in several X-ray structures in the presence of xylitol the metal ion was not observed in the B* position.

In this regard the X-ray structure from Mg^{2+}-XylI with the potent inhibitor D-threonohydroxamic acid is interesting, since it is a linear open chain inhibitor in which a movement of the B-site metal ion was observed (see Fig. 4). For this complex only one position of the B-site metal was observed in which a deprotonated O-2 is bridging the two metal sites. The metal position in the B site was similar to the respective B* position in the substrate structures (the metal–metal distance was shortened from 5.1 to 4.1 Å in the THA structure). Since hydrox-

---

FIG. 12.   Schematic representation of the binding of substrate and inhibitor to the binuclear metal center in XylI. Scheme I (derived from pdb-structure file 1xis [7]) shows the Mn^{2+} ions in site A and B as shaded spheres at a distance of 4.9 Å. The water at site B is deprotonated. Binding of the inhibitor xylitol displaces the two water molecules at site A, but the two metal ions remain in their positions (scheme II, from pdb-structure file 1xig). When substrate is bound the metal in site B (small shaded sphere in scheme III) is moving to its new position B* at 3.5 Å from site A. EPR data indicate that the metal shift may occur already upon binding the cyclic substrate. In scheme III the cyclic substrate xylose was modeled to the active site of the pdb-structure file 4xis [7] showing the binding to the A-site metal via hydroxyl groups at C3 and C4. Upon ring opening the metal in site A is ligated to the hydroxyl groups at C2 and C4 of the extended form, which was fit to the pdb-structure file 4xis (scheme IV). In that configuration the deprotonation of the C-2 hydroxyl group by the OH$^-$ at the shifted B*-site metal is suggested to occur, which then initiates the hydride shift step of the isomerization reaction.

amic acids have a lower p$K_a$as the extended form of xylose and in one tautomer of THA the deprotonated form has a negative charge on the C-2 oxygen it was proposed that this inhibitor is mimicking the deprotonated state of the linear substrate. Thus, in contrast to xylitol, the exceptional strong binding of THA together with the electrostatic interaction of the partial negative charge at the C-2 oxygen seems to be the major driving force for the metal shift in this case. The metal shift may be additionally initiated and enhanced upon binding of the cyclic substrate, which would be an explanation for the larger shift (4.9 to 3.5 Å) found in the enzyme–xylose complex in comparison to the shift in the enzyme-THA structure. In our proposed model (Fig. 12, III) the binding of the cyclic substrates is sufficient to induce the metal shift, but the ring opening has to occur rapidly to rearrange the substrate in the linear form, which then places the C-2 hydroxyl group of the substrate in the proper position for deprotonation by a metal-bound hydroxide (Fig. 12, IV). In summary, it has to be stated that there are still some conflicts between the spectroscopic data and the crystallographic work. Whereas in the X-ray structure with the cyclic substrate analog 5-thio-α-D-glucose no second position of the metal was observed [5,11], the EPR clearly indicates a metal movement. Therefore, the identification of the driving force for the metal ion movement appears to be a subject for further investigations.

From this linear arrangement of the xylose shown in scheme IV of Fig. 12 the metal-mediated hydride shift mechanism for the isomerization of the substrates can then proceed with the following steps, which have been described in detail by several groups [7,8,11]: The OH^- ion bound to the B site initiates the isomerization by removal of the O-2 hydrogen. The resulting negative charge on the O-2 is stabilized by both metal ions, and in the transition state of the reaction, both metal ions are bridged by the O-2 oxygen (see Fig. 4 with THA). Isomerization can then proceed by a hydride shift promoted by electrophilic catalysis of the metal ions (cf. Fig. 1b). In the xylose to xylulose direction the metal in the B* site is binding to the O-2 and, in addition, can polarize the carbonyl at C-1. This polarization will induce a partial positive charge on C-1 which facilitates the hydride shift from C-2 to C-1 and either a water molecule bound to the B site or the NZ of Lys183 protonates the O-1. In the last step, considered as the reverse of the ring opening reaction, the ring can be closed resulting in the cyclic xylulose form. Recently, a different mechanism with the hydride shift occurring in the cyclic form has been proposed by Meng et al. [47] to unify the following observations: (1) the rate limiting step of the reaction is the C-2/C-1 hydride shift, (2) both the wild-type and mutant xylose isomerases from *Clostridium thermosulforogenes* display a 2.5-fold difference in K_{cat} for α-D-glucose as compared to β-D-glucose. Because the ring opening of both anomers produces chemical identical molecules, Meng et al. [47] argued that the different K_{cat} values necessitate that the hydride shift must be concerted with ring opening. Such a hydride transfer mechanism with the cyclic form would in principle also be in agreement with the spectroscopic data. It should be mentioned that EPR spectroscopy alone cannot establish if the cyclic or the linear chain is prevailing, in the case of 5-thioglucose it is clear from other data that the cyclic form is bound. However, a major problem in the mechanism proposed by Meng et al. [47] is that the metal ion in the B site would not play any significant role and no metal shift would be necessary for catalysis. This is not consistent with the majority of the kinetic and metal binding studies which clearly demonstrate the importance of both metal sites and therefore the metal-mediated hydride shift mechanism is favored.

5.2.   Role of the Binuclear Manganese(II) Center

As described above, the two metal ions in XylI have multiple roles in substrate binding, activation, and catalysis. Binuclear sites in enzymes in general appear to have several potentially useful properties either not found or deficiently expressed in mononuclear centers that could be important for catalysis [15]. One central point is that the electrostatic activation of a substrate or the ionization of a proton from an active site water molecule will occur more readily in binuclear centers than at a corresponding mononuclear center. Thus, the involvement of a metal-bound hydroxide ion in catalysis as proposed for XylI is found in several enzymes with binuclear manganese(II) sites [15]. Furthermore, the binding of polyatomic substrates that bind with more than one atom to the metal ion can also be better achieved in binuclear sites. In the case of XylI, the metal ion in the A site is the major determinant for substrate binding and both metals ion are involved in reorientation, activation, and isomerization of the substrate. A unique feature of the binuclear center in XylI seems to be flexibility of the B-site coordination and the significant shift of this metal ion during substrate binding and catalysis. Although much work has been done in the last decade and important progress achieved in elucidating the structure and mechanism of the enzyme, as well as in understanding the spectroscopic properties, many details are not entirely clear. Thus the field is open for further investigation.

ACKNOWLEDGMENTS

The spectroscopic work of the authors (Secs. 3 and 4) was supported by the Bundesministerium für Forschung und Technologie and by the Deutsche Forschungsgemeinschaft within the Priority Programme: "Bioanorganische Chemie: Übergangsmetalle in der Biologie und ihre Koordinationschemie." We want to commemorate the initiator of the project, Professor Herbert Witzel, who died in 1997. We gratefully acknowledge helpful discussions with Dr. C. Sudfeldt and technical assistance of S. Wulff and J. Marx.

ABBREVIATIONS

CD	circular dichroism
EDTA	ethylenediamine-N,N,N',N'-tetraacetate
ENDOR	electron nuclear double resonance
EPR	electron paramagnetic resonance
MCD	magnetic circular dichroism
pdb	protein database
THA	D-threonohydroxamic acid
XylI	xylose isomerase
zf	zero field
zfs	zero field splitting

REFERENCES

1. H. F. Verhoff, G. Bogulawski, O. J. Lantero, S. T. Schlager, and Y. C. Jao, in *Comprehensive Biotechnology*, Vol. 3 (H. W. Balanch, S. Drew, and D. L. C. Wang, eds.), Pergamon Press, Oxford, 1985, p. 837f.

2. W. P. Chen, *Process Biochem.*, *15*, 30–41 (1980).

3. H. J. Carrell, B. H. Rubin, T. J. Hurley, and J. P. Glusker, *J. Biol. Chem.*, *259*, 3230–3236 (1984).

4. H. L. Carrell, J. P. Glusker, V. Burger, F. Manfre, D. Tritsch, and J.- F. Biellmann, *Proc. Natl. Acad. Sci. USA*, *86*, 4440–4444 (1989).

5. R. D. Whitaker, Y. Cho, J. Cha, H. L. Carrell, J. P. Glusker, P. A. Karplus, and C. A. Batt, *J. Biol. Chem.*, *270*, 22895–22906 (1995).

6. Z. Dauter, M. Dauter, J. Hemker, H. Witzel, and K. S. Wilson, *FEBS Lett.*, *247*, 1–8 (1989).

7. M. Whitlow, A. J. Howard, B. C. Finzel, T. L. Poulos, E. Winborne, and G. L. Gilliland, *Proteins*, *9*, 153–173 (1991).

8. A. Lavie, K. N. Allen, G. A. Petsko, and D. Ringe, *Biochemistry*, *33*, 5469–5480 (1994).

9. K. N. Allen, A. Lavie, G. A. Petsko, and D. Ringe, *Biochemistry*, *34*, 3742–3749 (1995).

10. K. Henrick, C. A. Collyer, and D. M. Blow, *J. Mol. Biol.*, *208*, 129–157 (1989).

11. C. A. Collyer, K. Henrick, and D. M. Blow, *J. Mol. Biol.*, *212*, 211–235 (1990).

12. A.-M. Lambeir, M. Lauwereys, P. Stanssens, N. T. Mrabet, J. Snauwaert, H. van Tilbeurgh, G. Matthyssens, I. Lasters, M. De Maeyer, S. J. Wodak, J. Jenkins, M. Chiadmi, and J. Janin, *Biochemistry*, *31*, 5459–5466 (1992).

13. J. Jenkins, J. Janin, F. Rey, M. Chiadmi, H. van Tilbeurgh, I. Lasters, M. De Maeyer, D. vanBelle, S. J. Wodak, M. Lauwereys, P. Stanssens, N. T. Mrabet, J. Snauwaert, G. Matthyssens, and A.-M. Lambeir, *Biochemistry*, *31*, 5449–5458 (1992).

14. G. K. Farber and G. A. Petsko, *Trends Biochem. Sci.*, *15*, 228–234 (1990).

15. G. C. Dismukes, *Chem. Rev.*, *96*, 2906–2926 (1996).

16. I. A. Rose, *Philos. Trans. R. Soc. Lond. B Biol. Sci.*, *293*, 131–143 (1981).

17. W. L. Albery and J. R. Knowles, *Biochemistry*, *15*, 5627–5631 (1976).

18. C. A. Collyer and D. M. Blow, *Proc. Natl. Acad. Sci. USA*, *87*, 1362–1366 (1990).

19. G. A. Farber, A. Glasfeld, G. Tiraby, D. Ringe, and G. A. Petsko, *Biochemistry*, *28*, 7289–7297 (1989).

20. K. J. Schray and I. A. Rose, *Biochemistry*, *10*, 1058–1062 (1971).

21. M. S. Feather, V. Deshpande, and M. J. Lybyer, *Biochem. Biophys. Res. Commun.*, *38*, 859–863 (1970).

22. K. Bock, M. Meldal, B. Meyer, and L. Wiebe, *Acta Scand. Series B37*, 101–108 (1983).

23. P. van Bastelaere, W. Vangrysperre, and H. Kersters-Hilderson, *Biochem. J.*, *278*, 285–292 (1991).

24. M. Rangarajan and B. S. Hartley, *Biochem. J.*, *283*, 223–233 (1992).

25. O. S. Smart, J. Akins, and D. M. Blow, *Proteins Struct. Funct. Genet.*, *13*, 100–111 (1992).

26. C. Lee, M. Bagdasarian, M. Meng, and J. G. Zeikus, *J. Biol. Chem.*, *265*, 19082–19090 (1990).

27. Y. Takasaki, Y. Kosugi, and A. Kanjabashi, *Agric. Biol. Chem.*, *33*, 1527–1534 (1969).

28. M. Suekane, M. Tamura, and C. Tomimura, *Agric. Biol. Chem.*, *42*, 909 (1978).

29. P. van Bastelaere, M. Callens, W. Vangrysperre, and H. Kersters-Hilderson, *Biochem. J.*, *286*, 729–735 (1992).

30. M. Callens, H. Kersters-Hilderson, O. Van Opstale, and C. K. De-Bruyne, *Enzyme Microb. Technol.*, *8*, 696–700 (1986).

31. C. Sudfeldt, A. Schäffer, J. Kägi, R. Bogumil, H.-P. Schulz, S. Wulff, and H. Witzel, *Eur. J. Biochem.*, *193*, 863–881 (1990).

32. R. Bogumil, R. Kappl, J. Hüttermann, C. Sudfeldt, and H. Witzel, *Eur. J. Biochem.*, *213*, 1185–1192 (1993).

33. M. Callens, P. Tomme, H. Kersters-Hilderson, R. Cornelis, W. Vangrysperre, and C. K. DeBruyne, *Biochem. J.*, *250*, 285–290 (1988).

34. R. Bogumil, R. Kappl, J. Hüttermann, and H. Witzel, *Biochemistry*, *36*, 2345–2352 (1997).

35. R. Bogumil, J. Hüttermann, R. Kappl, R. Stabler, C. Sudfeldt, and H. Witzel, *Eur. J. Biochem.*, *196*, 305–312 (1991).

36. S. A. Dikanov, A. M. Tyryshkin, J. Hüttermann, R. Bogumil, and H. Witzel, *J. Am. Chem. Soc.*, *117*, 4976–4986 (1995).

37. G. H. Reed and G. D. Markham, in *Biological Magnetic Resonance*, Vol. 6 (J. L. Berliner and J. Reuben, eds.), Plenum Press, New York, 1984, pp. 73–142.

38. A. Abragam and B. Bleaney, in *Electron Paramagnetic Resonance of Transition Ions*, Clarendon Press, Oxford, 1970.

39. G. D. Markham, B. D. N. Rao, and G. H. Reed, *J. Magn. Res.*, *33*, 595–602 (1979).

40. H. W. de Wijn and R. F. van Balderen, *J. Chem. Phys.*, *46*, 1381–1387 (1967).

41. G. H. Reed and W. R. Ray, *Biochemistry*, *10*, 3190–3197 (1971).

42. G. H. Reed and M. Cohn, *J. Biol. Chem.*, *248*, 6436–6442 (1973).

43. G. H. Reed and S. D. Morgan, *Biochemistry*, *13*, 3537–3541 (1974).

44. R. S. Levy and J. J. Villafranca, *Biochemistry*, *16*, 3293–3301 (1977).

45. E. Meirovich and R. Poupko, *J. Phys. Chem.*, *82*, 1920–1925 (1978).

46. R. D. Shannon, *Acta Crystallogr. A*, *32*, 751–767 (1976).

47. M. Meng, M. Bagdsarian, and G. J. Zeikus, *Proc. Natl. Acad. Sci. USA*, *90*, 8459–8463 (1993)

13

Arginase: A Binuclear Manganese Metalloenzyme

David E. Ash,[1] J. David Cox,[2] and David W. Christianson[2]

[1]Department of Biochemistry,
Temple University School of Medicine,
Philadelphia, PA 19140, USA

[2]Roy and Diana Vagelos Laboratories,
Department of Chemistry, University of Pennsylvania,
Philadelphia, PA 19104-6323, USA

1. INTRODUCTION

Arginase catalyzes the divalent cation–dependent hydrolysis of L-arginine to form the nonprotein amino acid L-ornithine and urea:

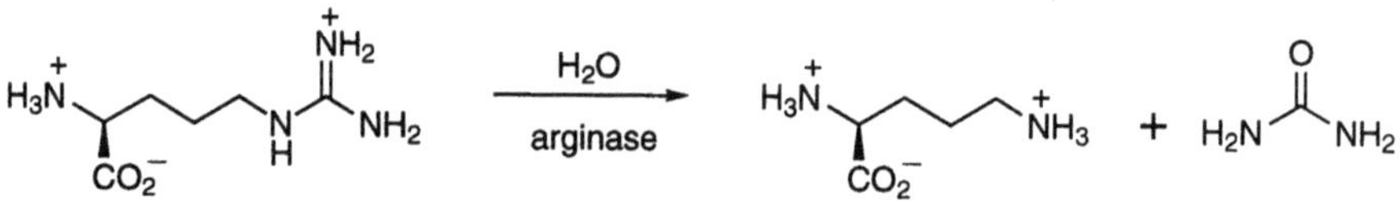

Enzyme activity is found at highest levels in mammalian liver [1], where
this reaction constitutes the final step of the urea cycle. The flux of substrate through this step is considerable, since the average adult excretes
about 10 kg of urea per year. In addition to its presence in liver, arginase
activity has been detected in a number of extrahepatic tissues that lack
a complete urea cycle, such as lactating mammary gland [2,3], kidney
[4–7], prostate [6], and activated macrophages [5]. In most of these tissues, the arginase present represents a second isozyme (arginase II)
that is distinct in immunological properties, amino acid sequence, and
subcellular location from the more abundant liver isozyme (arginase I).
The biological function of arginase II has been the subject of considerable interest; current thinking is that this isozyme provides a supply of
L-ornithine for proline and polyamine biosynthesis, and along with
arginase I it also serves to regulate the levels of L-arginine available for
nitric oxide production. The comparative properties of the two arginase
isozymes are discussed in a number of recent reviews [8–10]. Arginase
I is the more abundant isozyme of the two, and it has been extensively
characterized in terms of its biochemistry, enzymology, and three-dimensional structure. Arginase I is a 105-kDa homotrimer, and each 35-
kDa protomer contains a binuclear manganese cluster required for catalytic activity. The remainder of this chapter outlines the catalytic
mechanism and structure–function relationships for this well-studied
isozyme.

2. ENZYMOLOGY AND BIOINORGANIC CHEMISTRY

2.1. Metal Activation and Identification of the Binuclear Manganese Cluster

A common feature of arginases thus far studied, whether of eukaryotic or prokaryotic origin, is the critical catalytic requirement for divalent cations. Mn^{2+} is the physiological activator, although the divalent cation requirement for some arginases is reportedly satisfied by Co^{2+} and Ni^{2+} [11–13] and in some instances by Fe^{2+}, VO^{2+}, and Cd^{2+} [14,15]. Arginases from the *Agrobacterium* TiC58 plasmid [16] and *Neurospora crassa* [17] are specifically activated by Mn^{2+}, and the enzyme from the thermophile *Bacillus caldovelox* contains ≥ 1 Mn/subunit [18]. The enzyme from rat liver contains tightly bound Mn^{2+}, and marginal activation of the partially manganese-depleted enzyme is observed only with Cd^{2+} [19]. Manganese binding experiments demonstrate that fully metal-activated rat liver arginase contains 2 Mn^{2+}/subunit; moreover, these Mn^{2+} ions form electron paramagnetic resonance (EPR) spin-coupled binuclear clusters (Fig. 1) [20]. Curiously, human liver arginase is reported to contain only 1 Mn^{2+}/subunit in its fully active state, despite 87% sequence identity with the rat liver enzyme and conservation of all metal ligands [21].

Multicomponent analysis of the EPR spectra for metal-loaded rat liver arginase yields the spectral properties of the triplet and quintet electronic states, and the resultant zero field splitting of the quintet state indicates Mn^{2+}–Mn^{2+} separations of 3.36–3.57 Å in the native enzyme (multiple forms), and 3.5 Å in the arginase–borate complex [22]. Similar EPR spectra measured for the binuclear manganese catalase from *T. thermophilus* suggested that arginase might likewise catalyze the disproportionation of hydrogen peroxide. Although this reaction is indeed catalyzed by rat liver arginase, the kinetic constants of $K_M = 2.75$ M and $k_{cat} = 30$ s^{-1} suggest that this reaction is unlikely to be physiologically significant [19].

2.2. Kinetics and pH Dependence of Catalysis

The reaction catalyzed by arginase is effectively a uni-bi reaction, since water is a nonlimiting substrate in the forward direction. The compet-

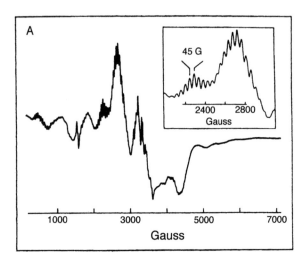

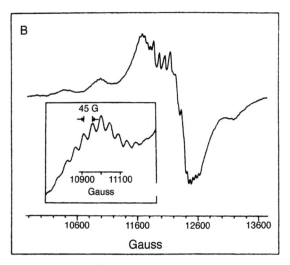

FIG. 1.   EPR spectra for Mn^{2+}-activated arginase. (A) X-band spectrum at 20 K for a 51 mg/mL arginase solution. (B) Q-band spectrum at 155 K for a 54 mg/mL arginase solution. The 45-gauss hyperfine coupling constant in each spectrum is diagnostic for the presence of a binuclear manganese cluster. (Reprinted with permission from [20]. Copyright 1992 American Chemical Society.)

itive inhibition of the enzyme by both products, ornithine (K_i = 1 mM) and urea (K_i = 880 mM), is consistent with a rapid equilibrium-random mechanism (Fig. 2) [23]. Under the assay conditions employed in these experiments, the K_M for substrate arginine is 1 mM.

Arginase-catalyzed arginine hydrolysis exhibits an unusual pH dependence, with a pH activity optimum at about pH 9.0–9.5 [24]; furthermore, enzyme activity is extremely sensitive to minute changes in pH in the region of physiological pH (Fig. 3) [25]. The pK calculated from this plot is in the range of 7.8–8.0, similar to the pK values of 7.8 and 7.9 measured for the human liver [26] and mouse liver [27] enzymes, respectively. These pK values are consistent with the pK_a value expected for the ionization of a solvent molecule bridging the Mn^{2+}–Mn^{2+} cluster [28]. Work by Kuhn and colleagues [26] suggests that the pH sensitivity of enzymatic activity may arise in part from the pH dependence of Mn^{2+} binding to the enzyme.

2.3. Substrate and Inhibitor Specificity

Maximal arginase activity depends on three critical substrate features: (1) the presence of a guanidinium group, (2) the length of the side chain, and (3) the stereochemistry and chemical nature of the Cα substituents (Table 1) [23]. For example, D-arginine and guanidinobutyrate are not

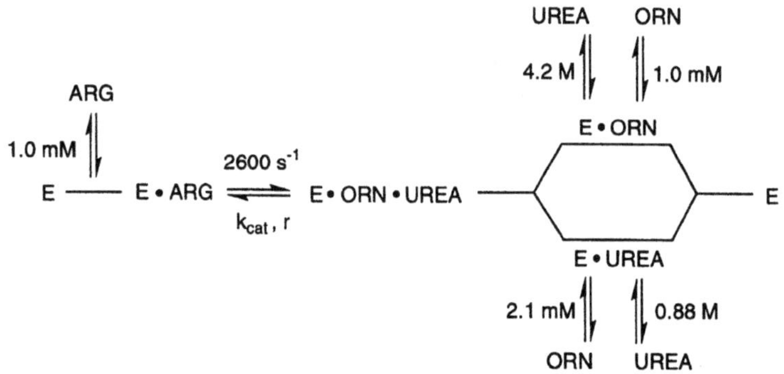

FIG. 2. Kinetic mechanism of rat liver arginase as determined by product inhibition studies. (Reprinted with permission from [23].)

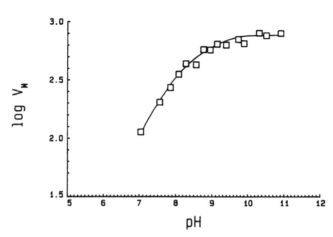

FIG. 3.   The pH-rate profile for rat liver arginase. The solid line drawn through
the data corresponds to the theoretical curve for a group ionizing with $pK_a = 8$.
(Reprinted with permission from [25].)

substrates for the enzyme. Alterations at the α-carbon of L-arginine (L-
argininamide, L-argininic acid, and agmatine) yield alternate substrates with significant changes in both K_M and V_{max}.

In addition to inhibition by the product ornithine, arginase is
weakly inhibited by a number of amino acids including lysine (a competitive inhibitor [23]), the branched chain amino acids, and proline
[29]. In fact, arginase appears to be weakly inhibited by most—if not
all—of the amino acids, with K_i values in the high millimolar range. Borate has long been known to be an inhibitor of the arginase reaction,
and as early as 1945 inhibition was thought to be due to interaction with
activating metal ions [30]. For the rat liver enzyme, borate is a non-
competitive inhibitor with $K_{is} = 1$ mM and $K_{ii} = 0.26$ mM; double-inhi-
bition experiments demonstrate that borate and ornithine bind simultaneously to arginase, whereas the binding of borate and urea is
mutually exclusive [23]. Reczkowski and Ash [23] postulate that borate
inhibition might result from the coordination of borate to Mn^{2+} in the
binuclear cluster, either by direct displacement of metal-bound solvent
or by nucleophilic attack of a metal-bound hydroxide. The structure of
the enzyme–ornithine–borate complex confirms this prediction [31].

The discovery of nitric oxide (NO) synthase, which catalyzes the
oxidation of arginine to form citrulline and nitric oxide, has motivated

TABLE 1

Arginase Substrates

	K_M (mM)	k_{cat}/K_M $(M^{-1} s^{-1}) \times 10^3$	V_{max} (μmol/min/mg)
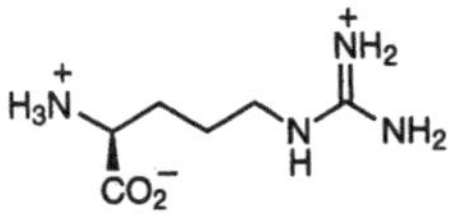 L-arginine	1.0	2600	4380
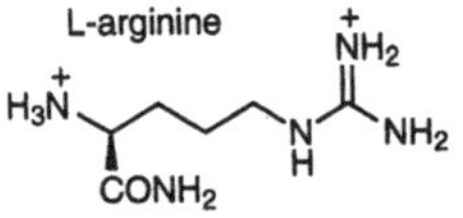 L-argininamide	12.4	150	315
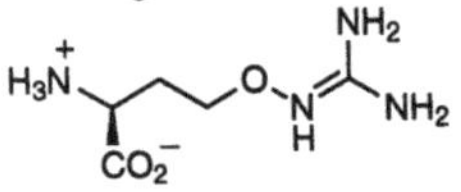 L-canavanine	12.0	7.4	153
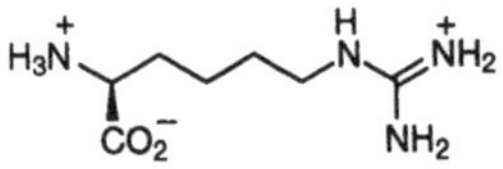 L-homoarginine	7.2	2.8	34
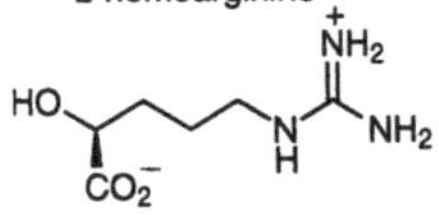 L-argininic acid	9.3	0.82	13
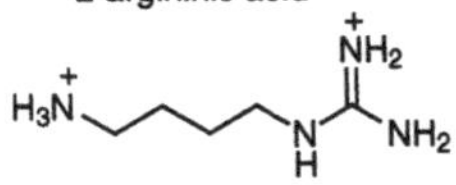 agmatine	10.8	0.048	0.9

significant research into the role of arginase as a regulator of NO synthase: arginase activity depletes the substrate pool of arginine that would otherwise be utilized for NO biosynthesis. Conversely, arginase inhibition promotes NO biosynthesis by sustaining the substrate pool of arginine. N^ω-Hydroxy-L-arginine, an intermediate in NO biosynthesis, is a potent inhibitor of both arginase isozymes [32–34]; the K_i for the inhibition of the rat liver enzyme is approximately 40 μM [32]. Intriguingly, sufficient concentrations of N^ω-hydroxy-L-arginine are produced in endothelial cells and activated macrophages to inhibit arginase [33,35].

Based on the inhibitory properties of N^ω-hydroxy-L-arginine, a number of N-hydroxy analogs have been synthesized and evaluated as arginase inhibitors. The most potent of these compounds include N^ω-hydroxy-D,L-indospicine ($K_i = 20\ \mu M$), N^ε-hydroxy-L-lysine ($K_i = 4\ \mu M$), and N^ω-hydroxy-nor-L-arginine ($K_i = 0.5\ \mu M$) (Table 2) [36–38]. Although the structures of enzyme inhibitor complexes have not yet been determined, it is suggested that these compounds either displace the metal-bridging solvent molecule or form a hydrogen bond with this solvent [32,37, 38]. An alternative binding mode is considered on the basis of the EPR spectral properties of the enzyme complexes with lysine and enzyme N^ω-hydroxy-L-arginine complex [39].

TABLE 2

Arginase Inhibitors

	K_i (μM)
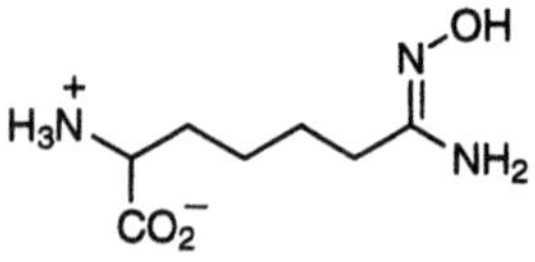 N^ω-hydroxy-D,L-indospicine	20
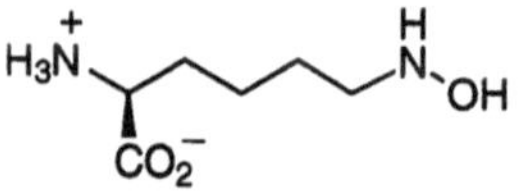 N^ε-hydroxy-L-lysine	4
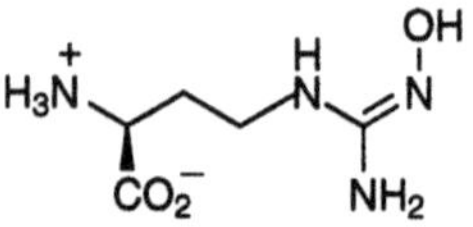 N^ω-hydroxy-nor-L-arginine	0.5
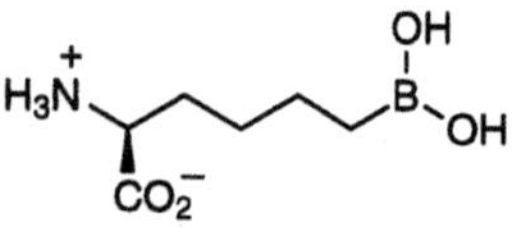 (S)-2-amino-6-boronohexanoic acid	0.1

The boronic acid-based arginine analog (S)-2-amino-6-borono-hexanoic acid is the most potent arginase inhibitor studied to date (Table 2) [31]. Isothermal titration calorimetry indicates a dissociation constant of 0.11 μM, and analysis of slow-binding kinetics yields K_i = 0.13 μM (unpublished results). The electron-deficient boron atom of a boronic acid invites the addition of a nucleophile, e.g., a protein-bound nucleophile or a solvent molecule, to yield a tetrahedral boronate anion. Accordingly, we postulate that the tight binding of (S)-2-amino-6-boronohexanoic acid arises from the binding of the tetrahedral boronate species to mimic the tetrahedral intermediate and its flanking transition states in the arginine hydrolysis reaction (Fig. 4) [31]. The X-ray structure determination of this enzyme inhibitor complex from crystals exhibiting perfect hemihedral twinning has confirmed this binding mode (unpublished results). Interestingly, in physiological studies of smooth muscle relaxation this arginase inhibitor promotes smooth muscle relaxation, probably by sustaining cellular arginine concentrations available for NO biosynthesis and subsequent NO-dependent relaxation (unpublished results).

2.4.   A Functional Biomimetic

The first functional model of the arginase reaction, the hydroxo-bridged binuclear cobalt(II) complex $[Co_2(\mu\text{-OH})(\mu\text{-XDK})(bpy)_2(EtOH)](NO_3)$ (XDK = m-xylylenediamine bis(Kemp's triacid imide); bpy = 2,2′-bipyridine), was recently reported by He and Lippard [40]. Although this biomimetic employs a binuclear cobalt cluster instead of a binuclear manganese cluster (the binuclear manganese complex is inactive), it nevertheless achieves hydrolysis of the guanidinium cation (Fig. 5). In ethanol solutions this biomimetic catalyzes the single-turnover hydrolysis of aminoguanidine to form urea with a pseudo-first-order rate constant of 4.4×10^{-4} s^{-1}. Aminoguanidine is the assay substrate, rather than arginine, because binding of aminoguanidine directly to the metal center is expected to orient the guanidinium group close to nucleophilic metal-bridging hydroxide ion (arginine itself is not expected to bind with high affinity to the metal center). A stoichiometry of 1:1 urea formed per molecule of complex is observed, since the metal-bridging hydroxide ion is the only water-derived nucleophile available.

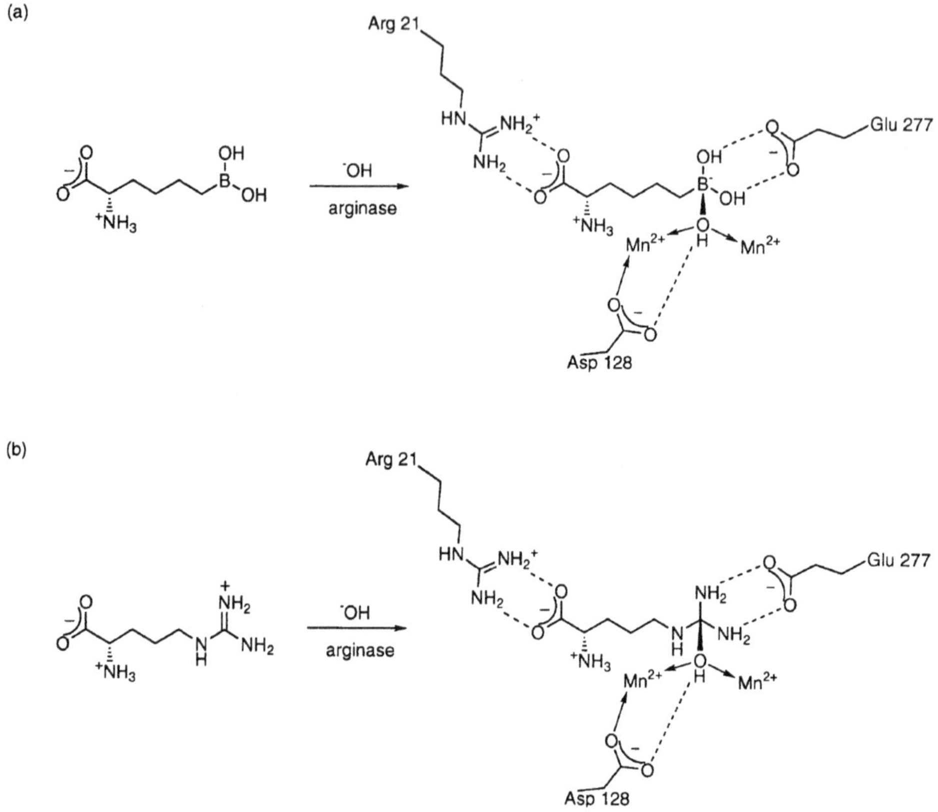

(a)

(b)

FIG. 4.   (a) The boronic acid-based arginine analog (S)-2-amino-6-borono-hexanoic acid inhibits arginase with a dissociation constant of 0.11 µM. High affinity arises from the binding of the hydrated boronic acid—a tetrahedral boronate anion—which mimics the tetrahedral intermediate (and its flanking transition states) in the arginine hydrolysis reaction (b).

3.   ARGINASE STRUCTURE AND MECHANISM

3.1.   Overall Fold and Trimer Assembly

The overall fold of the arginase monomer belongs to the α/β family, consisting of a parallel, eight-stranded, β-sheet flanked on both sides by numerous α helices (Fig. 6) [41]. The binuclear manganese cluster is located on one edge of the central β sheet. Trimer assembly is stabilized by a novel, S-shaped polypeptide tail at the C terminus of each monomer

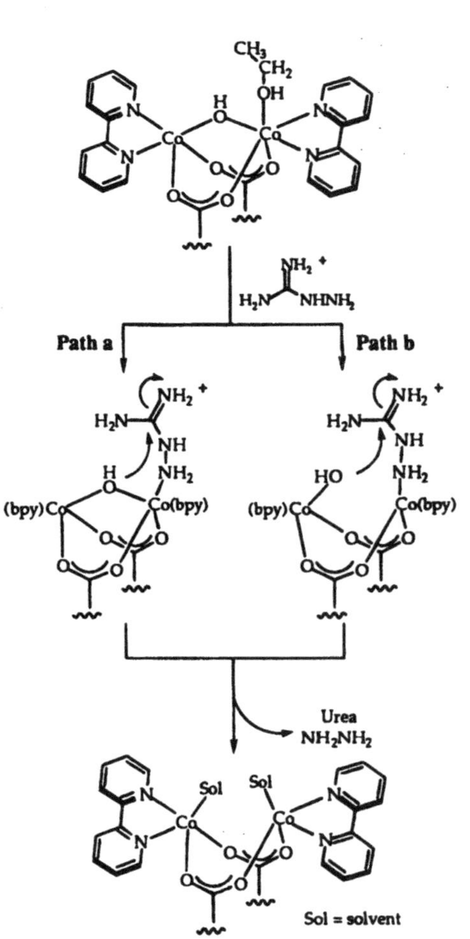

FIG. 5.   The binuclear cobalt(II) complex, $[Co_2(\mu\text{-OH})(\mu\text{-XDK})(bpy)_2(EtOH)]$ (NO_3) (XDK = m-xylylenediamine bis(Kemp's triacid imide); bpy = 2,2-bipyridine), hydrolyzes the aminoguanidinium cation to form urea through a metal-activated hydroxide mechanism. This is the first functional arginase biomimetic. (Reprinted with permission from [40]. Copyright 1998 American Chemical Society.)

(Phe304–Leu319). Each S-shaped tail wraps around helix E of the adjacent monomer to make multiple inter-subunit van der Waals and hydrogen bond interactions. The S-shaped tail appears to be critical for trimer assembly and stabilization since it contributes 54% of the total solvent-excluded surface area at each monomer–monomer interface.

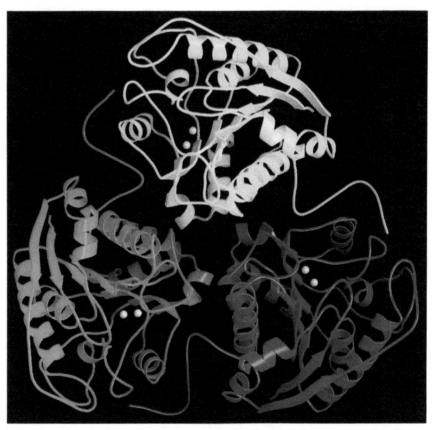

FIG. 6.   Ribbon plot of the arginase trimer. The binuclear manganese cluster
is represented by a pair of spheres in each monomer. (Reprinted with permission from [41]. Copyright 1996, MacMillan Magazines Ltd.)

3.2.   Manganese Coordination Polyhedra

The binuclear manganese cluster is located at the bottom of an approximately 15-Å-deep active site cleft in each monomer (Fig. 7) [41].
The Mn^{2+}-Mn^{2+} internuclear separation is 3.3 Å, which is consistent
with the results of EPR spectroscopic experiments [22]. The more deeply
situated metal is designated Mn_A^{2+}: square-pyramidal coordination
geometry is provided by terminal ligands His101 and Asp128, and bridging ligands Asp124 (*syn-syn*-bidentate), Asp232 (*anti*-monodentate),
and hydroxide ion. Metal ion Mn_B^{2+} is coordinated with distorted octa-

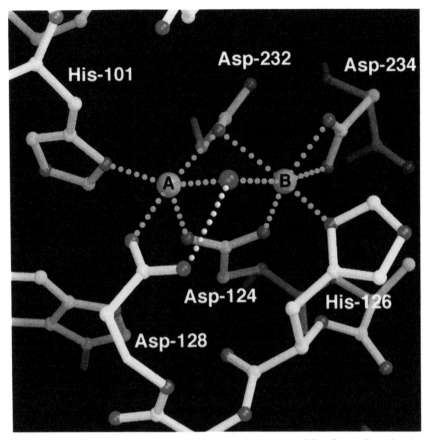

FIG. 7.   The binuclear manganese cluster of arginase. Metal coordination interactions are indicated by green dotted lines, and the hydrogen bond between the metal-bridging hydroxide ion and Asp128 is indicated by a white dotted line.

hedral geometry by terminal ligands His126 and Asp234 (bidentate), and bridging ligands Asp124 (*syn-syn*-bidentate), Asp232 (*syn*-monodentate), and hydroxide ion. Metal-bridging hydroxide ion donates a hydrogen bond to the noncoordinating carboxylate oxygen of Asp128.

Treatment of arginase crystals with the metal chelators dipicolinic acid and ethylenediaminetetraacetic acid results in the dissociation of Mn_A^{2+} [42]. That approximately 50% catalytic activity is retained in arginase containing about 3 Mn^{2+}/trimer [20,43] suggests that arginase may be capable of functioning as a mononuclear manganese hydrolase—in principle, a hydroxide ion coordinated to Mn_B^{2+} and hydrogen-bonded with Asp128 could still serve as a catalytic nucleophile. One manganese ion cannot polarize a solvent nucleophile as effectively as two manganese ions [28], so the approximately 50% loss of catalytic activity in the half-active state may reflect diminished activation of metal-bound hydroxide ion. However, using this rationalization it is difficult to explain the dramatic loss of catalytic activity in the His101 → Asn arginase variant, which exhibits only 0.17% activity relative to the wild-type enzyme [44]: this amino acid substitution weakens Mn_A^{2+} binding, but leaves an intact Mn_B^{2+} site identical in structure to that of Mn_A^{2+}-depleted native arginase [42]. Clearly, structure–function relationships in the binuclear manganese cluster of arginase are complex and remain the focus of ongoing site-directed mutagenesis and X-ray crystallographic studies.

3.3.   Substrate Binding and Catalytic Mechanism

The arginase mechanism proposed by Kanyo and colleagues [41] is most consistent with the available biochemical, enzymological, and structural data. The ionization of metal-bridging hydroxide probably reflects the apparent pK_a of 7.9 in the pH-rate profile [25–27], consistent with a metal-activated hydroxide mechanism in which substrate arginine does not coordinate to manganese prior to nucleophilic attack by hydroxide (Figs. 8 and 9) [41]. Accordingly, with metal-bridging hydroxide ion donating a hydrogen bond to Asp128, only one lone electron pair is available for nucleophilic attack at the substrate. The crystal structure of the enzyme reveals that this lone pair is oriented toward a postulated substrate binding site. Numerous examples from small molecule biomimetic systems as well as other hydrolytic enzymes support the proposed role of a metal-bridging solvent molecule as a catalytic nucleophile [45]. For example, Williams and colleagues have recently reported the hydrolysis of phosphate diesters by cobalt(III)-bridging hydroxide and oxide ions [46]. Therefore, the nucleophilic hydroxide ion appears to be fully activated by symmetrically bridging both Mn^{2+} ions in the binuclear manganese cluster [28].

We emphasize that enzymological measurements argue against a direct substrate–metal coordination interaction in the precatalytic Michaelis complex: the substrate K_M value (which reflects enzyme–substrate affinity) does not change significantly when the binuclear man-

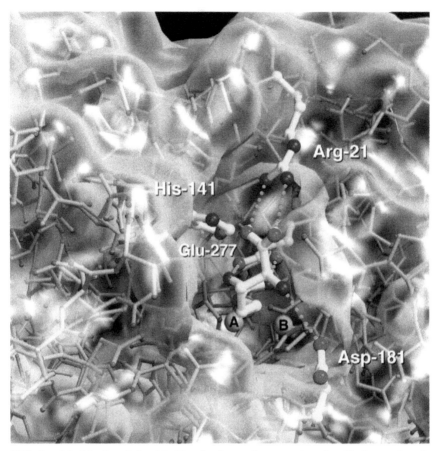

FIG. 8.   Model of arginine binding in the arginase active site. Hydrogen bonds
are indicated by green dotted lines. A salt link between Glu277 and the substrate guanidinium group likely orients the substrate for nucleophilic attack by
metal-bridging hydroxide ion (red sphere, partially occluded by the substrate).
Additional salt links indicated may contribute to substrate specificity. Located
about half-way out of the active site cleft, His141 likely serves as a proton shuttle in catalysis. (Reprinted with permission from [41]. Copyright 1996, MacMillan Magazines Ltd.)

ganese cluster is perturbed by site-directed mutagenesis [44], nor does
it change when Mn_A^{2+} is dialyzed out of the active site [42]. Instead, modeling studies indicate that Glu277 can make an ideal salt link with the
substrate guanidinium group; moreover, this interaction would position
the scissile guanidinium carbon directly adjacent to—and in-line with

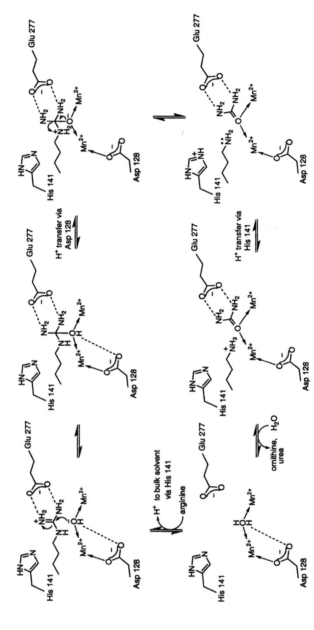

FIG. 9 Proposed mechanism of arginase-catalyzed arginine hydrolysis by metal-activated hydroxide. The α-amino and α-carboxylate groups of the substrate are omitted for clarity.

the nucleophilic lone electron pair of—the metal-bridging hydroxide ion (Fig. 8) [41].

The tetrahedral intermediate resulting from nucleophilic attack of metal-bridging hydroxide ion at substrate arginine (Fig. 9) is mimicked by the binding of (S)-2-amino-6-boronohexanoic acid as the tetrahedral boronate anion (Fig. 4). Subsequent to proton transfer to the leaving group of ornithine (perhaps mediated by Asp128), the tetrahedral intermediate collapses to yield products ornithine and urea. Implicated as catalytically important in site-directed mutagenesis and chemical labeling experiments [44,47], His141 may play a role in catalysis as a proton shuttle. Located about halfway out of the active site cleft, His141 is 4.2 Å away from the metal-bridging hydroxide ion of the native enzyme [41]. His141 may shuttle a proton from bulk solvent to the ε-amino group of ornithine prior to product dissociation. Additionally, His141 may facilitate the ionization of a metal-bridging water molecule by shuttling a proton to bulk solvent—this step is critical for the regeneration of nucleophilic metal-bridging hydroxide ion after each catalytic turnover. The proton shuttle role for His141 of arginase is analogous to that determined for His64 in the carbonic anhydrase II active site [48,49].

It should be noted that an alternative arginase mechanism is proposed by Dismukes based on EPR spectroscopic studies of arginase–inhibitor complexes [39]. Key differences of this alternative mechanism are (1) deprotonation of the substrate guanidinium group by His141; (2) coordination of the substrate guanidine to Mn_B^{2+}; and (3) nucleophilic attack of Mn_A^{2+}-bound hydroxide ion. This proposal is inconsistent with enzymological data suggesting a nonmetal binding site for substrate arginine, i.e., an invariant K_M despite perturbations in the metal binding site [42–44].

4.   RELATED BINUCLEAR MANGANESE METALLOENZYMES

Structural comparisons of arginase with the binuclear manganese metalloenzymes catalase and serine/threonine protein phosphatase-1 have been made recently [50] so these enzymes will not be discussed here. However, the recently reported structure of the proline-specific aminopeptidase P from *Escherichia coli* reveals a new binuclear manganese cluster bearing partial resemblance to that of arginase, and it is instructive to compare these two metallohydrolases.

Aminopeptidase P hydrolyzes N-terminal Xaa-Pro peptide bonds, and EPR measurements initially revealed the presence of a spin-coupled binuclear manganese cluster [51]. The recently determined X-ray crystal structure of aminopeptidase P indicates a tetrameric structure in which each monomer contains a single binuclear manganese cluster (Mn^{2+}–Mn^{2+} separation = 3.3 Å) located on a central β sheet [52]. As noted by Wilce and colleagues [52], aminopeptidase P shares these features with the binuclear manganese cluster of arginase; moreover, both metalloenzymes contain a metal-bridging solvent ligand that donates a hydrogen bond to one oxygen of a carboxylate group, the second oxygen of which coordinates to Mn_A^{2+} (Fig. 10). Accordingly, Wilce and colleagues [52] propose that metal-bridging hydroxide ion is the catalytic nucleophile that attacks the scissile Xaa-Pro peptide linkage. Structural and spectroscopic evidence is consistent with a nonmetal precatalytic binding site for the substrate [52], as has been proposed for arginase [41].

In aminopeptidase P, the imidazole group of His361 is located adjacent to the manganese cluster and hydrogen bonds to a water molecule coordinated to Mn_A^{2+}. It is conceivable that His361 serves a role as a proton shuttle in catalysis, much like the role proposed for His141 in the arginase mechanism. It is striking that histidine residues often dangle from the active site walls of hydrolytic metalloenzymes such as carbonic anhydrase II, arginase, and aminopeptidase P. This may reflect the broad requirement for an intermediary proton shuttle group to ensure the rapid regeneration of nucleophilic metal-bound hydroxide ion in catalytic turnover.

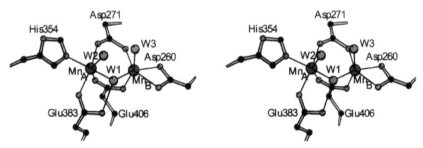

FIG. 10.   Binuclear manganese cluster of aminopeptidase P. (Reprinted with permission from [52]. Copyright 1988 National Academy of Sciences, U.S.A.)

5. CONCLUSIONS

Arginase is the prototypical binuclear manganese metalloenzyme and it is the most extensively studied in terms of biochemistry, enzymology, and structural analysis. The biological interest in arginase is growing rapidly due to its apparent biological role in the regulation of substrate pools for nitric oxide synthase in smooth muscle relaxation. This has potential pharmaceutical implications for the treatment of pulmonary hypertension, gastromotility disorders, and erectile dysfunction. Arginase catalyzes arginine hydrolysis through a metal-activated hydroxide mechanism in which a bridging solvent molecule is activated by both metal ions in the binuclear cluster; a nonmetal site is implicated for precatalytic substrate binding. The related metallohydrolase aminopeptidase P is likewise proposed to function through a metal-activated hydroxide mechanism involving a nonmetal binding site for the Xaa-Pro substrate, and it is striking that both enzymes contain an active site histidine residue serving a potential role as a catalytic proton shuttle.

ACKNOWLEDGMENT

We thank the NIH for grants GM49758 and DK44841 in support of this work.

REFERENCES

1. A. Herzfeld and S. M. Raper, *Biochem. J.*, *153*, 469–478 (1976).
2. M. C. M. Yip and W. E. Knox, *Biochem. J.*, *127*, 893–899 (1972).
3. C. P. Jenkinson and M. R. Grigor, *Biochem. Met. Metab. Biol.*, *51*, 156–165 (1994).
4. G. A. Kaysen and H. J. Strecker, *Biochem. J.*, *133*, 779–788 (1973).
5. T. Gotoh, T. Sonoki, A. Nagasaki, K. Terada, M. Takiguchi, and M. Mori, *FEBS Lett.*, *395*, 119–122 (1996).
6. J. G. Vockley, C. P. Jenkinson, H. Shukla, R. M. Kern, W. W. Grody, and S. D. Cederbaum, *Genomics*, *38*, 118–123 (1996).

7. S. M. Morris, Jr., D. Bhamidipati, and D. Kepka-Lenhart, *Gene*, *193*, 157–161 (1997).

8. C. P. Jenkinson, W. W. Grody, and S. D. Cederbaum, *Comp. Biochem. Physiol.*, *114B*, 107–132 (1996).

9. R. Iyer, C. P. Jenkinson, J. G. Vockley, R. M. Kern, W. W. Grody, and S. Cederbaum, *J. Inher. Metab. Dis.*, *21 (Suppl 1)*, 86–100 (1998).

10. J. Perozich, J. Hempel, and S. M. Morris, Jr., *Biochim. Biophys. Acta*, *1382*, 23–37 (1998).

11. L. Hellerman and M. E. Perkins, *J. Biol. Chem.*, *112*, 175–194 (1935).

12. J. Mora, R. Tarrab, J. Martuscelli and G. Soberon, *Biochem. J.*, *96*, 588–594 (1965).

13. G. W. Brown, Jr., *Arch. Biochem. Biophys.*, *114*, 184–194 (1966).

14. A. B. Anderson, *Biochem. J.*, *39*, 139–142 (1945).

15. S. Edlbacher and H. Baur, *Hoppe-Seyler's Z. Physiol. Chem.*, *254*, 275–284 (1958).

16. A. Shrell, J. Altmoerbe, T. Lanz, and J. Schroeder, *Eur. J. Biochem.*, *184*, 635–641 (1989).

17. K. A. Borkovich and R. L. Weiss, *J. Biol. Chem.*, *262*, 7081–7086 (1987).

18. M. L. Patchett, R. M. Daniel, and H. W. Morgan, *Biochem. Biophys. Acta*, *1077*, 291–298 (1991).

19. T. M. Sossong, Jr., S. V. Khangulov, R. C. Cavalli, D. R. Soprano, G. C. Dismukes, and D. E. Ash, *J. Biol. Inorg. Chem.*, *2*, 433–443 (1997).

20. R. S. Reczkowski and D. E. Ash, *J. Am. Chem. Soc.*, *114*, 10992–10994 (1992).

21. N. Carvajal, C. Torres, E. Uribe, and M. Salas, *Comp. Biochem. Physiol.*, *112B*, 153–159 (1995).

22. S. V. Khangulov, P. J. Pessiki, V. V. Barynin, D. E. Ash, and G. C. Dismukes, *Biochemistry*, *34*, 2015–2025 (1995).

23. R. S. Reczkowski and D. E. Ash, *Arch. Biochem. Biophys.*, *312*, 31–37 (1994).

24. O. A. Roholt and D. M. Greenberg, *Arch. Biochem. Biophys.*, *62*, 454–470 (1956).

25. R. S. Reczkowski, Ph.D. thesis, Temple University (1991).

26. N. J. Kuhn, S. Ward, M. Piponski, and T. W. Young, *Arch. Biochem. Biophys.*, *320*, 24–34 (1995).

27. N. J. Kuhn, J. Talbot, and S. Ward, *Arch. Biochem. Biophys.*, *286*, 217–221 (1991).

28. G. C. Dismukes, *Chem. Rev.*, *96*, 2909–2926 (1996).

29. N. Carvajal and S. D. Cederbaum, *Biochim. Biophys. Acta*, *870*, 181–184 (1986).

30. M. S. Mohamed and D. M. Greenberg, *Arch. Biochem. Biophys.*, *8*, 349–363 (1945).

31. R. Baggio, D. Elbaum, Z. F. Kanyo, P. J. Carroll, R. C. Cavalli, D. E. Ash, and D. W. Christianson, *J. Am. Chem. Soc.*, *119*, 8107–8108 (1997).

32. F. Daghigh, J. M. Fukuto, and D. E. Ash, *Biochem. Biophys. Res. Commun.*, *202*, 174–180 (1994).

33. M. Hecker, H. Nematollahi, C. Hey, R. Busse, and K. Racke, *FEBS Lett.*, *359*, 251–254 (1995).

34. J.-L. Boucher, J. Custot, S. Vadon, M. Delaforge, M. Lepoivre, J.-P. Tenu, A. Yapo, and D. Mansuy, *Biochem. Biophys. Res. Commun.*, *203*, 1614–1621 (1994).

35. G. M. Buga, R. Singh, S. Pervin, N. E. Rogers, D. A. Schmitz, C. P. Jenkinson, S. D. Cederbaum, and L. J. Ignarro, *Am. J. Physiol.*, *271*, H1988–H1998 (1996).

36. J. Custot, J.-L. Boucher, S. Vadon, C. Guedes, S. Dijols, M. Delaforge, and D. Mansuy, *J. Biol. Inorg. Chem.*, *1*, 73–82 (1996).

37. S. Vadon, J. Custot, J.-L. Boucher, and D. Mansuy, *J. Chem. Soc. Perkin Trans.*, *1*, 645–648 (1996).

38. J. Custot, C. Moali, M. Brollo, J. L. Boucher, M. Delaforge, D. Mansuy, J. P. Tenu, and J. L. Zimmermann, *J. Am. Chem. Soc.*, *119*, 4086–4087 (1997).

39. S. V. Khangulov, T. M. Sossong, Jr., D. E. Ash, and G. C. Dismukes, *Biochemistry*, *37*, 8539–8550 (1998).

40. C. He and S. J. Lippard, *J. Am. Chem. Soc.*, *120*, 105–113 (1998).

41. Z. F. Kanyo, L. R. Scolnick, D. E. Ash, and D. W. Christianson, *Nature*, *383*, 554–557 (1996).

42. L. R. Scolnick, Z. F. Kanyo, R. C. Cavalli, D. E. Ash, and D. W. Christianson, *Biochemistry*, *36*, 10558–10565 (1997).

43. H. Hirsch-Kolb, H. J. Kolb, and D. M. Greenberg, *J. Biol. Chem.*, *246*, 395–401, (1971).

44. R. C. Cavalli, C. J. Burke, S. Kawamoto, D. R. Soprano, and D. E. Ash, *Biochemistry*, *33*, 10652–10657 (1994).

45. D. W. Christianson and J. D. Cox, *Ann. Rev. Biochem.*, *68*, 33–57.

46. N. H. Williams, W. Cheung, and J. Chin, *J. Am. Chem. Soc.*, *120*, 8079–8087 (1998).

47. F. Daghigh, R. C. Cavalli, D. R. Soprano, and D. E. Ash, *Arch. Biochem. Biophys.*, *327*, 107–112 (1996).

48. D. N. Silverman and S. Lindskog, *Acc. Chem. Res.*, *21*, 30–36 (1988).

49. D. W. Christianson and C. A. Fierke, *Acc. Chem. Res.*, *29*, 331–339 (1996).

50. D. W. Christianson, *Prog. Biophys. Molec. Biol.*, *67*, 217–252 (1997).

51. L. Zhang, M. J. Crossley, N. E. Dixon, P. J. Ellis, M. L. Fisher, G. F. King, P. E. Lilley, D. MacLachlan, R. J. Pace, and H. C. Freeman, *J. Biol. Inorg. Chem.*, *3*, 470–483 (1998).

52. M. C. J. Wilce, C. S. Bond, N. E. Dixon, H. C. Freeman, J. M. Guss, P. E. Lilley, and J. A. Wilce, *Proc. Natl. Acad. Sci. USA*, *95*, 3472–3477 (1998).

14

The Use of Model Complexes to Elucidate the Structure and Function of Manganese Redox Enzymes

Vincent L. Pecoraro* and Wen-Yuan Hsieh

Department of Chemistry, University of Michigan,
Ann Arbor, MI 48109-1055, USA

*To whom correspondence should be addressed.

1. INTRODUCTION

This chapter, completed in March 1999, summarizes research literature published through late January of that year. The purpose of the chapter is to illustrate where model compounds have been used to enhance our understanding of manganese redox enzymes. Particular emphasis will be placed on studies of the oxygen evolving complex (OEC) and manganese catalase. The general approach will be to present the available biophysical data on the enzymes and to show how model complexes have been useful in interpreting these studies. Therefore, it is not the intent of the authors to provide an exhaustive review of the literature. Rather we hope to highlight how synthetic model studies, in conjunction with biochemical and biophysical investigations, can lead to reasonable proposals for structure and mechanism in these systems. The interested reader is directed to recent review articles on model compounds, manganese catalase, and the OEC that are found elsewhere in this book and in other reviews for more detailed coverage of these systems.

2. MANGANESE CATALASES

The catalases are a class of proteins that catalyze the disproportionation of hydrogen peroxide into dioxygen and water. Generally the need for such an enzyme has been ascribed to the necessity of removing hydrogen peroxide, which is cytotoxic. Most organisms carry out this reaction using heme enzymes. The heme catalases begin in the ferric oxidation level and proceed through a compound I intermediate, Fe(IV)=O(porphyrin$^{\bullet+}$), generated by the first equivalent of peroxide [1,2]. Dioxygen is liberated upon addition of the second peroxide equivalent. In the past two decades it has been realized that there are several species (e.g., thermophilic bacteria such as *Thermus thermophilus* [3,4] or the lactic acid-utilizing bacteria, *Lactobacillus plantarum* [5,6]) that substitute an enzyme containing a dinuclear manganese site to carry out this reaction. In addition, human arginase, which has an active site that is structurally similar to that found in the manganese catalases, can decompose hydrogen peroxide. These manganese enzymes do not contain an organic cofactor; instead they cycle between the Mn(II)$_2$ and Mn(III)$_2$ oxidation levels. There is also a superoxidized form [Mn(III)Mn(IV)] that is catalytically inactive, but can be reactivated to the Mn(III)$_2$ form. While the heme enzymes are much more efficient than the corresponding Mn systems, the latter still show respectable activities. Because Chap. 16 provides a detailed analysis of the *T. thermophilus* and *L. plantarum* enzymes, we will focus exclusively on structural, spectroscopic, and reactivity model systems.

2.1. Structural Models

One of the first structural models for the manganese catalases was the binuclear complex shown in Fig. 1A that was reported by Wieghardt et al. [7]. This compound nicely matched the visible electronic spectra that

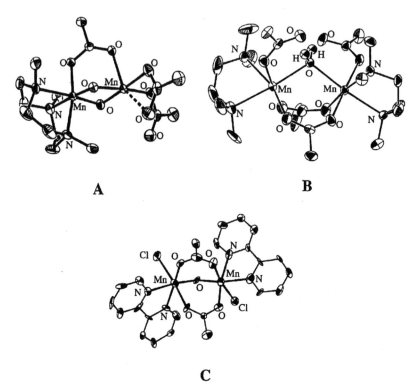

FIG. 1. Structure of [((CH$_3$)$_3$tacn)Mn^{IV}(μ-O$_2$)(μ-OAc)Mn^{III}(OAc)$_2$], (A); [Mn^{II}(*N,N,N',N'*-tetramethyl(ethylenediamine))]$_2$(OAc)$_2$(μ-OAc)$_2$(μ-OH$_2$), (B); [Mn^{III}(bipy)Cl$_2$]$_2$(μ-OAc)$_2$(μ-O), (C). (Reproduced with permission from [7], [8], [9]. Copyright 1992 the Royal Society of Chemistry, Copyright 1993 the American Chemical Society, and Copyright 1992 the American Chemical Society.)

had been reported for the oxidized enzyme. The important core of the molecule contained two manganese ions that were linked in a bis-oxo-monocarboxylato core. The oxo, carboxylato core is now recognized to be a generally important feature in binuclear iron and manganese enzymes. One can also find structures that have oxo-bis-carboxylato [8], aqua-bis-carboxylato [9], and (oxo, hydroxo, or aqua)-monocarboxylato cores [10]. Two of these are shown in Fig. 1B and C. There are also compounds that are known to contain solely bis-hydroxo [11] or bis-alkoxo [12] bridging ligand environments. In most cases, these structure elements support lower oxidation states of manganese with Mn(II)$_2$,

Mn(II)Mn(III), and Mn(III)$_2$ being the most common. Complexes with one oxo or hydroxo group and one or more bridging carboxylates typically have Mn-Mn separations that are on the order of 3.3 Å. Higher oxidation state dimers [Mn(III)Mn(IV) and Mn(IV)$_2$] are usually accessed with di-μ_2-oxo or oxo, hydroxo bridges [12,13]. These compounds have much smaller Mn-Mn separations, usually on the order of 2.7 ± 0.2 Å, depending on whether additional bridges are present. These models have been very useful in understanding the scattering properties and detectability of manganese at long Mn-Mn distances using X-ray absorption spectroscopy (XAS). From a combination of these studies, as well as electron paramagnetic resonance (EPR) experiments described below, the general environments of the Mn catalases in several oxidation states were correctly predicted.

Since the preparation of these molecules, X-ray structures of three related enzymes have appeared. The *T. thermophilus* manganese catalase has recently been solved at 1.6 Å resolution [14]. The active site is shown in Fig. 2A. This can be compared to the structures of the Mn-substituted ribonucleotide reductase [15] (Fig. 2B) and arginase [16] (Fig. 2C). The structures are remarkably similar. One key component is the utilization of the carboxylate as a metal complexing ligand. Lippard has commented for iron enzymes on the versatility of carboxylate ligation due to the ability of this unit to adopt several different coordination modes [17,18]. This is known as the carboxylate shift. One example of this phenomenon in manganese model compounds [19,20] is shown for the trinuclear complexes presented as Fig. 3. One can see that carboxylate ligational versatility is operative between these enzymes. It is also very likely that the carboxylate shift is mechanistically important during the catalytic cycle of all of these enzymes.

While we now have confirmation of the core structures in these manganese enzymes, it is important to realize that many of the features of the active sites were correctly predicted using XAS (see Chap. 16) and EPR spectroscopy. Binuclear manganese complexes have characteristic EPR spectra [21]. Examples of Mn(II)$_2$ dimers [21,22] are shown in Fig. 4. The Mn(II) dimers are always weakly antiferromagnetically exchanged coupled (|J| < 10 cm^{-1}), which means that low-lying excited states can be populated even at very low temperatures. Although integral spin systems are often not observed with perpendicular mode detection, Mn(II)$_2$ complexes are a common exception to this rule. Typi-

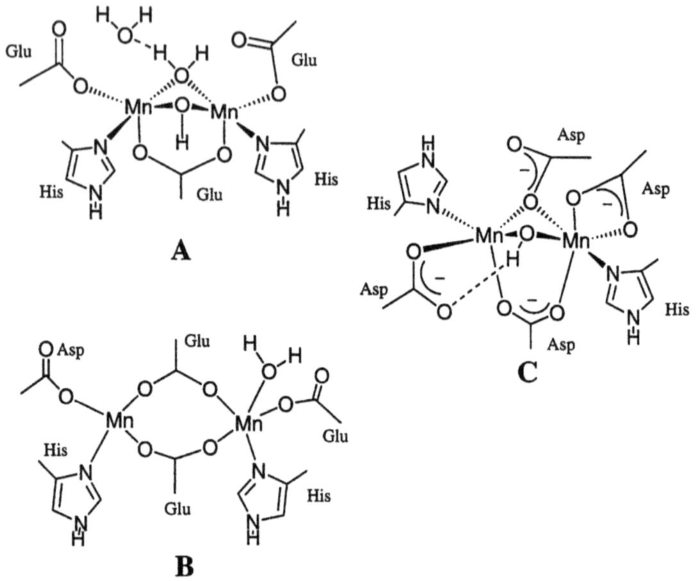

FIG. 2.   Structure of the active sites of *T. thermophilus* manganese catalase
(A), Mn^{II}-substituted ribonucleotide reductase (B), and arginase (C) based on
[14], [15], and [16].

cally one sees one or two groups of 11 line features that arise from the
coupling of the electron spin with the angular momentum of the manganese nucleus. Manganese with a nuclear spin, I, equal to 5/2 will show
a six line signal for mononuclear species. For homovalent dimers with
nearly equivalent coordination environments, 11 lines are predicted. As
one will see below, the situation becomes more complex for mixed-valent species. The spectroscopic signature shown in Fig. 4 uniquely identifies an enzyme as having a binuclear Mn(II) core. A visual comparison
to the EPR spectra for the Mn(II)$_2$ form of the manganese catalase [22]
and arginase [23], shown in Fig. 5, underscores this point. Dismukes et
al. have shown that detailed analysis of the spectra can also provide
metrical information on the Mn-Mn separation [24]. This point is discussed in more detail in Chap. 16.

The catalytically active high valent form [Mn(III)$_2$] of the manganese catalases is typically EPR-silent; however, two other oxidation
levels have been detected using this technique. The *T. thermophilus* (but
apparently not the *L. plantarum*) enzyme can form a Mn(II)Mn(III)
state in the presence of reductants [25]. If antiferromagnetically cou-

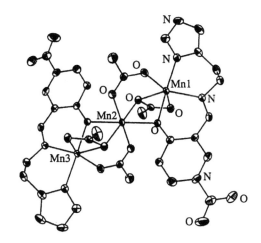

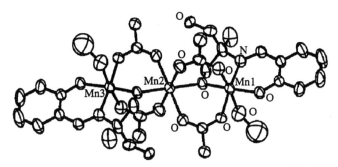

FIG. 3. Structure of $[Mn^{II}_3(5\text{-}NO_2\text{salim})_2(OAc)_4]$ and $\beta\text{-}[Mn^{III}_2Mn^{II}(sal\text{-}adhp)_2(OAc)_4(CH_3OH)_2$. (Reproduced with permission from [19], [20]. Copyright 1995 the American Chemical Society and Copyright 1989 the Royal Society of Chemistry.)

pled to give an $S = 1/2$ ground state, such a compound has a characteristic EPR spectrum which is shown for model compounds [22] in Fig. 6. Unlike the $Mn(II)_2$ forms, there are more than 11 lines (typically between 16 and 36 hyperfine lines) with a spectral range on the order of 1350 gauss. In contrast, the two-electron, more oxidized dimers have similar yet distinct spectra. In most cases, Mn(III)Mn(IV) compounds are strongly antiferromagnetically coupled ($|J| < 100$ cm^{-1}), assuring an $S = 1/2$ ground state and making most excited states too high to be pop-

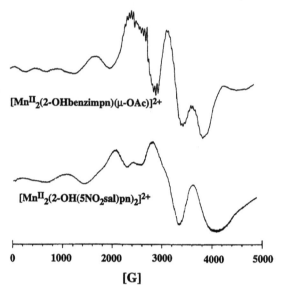

FIG. 4.   Examples of the EPR spectra of $Mn_2(II/II)$ dimers, $[Mn^{II}_2(2\text{-OHbenz-}$
$impn)(\mu\text{-OAc})]^{2+}$ (top); $[Mn^{II}_2(2\text{-OH}(5\text{-NO}_2sal)pn)_2]^{2+}$ (bottom). (Reproduced
with permission from [21], [22]. Copyright 1997 the American Chemical Soci-
ety and Copyright 1994 the American Chemical Society.)

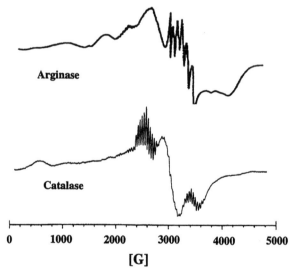

FIG. 5.   Comparison of the EPR spectra of arginase and Mn(II/II)catalase. (Reproduced with permission from [22], [23]. Copyright 1994 the American Chemical Society and Copyright 1997 Springer.)

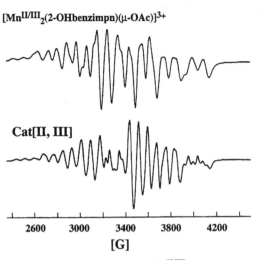

FIG. 6. Comparison of the EPR spectra of $[Mn^{II/III}_2(2\text{-OHbenzimpn})(\mu\text{-OAc})]^{3+}$ and Mn(II/III) catalase. (Reproduced with permission from [22]. Copyright 1994 the American Chemical Society.)

ulated significantly at liquid helium temperatures where spectra are usually recorded. Because the inherent hyperfine coupling constant for Mn(IV) is less than that for Mn(II) the spectral range (1150 gauss) for Mn(III)Mn(IV) dimers is typically significantly smaller than for the Mn(II)Mn(III) species, providing a convenient way of distinguishing between Mn(II)Mn(III) and Mn(III)Mn(IV). For many years it was assumed that all Mn(III)Mn(IV) dimers would provide the hallmark multiline spectra shown in Fig. 7A–C for models and the superoxidized Mn catalase [26]. This "dogma" was overturned by the production of a compound with $J \approx -8$ cm^{-1} ($[Mn^{III}Mn^{IV}(2\text{-OH-salpn})_2]^+$), which gave a unique 12-line spectrum shown as Fig. 7D. A satisfying explanation for the spectral modification exhibited by this compound has been provided by Dismukes et al. [27]. To date, there are no biological samples exhibiting this modified multiline signal. Thus, the EPR spectral data for the superoxidized manganese catalase are most consistent with a strongly coupled Mn(III)Mn(IV)(di-μ_2-oxo) core. Magnetic circular dichroism spectroscopy (MCD) has recently been used to probe the superoxidized Mn catalase [28]. A comparison of the spectra that were obtained for model compounds and that of the enzyme have been interpreted to suggest a third bridging ligand. Given the knowledge from the X-ray structure of the *T. thermophilus* enzyme, a reasonable proposal

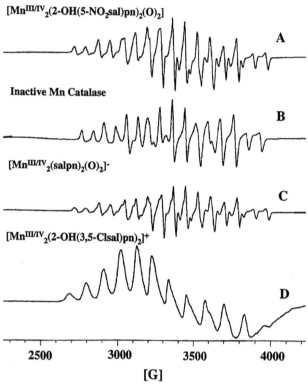

FIG. 7.   Comparison of EPR spectra for various Mn(III/IV) species. Spectrum
A is the oxidized product from the reaction of $[Mn^{III/IV}_2(2\text{-OH}(5\text{-NO}_2)salpn)_2]^-$ by
hydrogen peroxide. B is the "superoxidized" inactive Mn catalase from *L. plan-
tarum*. C is the dioxo-bridged dimer $[Mn^{III/IV}(salpn)_2O_2]^-$ and D is $[Mn^{III/IV}(2\text{-}$
$OH(3,5\text{-Cl}_2)salpn)_2]^+$. (Reproduced with permission from [26].)

for the active site structure is a di-μ_2-oxo-monocarboxylato site with a
core that is similar to $[(Me_3tacn)Mn^{IV}(\mu_2\text{-O})_2(\mu\text{-OAc})Mn^{III}(OAc)_2]$ shown
in Fig. 8.

2.2.   Reactivity Models

Given the recent structural resolution of the manganese catalases, a
greater emphasis by synthetic chemists has been focused on preparing
reactivity models for the manganese catalases. Examples of binuclear

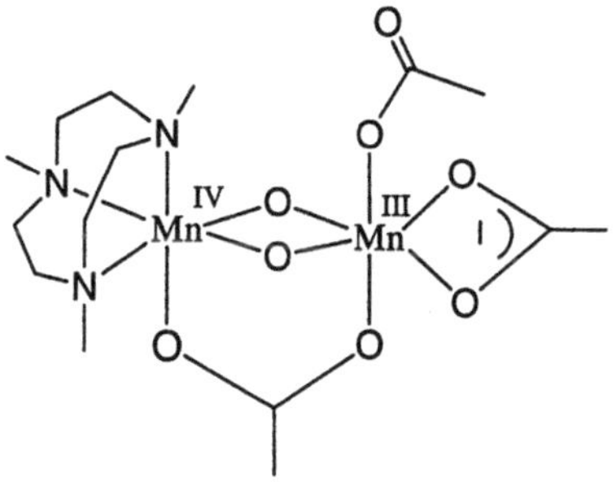

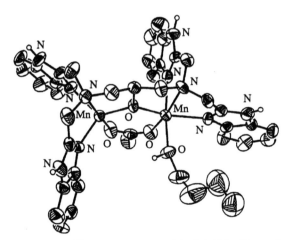

FIG. 8. $[(\text{Me}_3\text{tacn})\text{Mn}^{IV}(\mu_2\text{-}O)_2(\mu\text{-OAc})\text{Mn}^{III}(\text{OAc})_2]$.

[7,24,29–32] and tetranuclear species [33,34] capable of disproportionating hydrogen peroxide are known. Typically, these materials cycle between either the Mn(II)_2 and Mn(III)_2 oxidation levels or the Mn(III)_2 and Mn(IV)_2 states. Figure 9 shows the first effective model for the disproportionation reactions, $[\text{Mn}^{II}_2(\text{2-OHbenzimpn})(\mu\text{-OAc})]^{2+}$ [22]. This compound actually appears to be a precatalyst which, when dissolved in methanol/water mixtures, becomes the active species $[\text{Mn}^{II}_2(\text{2-OHbenzimpn})(\text{H}_2\text{O})_2]^{3+}$. The first step of the reaction has been proposed to be inner sphere coordination of peroxide followed by oxidation of the dimer to the Mn(III)_2 oxidation level. Rereduction of the Mn(III)_2 com-

FIG. 9.   Structure of $[\text{Mn}^{II}_2(\text{2-OHbenzimpn})(\mu\text{-OAc})]^{2+}$. (Reproduced with permission from [22]. Copyright 1994 the American Chemical Society.)

pound may proceed through an outer sphere, hydrogen-bonded complex. This system exhibited rates (k_{cat}) of 1.2 s^{-1}. For comparison, the T. thermophilus enzyme has k_{cat} = 2.6 × 10^5 s^{-1} and k_{cat}/K_m = 3.2 × 10^6 M^{-1} s^{-1} [3]. Nonetheless, this catalyst leads to a nearly 200-fold rate enhancement with respect to free Mn(II) in solution and is expected to be tens to hundreds of thousands fold faster than noncatalyzed peroxide disproportionation.

The most active model that cycles between the Mn(II)$_2$ and Mn(III)$_2$ oxidation levels is the [Mn(2-OH-salpn)]$_2$ system [31]. This is also the first compound that exhibited saturation kinetics with hydrogen peroxide. The k_{cat} for this system is 22 s^{-1} and k_{cat}/K_m = 350 M^{-1} s^{-1}. This places this system approximately 10 000-fold slower than the T. thermophilus enzyme; however, since the ratio for k_{cat}/K_m is also approximately 10 000, the K_m for the model system is nearly identical to that of the enzyme. The T. thermophilus enzyme is the most active manganese catalase. If one uses the kinetic constants for either the L. plantarum enzyme (k_{cat} = 2.0 × 10^5 s^{-1}; k_{cat}/K_m = 5.7 × 10^5 M^{-1} s^{-1}) [35] or the Thermoleopilum album catalase (k_{cat} = 26 000 s^{-1}; k_{cat}/K_m = 1.7 × 10^6 M^{-1} s^{-1}) [36], the success seems more impressive. Also, this model compound is as good a catalase as rat liver arginase [23]. Isotope effects on the rate (D$_2$O$_2$ vs. H$_2$O$_2$) demonstrated that hydrogen ions, either through equilibrium or kinetic isotope effects, are important for determining the rate of reaction. Unlike the previous model system, inner sphere ligation of the peroxide to both the Mn(II)$_2$ and Mn(III)$_2$ complex has been proposed. The reaction proceeds via an alkoxide shift, shown in Fig. 10, where a previously six-coordinate manganese ion can add a ligand by displacing a bridging ligand. This is directly analogous to what may occur in the enzyme where either a bridging OH$^-$, water, or carboxylate reorganizes its binding for substrate complexation. We will come back to this system later when we consider how the superoxidized Mn(III)Mn(IV) enzyme may be formed.

Wieghardt et al. have reported two different binuclear systems that have structural features that best match the enzyme [7]; however, the oxidation states of the complexes are one electron too oxidized to mimic the biological reaction. Neither compound has been reported to show saturation kinetics and therefore, comparison of k_{cat}/K_m is impossible. The rates for the system (k_{cat} = 5–13 s^{-1}) are only slightly slower than that for [Mn(2-OH-salpn)]$_2$. Other binuclear synthetic catalases are known such as an anthracene diporphyrin [32,37]. Once again, these

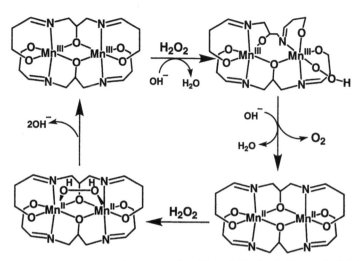

FIG. 10. Catalytic cycle between $[Mn^{II}_2(2\text{-}OHsalpn)_2]^{2-}$ and $[Mn^{III}_2(2\text{-}OHsalpn)_2]$, proposed mechanism for $[Mn^{III}_2(2\text{-}OHsalpn)_2]$ to disproportionate hydrogen peroxide to oxygen and water. (Reproduced with permission from [31]. Copyright 1998 the American Chemical Society.)

complexes do not reach the efficiency for peroxide disproportionation of $[Mn(2\text{-}OH\text{-}salpn)]_2$.

The most efficient manganese catalase mimic actually is a compound that cycles between the $Mn(IV)_2$ and $Mn(III)_2$ oxidation levels [12]. The complex is $[Mn^{IV}(salpn)(\mu_2\text{-}O)]_2$. The $k_{cat} = 250$ s^{-1} and recently it has been shown that this system can saturate $k_{cat}/K_m = 1.0 \times 10^3$ M^{-1} s^{-1}. Thus, one sees that models are now within 100–1000 of the enzymatic reactions on both k_{cat} and k_{cat}/K_m criteria. Unlike the [Mn(2-OH-salpn)]$_2$ system, which stays intact during the catalytic cycle, the first step of the reaction of $[Mn^{IV}(salpn)(\mu_2\text{-}O)]_2$ is probably outer sphere reduction to form two equivalents of $[Mn^{III}(salpn)(OH)_2]^-$ (or a related complex). The saturable intermediate is probably associated with the reformation of the Mn(IV) dimer. This mechanism was confirmed through competition experiments using isotopically labeled $H_2^{18}O_2$ [38]. While these studies are probably irrelevant for understanding the manganese catalases, this compound is potentially a model for the oxygen evolving complex (vide infra).

Before focusing on the mechanism of inactivation of the manganese catalases in the presence of hydroxylamine, we will consider the reactions of tetranuclear catalase models. The two most important are a tetramer prepared by Gorun and Stibrany, which is composed of an EDTA analog [34], bridging carboxylates and Ba^{2+} or Ca^{2+}, and a complex from our laboratory, $[Mn^{II}(2\text{-OH-picpn})]_4$. The Gorun molecule, shown as Fig. 11, is particularly interesting as it contains a central $(\mu_2\text{-}$ $O\text{-}H\text{-}\mu_2\text{-}O)^{3-}$ bridging ligand. It is tempting to speculate that these oxo and hydroxo ligands can be displaced in favor of peroxide to generate one of the catalytically active species. Despite this preformed cavity, the complex is only a moderate effective peroxide disproportionation catalyst with $k_{cat} = 1\ s^{-1}$. A far more effective tetranuclear catalyst is $[Mn^{II}(2\text{-}$ $OH\text{-picpn})]_4$ [33], shown as Fig. 12. This molecule also has a planar orientation of manganese ions and could be thought of as having the alkoxide bridges displaced during the reaction. This is the only tetramer that shows saturation behavior $(k_{cat}/K_m = 70\ M^{-1}\ s^{-1})$ and the $k_{cat} = 150$ s^{-1} is second only to $[Mn^{IV}(salpn)(\mu_2\text{-}O)]_2$.

The manganese catalase will become inactivated if the enzyme turns over in the presence of hydroxylamine [39]. It is also known that hydroxylamine in the absence of peroxide will reduce the enzyme, including the superoxidized form, to the $Mn(II)_2$ oxidation level [40]. The chemistry of both hydroxylamine and hydrogen peroxide can be quite

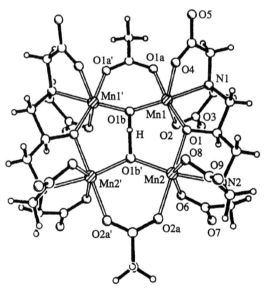

FIG. 11. Structure of $[Mn^{III}_3Mn^{II}(\mu\text{-}O)(\mu\text{-}OH)(\mu\text{-}OAc)_2(L)_3]^{2-}$, L=1,3-diamino-propan-2-ol-N,N,N',N',-tetraacetic acid. (Reproduced with permission from [34]. Copyright 1990 Wiley-VCH Verlag.)

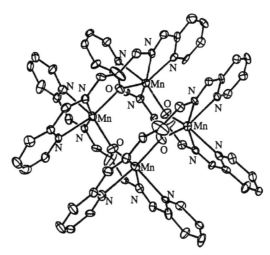

FIG. 12.   Structure of $[Mn^{II}_4(2\text{-OHpicpn})_4]^{4+}$, 2-OHpicpn is the condensation product of pyridine-2-carboxaldehyde with 1,3-diaminopropan-2-ol. (Reproduced with permission from [33]. Copyright 1996 the American Chemical Society.)

complex. In these systems, it is likely that hydrogen peroxide behaves as a two-electron oxidant or reductant while hydroxylamine functions as a one-electron reducing agent. Considering this perspective, we have used $[Mn(2\text{-OH-salpn})]_2$ to try to understand the formation of the superoxidized Mn catalase. By analogy to the enzyme, the complexes $[Mn^{III}Mn^{IV}(2\text{-OH-salpn})_2]^+$, $[Mn^{III}(2\text{-OH-salpn})]_2$ and $[Mn^{II}Mn^{III}(2\text{-OH-salpn})_2]^-$ can all be reduced by hydroxylamine to form $[Mn^{II}(2\text{-OH-salpn})]_2^{2-}$. While $[Mn^{III}(2\text{-OH-salpn})]_2$ and $[Mn^{II}(2\text{-OH-salpn})]_2^{2-}$ will react with H_2O_2 in a catalase reaction, $[Mn^{II}Mn^{III}(2\text{-OH-salpn})_2]^-$ undergoes a two-electron oxidation to form a new di-μ_2-oxo $Mn^{III}Mn^{IV}$ compound that does not carry out catalase reactions but that also can be reduced by hydroxylamine. Based on these observations, we have proposed that inactivation of the Mn catalase occurs because hydroxylamine, being a hydrogen peroxide analog, can intercept the $Mn(III)_2$ enzyme to form the Mn(II)Mn(III) form. If a second equivalent of hydroxylamine reacts with this mixed-valent protein the low oxidation state resting enzyme is recovered and the system is primed to continue turnover. However, if hydrogen peroxide reacts with the Mn(II)Mn(III) enzyme, a di-μ_2-oxo $Mn^{III}Mn^{IV}$ superoxidized enzyme, which is trapped in the higher oxidation state, results. Because reduction of the Mn(III)Mn(IV) catalase by hydroxylamine is slow, the superoxidized form accumulates and enzyme activity plummets [31].

The examples discussed above show how model compounds have made an essential contribution to our understanding of active site topology and oxidation levels, electronic structure, and chemical reactivity of the manganese catalases. The following section focuses on a more daunting challenge: photosynthetic water oxidation catalyzed by four manganese ions in the OEC.

3. THE OXYGEN EVOLVING COMPLEX

Chapters 19 and 20 provide excellent coverage of the state-of-the-art for the biophysical studies of the OEC. Readers may wish to read these chapters prior to embarking on the subsequent discussion, or at least be prepared to visit these sections in order to fortify their understanding of this complex subject. In this chapter we will attempt to address many of the major controversial issues dealing with the structure, physical properties, and reaction mechanisms that have arisen over the past 5 years. Individuals interested in the more historical development of the field since the mid-1980s should refer to references [41–45].

We can categorize the primary controversial issues in water oxidation chemistry into four main groups. *The first issue is the nuclearity and topology of the manganese cluster* that is responsible for water oxidation. Several topics are contained in this category. Is the structure of the manganese cluster invariant upon each photooxidation of the enzyme? Are the manganese ions arranged in a "dimer of dimers" motif or some other topological structure? Are chloride or calcium ions part of the structure? *The second major issue deals with cluster oxidation levels.* Here we must consider the evidence supporting or contradicting the assignment of an $Mn(III)_2Mn(IV)_2$ oxidation level for the S_1 state of the enzyme. Furthermore, there is a disagreement on the site of enzyme oxidation for at least one S-state transition. There is some support for manganese-localized oxidations; however, other workers support either protein oxidation or substrate oxidation on some of the transitions. The third subject for consideration is *the role of the redox active tyrosine Y_z and the movement of protons/H atoms during each S-state transition.* Finally, *one must assess reasonable mechanisms for forming O–O bonds using moderate valency manganese clusters.* We will discuss each topic consecutively using model compounds as a vehicle to obtain insight on these essential issues.

3.1. Manganese Oxidation Levels in the OEC

3.1.1. The S_1 Oxidation Level

The oxidation levels of the manganese in the S_1 state have been interrogated using a specific type of XAS known as XANES. The technique of XANES (X-ray absorption near-edge structure) spectroscopy provides information on oxidation state and local site symmetry by looking at the energy required to eject a core electron from a specific element of interest. Model compounds are required to calibrate the energy scale, which produces an edge energy in order to determine the oxidation states for metal centers in proteins. Figure 13 illustrates the XANES spectra of four structurally related dimeric compounds that increase in oxidation level from $Mn(II)_2$ to $Mn(III/IV)$ [data are now available for $Mn(IV)_2$ and the progression continues as predicted]. We can notice

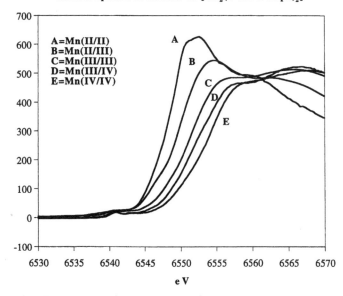

FIG. 13.   XANES spectra of the families of $[Mn_2(2\text{-OH-}x\text{-salpn})_2]^n$ ($n = 2-, 1-,$ 0, 1+, 2+).

three interesting features in the spectra. First, are the very small "bumps" in the pre-edge region. If examined closely, one would see varying energies for absorptions due to core electron to valence electron transitions. From this information one can, in theory, extract information regarding coordination number/symmetry of the Mn ions and oxidation state. We will not dwell on the information provided in this region of the XANES spectrum because often it is not analyzed in the oxygen evolution literature. The second and probably most important feature is the progressive shift to higher energy for the edge as the models are oxidized. It is the value of this edge energy that is used to assign oxidation levels for the enzyme. The way in which the edge energy is extracted from the data varies from group to group. These techniques will be commented on more fully below. The third feature of the spectrum is the progressive decrease in intensity of the edge upon a rise in oxidation state of the manganese. Compounds containing Mn(II) always contain a strong absorption at the edge. In contrast, higher oxidation states of manganese have a smoother and less intense absorption profile. While not used quantitatively, an inspection of the XANES spectrum can reveal whether Mn(II) is likely to be present in a sample.

There are at least four general methods used for extracting edge energies from a XANES spectrum [46,47]. In the integral method, the mean energy, E_{mean}, is determined using Eq. (1). Edge energy is determined by fitting the increase in the inverse of the normalized absorption $E(\mu)$ over the integration range μ_1 to μ_2. This method has the advantage of taking the shape of the edge into account.

$$E_{mean} = (\mu_2 - \mu_1) \int_{\mu_1}^{\mu_2} E(\mu)\, d\mu \tag{1}$$

An alternative approach is to calculate the second derivative spectrum and then to assign the edge energy as the first zero crossing of this plot. This method is very dependent on the smoothing functions that are required for the calculation of the second derivative. The third method frequently employed is calculating the edge energy at half-height of the normalized spectrum. Finally, there is also a report of defining the edge as the energy that corresponds to half the maximal absorption. Each method has advantages and disadvantages. Analysis of model compounds using any approach is rather straightforward; however, application to the more demanding biological samples requires greater skill.

It should be noted that workers rarely compare the absolute values of the edge energies obtained between laboratories. Rather, oxidation assignments are made with respect to structurally well-defined model compounds that have been independently subjected to XANES analysis by the same workers using the same fitting techniques as for the enzyme.

To validate this oxidation state assignment approach one must evaluate certain special cases that might cause unexpected changes in edge energies. As an example, if the XANES energy reflects average bond length rather than metal oxidation state, one might expect that an ion with lower coordination number would have an abnormally high edge energy. (In general, as one decreases the coordination number the average bond length decreases.) Thus, a five-coordinate Mn(III) might have an edge energy that more closely resembles a six-coordinate Mn(IV) than a six-coordinate Mn(III). One flaw with the early database of model compounds is that the vast majority of examined compounds had a limited range of coordination numbers for the manganese ions. There are cases now available that allow this hypothesis to be evaluated. In particular, if one looks at a five-coordinate Mn(III) model [48], shown as Fig. 14, the edge energy actually *decreases slightly* rather than increasing. Furthermore, if one considers the Mn catalase as a model for the OEC, one realizes that the oxidation levels of the catalase were correctly determined using XANES even though a recent X-ray structure has revealed that some of the Mn are five-coordinate [14]. Another potentially complicating factor for edge energy assignment is protona-

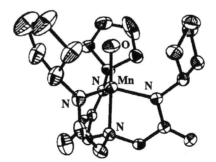

FIG. 14. Example of Mn(III)-OH five coordinate complex: [Mn^{III}(tris(cyclopropylcarbanoylmethyl)amine)OH]$^-$. (Reproduced with permission from [48]. Copyright 1997 the Royal Society of Chemistry.)

tion/deprotonation of oxo bridges. Once again, this type of reaction might change bond lengths without changing oxidation states. A detailed analysis of isostructural di-μ_2-oxo compounds that have been protonated and/or alkylated at the bridging oxo groups (i.e., [Mn^{IV}(salpn)(μ_2-O)]$_2$, {[Mn^{IV}(salpn)]$_2$(μ_2-O)(μ_2-OH)]}$^+$, and [Mn^{IV}(salpn)(μ_2-OH)]$_2^{2+}$) has shown unambiguously that the protonation state of the bridges does not significantly alter the edge energies [49].

Given the caveats described above, the different methods of analysis of edge spectra and the widely different sample preparations that have been examined, it is nothing short of miraculous that there is near-unanimity among the XAS community that the Mn oxidation states in the dark-adapted, resting form of the enzyme (S$_1$) are Mn(III)$_2$Mn(IV)$_2$. Very recently, XAS L edge spectra of models and the OEC have been acquired and these data also support this oxidation state assignment. At this point one could feel that one of the foundations of our understanding of this complex system is the oxidation state of the manganese; however, as one reads below, the clarity disappears as other S states are probed.

3.1.2. S-State Advancement: The S$_2$ Oxidation Level of the OEC

All S states other than S$_1$ are prepared by illumination or chemical reduction. Therefore, it is essential to emphasize that sample quality is an important issue when evaluating the biophysical data for the OEC. Data have been collected over the past two decades on samples as primitive as intact thylakoid membranes to highly refined core particles that contain only the essential components for water oxidation chemistry. Furthermore, with the advent of molecular biology, it has sometimes been more convenient to examine the PS II in blue-green algae, where cloning and expression is far simpler than in higher plants, rather than spinach. Not surprisingly, samples from varying organisms or obtained through alternate preparations often behave somewhat differently. Often investigators "salt-wash" their samples or extract calcium using chelating agents [42,50,51]. In other cases, reagents are added to block electron transfer and/or inhibit the enzyme (e.g., acetate or ammonia) [52–54]. Even the use of different cryoprotectants or solvents has led to perturbations of the system that are easily discernible using EPR spectroscopy [55]. The reader who is new to this field must assess whether the conclusions reached by the authors of an article rely not only on high-quality spectroscopic analysis but also with high-quality sample preparation. Even the best preparations suffer from the phenomena of double hits (advancement of two steps on a single flash) and misses (no S-state advancement upon illumination). Relatively simple formulas have been derived to account for the resultant S-state scrambling, but these are at best approximate. The use of lasers rather than xenon lamps diminishes some of these problems but they never are entirely absent. Because of double hits and misses, one often needs to subtract a background from the S state under observation. Some techniques are more sensitive to these problems. For example, XAS samples all manganese in the sample, so edge energies or Mn-Mn distances can become muddled if there is too much scrambling of S states. EPR spectra, on the other hand, may only sample a small fraction of centers that are in the appropriate oxidation level. It is our opinion that much of the controversy in the field of S-state advancement will ultimately be shown to originate from issues of sample preparation.

There is nearly universal agreement that photooxidation of the OEC leads to a manganese-centered oxidation to form the S_2 state. This statement is supported by XANES, EPR, and difference ultraviolet (UV) spectroscopies. The X-ray edge shifts by approximately 0.8 eV, which is consistent with an increase of one oxidation level for one of the four manganese ions [56]. Using the XANES assignment for S_1 [57], S_2 can be formulated as $Mn(III)Mn(IV)_3$. The S_1 state is EPR-silent at 4 K when looking at X-band frequencies with perpendicular mode detection. Depending on the temperature of illumination and/or the presence of certain anions (e.g., fluoride) [58], two different signals are observed in S_2. The first signal, which was discovered by Siderer and Dismukes [59], is centered around $g = 2$ and has greater than 16 hyperfine lines. The g value and number of hyperfine lines are suggestive of a mixed-valence manganese cluster with a spin doublet ground state. A second signal centered around $g = 4.1$ [58,60], which can be generated at the expense of the multiline intensity, has a broad derivative shape that is usually devoid of hyperfine structure. This feature has been assigned to an $S = 5/2$ spin manifold [61]. Either the $g = 2$ or $g = 4.1$ signals can, in theory, be explained by a $Mn(III)Mn(IV)_3$ assignment. It has been suggested, however, that the best way to simulate the $g = 2$ multiline EPR spectrum is to use a lower oxidation state assignment which corresponds to $Mn(III)_3Mn(IV)$ [62]. Such a formulation requires that S_1 be $Mn(III)_4$.

Many compounds have been prepared as monomers, dimers, and

tetramers to model the S_2-state EPR signals. In the mid 1980s, Vänn-gård suggested that the $g = 4.1$ and the $g = 2$ mulitline might arise from a monomeric Mn(IV) with an $S = 3/2$ electronic ground state that was isolated from a Mn dimer with an $S = 1/2$ ground state [63]. To test this hypothesis, we and others prepared monomeric Mn(IV) compounds [12,64–69] (two of which are shown in Fig. 15) and studied the EPR spectra of these complexes (Fig. 16). While all of the spin quartet systems showed features near $g = 4$ (in general, between $g = 4$ and 6), the shape and relative intensities of the monomeric Mn(IV) signals were incompatible with the $g = 4.1$ signal. Subsequently, Haddy et al. reported multifrequency EPR spectra of the $g = 4.1$ signal and concluded that this

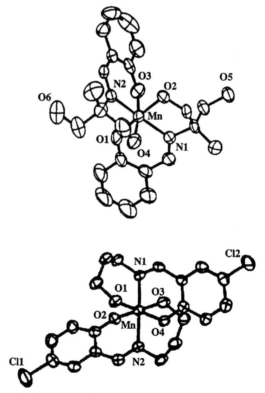

FIG. 15. Example of mononuclear Mn(IV) complexes: Mn(saladhp)$_2$ (top), sal-adhp is the condensation product of salicylaldehyde and 2-amino-2-methyl-1,3-propanediol, and Mn(5-Cl-salahp)$_2$ (bottom). (Reproduced with permission from [69]. Copyright 1989 International Union of Crystallography.)

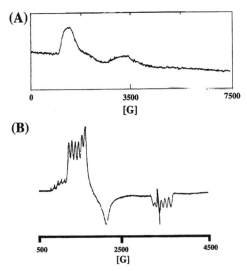

FIG. 16.   EPR spectrum of (A) Mn(saladhp)$_2$ and (B) Mn(5-Cl-salahp)$_2$.

component was due to a spin 5/2 system [61] (although there is a recent report suggesting that there are two $g = 4.1$ signals that are both generated by $S = 3/2$ centers [70]). Britt et al. later showed that this feature probably arises from a cluster of manganese ions [71] but did not specify the oxidation states for the cluster. In fact, there are many Mn clusters, with varying oxidation levels, that can give features at $g = 4.1$. Therefore, it may be difficult to assign the oxidation level of the system from this approach. In contrast, Zheng and Dismukes have used model compounds as a basis for contending that a unique coordination environment for the Mn cluster could give spin parameters [consistent with Mn(III)$_3$Mn(IV)] that simulate the $g = 2$ multiline very well [62].

3.1.3.   An Assessment of S_3 and "Split S_3" Oxidation Levels

The assignment of oxidation states for S_3 is even more contentious than that for S_2. The origin for this disagreement comes from interpretation of the XANES data. Klein et al. have reported that there is virtually no change in the XANES spectrum on the transition from S_2 to S_3 [45]. Since enzyme oxidation is occurring on this transition, this implies either that a protein residue is oxidized or that the substrate is oxidized (supporting speculation that an intermediate peroxo species could be formed in S_3). This interpretation is opposed by several scientists who claim either that the Berkeley group has not correctly accounted for hits and misses, or that their procedure for smoothing the XANES spectrum artificially overestimates the energy for the S_1-to-S_2 transition and, therefore, underestimates the S_2-to-S_3 transition. A summary of the transition energies reported by Klein et al. [72], Ono et al. [73,74], and Dau et al. [46] are given in Table 1. The most interesting observation in this table is that the greatest total edge shift ($S_0 \rightarrow S_3$) is that reported by the Berkeley group. Also provided in this table and graphically represented in Fig. 13 are edge shifts for isostructural model compounds prepared by our group, and collected and analyzed by Jim Penner-Hahn's group in Michigan, which provide a basis for comparison to the PS II. The best fit for the slope of the line for these data is 2.97 eV per oxidation state change. Since these data were obtained by examining dimers, the average change per oxidation state of the dimer is half this value (i.e., 1.49 eV) and would predict that for the tetrameric Mn center of the OEC one should see a change of ≈0.75 eV/S state change. Thus, one would predict that the total edge energy shift between S_0 and S_3 would be ≈2.25 eV. These values are in reasonable agreement with the data reported by Ono and Dau. In contrast, the early S-state energy changes reported by the Berkeley group would appear too large to correspond to a single manganese oxidation. The total change also is greater than would be predicted using this analysis.

Obviously proper assignments of cluster oxidation states is of major importance for understanding the mechanism of water oxidation. Unfortunately, this controversy has not been resolved using EPR spectroscopy. Those workers supporting a manganese-centered oxidation emphasize that the $g = 2$ multiline is not apparent in S_3, suggesting that a nonintegral, EPR-silent state is formed. Proponents of substrate or protein oxidation counter that a protein or substrate radical in close proximity to the manganese cluster could enhance the relaxation of the paramagnet responsible for the multiline, making it invisible. There is a recent report of an S_3 EPR signal detected in parallel mode, suggesting that the center responsible for the feature is a non-Kramer ion [75]. If true, this would provide additional support for a manganese-centered oxidation since it is unlikely that a multiline signal would be relaxed under these conditions whereas a metal-centered low-field signal would be unperturbed. Difference UV experiments also support the notion that

TABLE 1

Perturbation of Edge Energies (in eV) upon Mn Oxidation

OEC

S_{-1}	Δ	S_0 6550.1	Δ	S_1 6551.7	Δ	S_2 6553.5	Δ	S_3 6553.8	Interpretation	Ref.
			1.6		1.8		0.3		No oxidation of Mn on $S_2 \to S_3$	Klein et al. [72]
			1.0		0.8		1.2		Δ_{Total} $S_0 \to S_3$ = 3.7 eV. Mn-centered oxidation on each S-state transition	Ono et al. [73,74]
			0.8–1.5		0.5–0.9		0.6–1.3		Δ_{Total} $S_0 \to S_3$ = 3.0 eV. Mn-centered oxidation on each S-state transition	Dau et al. [46]
	6546.2	6546.9	0.7	6547.4	0.5	6547.9	0.5		Δ_{Total} $S_0 \to S_3$ = 2.3–3.1 eV. Mn-centered oxidation on each S-state transition measured. Δ_{Total} $S_0 \to S_3$ = 1.7 eV	Yocum/Penner-Hahn [95]

Isostructural dimeric model compounds

II_2	Δ	II/III	Δ	III_2	Δ	III/IV	Δ	IV_2	Interpretation	Ref.
	1.53		1.69		0.95		1.97		Predicted magnitude for tetramer	Pecoraro/Penner-Hahn [95]
	0.76		0.84		0.48		0.98			

Mn is oxidized in S_3 [76]. Comparison of the electronic spectra of model compounds in different oxidation states is consistent with this interpretation of S-state transitions.

There are model compounds that address many of the possible structures associated with S_3. These will be presented in more detail below; however, one that is particularly relevant at this juncture is shown in Fig. 17. Assuming that a peroxo intermediate is formed upon formation of S_3, one can examine the peroxo dimer (Fig. 17) reported by Wieghardt et al. as a model for such a structure within a "dimer of dimers" motif [77]. The bridging peroxide in this molecule causes a shortening of the Mn-Mn vector to 2.531 Å. As we will see in the following section on nuclearity of the cluster, this is inconsistent with EXAFS data for S_3. This work shows that if a peroxo intermediate is formed, it is highly unlikely that it forms across the face of a di-μ_2-oxo dimer.

Proper S-state advancement can be blocked on the $S_2 \rightarrow S_3$ transition by treatment of samples with high levels of EGTA or acetate to inhibit electron transfer [78–81]. Under these circumstances an EPR feature known as the "split S_3" signal appears that is assigned to an organic radical [76,82]. This signal was initially thought to be an imidazole radical but was subsequently shown to be the redox-active tyrosine (Y_z) that is responsible for the initial oxidation step of the manganese cluster [83–85]. Analysis of the signal has now placed Y_z within approximately 8 Å of the Mn cluster [86]. The proximity of Y_z to the manganese ions has led to the suggestion that the OEC is one of a growing

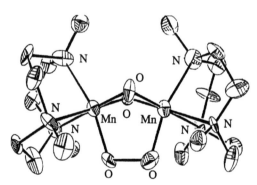

FIG. 17.   Structure of $\{[Mn^{IV}(tacn)_2](\mu\text{-}O)_2(\mu\text{-}O_2)\}$. (Reproduced with permission from [77]. Copyright 1990 the American Chemical Society.)

class of metalloradical enzymes. It has also encouraged research into model compounds that have imidazole or phenolate radicals that are bound directly to manganese. In every case studied, models with phenolate radicals bound to manganese have a strong absorption in the 400-nm region of the visible spectrum [87]. Such a feature is not observed in the PS II, which further demonstrates that the tyrosyl radical generated through oxidation by the reaction center is not forming an inner sphere complex with the manganese cluster. Imidazole radicals bound to manganese are much more difficult to synthesize and it is unclear if any models have truly been prepared for these systems. There is now some interest in developing model compounds that contain manganese and a pendent phenol that might be independently oxidized to a phenolate radical to test many of the ideas for electron and proton flow in the PS II.

It should be emphasized that all of the biophysical studies on this "split S_3" state do not correspond to functional enzyme and, therefore, do not provide support for the idea that a protein radical is generated in S_3. The authors of this article presently prefer the argument that oxidation of the OEC to form S_3 occurs at the manganese center.

3.1.4. S States Below S_1: S_0 and S_{-1}

Lower S states can be prepared by chemical reduction or by trapping S_0 after dioxygen is released [88–90]. The addition of hydroxylamine or hydrazine to the S_1 state of the OEC leads to a two-electron reduced enzyme referred to as the S_{-1} state [91–93]. Under certain conditions when S_{-1} is generated [94], the resultant XANES energy and EPR spectra are inconsistent with the formation of Mn(II). This observation is of profound importance since it should be impossible to reduce an S_1 state with oxidation levels Mn(III)$_3$Mn(IV) to the S_{-1} level without generating at least one Mn(II) ion. This provides strong evidence supporting the S_1 oxidation state assignment of Mn(III)Mn(IV)$_3$. Another interesting conclusion from these studies is that hydroxylamine apparently reduces a different set of manganese ions than does hydroquinone. This differential reactivity of the manganese ions has been taken as supporting a dimer-of-dimers structure for the active site cluster; however, this observation can easily be consistent with other manganese topologies.

In the past 2 years, EPR signals have been observed for the S_0 enzyme oxidation level. In the presence of methanol, a multiline feature at $g = 2$ can be detected [88,89]. The breadth of the S_0 signal is significantly greater than the multiline feature found in S_2, which is consistent with a more reduced manganese cluster. XANES studies of this enzyme level indicate that Mn(II) is present in the catalytically active form of S_0 [95]. This leads to an interesting conundrum since a one-electron reduction of S_1 should lead to 13 positive charges distributed among 4 manganese ions. The simplest case would give Mn(III)$_3$Mn(IV). However, Mn(II) is not included in the formulation; therefore, the required alternative is Mn(II)Mn(III)Mn(IV)$_2$. This triple-valence cluster has fueled speculation that possibly only two of the four manganese ions are oxidized over the entire catalytic cycle. Also, it has been suggested that there are spatially separated but magnetically communicating Mn(II)Mn(III) and Mn(IV)Mn(IV) dimers in S_0.

Conclusions drawn from the study of model compounds have the capability of resolving some of these issues. It is well known that the multiline features associated with Mn(II)Mn(III) dimers have a larger spectral width than for the more oxidized Mn(III)Mn(IV) species. Different Mn(III)Mn(IV) dimers (shown previously in Fig. 7) can have very different Heisenberg exchange parameters and chemical structures. The one constant is that the spectral range covers from 1100 to 1250 G. In contrast, Mn(II)Mn(III) dimers typically have spectral widths on the order of 1450 G. These observations are consistent with the formulation of a lower oxidation state for S_0; however, they also indicate that the large spectral width of the S_0 state is unlikely to result from an isolated Mn(II)Mn(III) dimer. Therefore, one minimally will need a trimeric arrangement of manganese to begin simulating the S_0 multiline. The EPR spectrum of a Mn(III)Mn(II)Mn(III) trimeric compound [20] is compared to the S_0 multiline in Fig. 18. There is remarkable agreement between both the total spectral width and the individual hyperfine spacings. This is the first model compound to accurately reproduce the spectral features of S_0; however, it may be possible that other nuclearities or oxidation state combinations will also lead to reasonably similar spectra. Nonetheless, this once again shows the apparent inconsistencies with which one is faced when comparing conclusions based on EPR and XANES measurements.

Another possible inconsistency that one encounters using the XANES-determined oxidation states for S_1 and the requirement of a

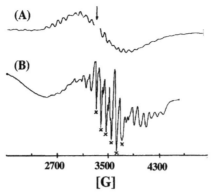

FIG. 18. Comparison of the EPR spectra of OEC S_0-state (A) and β-[$Mn^{III}_2Mn^{II}$(saladhp)$_2$-(OAc)$_4$](CH$_3$OH)$_2$ (B). Resonances identified with an × are due to a small amount of Mn(II) impurity.

cluster containing four manganese to give the appropriate S_0 EPR signal is that Mn(II), Mn(III), and Mn(IV) must all exist within the same structure. There are many examples of small-molecule manganese systems that engage in either disproportionation [i.e., 2 Mn(III) → Mn(II) + Mn(IV)] or comproportionation [Mn(II) + Mn(IV)) → 2 Mn(III)] chemistries. There is only one stable compound known to contain manganese where the Mn(II), Mn(III), and Mn(IV) oxidation levels coexist. This molecule, prepared by the Armstrong group [96], is shown in Fig. 19. The core is a mixed-valence Mn(III)Mn(IV) dimer that has Mn(II) ions bound to either end of the molecule. This demonstrates that such a triple-valence compound can exist; however, one must be careful when extrapolating this result to the PS II. The Armstrong tetramer has distinct environments for the Mn(II) ions that do not allow for further oxidation, which leads to stabilization of the three oxidation levels. There is no evidence that the Mn(II) in this model complex can be oxidized to form a related higher oxidation state assembly. In contrast, the Mn(II) in the OEC must be oxidized minimally to the Mn(III) level and possibly as high as Mn(V)! This means that the chemical environment of the Mn(II) in the OEC must be capable of supporting at least one, probably two, and possibly three oxidations at this site. Thus, it would seem unlikely that such a site in the PS II would not be susceptible to a comproportionation reaction generating the Mn(III)$_3$Mn(IV) oxidation level (this is especially true since reduction of Mn(IV)$_2$ → Mn(III)Mn(IV) dimers occurs with little structural reorganization). This might then

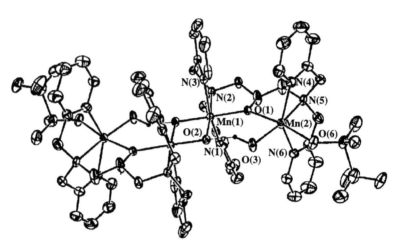

FIG. 19. Structure of the tetranuclear manganese-oxo complex, $[Mn_4O_2(tphpn)_2(H_2O)_2(CF_3SO_3)_2]^{3+}$, tphpn = N,N,N',N',-tetrakis(2-pyridyl-methyl)-2-hydroxypropane-1,3-diamine. (Reproduced with permission from [96]. Copyright 1990 the American Chemical Society.)

argue for the lower oxidation state assignment or for separated redox centers in S_0.

To summarize this section on cluster oxidation state, we see that the two major issues of contention are the absolute oxidation level of the cluster and the site of oxidation upon S state progression. XAS and biochemical studies support an oxidation state for S_1 that is $Mn(III)_2Mn(IV)_2$. EPR spectra are often better interpreted to give $Mn(III)_4$ for S_1. Both workers in XAS and EPR spectroscopies agree that S_0 contains Mn(II); however, this provides certain limitations relating to structure or redox state of this lowest catalytically active enzyme oxidation level. While there is universal agreement that the transitions from S_0 to S_1 to S_2 are manganese-centered, debate continues on the S_2 → S_3 transition. Our research group, while still open to discussion, favors an oxidation state progression as shown below. The following section will attempt to combine this oxidation state framework with a manganese topology to provide a unified view of the water-oxidizing catalyst.

S_0:Mn(II)Mn(III)Mn(IV)$_2$ S_1:Mn(III)$_2$Mn(IV)$_2$
S_2:Mn(III)Mn(IV)$_3$ S_3:Mn(IV)$_4$ S_4:Mn(IV)$_3$Mn(V)

3.2. Nuclearity and Topology of the Manganese Cluster

3.2.1. A Brief Background

The previous section described attempts to define the oxidation levels of manganese in the OEC. In this section, the specific orientations and distances between the manganese atoms will be considered. The reader should be warned that many of the conclusions from the previous section were dependent on assumptions for the nuclearity and organization of the manganese. For example, if there were two separate dimers or a monomer and a trimer organization of metal centers, then the necessary restrictions on oxidation state to form $S = 1/2$ or $S = 5/2$ would be altered. However, just as one cannot talk intelligently about oxidation state without having a model for nuclearity, many of the nuclearity models are in fact dependent on the chosen oxidation states. This interrelatedness between electron count and structure is often at the heart of debates on the functioning of the OEC. Thus, the reader may gain deeper insight into this problem by rereading the previous section after the following section has been digested.

3.2.2. Manganese Topology in S_1

In the previous section we saw the important application of XANES spectroscopy to provide oxidation state for the manganese in the active site cluster. The technique of EXAFS (extended X-ray absorption fine structure) spectroscopy provides metrical information and the number and types of ligands bound to manganese. As in XANES spectroscopy, one obtains an average over all of the manganese centers. While XANES has been the preferred method to establish oxidation states of the manganese ions, EXAFS has been the primary tool to establish the topology of atoms in the Mn cluster. Just as with XANES, EXAFS requires a range of appropriate model compounds to interpret the scattering. Many of these compounds have been reviewed previously and so will not be described in detail herein.

The EXAFS values of S_1 have variously been interpreted to show three shells of scatterers [45,95,97,98]. The first shell corresponds to light atom scatterers found at distances (1.75–1.9 Å) that are consistent with inner sphere oxygen or nitrogen ligation. The EXAFS values are inconsistent with a bound sulfur atom and are inconclusive when evaluating chloride ligands. The second shell has approximately 1.3 Mn-metal scatterers at 2.71 Å. This 2.7-Å distance is the hallmark of $Mn(III)Mn(IV)(\mu_2-O)_2$ or $[Mn(IV)(\mu_2-O)]_2$ diamond cores. Because no other transition metals are thought to be part of the manganese cluster, because calcium is too light a scatterer to provide the appropriate intensity, and because of the excellent correlation of this distance to model manganese compounds with the di-μ-oxo core, most workers in the field have accepted the proposition that there are two $Mn_2(\mu_2-O)_2$ dimers in S_1. A third shell at 3.3 Å (0.5 metals/Mn) has been reproduced by all of the EXAFS groups studying the OEC. This scatterer has been associated with another Mn at 3.3 Å, as well as carbon atoms from ligands such as imidazole and/or Ca(II).

An important lesson learned from model chemistry is that it is very difficult to obtain an Mn-Mn separation as short as 2.7 Å without accommodating both structural and oxidation state constraints. First, there are no known molecules with an Mn-Mn separation at 2.73 Å or below that have Mn in an oxidation state below Mn(III) and that do not contain at least one of the metals as a Mn(IV). Given this observation, it seems highly unlikely that the EPR-derived oxidation levels for S_1 [Mn(III)$_4$] can be correct. Second, all Mn compounds with a distance of 2.7 Å or shorter contain at least two μ_2-O^{2-} or μ_3-O^{2-} bridges. Also based on model chemistry, for the oxo bridges to be protonated (μ_2-OH^-) one would expect that a third bridging group would be necessary to reach the very short observed Mn-Mn distances. The Mn-Mn 3.3-Å distance is best achieved using the μ_2-O^{2-}, bis-carboxylato motif that is well established in the Mn catalases and many binuclear iron enzymes such as hemerythrin, methane monooxygenase, and ribonucleotide reductase [3,5,99,100].

When interpreting EXAFS results, it is important to look both at the Mn-scatterer distance and the average number of scatterers at that distance. Because the distances come from the frequency of the EXAFS, one can obtain high-precision values for Mn-X distances; however, since the number of scatterers comes from the amplitude of the scattering, the error associated with the number of scatterers at a distance is much greater [101]. Figure 20 is provided to explain the implication of the number of scatterers at a specified distance. Eight distinct structures are shown that either have been or could be considered as appropriate

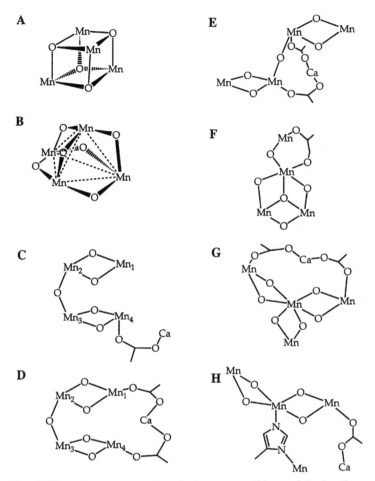

FIG. 20.   Different manganese topologies as possible models for the oxygen evolving complex.

topologies for the manganese ions. It should be realized that many other topologies will satisfy the EXAFS requirements. Furthermore, the eight given in Fig. 20 are written in two dimensions, a necessity not imposed on the protein.

Figure 20A–D have all appeared as possible models for the OEC. The first tetranuclear model was the cubane [102] shown as structure A. In a symmetric cubane, there are six edges of an inscribed tetrahedron that relate the Mn ions at 2.7 Å. It is obvious that each Mn ion sees three other Mn atoms, not 1.3/Mn as is observed experimentally, which excludes the symmetric cubane as a viable structure. A similar argument can be made for the adamantane structure [103] shown as structure B since the Mn ions are again arranged according to a tetrahedron. In this case, there are six μ_2-O^{2-} bridges that connect the four Mn across the tetrahedral edges. The number of scatterers per Mn becomes a bit harder to calculate when one considers the dimer-of-dimers model. To obtain an accurate count, we must account for the number of Mn atoms at a specified distance from all other manganese atoms and then divide by the total number of manganese atoms. Thus, in structure C Mn_1 is 2.7 Å from Mn_2 and 3.3 Å from Mn_3. This accounting of the scatterers from Mn_1 gives one scatterer at 2.7 Å and one at 3.3 Å. There is only one relevant scatterer (Mn_1) near Mn_2 at 2.7 Å. Looking at Mn_3, there is Mn_1 at 3.3 Å and Mn_4 at 2.7 Å. Finally we evaluate Mn_4 to see a single 2.7-Å vector to Mn_3 and an Mn-Ca vector at 3.3 Å. Although the scattering power is different between Ca and Mn, the calcium will contribute significantly to the EXAFS. Notice that we do not count scatterers from calcium for evaluating Mn EXAFS. This totals to four Mn-Mn scatterers at 2.7 Å and three Mn-M (Mn or Ca) scatterers at 3.3 Å. Since EXAFS provides an average value, we must divide by 4 yielding the final values of 1.0 Mn at 2.7 Å and 0.75 metals at 3.3 Å. The errors associated with this stoichiometry are usually within about 25%, putting these values at the edge of the acceptable range. This approach works, as it must, for models 20A and 20B, which was the basis for excluding these structures. Structure D, the most recent offering for cluster structure from the Berkeley group [104], gives the same number of scatterers at 2.7 Å (1.0) but increases the number of scatterers at 3.3 Å (1.0), which would suggest that this is actually a poorer fit to the data. Structure E is a rotational isomer in which the dimer of dimers is rotated 180° out of phase. The structures that have yet to be considered seriously by the PS II community are shown as Fig. 20F–H. These structures have the virtue of satisfying the EXAFS parameters equivalently as well as the dimers-of-dimers model while providing an opportunity to explain the magnetic properties of the system better. Both structures F and G give 1.5 scatterers at 2.7 Å and predict 0.5 scatterer at 3.3 Å. These values are equal to or better than the other models being considered. Figure 20H provides a very speculative topology that has one 2.7-Å distance and 0.25 scatter at 3.3 Å.

Our understanding of the EPR spectra of S_1 is still in its infancy. In 1992, Dexheimer and Klein reported a new EPR signal ($g \approx 5$) that was observed at this enzyme oxidation level using parallel mode detection [105], a technique that interrogates integral spin systems. While this broad, low-field signal could not provide information capable of resolving oxidation states of the cluster, it may provide insight for cluster nuclearity. Armstrong and Chan have prepared a tetranuclear species that has the same breadth as the S_1 signal [106]. In addition, we have made monomeric model compounds recently that also show similar spectra. Upon illumination of the sample that contains this broad EPR signal, the S_2 state is formed. In theory, the Dexheimer S_1 signal could be a precursor to either the $g = 4.1$ multiline or the $g = 2$ multiline. Dexheimer showed that the S_1 signal could coexist with the $g = 4.1$ signal but not the multiline feature, suggesting that the S_1 signal was a precursor to the multiline. The implications of this observation are profound because they require that the centers that generate the $g = 4.1$ and $g = 2$ multiline are not the same. Furthermore, the centers must be sufficiently separated so as not to perturb one another. If this is true, the manganese cluster cannot be tetranuclear! These experiments have been criticized as being nonreproducible or resulting from a dioxygen impurity. However, Kawamori et al. have recently reproduced these results, suggesting that more merit must be placed on this observation and its implications [107].

In 1997, Britt and co-workers discovered yet another parallel mode-detected EPR signal in *Synechocystis*, a photosynthetic blue-green algae [108]. The spectrum is shown in Fig. 21. In this case, the multiple hyperfine lines and the magnitude of the hyperfine separations conclusively implicate a manganese cluster as the origin of the resonance. An issue that has not yet been addressed is whether the same discrimination between the production of the S_2 $g = 2$ multiline vs. $g = 4.1$ signal is seen as for the Dexheimer S_1 signal. In collaboration with the Britt group, we are now examining model compounds that have spectra that are closely similar to that shown here. Through model studies such as these, it is hoped that the oxidation state and topology of the manganese cluster in S_1 will be elucidated.

3.2.3. Manganese Topology in S_2

The EXAFS spectra of S_2 are virtually unchanged from that of S_1 [109,110]. Furthermore, there is little difference between the EXAFS of an S_2, $g = 2$ multiline sample and an S_2, $g = 4.1$ signal [111]. Thus, the same structural arguments that were outlined in the previous section

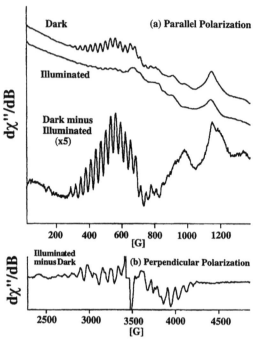

FIG. 21.   (a) Parallel polarized EPR spectrum of the S_1-state multiline signal.
Dark represents a dark-adapted PS II sample, S_1 state. Followed by illumination, the S_1 state oxidized to S_2 state. The Dark minus illuminated difference
spectrum yielded a well-resolved multiline signal arising from a multinuclear
exchange coupled paramagnetic Mn cluster. (b) Perpendicular polarized EPR
difference spectrum of the illuminated minus Dark spectra (the S_2-state multiline is observed). (Reproduced with permission from [108]. Copyright 1998 the
American Chemical Society.)

for S_1 apply to both forms of S_2. However, unlike S_1 where EPR signals
have only recently been discovered, it has been nearly two decades since
the $g = 2$ multiline was discovered. Therefore, tremendous effort has
been expended to simulate this signal and to prepare model compounds
that reproduce the EPR spectrum. There have been reported excellent
simulations of the spectra [62,112]; however, the best either require oxidation states that contradict XAS and biochemically derived oxidation
states or require very special sets of hyperfine parameters to match the
spectrum well. Furthermore, we know from a comparison of the EXAFS
that the configuration that leads to the multiline is very similar to that

for the $g = 4.1$ signal [111]. Since there are no major structural changes upon this spectroscopic conversion, the metal topology and oxidation states of the cluster must also be able to rationalize the $g = 4.1$ signal.

While one often sees models for water oxidation presented using the dimer of dimers as the structural basis for discussion, it is highly unlikely that this organization of manganese ions accurately describes the active site of the OEC. This somewhat controversial statement is based on the simple consideration of magnetic properties of the cluster. The standard coupling scheme used to explain the $S = 1/2$ ground state of the S_2 dimer-of-dimers topology is shown as Fig. 22. The first dimer has Mn(III) strongly antiferromagnetically coupled to a Mn(IV) giving an $S = 1/2$ ground state. The second dimer contains two Mn(IV) ions that are presumed to be strongly antiferromagnetically coupled. Many model compounds support this contention. In fact, we have recently shown that there is a reasonable correlation between the Mn-O-Mn angle and the Heisenberg exchange coupling constant for Mn(IV) compounds that have metal-metal separations between 2.65 and 2.78 Å [113]. This Mn-Mn separation completely brackets the distances reported for the Mn ions in the OEC. What we have seen is that these compounds will always be antiferromagnetically coupled to give an $S = 0$ ground state. Because it is expected that exchange interactions between Mn connected in an oxo-carboxylato bridging motif are smaller than that of the di-μ_2-oxo dimers, one has the resultant $S = 1/2$ system by coupling $S = 1/2$ of dimer 1 with $S = 0$ of dimer 2. While this analysis works exceptionally well to explain the doublet state that gives the multiline signal, it does not allow for a ground state $S = 5/2$ formulation that is needed to generate the $g = 4.1$ signal. This conclusion is reached because dimer 2 will always have an $S = 0$ ground state. An $S = 5/2$ can only result from this topology if the dimer 2 has two Mn(IV) ions that are fer-

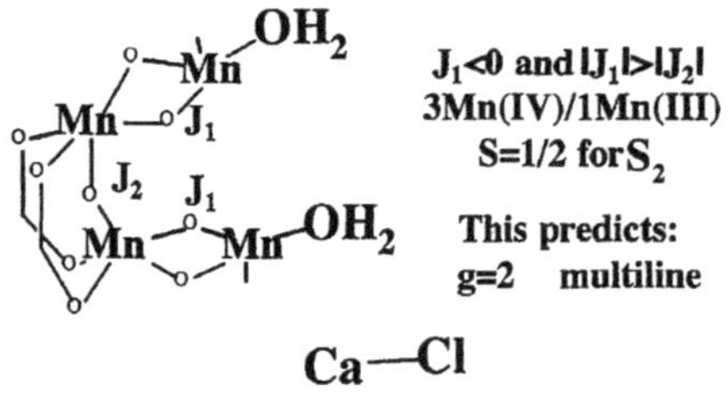

$J_1 < 0$ and $|J_1| > |J_2|$
3Mn(IV)/1Mn(III)
$S = 1/2$ for S_2

This predicts:
$g = 2$ multiline

Ca—Cl

FIG. 22.   A magnetic model for the S_2 state of the OEC.

romagnetically coupled forming an $S = 3$ system. This $S = 3$ could couple with dimer 1 antiferromagnetically to give an $S = 5/2$ ground state. The model compounds described above strongly refute this possibility. Therefore, we conclude that the cluster topology that gives the $g = 4.1$ signal cannot be a dimer-of-dimers containing Mn(III)Mn(IV)$_3$. Furthermore, the fact that the EXAFS of the cluster in the forms giving the $g = 2$ multiline and $g = 4.1$ are essentially identical suggests that the topology for the $g = 2$ multiline form also is not a dimer of dimers. One should recognize that the newest dimer of dimers model (see Fig. 27 below) that contains a calcium ion bridging the two di-μ_2-O dimers [104] is also fatally flawed for identical reasons (the coupling between the outer manganese will for all practical purposes be zero).

There are now two obvious questions to consider. The first is whether the dimer-of-dimers topology can be salvaged if the oxidation states are Mn(III)$_3$Mn(IV) rather than Mn(III)Mn(IV)$_3$. If not, then what is the proper topology? We have already commented on the problems with this oxidation level assignment in the previous section; however, we will spend a moment to reconsider some important issues here. Model compounds have demonstrated that it is very difficult, if not impossible, to place two Mn atoms at less than 2.8 Å unless one of the manganese ions is in the Mn(IV) oxidation level. Therefore, a low oxidation state assignment does not make sense (this is particularly true when the lower S states are considered). If one assumes that the Mn(III)Mn(IV) dimer is again antiferromagnetically coupled, one retains one dimer with an $S = 1/2$ spin. A diamagnetic dimer formed by antiferromagnetically coupled Mn(III) ions ($S = 2$) would reproduce the $g = 2$ multiline ground state. Zheng and Dismukes have shown that this oxidation set can be used to give excellent simulations of the multiline EPR signal [62], albeit with rather nonstandard single-ion hyperfine coupling constants. If the Mn(III) dimer is ferromagnetically coupled, then interaction with the $S = 1/2$ dimer should lead to $S = 7/2$ (antiferromagnet interaction) or $S = 9/2$ (ferromagnetic) interaction. Once again, neither is consistent with an $S = 5/2$ ground state. The only way to obtain an $S = 5/2$ state is to propose an intermediate spin dimer, yet this is unlikely to give a ground state signal and has never been observed in models. Therefore, we conclude that the dimer-of-dimers model also fails with the lower oxidation state assignments.

There is no unique topological answer to our question even when considering the EXAFS results and the magnetic behavior of the cluster. Many tetrameric formulations would satisfy these criteria. The minimal topology is probably a spin-frustrated trimeric center that is exchange-coupled to a monomeric species. The trimer of $Mn(III)Mn(IV)_2$ could be $S = 1$ which, when coupled appropriately to a $Mn(IV)$ ion ($S = 3/2$), yields either an $S = 1/2$ (antiferromagnetic) or $S = 5/2$ (ferromagnetic) cluster.

3.2.4.   Manganese Topology in S_0 and S_3

EXAFS data are now being accumulated on other S states including S_3 and S_0 [45]. Before discussing these results, it is important to reiterate how these data are obtained. Since S_3 cannot be prepared in 100% purity, one must use a subtraction process to extract the EXAFS for this oxidation level. The magnitude of the extraction depends on functional centers and the number of double hits/misses using the $g = 2$ multiline as an estimate of the proportion of centers that have reached S_2. Thus, it is quite possible to have a mixture of three oxidation levels that must be deconvoluted. Under such daunting circumstances, it is difficult to truly evaluate the meaning of increased disorder that is observed. With this caveat in mind, it appears that there is an increase (2.87 Å) in at least one of the Mn-Mn vectors upon oxidation to S_3. This is completely counterintuitive since Mn-Mn separations generally decrease as the oxidation state is increased. The only obvious way to account for this change is to suggest a major cluster structural change. This 2.87-Å separation is a curious distance since most manganese model compounds have Mn-Mn separations that fall in the range of distances 2.75 Å or less or 3.0 Å or greater. One group of compounds in the 2.85-Å range are the singly protonated di-μ_2-oxo dimers. However, it is difficult to reconcile both the oxidation of the manganese cluster and accumulation of a second positive charge by protonation of an oxo bridge. Because these data are at their early stage, it is probably best to leave any further interpretation for the future.

The EXAFS of S_0 (and lower oxidation states) have usually been collected on chemically treated samples using reductants such as hydroxylamine or hydroquinone. Because treating samples with these reagents can lead to overreduction, the data that have been accumulated are often controversial. The S_0^* Mn EXAFS were reported in 1990 by Klein and coworkers on PS II samples treated with hydroxylamine [114]. The S_0^* refers to a hydroxylamine-induced state that is at the same oxidation level as the normal S_0. The authors see a change in the two 2.7-Å distances to one 2.7-Å and one 2.87-Å. This is consistent with Mn(II) being present in S_0. A 1996 paper by Yocum, Penner-Hahn, et al. demonstrated differential reduction of S_1 by hydroquinone and hydroxylamine [95]. Under appropriate conditions, both reductants could reduce the OEC to S_{-1}; however, the resulting oxidation states of the manganese, and the corresponding EXAFS, are markedly different. Hydroquinone reduction yielded a sample that was best described as an $Mn(II)_2Mn(IV)_2$. The 2.7-Å scatterer was diminished by half, which is consistent with the destruction of one di-μ_2-O dimer. In contrast, hydroxylamine reduction leads to a state best described as $Mn(III)_4$ with no perturbation in the 2.7-Å scatterer. Possibly the most important aspect of this work is that both samples can be illuminated to regenerate active enzyme. The differential reduction properties described here support a dimer-of-dimers model. However, due to the wide range in EXAFS precision for coordination number, other structural models can be made consistent with these data.

3.2.5. Protein Ligands Bound to Manganese

The D1 and D2 polypeptides were originally thought to form the locus of manganese binding sites to the enzyme [115–120]. Several groups have been involved in preparing site-directed mutations in both of these proteins. Extensive mutagenesis studies have now shown that D2 probably does not provide any of the ligands to the manganese cluster. However, site mutations in D1 have led to several reasonable candidates that are implicated either in cluster assembly or directly as Mn ligands. Chief among these is imidazole, although it is likely that carboxylates are also metal ligands (especially to calcium). Recent Fourier transform infrared (FT-IR) studies provide direct evidence for carboxylate coordination to manganese [121]; however, the analysis has not discerned whether these ligands are monodentate/bidentate or, in the latter case, whether they bridge two manganese ion and, if so, how? Because manganese carboxylate chemistry is rather well defined in other reviews [122,123], we will focus herein primarily on models for imidazole ligation. It should also be remembered that tyrosine Y_z is probably very close (approximately 8 Å) [86] to the manganese cluster and may form an outer sphere interaction with water coordinated to manganese. While many workers are attempting to append noncoordinated tyrosines or phenols to manganese clusters, this work has not developed sufficiently to warrant inclusion here. Those readers interested in phenolate radicals bound directly to metal ions are encouraged to examine the recent papers by Wieghardt et al. on this subject [87].

Experiments that demonstrated imidazole ligation to the manganese ions used a combination of approaches including site-directed mutagenesis, isotopic enrichment, and spectroscopic studies. The ENDOR studies demonstrated that two chemically different nitrogens were bound to manganese, suggesting one of two chemical models [124]. In the first, manganese would be bound using two different histidine ligands that used γ and ε N of the imidazole ring, respectively. An alternative interpretation is that a single histidine is involved in metal complexation. In this model, the ligand is imidazolate and binds in a manner analogous to the Cu/Zn superoxide dismutases [125]. The model utilizing two different histidines would suggest a more common ligation type that is found in many nonheme dinuclear iron and manganese enzymes. The bridging imidazolate model has the virtue of clarifying many of the magnetic properties that have so far defied explanation. For example, one could have a monomeric ion linked to a trinuclear manganese oxo aggregate. Such a species could explain the magnetic properties of the system and also explain the presence of multiple EPR features at different S states.

While there are relatively few manganese compounds that have coordinated imidazole groups, many complexes have been prepared with aromatic nitrogen donors such as pyrazoles or pyridine. One example of a manganese cluster with bound imidazole, prepared by Christou's group [126], is shown in Fig. 23. Generally speaking, imidazole compounds tend to favor lower oxidation states of manganese and are poorer ligands than oxo anions from oxide-, hydroxide-, phenolate-, or alkoxide-bearing ligands. Imidazole appears to be a slightly better ligand than water for manganese. The bond lengths of these compounds are unremarkable compared with those of other nitrogen donors. In no case has nitrogen superhyperfine been observed in a continuous wave EPR experiment for model complexes containing imidazole or other nitrogenous ligands. Thus, unlike copper complexes, facile identification of nitrogen ligands to manganese using EPR spectroscopy requires pulsed EPR technology. Until recently, there were no reports of bridg-

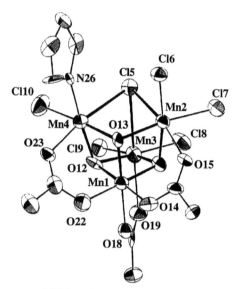

FIG. 23.   Structure of $(H_2Im)_2[Mn_4O_3Cl_6(O_2CCH_3)_3(HIm)]$, an example of imidazole bound to a manganese cluster. (Reproduced with permission from [126].
Copyright 1992 the American Chemical Society.)

ing imidazolate complexes with manganese. Figure 24 illustrates the
first example of this molecular class of compound using the dicarboxy-
imidazole ligand [127]. This compound was the first EPR-active Mn(IV)$_2$
which dispelled the dogma that all Mn(IV) dimers would be highly exchange-coupled and, therefore, EPR-silent. Analysis of subsequent vari-
able-temperature magnetic measurements allowed a model for the
magnetic behavior to be developed which utilized a small, antiferromagnetic Heisenberg exchange parameter. This system shows that coupled Mn(IV) cluster can, with the proper ligand set, exhibit the weak
magnetic exchange that may be requisite to explain the magnetic phenomena of the OEC Mn cluster. We have now prepared dimers with
bridging imidazole with Mn(III)$_2$ and Mn(III)Mn(IV) oxidation levels.
Once again, these compounds are weakly exchange-coupled and exhibit
EPR spectra that are distinct from the large catalogue of spectra
amassed with other bridging ligands.

3.2.6.   Substrate Binding to the Manganese Cluster

The first evidence for direct water ligation to the manganese cluster
came from kinetic studies [128,129]. Among the most important of these

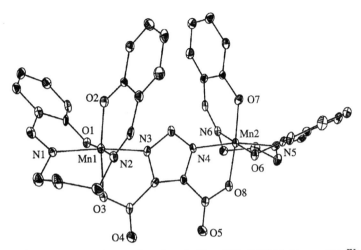

FIG. 24. Structure of the imidazolate-bridged Mn(IV/IV) dimer, [Mn^{IV}(3,5-di-t-busalpn)]$_2$(DCBI). (Reproduced with permission from [127]. Copyright 1997 the American Chemical Society.)

was the observation that ammonia could act as a competitive inhibitor of water oxidation [130,131]. Spectroscopists next learned that ammonia binding could perturb the S_2 EPR signals in two ways [54]. First, the hyperfine structure of the g = 2 multiline signal was modified. Second, the g = 4.1 signal could be enhanced at the expense of the multiline feature. These observations led to two very important experiments that have been cited to explain both the nuclearity of the cluster and substrate binding. In Sec. 3.2.3, we described the perpendicular mode EPR experiments on oriented PS II samples that had been treated with ammonia. The resultant signal gave a multiline feature on the g = 4.1 component. As discussed above, this experiment is one of the strongest pieces of evidence supporting the formulation as a tetranuclear cluster. The second important study utilized pulsed EPR spectra sampling the g = 2 region. In these studies, ^{15}N derived from ammonia modulated the ^{55}Mn ENDOR spectrum, which demonstrated that ammonia bonded to the Mn ions that are responsible for the S_2 multiline signal [53]. It was further suggested that an imidazo bridge between Mn ions might form.

Unfortunately, there is a paucity of manganese model compounds to test these issues. Nonbridging Mn(V)nitrido molecules have been prepared either by azide photodissociation [132] from a Mn(III) precursor or by ammonia exchange into an Mn(V)=O precursor [133,134]. While bridging imidazo compounds are well known in cobalt chemistry, the only such bridging motif for manganese contains a bridging trimethylsi-lylamide species. Because manganese is so oxophilic, ammonia will nor-mally not bind if oxygen donor ligands are available. The more highly charged nitrido and imidazo complexes are predicted to be stable; how-ever, they are only now being reported.

A more indirect method for looking at water binding to the OEC is through ^{18}O exchange studies [129,135]. While these experiments do not directly address whether water is bound to manganese, they do ad-dress whether the oxygen atoms that ultimately form dioxygen are ex-changeable with bulk water. The most recent determination of water ex-change suggests that there are two rates that differ by approximately a factor of 5 [135]. Both exchange rates are fast, especially when one considers that bulk water must minimally diffuse to the enzyme active site (and possibly exchange with water bound to a metal). These rates have been determined for water exchange in the S_2 and S_3 states. These studies lead to some interesting conclusions. It is unlikely that an irre-versible, intermediate substrate oxidation level is formed in S_2 or S_3 since water exchange would be excluded. This suggests that water is not oxidized on the $S_2 \rightarrow S_3$ transition. The copper complex of Tolman et al. [136] that reversibly converts between a $[Cu^{III}(\mu_2\text{-O})]_2$ and $[Cu^{II}_2(\eta_{1,1,2,2}\text{-}O_2)]$ is sometimes invoked as an example of a way that ^{18}O from water might be incorporated into such an oxidized system. However, this would correspond for manganese to the oxidation levels $[Mn^{IV}(\mu_2\text{-O})]_2$ and $[Mn^{III}_2(\eta_{1,1,2,2}\text{-}O_2)]$. We believe that this is unlikely for two reasons. The only report for hydrogen peroxide formation from an $[Mn^{IV}(\mu_2\text{-O})]_2$ dimer is that by Boucher and Coe [137,138] using the model compound $[Mn^{IV}(\text{di-}t\text{-butyl-salpn})(\mu_2\text{-O})]_2$. We have examined this reaction ex-haustively and conclude that while it is true that Mn(III) products are formed under the reported conditions, hydrogen peroxide or more oxi-dized oxygen species are not realized. Instead, it appears that ligand ox-idation products are the reducing agent for manganese. This suggests that it is unlikely that an equilibrium between levels of $[Mn^{IV}(\mu_2\text{-O})]_2$ and $[Mn^{III}_2(\eta_{1,1,2,2}\text{-}O_2)]$ will occur. If such an equilibrium were to be vi-able, ^{18}O exchange should only proceed through the $Mn(IV)_2$ form since the coordinated peroxide should be stable to exchange. We have deter-mined the rate of exchange of oxo bridges using $[Mn^{IV}(\text{di-}t\text{-butyl-salpn})(\mu_2\text{-}^{18}O)]_2$ in a medium dielectric solvent (acetonitrile). It takes days for water to incorporate into the bridges. In the presence of amines, the reaction speeds up dramatically; however, this is because the

$Mn(IV)_2$ dimer is reduced to a more labile $Mn(III)Mn(IV)$ system. Generally speaking, model $Mn(III)Mn(IV)$ species will show more rapid exchange than $Mn(IV)_2$ complexes. This is in part because they are susceptible to very rapid disproportionation/comproportionation reactions. The water can exchange rapidly from the resultant $Mn(III)_2$ [Mn(III) has rapid exchange of ligands] and then be trapped in the reoxidized $Mn(III)Mn(IV)$ dimer leading to the incorrect conclusion that the $Mn(III)Mn(IV)$ or $Mn(IV)_2$ dimers are labile. A sequestered manganese active site in a protein will not be susceptible to disproportionation reactions that are prevalent in millimolar solutions of model compounds. Therefore, we feel that water exchange with the oxo groups are prohibited for $Mn(IV)_2$ dimers. This again excludes the peroxide intermediate described above. In fact, based on these results it is unlikely that the resulting dioxygen is formed from bridging oxo groups in general.

There is now direct spectroscopic evidence for water binding to the S_2 state [139]. Davies ENDOR of the $g = 2$ multiline suggested that water and small alcohols such as methanol and ethanol can bind to the manganese cluster [140]. Model compounds were very useful in validating this approach. The mixed-valence dimer $[Mn^{III}Mn^{IV}(2\text{-OH-salpn})_2]^+$ can be reacted with water (or hydroxide or methanol) to form $[Mn^{III}Mn^{IV}(2\text{-OH-salpn})_2(H_2O)]^+$ [141]. This complex has a single solvent molecule bound to the Mn(III) ion. The ^{55}Mn ENDOR allowed for determination of distances of protons/deuterons from the manganese center and verified that the dipole model used to interpret the spectra was valid [142]. Based on all of the studies described in this section, we believe that at least one water is bound to the manganese cluster minimally from the S_2 state. Water exchange studies suggest that water remains bound in S_3 and provide strong arguments against the intermediacy of peroxide in S_3.

3.3. Other Inorganic Cofactors

3.3.1. Role of Chloride in Photosynthetic Water Oxidation

While most of the attention paid by bioinorganic chemists to the oxygen evolving complex focuses on the structure and function of the manganese cofactor, it should be realized that both calcium and chloride are thought to be essential for the water splitting reaction. Sandusky and Yocum definitively demonstrated that chloride was an essential anion that might bind to the manganese cofactor [130,131,143]. While other anions may substitute for chloride [144], no other anion is as effective in water oxidation chemistry. Sandusky and Yocum proposed that chloride might act as a bridge between manganese ions that could facilitate electron transfer reactions between manganese ions of the cluster [130,143]. While this proposal is reasonable, other alternative explanations have been presented which include (1) stabilizing higher oxidation states of manganese; (2) preventing early, unproductive oxidation chemistry (to form peroxide) by blocking a substrate binding site in the early S states (S_2 or S_3); (3) direct oxidation of chloride to form a hypochlorite intermediate (as proposed for water splitting reactions using ruthenium catalysts); (4) acting to provide charge balance; and (5) helping to shuttle protons to the manganese center in order to facilitate H-atom abstraction chemistry.

Model chemistry has been of some utility in evaluating these hypotheses. Probably the most significant debate regarding chloride is whether this anion is a manganese ligand in any or all of the S states. While there are studies that show that chloride binds to the OEC and has differential affinity at different S states, the location on the enzyme has not been established definitively. It is also known that chloride is only essential for the $S_2 \rightarrow S_3$ and $S_3 \rightarrow S_0$ transitions [145], implicating the element in electron transfer chemistry. Early spectroscopic and kinetic data supported the proposal that chloride binds directly to manganese [130,143,144]. In fact, it is believed that at least one chloride binding site is competitive with ammonia or acetate binding sites that are known through EPR studies to be very near the $Mn/Y_z^{\cdot}$ center. Because an X-ray structure of the enzyme is not available, spectroscopic techniques such as EXAFS have provided the most precise structural details for the cluster assembly. Unfortunately, detecting one chloride ion is not trivial even in manganese EXAFS since there are four manganese ions to consider. Assuming the chloride is not bridging and that the average coordination sphere for each manganese atom is 5.5, one expects chloride to contribute as 1 of 22 ligands. While it is true that the scattering power of chloride is different from that of oxygen or nitrogen and that the phase of the scattered wave is different, it is also true that EXAFS is a spectroscopic technique that generates a model from an underdetermined data sampling. As Penner-Hahn et al. have commented, the fit to the parameters improves as parameters are added; however, it is unclear as to whether the use of more parameters is justified. It is our conclusion that chloride may be bound to the manganese cluster and chemically this is very reasonable; however, we do not believe that the available data demonstrate this Mn–Cl interaction. An alternative EXAFS approach is to probe chloride directly. This strategy is also limited since the sensitivity of chloride EXAFS is much lower than that for manganese. Furthermore, there is a very high level of chloride in a functional OEC preparation, which leads to significant background scattering. Given these caveats, the first Cl EXAFS of manganese containing model compounds has recently appeared [146]. The authors conclude that one can distinguish chloride bound to Mn(III) vs. Mn(IV) and show that spatially proximal, but uncoordinated, chloride does not lead to a short Cl-Mn scatterer. It is hoped that future experiments on high-purity preparations will put the issue of chloride ligation to rest.

It is sometimes forgotten that whether a ligand provides stabilization of one oxidation state over another is a relative question. That is, it is inappropriate to ask if chloride stabilizes the Mn(IV) or Mn(III) oxidation states since we must by the nature of the question know what ligand the chloride will displace upon coordination. If we are interested in comparing water or alcohols vs. chloride we might expect that the neutral donors might not provide sufficient charge to mitigate the loss of an electron from Mn(III) while chloride could satisfy charge neutralization better. If we examine the $Mn(salen)R_2$ or $Mn(salpn)R_2$ systems (where $R = H_2O$, CH_3OH, or Cl^-), we see that this is precisely the observation [147]. Compounds such as $Mn(III)(salpn)(CH_3OH)_2$ can easily be reduced to the Mn(II) compounds (which usually are air-sensitive). In contrast, ligand oxidation is usually observed rather than formation of the Mn(IV) species. Compare these observations with the reports of stable $Mn(IV)(salen)Cl_2$ or $Mn(IV)(salpn)Cl_2$ [64]. These dichlorides can be reduced to Mn(III) at approximately +0.8 V vs. SCE. They are still highly reactive because they are reagents that carry out caged radical chlorination of alkenes and can react with water to liberate dioxygen! Thus, one realizes that chloride stabilizes the Mn(IV) oxidation level with respect to water or methanol (both of which are known to bind to the Mn cluster of the OEC).

In contrast, chloride is an inferior ligand to hydroxide or methoxide for stabilization of Mn(IV). If one adds base to $Mn(III)(salpn)(H_2O)_2$, then the dimer of $[Mn^{III}(salpn)(\mu_2\text{-OH})]_2$ is rapidly formed [12]. This compound is air-sensitive and will ultimately form $[Mn^{IV}(salpn)(\mu_2\text{-}O)]_2$. While it is true that the oxidation of manganese is driven by the formation of the di-μ_2-O bridged dimer, it is also true that higher oxidation states are immediately accessed by deprotonation. From this analysis we conclude that for stabilizing Mn(IV) with respect to Mn(III), the following order for unidentate ligands is maintained: $O^{2-} > OH^- > Cl^- >$ H_2O, CH_3OH. With respect to the OEC, this suggests that chloride should bind preferentially to water, especially at lower S states; however, it is likely that hydroxide or oxide ligands can displace chloride and these are most likely at higher S states.

While there is no direct evidence for chloride bridges in the OEC, this possibility has been suggested [143]. The chloride would serve as a mediator of electron transfer through the cluster. Models provide supportive precedents for this viewpoint. For example, Christou et al. have prepared tetramers that have μ_3- bridging chlorides [148]. There is also no doubt that chloride can act as an efficient facilitator for inner sphere electron transfer. One example is the comproportionation reaction of Mn(IV)(salpn)Cl$_2$ with Mn(II)(salpn)(CH$_3$OH)$_2$, which is too fast to measure even on stopped-flow time scales, but which occurs at a much slower rate if chloride is substituted with ligands incapable of forming an inner sphere complex.

Finally, we will consider the possible functional roles of chloride. Because S_1 and S_2 are stable in the absence of chloride and chloride is needed for S-state advancement above S_2 [145], the protective aspect of chloride with respect to peroxide formation is certainly ruled out for the lower S states. However, it is possible that chloride protects the S_3 state from early reductive chemistry. Models have been presented that indicate how adjacent aqua/chloro ligation could be used to block sites through which peroxide formation might occur. It is also clear that chloride is essential for allowing the manganese ions to attain higher oxidation states (S_3 and S_4), although it is unclear if this is the only role of the anion. Because other anions can facilitate water oxidation, the role of chloride as forming an intermediary hypochlorite species would appear to be ruled out. However, Meyer et al. have shown that this is an attractive mechanism for water oxidation catalyzed by Ru complexes [149]. Furthermore, there is a documented example of Mn(IV)salenCl$_2$ reacting with water to form dioxygen [150,151]. Thus, exclusion of this mechanism rests on the ability to completely remove chloride from the

PS II preparations. It is certain that chloride will serve, at least in part, to provide charge balance to the cluster. There is no model evidence that addresses whether chloride is particularly effective in shuttling protons within the enzyme as has been proposed in the Babcock H-atom abstraction mechanism [152].

3.3.2. Role of Calcium in Photosynthetic Water Oxidation

It is fair to conclude that the location and function of calcium is even more contentious than that of chloride. This conclusion is drawn in part from the different ways that individuals have used to address calcium ligation and function. One approach has been to deplete PS II preparations of calcium by carrying out a wash of the membranes using a good calcium chelator such as EGTA [50,51]. Depending on pH, salt conditions, type of PS II preparation, and amount of added chelator, differing degrees of calcium depletion can be achieved. Furthermore, in some cases, one must be careful not to deplete manganese simultaneously. All systems carefully depleted of calcium are devoid of oxygen evolving activity and appear to have photooxidation of the manganese center blocked beyond S_2. An alternative approach has been to reconstitute calcium-depleted preparation with another metal [153]. To date, the only metal that leads to recovery of activity is strontium, although many metals (including lanthanides) have been investigated. Most other metals such as monovalents, divalents, and trivalents [e.g., Na(I), Cd(II), La(III), but surprisingly not Mg(II)] are competitive inhibitors of enzymatic activity vs. calcium. Water oxidation rates are diminished with Sr(II) substitution and the $g = 2$ multiline signal is perturbed [154,155]. It was shown a decade ago that the manganese cluster could be removed and then reconstituted [156,157]. The use of calcium is required to regain activity and assemble the manganese cluster properly. There is an interesting and important synergy in this system since the presence of manganese is required to generate the calcium binding site. While these observations directly demonstrate the interrelationship between and essential requirement for both Mn and Ca(II), they do not resolve the location of the alkaline earth cation with respect to the manganese cluster.

Quantitative estimates for the manganese calcium distance have come from EXAFS. The Mn EXAFS include a scatterer at 3.3–3.5 Å from the manganese [45,95,97,98]. This shell can be fit with various combinations of manganese, carbon, and calcium; however, the fits are not unique. Therefore, one can interpret the data in several ways. Calcium depletion leads to apparent changes in the EPR spectrum [78,158], again suggesting that the manganese cluster is perturbed. Unfortunately, these data can be interpreted in several ways, especially since the PS II preparations are now catalytically inactive. Thus, there is no way to assess whether the sample has undergone major changes not associated with the simple loss of calcium. Because of these ambiguities, workers have shifted to examining Sr(II)-substituted samples.

Strontium-substituted materials have the advantages of retaining some activity, causing a perturbation in the S_2-state multiline signal and also providing a stronger scatterer for the Mn EXAFS experiments [154]. Despite these apparent advantages, the verdict is still out regarding the presence of Sr (and by extension Ca) near the manganese cluster. One group claims that Sr substitution leads to a new scatterer at slightly longer distances (about 3.6 Å) [45,159], while another group claims that there are no discernible differences between native and strontium substituted samples [160,161]. Apparently, the definitive experiment regarding the location of calcium was recently performed by Klein's group [104]. In these studies, Sr EXAFS was used to detect heavy atom scatterers (presumably Mn). Two manganese scatterers were detected at approximately 3.6 Å suggesting that the divalent cation is in close proximity to the manganese cluster. One ambiguity still remains with these experiments as the samples that were used for EXAFS analysis did not show a perturbed $g = 2$ multiline, which could indicate that Sr(II) did not access the catalytically relevant binding site. Based on these studies, it is highly likely that calcium is near to the manganese cluster, but there are still reasonable doubts about its presence.

There are few model compounds that have been prepared that include both manganese and calcium [34,162–165]. In some ways, concanavalin A represents a model for Mn-Ca interactions in proteins (see Chap. 9). The pertinent structural features of this protein are that there is a direct bridging carboxylate between the Mn and Ca ions and that the Mn–Ca distance is much greater than 3.5 Å. Horwitz et al. have been preparing compounds that include crown ether ligands linked to more conventional manganese binding ligands [162,163]. The idea is to append a calcium (or strontium) ion close to a manganese cluster by taking advantage of the high affinity of crown ethers for divalent alkaline earth cations. Structural information is available for sodium ions bridging Mn(III) and Mn(IV) ions in linear arrays. These could represent models for the sodium-inhibited form of the enzyme.

Because there is a paucity of good heterologous models for manganese and calcium interactions in proteins, one must rely on first principles to evaluate the possible functional role(s) of calcium. It is well known that calcium can stabilize specific protein conformations. While there are no E-F hand-type structures in the OEC (as assessed by sequence gazing of the gene sequences), it is possible that a specific structure is strongly stabilized by calcium. Support for this notion is the dramatic destabilization of the Mn cluster with respect to reduction upon depletion of calcium. Thus, there is no doubt that calcium stabilizes the water oxidation center; however, there may be additional aspects of water oxidation chemistry that are enhanced by calcium. Certainly, the addition of a +2 cation to the manganese cluster will change the number of anions to achieve charge neutrality. By extension, this means that the presence of calcium can perturb the redox potential locally (i.e., a single Mn ion) or more globally (i.e., the entire Mn cluster). In so doing, calcium could help define the proper potential for cluster oxidation. This property could be very sensitive to the type of ion and may partially explain why only strontium can substitute productively for calcium while sodium would be an inhibitor. It is also well known that alkaline earth and alkaline metal cations are often used by enzymes to lower the pK_a of water in order to generate a stronger nucleophile at the active site. It might be possible that a substrate water could bind to calcium forming a hydroxide ion that would be a better nucleophile to attack an electrophilic Mn(V)=O species. A very recent theoretical article provides calculations suggesting that calcium may stabilize a highly reactive Mn(IV)=O species [166]; however, there is no experimental evidence to support this notion. It is our opinion that significantly more attention by the biophysical, biochemical, and modeling community is necessary to understand the essential role of calcium in PS II.

3.4. Summary of Manganese Topology

Said simply, the field of oxygen evolution is in dire need of an X-ray crystal structure to resolve the present topological models. Witt provided encouraging progress to this end at the 1998 International Congress on

Photosynthesis [167]. Thus, all workers in the field are hopeful that this toughest of metalloenzymes will succumb to X-ray analysis very early in the next millennium. Until then we are left with an unsolved riddle. The manganese cluster is probably tetranuclear in all of the S states. It is unlikely that it is a dimer of dimers but an associated monomer/trimer topological organization may explain many of the apparent inconsistencies that we are left with.

4. THE ENERGETICS OF WATER OXIDATION AND THE ROLE OF PROTONS

Photosystem II is replete with organic cofactors that are responsible for irreversible charge separation [42]. Until recently, the portion of PS II that contains the OEC had been considered as being devoid of organic cofactors. The picture that is now emerging directly implicates a redox-active tyrosine, Y_z, in the chemical steps of water oxidation. Babcock has written extensively on the hypothesis that Y_z functions not only as an intermediary electron transfer agent that facilitates electron flow between the Mn cluster and P680$^+$, but also is directly engaged in water oxidation chemistry by abstracting H atoms from water bound to the manganese cluster [152,168,169]. It is now recognized that there are many metalloradical enzymes including ribonucleotide reductase (RR) [170]. In particular, the RRs from brevibacteria contain a binuclear manganese center and presumably the same redox-active tyrosine that has been studied extensively for the iron enzyme. Attractive features of the Babcock mechanism, which is shown as Fig. 25, include having a charge neutral cluster that is charge invariant upon each S-state transition, a process for proton translocation, and minimal movement of atoms through the catalytic cycle.

4.1. H Atom Bond Dissociation Energies

There are many criteria that must be met in order for the H atom abstraction proposal to be viable. The first issue is the proximity of the tyrosine to the water bound to the manganese. This distance has oscillated between being very long (≈ 14 Å) to very short (≈ 4.5 Å) [171]. The most recent determinations are placing the tyrosine ≈ 8 Å from the mag-

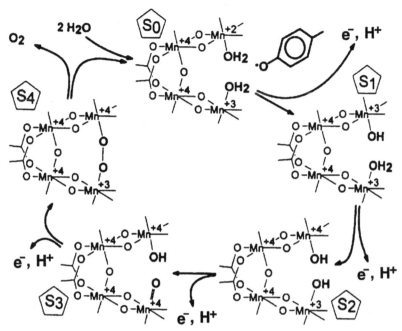

FIG. 25. A mechanism proposed by Hoganson and Babcock for dioxygen evolution from OEC via hydrogen atom abstraction theory. (Reproduced with permission from [152]. Copyright 1997 American Association for the Advancement of Science.)

netic center of the manganese cluster [86]. This is probably a reasonable distance for the tyrosine oxygen to interact with a coordinated water molecule. Therefore, the criterion for the proximity of the radical to the manganese cluster is likely satisfied. Another essential feature is that S-state advancement (below S_4) should be associated with kinetic oxidation of the cluster and likely thermodynamic oxidation of the cluster. This issue is best satisfied if one chooses to believe the data supporting manganese oxidation upon S_3 formation. A third criticism of this model comes from electrochromic shifts reported by Junge et al. [172]. These data suggest that protons do not leave the vicinity of the manganese cluster on S-state transitions and therefore are not pumped out of the active site by a hydrogen bond relay mechanism that was originally proposed by Babcock. As we discuss below, we feel that protons must be removed from the active site in order to ensure high-yield oxidation of the manganese cluster.

Another important concern is the thermodynamic criterion for H atom abstraction. The tyrosine radical in RR has an estimated homolytic bond dissociation energy (HBDE) of 86.5 kcal/mol [173,174]. In comparison, the HBDE for an O–H bond in water is 119 kcal/mol [175]. Therefore, one would not expect that abstraction of an H atom by a neutral tyrosine radical would be viable from bulk water. However, the Babcock hypothesis invoked H atom abstraction from a water terminally ligated to the manganese cluster. Unfortunately, at the time of this hypothesis, there were no data available for HBDE of water coordinated to manganese. In the past 5 years, however, there have been several studies with model compounds that now show that the HBDE for water (or hydroxide) bound to manganese is in the 73–95 kcal/mol range [176,177]. These values suggest that under the proper conditions, a neutral tyrosine radical may be capable of abstracting an H atom from a manganese-bound water or hydroxide ligand.

Gardner and Mayer performed the first study in this area by examining the rate of permanganate oxidation of organic substrates [178]. One can extract the value of the HBDE by comparing the rates of substrate oxidation by the desired oxidant using compounds with well-defined C–H bond energies. This paper also presented a straightforward methodology for calculating an HBDE from known reduction potentials and pK_a values as long as the potential for the formation of H$^\bullet$ and the energy of solvation of this species were known. This approach is summarized by Eqs. (2)–(5), which sum to give Eq. (6). The value obtained by both the kinetic and thermodynamic method was 76 kcal/mol.

The series of Mn dimers formed with 2-OH-salpn led to evaluation of the H atom abstraction proposal using more biologically relevant oxidation states. This dimer series, shown in Fig. 26, can be isolated in five oxidation levels beginning at Mn(II)$_2$ and proceeding to Mn(IV)$_2$ [21]. We also have evidence that a highly reactive Mn(IV)Mn(V) complex can be prepared transiently. Most important for this discussion is that the

$$(H_2O)M^n \text{ (sol)} \longrightarrow (H_2O)M^{n+1} \text{ (sol)} + 1e^- \text{ (sol)} \qquad E^0 \qquad (2)$$

$$(H_2O)M^{n+1} \text{ (sol)} \longrightarrow (OH)M^{n+1} \text{ (sol)} + H^+ \text{ (sol)} \qquad pK_a \qquad (3)$$

$$H^+ \text{ (sol)} + 1e^- \text{ (sol)} \longrightarrow 1/2H_2 \text{ (sol)} \qquad\qquad (4)$$

$$1/2H_2 \text{ (sol)} \longrightarrow H^\bullet \text{ (sol)} \qquad\qquad (5)$$

$$(H_2O)M^n \text{ (sol)} \longrightarrow (OH)M^{n+1} \text{ (sol)} + H^\bullet \text{ (sol)} \qquad HBDE \qquad (6)$$

Mn(III)$_2$ through Mn(IV)$_2$ complexes can bind either water or hydroxide ligands to one of the manganese ions, making the asymmetric complexes on the right of Fig. 26. The reduction potentials and pK_a values for these compounds have been determined in acetonitrile. In these systems, the HBDE range from 83 to 92 kcal/mol depending on the phenolate ring substitution pattern (i.e., whether electron-donating or withdrawing groups are present) and oxidation state of the metals (there is a 3–4 kcal/mol increase as the oxidation state of the complex is increased) [177]. Most important, these values are within a range that would be energetically feasible for H atom abstraction in PS II. These studies focused solely on H atom abstraction from water bound to Mn(III). Further experiments are necessary to establish whether the conversion of hydroxide to oxide ligands is energetically permissible for this process and to establish whether water (or hydroxide) bound to Mn(IV) will have the similar energies.

The [Mn^{IV}salpn(μ_2-O)]$_2$ dimer can be protonated at the bridging oxo moiety [49]. This allows determination of the HBDE for the conversion of [Mn^{III}Mn^{IV}(μ_2-O)(μ_2-OH)] to [Mn^{IV}salpn(μ_2-O)]$_2$. Values for this process are around 76 kcal/mol [176]. An HBDE of this magnitude may be too small for efficient energy transfer from Y$_z$ to the manganese cluster and is unlikely to be a significant process for more than one or two steps. Since these initial HBDE determinations, other reports have appeared in the manganese and iron literature supporting these conclusions. Furthermore, Mn-OH$_2$ and Mn-OH HBDEs have now been reported from calculational studies and these too are in agreement with the experimentally determined values [166,179].

The H atom abstraction mechanism is an attractive model; however, simple proton-coupled electron transfer (i.e., unconcerted electron and proton movement) is also thermodynamically viable. Such a proposal was made by Britt et al. [84] at around the same time that Babcock suggested H atom abstraction chemistry as being essential for water oxidation. We make this distinction since the energetic arguments for water oxidation are equally valid if the proton does not move away from the manganese cluster toward Y$_z$ electron transfer. It is our belief that charge neutral transitions are an integral component of high-energy charge accumulation. Either H atom abstraction or proton-coupled electron transfer would satisfy this objective.

To understand the necessity for charge neutral transitions, one must consider the overall energetics of water oxidation [180]. At pH =

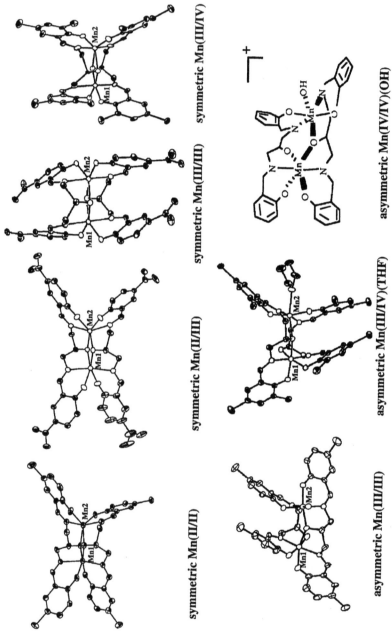

FIG. 26. Structures of the family of [Mn$_2$(2-OHsalpn)$_2$], ranging from Mn(II/II) to Mn(III/IV). (Reproduced with permission from [26].)

6, the oxidation of water to dioxygen requires ≈ 0.89 V/e$^-$. This amounts to accumulation of 3.6 V for this chemistry to occur. The oxidized P_{680} is poised at approximately 1.8 V; however, 0.6 V is transferred to the reducing side to generate, ultimately, NADPH. Of the remaining 1.2 V, approximately 100–200 mV is required to have high quantum yield oxidation of Y_z to $Y_z^\cdot$. Therefore, it is unlikely that more than 1.0–1.1 V is available for water oxidation on each step. Estimates for the $S_0 \rightarrow S_1$ potential are between 0.5 and 0.7 V. This puts biological water oxidation at the edge of success for the final three oxidation steps and suggests that there is at most 0.5 V of driving force that can be lost over the next three transitions. Therefore, the difference in redox potentials for the final three oxidations must be within approximately 200 mV of one another. Said differently, the $S_1 \rightarrow S_2$, $S_2 \rightarrow S_3$ and the $S_3 \rightarrow S_4$ transitions must all occur at 0.9 V or greater but never exceed 1.1 V. A striking realization occurs at once if one considers the redox behavior of polynuclear metal complexes.

Typically, for an isostructural complex that does not dissipate the accumulated charge, each subsequent oxidation of the complex will cost between 300 and 500 mV [21]. That is, for the series shown as Eq. (7), the reduction potentials will shift approximately 400 mV on each transition. While the magnitude of the potential shift is solvent dependent, the effect will occur in all solvents since it is the result of accumulating uncompensated charge on the cluster. Even considering the ability of proteins to generate electrostatic regions to compensate charge, it is not likely that a metal cluster would be able to overcome this large electrostatic penalty for further oxidation. In contrast, if the manganese cen-

$$Mn_4^n \longrightarrow Mn_4^{n+1} \longrightarrow Mn_4^{n+2} \longrightarrow Mn_4^{n+3} \qquad (7)$$
$$\quad 0\ V \qquad\qquad +0.4\ V \qquad\quad +0.8\ V$$

ter lost a positive charge equivalent at each oxidation, then the shifts in potential that have been observed for model compounds are more on the order of 100–150 mV [177]. Positive charge loss can occur through H atom abstraction or proton-coupled electron transfer. Alternatively, binding an anion such as chloride should cause a similar effect. Thus, it is our belief that for high-efficiency water oxidation, the catalytic center must be able to disperse charge away from the manganese aggregate during S-state advancement. H atom abstraction and proton-coupled electron transfer are the most appealing ways to achieve this end.

5.   TOWARD A UNIFIED VIEW OF BIOLOGICAL WATER OXIDATION CHEMISTRY

5.1.   A Structural and Oxidation State Perspective

The consensus view of the manganese cluster in PS II presents a tetranuclear cluster that is likely arranged in a dimer-of-dimers metal topology. The dimers would be arranged in the C clamp model shown in Fig. 27. While controversial, it is likely that the S_1 enzyme has an oxidation level of $Mn(III)_2Mn(IV)_2$. Each S-state conversion that has been investigated probably leads to oxidation of manganese. The $S_3 \rightarrow S_4 \rightarrow S_0$ transition has not been interrogated so any oxidation state assignment for S_4 can only be classified as speculative. Our view is that S_4 has the formal oxidation level of $Mn(IV)_3Mn(V)$; however, there may be ambiguity in the assignment in the same way that one may argue as to whether Compound I intermediates in heme enzymes are really Fe(V)=O(porphyrin), Fe(IV)=O(porphyrin·+) or Fe(IV)=O(porphyrin) (protein·+) [1,2]. Mounting evidence suggests that the S_0 state is best described as having $Mn(II)Mn(III)Mn(IV)_2$ [46,88–90]. Within the dimer-of-dimers structural model, one might best consider this as an assembly of an Mn(II)Mn(III) dimer with an $[Mn^{IV}(\mu_2\text{-O})]_2$ dimer. Such an

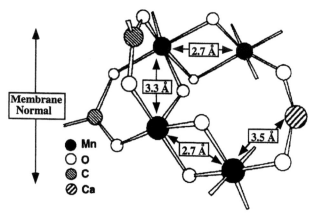

FIG. 27.   A model proposed for the active site for the oxygen evolving complex in PS II. (Reproduced with permission from [104]. Copyright 1998 the American Chemical Society.)

oxidation state and structural model could be attractively interpreted as having one structural dimer that always remained as an $[Mn^{IV}(\mu_2-O)]_2$ and a second dimer turning over all four oxidizing equivalents. This model is attractive from the perspective of the symmetry of the OEC. Charge separation only occurs on one polypeptide of PS II although all of the cofactors necessary for electron transfer are available in a pseudo-C_2-related subunit (which also contains a redox-active tyrosine designated Y_D). Thus, one could consider a gene duplication that started with a peptide that had a single dimer and then generated a second, normally redox-inactive, dimer that was in close proximity to the first.

What bothers us about this apparently reasonable model is that it is difficult to reconcile the growing spectroscopic and magnetic data for the enzyme with a dimer-of-dimers motif. As was discussed above, it is challenging at best to explain the different S_2 state EPR spectral features with a dimer-of-dimers topology. Furthermore, if the observation of Dexheimer and Klein [105] that the S_1 EPR signal correlates with production of the $g = 2$ multiline and not the $g = 4$ signal in S_2 is correct, then one must exclude an interacting dimer-of-dimers as a reasonable model.

One alternative that seems to fit the available data is a trimer coupled to a monomeric center. Depending on the conditions, one could generate both the $g = 2$ and $g = 4.1$ signal in S_2. If the bond between the monomer is not formed in S_1, then one could obtain S_1 EPR spectra that would exhibit the behavior described by Dexheimer and Klein. The problem with this topology is that it is difficult to explain the S_{-1} data of Yocum, Penner-Hahn, and co-workers which suggest that only one dimer is reduced with hydroquinone treatment [95]. It should be noted that a tetrameric cluster that has multiple exchange pathways will also work for explaining the origin of $g = 2$ and $g = 4.1$ features. However, such an organization cannot be consistent with the Dexheimer two-site precursor to S_2 model.

5.2.   Oxygen Bond Formation

The final issue that will be raised in this chapter is how the oxygen bond is made. Here synthetic chemistry is starting to provide some answers that are very difficult to glean from biophysical studies on the enzyme. One can segregate the mechanism into several categories depending on how we choose to view the reaction. If an intermediate substrate oxidation is invoked, then the O–O bond could form through two 2-electron reactions with the peroxide oxidation level as an intermediate. This view is often proposed as an explanation by workers that believe that manganese is not oxidized on the $S_2 \rightarrow S_3$ transition. Alternatively, a single 4-electron concerted process with no partially oxidized intermediate before S_4 has its proponents. Alternatively, we could consider not so much the number of electrons associated with the process, but rather where the oxygen atoms that form dioxygen might originate. The H atom abstraction proposal [152,168] predicts that both equivalents of oxygen atoms are derived from substrate water. In contrast, several proposals have appeared that invoke the oxo bridges condensing to form first peroxide and, essentially immediately, dioxygen [45,102,181]. Because both calcium and chloride are essential for water oxidation, one might reasonably ask if either of these elements plays a direct role in water oxidation. For example, it is known that HOCl can, under certain circumstances, generate dioxygen. Finally, one may take the perspective of analyzing the chemistry based on the highest available oxidation level that manganese can achieve. Here workers argue whether Mn(IV) is the limit or whether Mn(V) can be transiently formed.

Model compounds are beginning to address several of these issues. First we will consider the condensation of two oxo bridges to form peroxide. There are two very important papers that provided support for this idea. The first was that reported by Boucher and Coe [138] in which $[Mn^{IV}salpn(\mu_2\text{-}O)]_2$ was reported to form dioxygen and Mn(III) in acidic acetone solution. The second observation came from copper chemistry. Tolman et al. showed that certain copper dimers can reversibly convert between $Cu(II)(\eta_1,\eta_1,\eta_2,\eta_2\text{-}O_2^{2-})Cu(II)$ and $Cu(III)(di\text{-}\mu_2\text{-}O)_2Cu(III)$ [136]. Taken together, these data provide a strong precedent for a condensation type of mechanism. Because of the importance of these observations, we have attempted to reproduce the experiments of Boucher and Coe. While we confirm that Mn(III) is a product of the addition of very acidic protons to $[Mn^{IV}salpn(\mu_2\text{-}O)]_2$, we see no evidence for the production of hydrogen peroxide. We favor the reductant in this system being the Schiff base ligand itself. Therefore, while this is an attractive proposal, we feel that the strongest precedent supporting the mechanism is artifactual. The water exchange range studies of Wydrzynski et al. also speak against this proposal [129,135]. These data show relatively fast water exchange into the liberated dioxygen up through S_3. If dioxygen is being formed via the bridging oxo ligands, then water must be able to exchange into these bridges. We have shown that oxo exchange in $[Mn^{IV}salpn(\mu_2\text{-}O)]_2$ is extremely slow unless the environment is very acidic or there is a reductant present that will generate $[Mn^{III}Mn^{IV}salpn (\mu_2\text{-}O)_2]$ [29]. Thus, we conclude that such a mechanism is not kinetically competent given the measured ^{18}O incorporation rates.

The direct participation of chloride in water oxidation is an interesting mechanism to consider. Meyer et al. have shown that Ru complexes can oxidize through an HOCl type of intermediate [149]. Additionally, $Mn(IV)(salpn)Cl_2$ will react with water to form dioxygen, again through a proposed HOCl intermediate. Speaking against this mechanism is that Cl_2 gas is often observed under conditions that lead to O_2 generation by hypochlorite, yet neither Cl_2 nor HOCl has ever been detected in PS II preparations. However, the most compelling argument refuting this mechanism is that anions other than chloride can activate the OEC to undergo water oxidation. Thus, it is the presence of a certain anion (not just chloride) that is required for activity.

We and others have recently been focusing on the possible role of Mn(V) in the catalytic process. The first structurally characterized Mn(V) species were the mononuclear Mn(V)=O species reported by Collins et al. [182, 183] and O'Halloran et al. [184]. The Collins compound is remarkably stable and does not appear to generate dioxygen if challenged by the presence of water. Two other mononuclear Mn(V) species include the nitrido complexes. One of these molecules has been crystallized [132], and the second appears to carry out amination of organic substrates [133,134]. Kochi showed that m-CPBA or HOCl could be used to convert $Mn(III)(salen)(pyridine)_2^+$ to a reagent that could epoxidize olefins [185]. While the nature of this material is under debate, it is usually formulated as the $[Mn^V=O(salen)]^+$. Based on this observation, we have attempted oxo group transfer from m-CPBA to $[Mn^{III}Mn^{IV}(2\text{-}OH\text{-}salpn)_2]^+$ in acetone at $-78°C$ in order to prepare $[Mn^{IV}Mn^V=O(2\text{-}OH\text{-}salpn)_2]^+$. While we have been unable to isolate this complex as a pure solid, initial reactivity studies show that this compound epoxidizes olefins (but does not form alcohols or ketones) while $[Mn^{IV}(2\text{-}OH\text{-}salpn)]_2^{2+}$ or $[Mn^{IV}Mn^{IV}(OH)(2\text{-}OH\text{-}salpn)_2]^+$) do not.

Over the past few years there have been several reports of water oxidation by Mn(V)=O dimers [186–188]. A linked porphyrin system was the first to report dioxygen activity using electrocatalyzed reaction at high pH [32,186]. Related porphyrin dimers were also competent for carrying out catalase reactions. There was little direct evidence for the formation of the Mn(V) oxidation level in these systems, although it is reasonable that a such a formal oxidation could be achieved. While these studies represented a significant advance in reactivity modeling, workers have been attempting to oxidize water using nonporphyrin systems since the manganese cluster does not contain this organic cofactor.

The Yale group of Gary Brudvig, Bob Crabtree, and their students has made two interesting and important recent reports on dioxygen production with nonporphyrin dimers [187,188]. By using good oxo transfer agents such as peroxydisulfate or hypochlorous acid, these investigators have shown that ^{18}O can be incorporated into dioxygen. It is proposed that a Mn(V) dimer is the active catalytic species. Two Mn(V) Mn(V)=O dimers are thought to condense the terminal oxo atoms generating dioxygen. It is not yet known whether this is a four-electron concerted reaction or whether peroxide might form as an intermediate step in the reaction. This reaction is interesting as it is contradictory to recent theoretical predictions that suggesting that Mn(V) is not sufficiently reactive to form dioxygen. Further work is necessary to explore this exciting system; however, in terms of modeling the OEC the system has at least one drawback. The problem is that this model system is overoxidized as compared to the OEC. The maximum oxidation level for S_4 is $Mn(IV)_3Mn(V)$ while the model system would require the two dimers to be at the oxidation level $Mn(V)_4$.

Figure 28 provides a model [180] for water oxidation that uses the dimers-of-dimers structure as a framework although the mechanism is not unique to this topology. The major concern here is how the O–O bond may be formed. It is our belief that this reaction best proceeds by the nucleophilic attack of a manganese (or calcium) coordinated hydroxide (or oxide) from a metal adjacent to an electrophilic Mn(V)=O. In some ways, this is reminiscent of halide attack on a terminal oxo of compound I in heme systems. Figure 29 shows an alternative metal topology that would also foster dioxygen production. In this case, the trinuclear manganese would serve primarily as a sink for oxidizing equivalents while a chemical distinct manganese would form the terminal Mn(V)=O, which could be attacked by the hydroxide (or oxide). Of

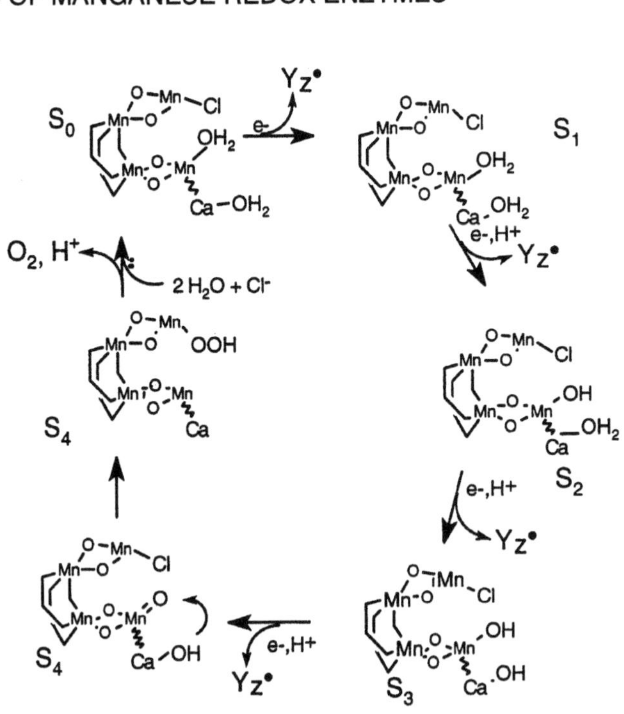

FIG. 28. A mechanism for dioxygen evolution by the OEC involving hydrogen atom abstraction as proposed by Pecoraro. (Reproduced with permission from [180]. Copyright 1998 IUPAC.)

course, there are other topologies that could be drawn that do not require Ca(II) near the cluster and put the nucleophilic oxygen on a manganese atom of the cluster. A density functional calculation study by Siegbahn and Crabtree prefer the Mn(IV)=O as the reactive unit to form dioxygen [166]. It is our belief that Mn(V) is the more likely candidate although just what oxidation state is formed in S_4 may be more a philosophical than scientific issue at our present level of study.

6. CONCLUSION

In this chapter, we have tried to present a comprehensive picture of two interesting manganoenzymes and the chemical model systems that as-

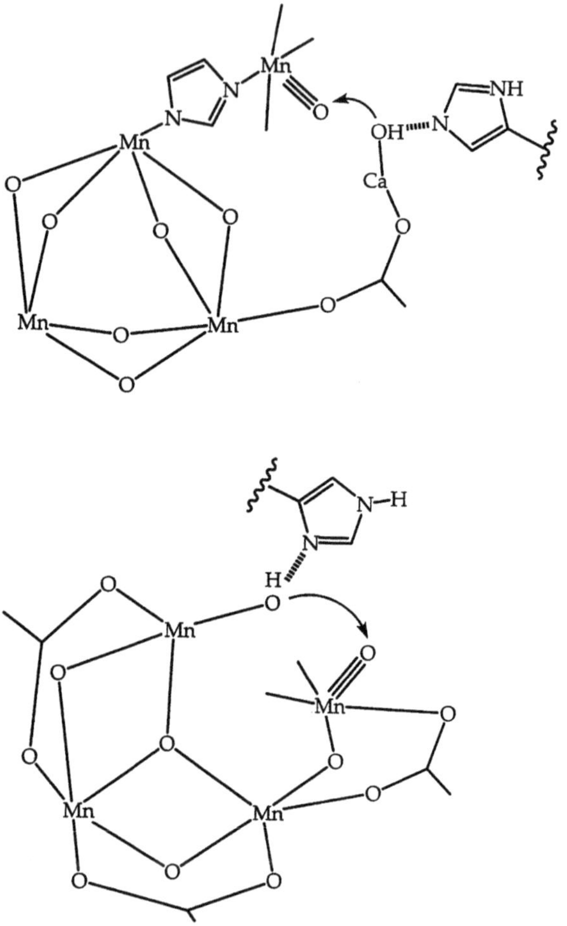

FIG. 29.   The calcium dependence of hydroxide attacking Mn(V)=O in the oxygen evolving complex (top). An alternative mechanism of hydroxide attacking Mn(V)=O in the OEC without calcium (bottom).

sisted developing the modern understanding of structure and function. Clearly, small-molecule compounds have been invaluable to the development of models for enzymatic oxidation states and structure. Ultimately, these biomimetic systems may present the best way to address the details of the chemical mechanism of these complex biomanganese systems.

ACKNOWLEDGMENTS

The authors acknowledge many useful conversations with Professors James E. Penner-Hahn, Charles F. Yocum, Gerald Babcock, and R. David Britt and Drs. Neil Law, Mike Baldwin, and Ty Caudle. This work was sponsored by the NIH (GM 39406).

ABBREVIATIONS AND DEFINITIONS

bipy	2,2′-bipyridine
HDCBI	4,5-dicarboxyimidazole
EDTA	ethylenediamine-N,N,N',N'-tetraacetic acid
EGTA	ethylene glycol-bis(2-aminoethyl)-N,N,N',N'-tetraacetic acid
ENDOR	electron nuclear double resonance
EPR	electronic paramagnetic resonance
ESEEM	electron spin-echo envelope modulation
EXAFS	extended X-ray absorption fine structure
FT-IR	Fourier transform infrared
HBDE	Homolytic bond dissociation energy
Im	imidazole
m-CPBA	$meta$-chloroperbenzoic acid
MCD	magnetic circular dichroism
Me	methyl
NADPH	nicotinamide adenine dinucleotide phosphate, reduced form
OAc	acetate
OEC	oxygen evolving complex
2-OHbenzimpn	N,N,N',N'-tetrakis(2-methylenebenzimidazole)-1,3-diaminopropan-2-ol
2-OHsalpn	N,N'-(salicylidenimine)-1,3-diaminopropan-2-ol
PS II	photosystem II
pic	picolinic acid
RR	ribonucleotide reductase
saladhp	2-(salicylideneaminato)-1,3-dihydroxy-2-methylpropane

5-Cl-salahp	3-(5-chlorosalicylideneamino)propanol
salen	N,N'-(salicylidenimine)-1,2-diaminoethane
salpn	N,N'-(salicylidenimine)-1,3-diaminopropane
SCE	saturated calomel electrode
tacn	1,4,7-triazacyclononane
XANES	X-ray absorption near-edge spectroscopy
XAS	X-ray absorption spectroscopy

REFERENCES

1. A. Deisseroth and A. L. Dounce, *Physiol. Rev.*, *50*, 319–375 (1970).

2. G. R. Schoenbaum and B. Chance, in *The Enzymes* (P. Boyer, ed.), Academic Press, New York, 1976, pp. 363–408.

3. V. V. Barynin and A. I. Grebenko, *Dokl. Akad. Nauk. SSSR*, *286*, 461–464 (1986).

4. V. V. Barynin, A. A. Vagin, V. R. Melik-Adamyan, A. I. Grebenko, S. V. Khangulov, A. N. Popov, M. E. Andrianova, and B. K. Vainshtein, *Dokl. Akad. Nauk. SSSR*, *288*, 877–880 (1986).

5. Y. Kono and I. Fridovich, *J. Biol. Chem.*, *258*, 6015–6019 (1983).

6. W. F. Beyer, Jr. and I. Fridovich, *Biochemistry*, *24*, 6460–6467 (1985).

7. U. Bossek, M. Saher, T. Weyhermüller, and K. Wieghardt, *J. Chem. Soc. Chem. Commun.*, 1780–1782 (1992).

8. J. B. Vincent, H.-L. Tsai, A. G. Blackman, S. Wang, P. D. W. Boyd, K. Folting, J. C. Huffman, E. B. Lobkovsky, D. N. Hendrickson, and G. Christou, *J. Am. Chem. Soc.*, *115*, 12353–12361 (1993).

9. S.-B. Yu, S. J. Lippard, I. Shweky, and A. Bino, *Inorg. Chem.*, *31*, 3502–3504 (1992).

10. K. J. Oberhausen, R. J. O'Brien, J. F. Richardson, R. M. Buchanan, R. Costa, J.-M. Latour, H.-L. Tsai, and D. N. Hendrickson, *Inorg. Chem.*, *32*, 4561–4565 (1993).

11. N. Kitajima, U. P. Singh, H. Amagai, M. Osawa, and Y. Moro-oka, *J. Am. Chem. Soc.*, *113*, 7757–7758 (1991).

12. E. J. Larson and V. L. Pecoraro, *J. Am. Chem. Soc.*, *113*, 3810–3818 (1991).

13. A. F. Jensen, Z. Su, N. K. Hansen, and F. K. Larsen, *Inorg. Chem.*, *34*, 4244–4252 (1995).

14. V. V. Barynin, P. D. Hempstead, A. A. Vagin, S. V. Antonyuk, W. R. Melik-Adamyan, V. S. Lamzin, P. M. Harrison, and P. J. Artymiuk, *J. Inorg. Biochem.*, *67*, 196 (1997).

15. M. Atta, P. Nordlund, A. Aberg, H. Eklund, and M. Fontecave, *J. Biol. Chem.*, *267*, 20682–20688 (1992).

16. Z. F. Kanyo, L. R. Scolnick, D. E. Ash, and D. W. Christianson, *Nature*, *383*, 554–557 (1996).

17. R. L. Rardin, A. Bino, P. Poganiuch, W. B. Tolman, S. Liu, and S. J. Lippard, *Angew. Chem. Int. Ed. Eng.*, *29*, 812–814 (1990).

18. R. L. Rardin, W. B. Tolman, and S. J. Lippard, *N. J. Chem.*, *15*, 417–430 (1991).

19. M. J. Baldwin, J. W. Kampf, M. L. Kirk, and V. L. Pecoraro, *Inorg. Chem.*, *34*, 5252–5260 (1995).

20. D. P. Kessissoglou, M. L. Kirk, C. A. Bender, M. S. Lah, and V. L. Pecoraro, *J. Chem. Soc. Chem. Commun.*, 84–86 (1989).

21. A. Gelasco, M. L. Kirk, J. W. Kampf, and V. L. Pecoraro, *Inorg. Chem.*, *36*, 1829–1837 (1997).

22. P. J. Pessiki, S. V. Khangulov, D. M. Ho, and G. C. Dismukes, *J. Am. Chem. Soc.*, *116*, 891–897 (1994).

23. T. M. Sossong, Jr., S. V. Khangulov, R. C. Cavalli, D. R. Soprano, G. C. Dismukes, and D. E. Ash, *J. Biol. Inorg. Chem.*, *2*, 433–443 (1997).

24. P. Mathur, M. Crowder, and G. C. Dismukes, *J. Am. Chem. Soc.*, *109*, 5227–5233 (1987).

25. S. V. Khangulov, V. V. Barynin, and S. V. Antonyuk-Barynina, *Biochim. Biophys. Acta*, *1020*, 25–33 (1990).

26. A. K. Gelasco, Low Valent Manganese as Functional Models for the Mn Catalases and the Alternate Catalase Reaction of the Oxygen Evolving Complex, PhD. dissertation, University of Michigan, 1995.

27. M. Zheng, S. V. Khangulov, G. C. Dismukes, and V. V. Barynin, *Inorg. Chem.*, *33*, 382–387 (1994).

28. D. R. Gamelin, M. L. Kirk, T. L. Stemmler, S. Pal, W. H. Armstrong, J. E. Penner-Hahn, and E. I. Solomon, *J. Am. Chem. Soc.*, *116*, 2392–2399 (1994).

29. E. J. Larson and V. L. Pecoraro, *J. Am. Chem. Soc.*, *113*, 7809–7810 (1991).

30. P. J. Pessiki and G. C. Dismukes, *J. Am. Chem. Soc.*, *116*, 898–903 (1994).

31. A. Gelasco, S. Bensiek, and V. L. Pecoraro, *Inorg. Chem.*, *37*, 3301–3309 (1998).

32. Y. Naruta and K. Maruyama, *J. Am. Chem. Soc.*, *113*, 3595–3596 (1991).

33. A. Gelasco, A. Askenas, and V. L. Pecoraro, *Inorg. Chem.*, *35*, 1419–1420 (1996).

34. R. T. Stibrany and S. M. Gorun, *Angew. Chem. Int. Ed. Engl.*, *29*, 1156–1158 (1990).

35. J. E. Penner-Hahn, in *Manganese Redox Enzymes* (V. L. Pecoraro, ed.), VCH, New York, 1992, pp. 29–45.

36. G. S. Algood and J. J. Perry, *J. Bacteriol.*, *168*, 563–567 (1986).

37. Y. Naruta and M. Sasayama, *J. Chem. Soc. Chem. Commun.*, 2667–2668 (1994).

38. V. L. Pecoraro, in *Manganese Redox Enzymes* (V. L. Pecoraro, ed.), VCH, New York, 1992, pp. 197–231.

39. S. V. Khangulov, N. V. Voyevodskaya, V. V. Barynin, A. I. Grebenko, and V. R. Melik-Adamyan, *Biofizika*, *32*, 960–966 (1987).

40. G. S. Waldo, R. M. Fronko, and J. E. Penner-Hahn, *Biochemistry*, *30*, 10486–10490 (1991).

41. D. F. Ghanotakis and C. F. Yocum, *Annu. Rev. Plant Physiol. Plant Mol. Biol.*, *41*, 255–276 (1990).

42. R. J. Debus, *Biochim. Biophys. Acta*, *1102*, 269–352 (1992).

43. D. R. Ort and C. F. Yocum, eds., *Oxygenic Photosynthesis: The Light Reactions*, Kluwer Academic, Boston, 1996.

44. P. Mathis, ed., *Photosynthesis: From Light to Biosphere, Proceedings of the Congress on Photosynthesis*, Kluwer Academic, Amsterdam, 1995.

45. V. K. Yachandra, K. Sauer, and M. P. Klein, *Chem. Rev.*, *96*, 2927–2950 (1996).

46. L. Iuzzolino, J. Dittmer, W. Dörner, W. Meyer-Klaucke, and H. Dau, *Biochemistry*, *37*, 17112–17119 (1998).

47. J. E. Penner-Hahn, in *Structure and Bonding*, Vol. 90 (H. A. O. Hill, P. J. Sadler, and A. J. Thomson, eds.), Springer-Verlag, Berlin, 1998, pp. 1–36.

48. Z. Shirin, V. G. Young, Jr., and A. S. Borovik, *J. Chem. Soc. Chem. Commun.*, 1967–1968 (1997).

49. M. J. Baldwin, T. L. Stemmler, P. J. Riggs-Gelasco, M. L. Kirk, J.

E. Penner-Hahn, and V. L. Pecoraro, *J. Am. Chem. Soc.*, *116*, 11349–11356 (1994).

50. D. F. Ghanotakis, J. N. Topper, G. T. Babcock, and C. F. Yocum, *FEBS Lett.*, *170*, 169–173 (1984).

51. D. F. Ghanotakis, G. T. Babcock, and C. F. Yocum, *FEBS Lett.*, *167*, 127–130 (1984).

52. W. F. Beck, J. C. de Paula, and G. W. Brudvig, *J. Am. Chem. Soc.*, *108*, 4018–4022 (1986).

53. R. D. Britt, J.-L. Zimmermann, K. Sauer, and M. P. Klein, *J. Am. Chem. Soc.*, *111*, 3522–3532 (1989).

54. H. Dau, J. C. Andrews, V. K. Yachandra, T. A. Roelofs, M. J. Latimer, W. Liang, K. Sauer, and M. P. Klein, *Biochemistry*, *34*, 5274–5287 (1995).

55. J. L. Zimmermann, A. Boussac, and A. W. Rutherford, *Biochemistry*, *25*, 4609–4615 (1986).

56. D. B. Goodin, V. K. Yachandra, R. D. Britt, K. Sauer, and M. P. Klein, *Biochim. Biophys. Acta*, *767*, 209–216 (1984).

57. V. K. Yachandra, V. J. Derose, M. J. Latimer, I. Mukerji, K. Sauer, and M. P. Klein, in *Research in Photosynthesis*, Vol. 2 (N. Murata, ed.), Kluwer Academic, Dordrecht, 1992, pp. 281–287.

58. J. L. Casey and K. Sauer, *Biochim. Biophys. Acta*, *767*, 21–28 (1984).

59. G. C. Dismukes and Y. Siderer, *Proc. Natl. Acad. Sci. USA*, *78*, 274–278 (1981).

60. J.-L. Zimmermann and A. W. Rutherford, *Biochim. Biophys. Acta*, *767*, 160–167 (1984).

61. A. Haddy, W. R. Dunham, R. H. Sands, and R. Aasa, *Biochim. Biophys. Acta*, *1099*, 25–34 (1992).

62. M. Zheng and G. C. Dismukes, *Inorg. Chem.*, *35*, 3307–3319 (1996).

63. O. Hansson, R. Aasa and T. Vänngård, *Biophys. J.*, *51*, 825–832 (1987).

64. N. A. Law, T. E. Machonkin, J. P. McGorman, E. J. Larson, J. W. Kampf, and V. L. Pecoraro, *J. Chem. Soc., Chem. Commun.*, 2015–2016 (1995).

65. S. M. Saadeh, M. S. Lah, and V. L. Pecoraro, *Inorg. Chem.*, *30*, 8–15 (1991).

66. S. K. Chandra and A. Chakravorty, *Inorg. Chem.*, *31*, 760–765 (1992).

67. P. Chaudhuri and K. Wieghardt, in *Progress in Inorganic Chemistry*, Vol. 35 (S. J. Lippard, ed.), Wiley Interscience, New York, 1987, pp. 329–436.

68. O. Schlager, K. Wieghardt, and B. Nuber, *Inorg. Chem.*, *34*, 6456–6462 (1995).

69. X. Li, M. S. Lah, and V. L. Pecoraro, *Acta Crystallographica, C*, 1517–1519 (1989).

70. K. A. Åhrling, P. J. Smith, and R. J. Pace, *J. Am. Chem. Soc.*, *120*, 13202–13214 (1998).

71. R. D. Britt, G. A. Lorigan, K. Sauer, M. P. Klein, and J. L. Zimmermann, *Biochim. Biophys. Acta*, *1140*, 95–101 (1992).

72. T. A. Roelofs, W. Liang, M. J. Latimer, R. M. Cinco, A. Rompel, J. C. Andrews, K. Sauer, V. K. Yachandra, and M. P. Klein, *Proc. Natl. Acad. Sci. USA*, *93*, 3335–3340 (1996).

73. T.-A. Ono, T. Noguchi, Y. Inoue, M. Kusunoki, T. Matsushita, and H. Oyanagi, *Science*, *258*, 1335–1337 (1992).

74. T. Ono, T. Noguchi, Y. Inoue, M. Kusunoki, H. Yamaguchi, and H. Oyanagi, *J. Am. Chem. Soc.*, *117*, 6386–6387 (1995).

75. A. Kawamori, H. Mino, and T. Matsukawa, Dual mode EPR study of S3-State manganese cluster in the oxygen evolving Photosystem II, *XIth International Congress on Photosynthesis*, Budapest, 1998, p. 72.

76. A. Boussac, J.-L. Zimmermann, A. W. Rutherford, and J. Lavergne, *Nature*, *347*, 303–306 (1990).

77. U. Bossek, T. Weyhermüller, K. Wieghardt, B. Nuber, and J. Weiss, *J. Am. Chem. Soc.*, *112*, 6387–6388 (1990).

78. A. Boussac, J.-L. Zimmermann, and A. W. Rutherford, *Biochemistry*, *28*, 8984–8989 (1989).

79. M. Baumgarten, J. S. Philo, and G. C. Dismukes, *Biochemistry*, *29*, 10814–10822 (1990).

80. D. J. MacLachlan and J. H. A. Nugent, *Biochemistry*, *32*, 9772–9780 (1993).

81. V. A. Szalai and G. W. Brudvig, *Biochemistry*, *35*, 1946–1953 (1996).

82. C. Berthomieu and A. Boussac, *Biochemistry*, *34*, 1541–1548 (1995).

83. B. J. Hallahan, J. H. A. Nugent, J. T. Warden, and M. C. W. Evans, *Biochemistry*, *31*, 4562–4573 (1992).

84. X.-S. Tang, D. W. Randall, D. A. Force, B. A. Diner, and R. D. Britt, *J. Am. Chem. Soc.*, *118*, 7638–7639 (1996).

85. J. M. Peloquin, K. A. Campbell, and R. D. Britt, *J. Am. Chem. Soc.*, *120*, 6840–6841 (1998).

86. P. Dorlet, M. D. Valentin, G. T. Babcock, and J. L. McCracken, *J. Phys. Chem. B*, *102*, 8239–8247 (1998).

87. B. Adam, E. Bill, E. Bothe, B. Goerdt, G. Haselhorst, K. Hildenbrand, A. Sokolowski, S. Steenken, T. Weyhermüller, and K. Wieghardt, *Chem. Eur. J.*, *3*, 308–319 (1997).

88. J. Messinger, J. H. A. Nugent, and M. C. W. Evans, *Biochemistry*, *36*, 11055–11060 (1997).

89. J. Messinger, J. H. Robblee, W. O. Yu, K. Sauer, V. K. Yachandra, and M. P. Klein, *J. Am. Chem. Soc.*, *119*, 11349–11350 (1997).

90. K. A. Åhrling, S. Peterson, and S. Styring, *Biochemistry*, *36*, 13148–13152 (1997).

91. J. Messinger, G. Seaton, and T. Wydrzynski, *Biochemistry*, *36*, 6862–6873 (1997).

92. J. Messinger and G. Renger, *Biochemistry*, *32*, 9379–9386 (1993).

93. J. Messinger, U. Wacker, and G. Renger, *Biochemistry*, *30*, 7852 (1991).

94. N. Ioannidis, J. Sarrou, G. Schansker, and V. Petrouleas, *Biochemistry*, *37*, 16445–16451 (1998).

95. P. J. Riggs-Gelasco, R. Mei, C. F. Yocum, and J. E. Penner-Hahn, *J. Am. Chem. Soc.*, *118*, 2387–2399 (1996).

96. M. K. Chan and W. H. Armstrong, *J. Am. Chem. Soc.*, *112*, 4985–4986 (1990).

97. V. K. Yachandra, V. J. DeRose, M. J. Latimer, I. Mukerji, K. Sauer, and M. P. Klein, *Science*, *260*, 675–679 (1993).

98. V. K. Yachandra, R. D. Guiles, A. McDermott, R. D. Britt, S. L. Dexheimer, K. Sauer, and M. P. Klein, *Biochim. Biophys. Acta*, *850*, 324–332 (1986).

99. L. Que, Jr., and A. E. True, in *Progress in Inorganic Chemistry*, Vol. 38 (S. J. Lippard, ed.), John Wiley and Sons, New York, 1990, pp. 97–200.

100. T. L. Stemmler, T. M. Sossong, Jr., J. I. Goldstein, D. E. Ash, T. E.

Elgren, D. M. Kurtz, Jr., and J. E. Penner-Hahn, *Biochemistry*, *36*, 9847–9858 (1997).

101. J. J. Rehr, J. Mustre de Leon, S. I. Zabinsky, and R. C. Albers, *J. Am. Chem. Soc.*, *113*, 5135–5140 (1991).

102. G. W. Brudvig and R. H. Crabtree, *Proc. Natl. Acad. Sci. USA*, *83*, 4586–4588 (1986).

103. K. Wieghardt, U. Bossek, and W. Gebert, *Angew. Chem. Int. Ed.*, *22*, 328–329 (1983).

104. R. M. Cinco, J. H. Robblee, A. Rompel, C. Fernandez, V. K. Yachandra, K. Sauer, and M. P. Klein, *J. Phys. Chem. B*, *102*, 8248–8256 (1998).

105. S. L. Dexheimer and M. P. Klein, *J. Am. Chem. Soc.*, *114*, 2821–2826 (1992).

106. M. K. Chan and W. H. Armstrong, *J. Am. Chem. Soc.*, *113*, 5055–5057 (1991).

107. T. Matsukawa, A. Kawamori, and H. Mino, *Spectrochim. Acta, Part A*, *55*, 895–901 (1999).

108. K. A. Campbell, J. M. Peloquin, D. P. Pham, R. J. Debus, and R. D. Britt, *J. Am. Chem. Soc.*, *120*, 447–448 (1998).

109. V. J. DeRose, I. Mukerji, M. J. Latimer, V. K. Yachandra, K. Sauer, and M. P. Klein, *J. Am. Chem. Soc.*, *116*, 5239–5249 (1994).

110. I. Mukerji, J. C. Andrews, V. J. DeRose, M. J. Latimer, V. K. Yachandra, K. Sauer, and M. P. Klein, *Biochemistry*, *33*, 9712–9721 (1994).

111. W. Liang, M. J. Latimer, H. Dau, T. A. Roelofs, V. K. Yachandra, K. Sauer, and M. P. Klein, *Biochemistry*, *33*, 4923–4932 (1994).

112. K. Hasegawa, M. Kusunoki, Y. Inoue, and T. A. Ono, *Biochemistry*, *37*, 9457–9465 (1998).

113. N. A. Law, J. W. Kampf, and V. L. Pecoraro, *Inorg. Chim. Acta*, submitted.

114. R. D. Guiles, V. K. Yachandra, A. E. McDermott, J. L. Cole, S. L. Dexheimer, R. D. Britt, K. Sauer, and M. P. Klein, *Biochemistry*, *29*, 486–496 (1990).

115. H.-A. Chu, A. P. Nguyen, and R. J. Debus, *Biochemistry*, *33*, 6137–6149 (1994).

116. H.-A. Chu, A. P. Nguyen, and R. J. Debus, *Biochemistry*, *33*, 6150–6157 (1994).

117. R. J. Debus, B. A. Barry, I. Sithole, G. T. Babcock, and L. McIntosh, *Biochemistry*, 27, 9071–9074 (1988).

118. R. J. Debus, B. A. Barry, G. T. Babcock, and L. McIntosh, *Proc. Natl. Acad. Sci. USA*, 85, 427–430 (1988).

119. C. Andronis, O. Kruse, Z. Deak, I. Vass, B. A. Diner, and P. J. Nixon, *Plant Physiol.*, 117, 515–524 (1998).

120. R. Hienerwadel, A. Boussac, J. Breton, B. A. Diner, and C. Berthomieu, *Biochemistry*, 36, 14712–14723 (1997).

121. T. Noguchi, T. Ono, and Y. Inoue, *Biochim. Biophys. Acta*, 1228, 189–200 (1995).

122. H. Ikura and T. Nagata, *Inorg. Chem.*, 37, 4702–4711 (1998).

123. H.-A. Chu, A. P. Nguyen, and R. J. Debus, *Biochemistry*, 34, 5859–5882 (1995).

124. K. A. Campbell, J. M. Peloquin, B. A. Diner, X.-S. Tang, D. A. Chisholm, and R. D. Britt, *J. Am. Chem. Soc.*, 119, 4787–4788 (1997).

125. P. J. Hart, M. M. Balbirnie, N. L. Ogihara, A. M. Nersissian, M. S. Weiss, J. S. Valentine, and D. Eisenberg, *Biochemistry*, 38, 2167–2178 (1999).

126. D. N. Hendrickson, G. Christou, E. A. Schmitt, E. Libby, J. S. Bashkin, S. Wang, H.-L. Tsai, J. B. Vincent, P. D. W. Boyd, J. C. Huffman, K. Folting, Q. Li, and W. E. Streib, *J. Am. Chem. Soc.*, 114, 2455–2471 (1992).

127. M. T. Caudle, J. W. Kampf, M. L. Kirk, P. G. Rasmussen, and V. L. Pecoraro, *J. Am. Chem. Soc.*, 119, 9297–9298 (1997).

128. R. Radmer and O. Ollinger, *FEBS Lett.*, 195, 285–289 (1986).

129. J. Messinger, M. Badger, and T. Wydrzynski, *Proc. Natl. Acad. Sci. USA*, 92, 3209–3213 (1995).

130. P. O. Sandusky and C. F. Yocum, *FEBS Lett.*, 162, 339–343 (1983).

131. P. O. Sandusky and C. F. Yocum, *Biochim. Biophys. Acta*, 849, 85–93 (1986).

132. A. Niemann, U. Bossek, G. Haselhorst, K. Wieghardt, and B. Nuber, *Inorg. Chem.*, 35, 906–915 (1996).

133. J. Du Bois, J. Hong, E. M. Carreira, and M. W. Day, *J. Am. Chem. Soc.*, 118, 915–916 (1996).

134. J. Du Bois, C. S. Tomooka, J. Hong, and E. M. Carreira, *Acc. Chem. Res.*, 30, 364–372 (1997).

135. W. Hillier, J. Messinger, and T. Wydrzynski, *Biochemistry*, *37*, 16908–16914 (1998).

136. J. A. Halfen, S. Mahapatra, E. C. Wilkinson, S. Kaderli, V. G. J. Young, L. Que, Jr., A. D. Zuberbühler, and W. B. Tolman, *Science*, *271*, 1397–1400 (1996).

137. L. J. Boucher and C. G. Coe, *Inorg. Chem.*, *15*, 1334–1340 (1976).

138. L. J. Boucher and C. G. Coe, *Inorg. Chem.*, *14*, 1289–1295 (1975).

139. S. Turconi, D. J. MacLachlan, P. J. Bratt, J. H. A. Nugent, and M. C. W. Evans, *Biochemistry*, *36*, 879–885 (1997).

140. D. W. Randall, A. Gelasco, M. T. Caudle, V. L. Pecoraro, and R. D. Britt, *J. Am. Chem. Soc.*, *119*, 4481–4491 (1997).

141. M. T. Caudle, P. Riggs-Gelasco, A. K. Gelasco, J. E. Penner-Hahn, and V. L. Pecoraro, *Inorg. Chem.*, *35*, 3577–3584 (1996).

142. D. W. Randall, B. E. Sturgeon, J. A. Ball, G. A. Lorigan, M. K. Chan, M. P. Klein, W. H. Armstrong, and R. D. Britt, *J. Am. Chem. Soc.*, *117*, 11780–11789 (1995).

143. P. O. Sandusky and C. F. Yocum, *Biochim. Biophys. Acta*, *766*, 603–611 (1984).

144. P. M. Kelly and S. Izawa, *Biochim. Biophys. Acta*, *502*, 198–210 (1978).

145. H. Wincencjusz, H. Van Gorkom, and C. F. Yocum, *Biochemistry*, *36*, 3663–3670 (1997).

146. A. Rompel, J. C. Andrews, R. M. Cinco, M. W. Wemple, G. Christou, N. A. Law, V. L. Pecoraro, K. Sauer, V. K. Yachandra, and M. P. Klein, *J. Am. Chem. Soc.*, *119*, 4465–4470 (1997).

147. X. Li and V. L. Pecoraro, *Inorg. Chem.*, *28*, 3403–3410 (1989).

148. M. W. Wemple, H.-L. Tsai, K. Folting, D. N. Hendrickson, and G. Christou, *Inorg. Chem.*, *32*, 2025–2031 (1993).

149. J. A. Gilbert, D. S. Eggleston, W.R. Murphy, Jr., D. A. Geselowitz, S. W. Gersten, D. J. Hodgson, and T. J. Meyer, *J. Am. Chem. Soc.*, *107*, 3855–3864 (1985).

150. M. Fujiwara, T. Matsushita, and T. Shono, *Polyhedron*, *4*, 1895–1900 (1985).

151. T. Matsushita, M. Fujiwara, and T. Shono, *Chem. Lett.*, 631–634 (1981).

152. C. W. Hoganson and G. T. Babcock, *Science*, *277*, 1953–1956 (1997).

153. C. F. Yocum, *Biochim. Biophys. Acta*, *1059*, 1–14 (1991).

154. A. Boussac and A. W. Rutherford, *Biochemistry*, *27*, 3476–3483 (1988).

155. A. Boussac and A. W. Rutherford, *Chem. Scripta*, *28A*, 123–126 (1988).

156. N. Tamura, Y. Inoue, and G. M. Cheniae, *Biochim. Biophys. Acta*, *976*, 173–181 (1989).

157. A. F. Miller and G. W. Brudvig, *Biochemistry*, *29*, 1385–1392 (1990).

158. M. Sivaraja, J. Tso, and G. C. Dismukes, *Biochemistry*, *28*, 9459–9464 (1989).

159. M. J. Latimer, V. J. DeRose, I. Mukerji, V. K. Yachandra, K. Sauer, and M. P. Klein, *Biochemistry*, *34*, 10898–10909 (1995).

160. J. E. Penner-Hahn, P. J. Riggs-Gelasco, E. Yu, P. Demarois, and C. F. Yocum, in *Photosynthesis: From Light to Biosphere* (P. Mathis, ed.), Kluwer Academic, Netherlands, 1995, pp. 241–246.

161. P. J. Riggs-Gelasco, R. Mei, D. F. Ghanotakis, C. F. Yocum, and J. E. Penner-Hahn, *J. Am. Chem. Soc.*, *118*, 2400–2410 (1996).

162. C. P. Horwitz and Y. Ciringh, *Inorg. Chim. Acta*, *225*, 191–200 (1994).

163. C. P. Horwitz, J. T. Warden, and S. T. Weintraub, *Inorganica Chimica*, *246*, 311–320 (1996).

164. S. M. Gorun, R. T. Stibrany, and A. Lillo, *Inorg. Chem.*, *37*, 836–837 (1998).

165. S. M. Rocklage, W. P. Cacheris, S. C. Quay, F. E. Hahn, and K. N. Raymond, *Inorg. Chem.*, *28*, 477–485 (1989).

166. P. E. Siegbahn and R. H. Crabtree, *J. Am. Chem. Soc.*, *121*, 117–127 (1999).

167. A. Zouni, P. Fromme, W. D. Schubert, W. Saenger, and H. T. Witt, Characterization of 3-dimensional crystals of Photosystem II from Synechococcus elongatus, *XIth International Congress on Photosynthesis*, Budapest, 1998, p. 64.

168. G. T. Babcock, in *Photosynthesis: From Light to Biosphere*, Vol. 11 (P. Mathis, ed.), Kluwer Academic, Netherlands, 1995, pp. 209–215.

169. C. W. Hoganson, N. Lydakis-Simantiris, X.-S. Tang, C. Tommos, K. Warncke, G. T. Babcock, B. A. Diner, J. McCracken, and S. Styring, *Photosynth. Res.*, *46*, 177–184 (1995).

170. S. J. Lippard and J. M. Berg, eds., *Principles of Bioinorganic Chemistry*, University Science Books, Mill Valley, CA, 1994.

171. M. L. Gilchrist, J. A. Ball, D. W. Randall, and R. D. Britt, *Proc. Nat. Acad. Sci. USA*, *92*, 9545–9549 (1995).

172. M. Haumann, A. Mulkidjanian, and W. Junge, *Biochemistry*, *38*, 1258–1267 (1999).

173. F. G. Bordwell and J.-P. Cheng, *J. Am. Chem. Soc.*, *113*, 1736–1743 (1991).

174. J. Lind, X. Shen, T. E. Ericksen, and G. Merényi, *J. Am. Chem. Soc.*, *112*, 479–482 (1990).

175. D. F. McMillen and D. M. Golden, *Annu. Rev. Phys. Chem.*, *33*, 493 (1982).

176. M. J. Baldwin and V. L. Pecoraro, *J. Am. Chem. Soc.*, *118*, 11325–11326 (1996).

177. M. T. Caudle and V. L. Pecoraro, *J. Am. Chem. Soc.*, *119*, 3415–3416 (1997).

178. K. A. Gardner and J. M. Mayer, *Science*, *269*, 1849–1851 (1995).

179. M. R. A. Blomberg, P. E. M. Siegbahn, S. Styring, G. T. Babcock, B. Akermark, and P. Korall, *J. Am. Chem. Soc.*, *119*, 8285–8292 (1997).

180. V. L. Pecoraro, M. J. Baldwin, M. T. Caudle, W.-Y. Hsieh, and N. A. Law, *Pure Appl. Chem.*, *70*, 925–929 (1998).

181. J. B. Vincent and G. Christou, *Inorg. Chim. Acta*, *136*, L41–L43 (1987).

182. T. J. Collins and S. W. Gordon-Wylie, *J. Am. Chem. Soc.*, *111*, 4511–4513 (1989).

183. T. J. Collins, R. D. Powell, C. Slebodnick, and E. S. Uffelman, *J. Am. Chem. Soc.*, *112*, 899–901 (1990).

184. F. M. MacDonnell, N. L. P. Fackler, C. Stern, and T. V. O'Halloran, *J. Am. Chem. Soc.*, *116*, 7431–7432 (1994).

185. K. Srinivasan, P. Michaud, and J. K. Kochi, *J. Am. Chem. Soc.*, *108*, 2309–2320 (1986).

186. Y. Naruta, M. Sasayama, and T. Sasaki, *Angew. Chem. Int. Ed. Engl.*, *33*, 1839–1841 (1994).

187. J. Limburg, G. W. Brudvig, and R. H. Crabtree, *J. Am. Chem. Soc.*, *119*, 2761–2762 (1997).

188. J. Limberg, J. S. Vrettos, L. M. Liable-Sands, A. L. Rheingold, R. H. Crabtree, and G. W. Brudvig, *Science*, *283*, 1524–1527 (1999).

15

Manganese(II)-Dependent Extradiol-Cleaving Catechol Dioxygenases

Lawrence Que, Jr. and Mark F. Reynolds

Department of Chemistry
and Center for Metals in Biocatalysis,
University of Minnesota, Minneapolis, MN 55445, USA

1. INTRODUCTION

Nature employs the catechol dioxygenases as an element of her strategy for degrading aromatic molecules in soil [1–3]. These enzymes catalyze the oxidative cleavage of dihydroxybenzene rings with the incorporation of both atoms of dioxygen into the aliphatic products. Two
families of catechol dioxygenases have been identified based on the position of ring cleavage (Fig. 1): intradiol, where the carbon-carbon bond
of the enediol unit is cleaved, and extradiol, where the carbon-carbon
bond adjacent to the enediol moiety is cleaved. Although they share
many substrates, the intra- and extradiol-cleaving enzymes exhibit
near-exclusivity in the regiospecificity of oxidative cleavage, indicating
the existence of two distinctly different catalytic mechanisms [2,3]. Furthermore, the intradiol-cleaving enzymes invariably require Fe(III),
while the extradiol-cleaving enzymes usually require Fe(II). However,
there are examples of extradiol-cleaving enzymes that require Mn(II)
[4–6] and one that requires Mg(II) [7].

2. THE INTRADIOL CLEAVAGE PRECEDENT

Every intradiol-cleaving dioxygenase has thus far been found to contain
Fe(III) as the active metal center. The elegant and comprehensive crystallographic studies of Ohlendorf and Lipscomb [8–12] on the protocatechuate 3,4-dioxygenase (PCD) from *Pseudomonas putida* have provided a very detailed picture of the enzyme active site and the
significant changes that occur when substrate binds and becomes acti-

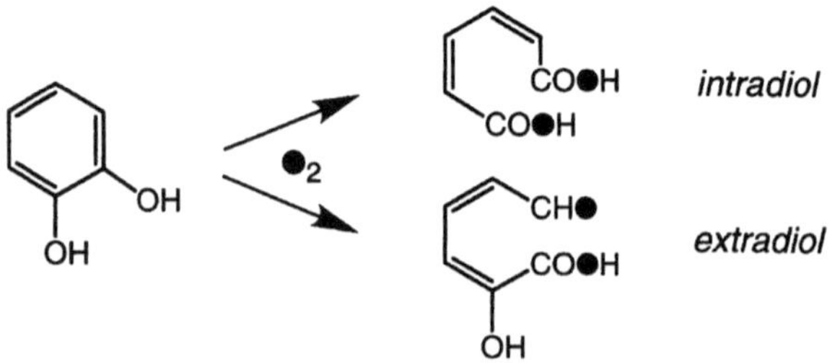

FIG. 1.   Modes of catechol cleavage.

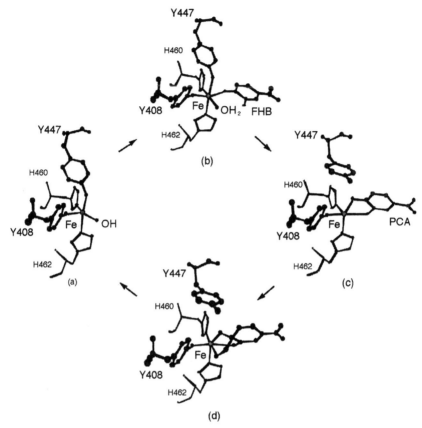

FIG. 2.   PCD reaction cycle based on coordinates from Orville et al. [10].

vated for dioxygen attack. As shown in Fig. 2a, the iron(III) center in the as isolated PCD is in a trigonal bipyramidal environment [8,9]. Tyr447 and His462 serve as the axial ligands, while Tyr408 and His460 act as equatorial ligands. The third equatorial ligand is a solvent molecule, deduced to be a hydroxide from an EXAFS study [13]. It is proposed that substrate binding occurs in stages, on the basis of the structures of several hydroxybenzoate complexes and the enzyme–substrate complex [10,11]. The initial phase of substrate binding entails the coordination of the 4-OH moiety to the metal center and the transfer of its proton to the bound hydroxide, as illustrated by the structure of the PCD–3-fluoro-4-hydroxybenzoate complex (Fig. 2b) [10]. The 3-OH group then binds to the metal center, resulting in a bidentate catecholate complex. The second catecholate proton is transferred to the axial Tyr447, which is then displaced from the iron coordination sphere, as shown in Fig. 2c for the PCD–protocatechuate complex [11]. The enzyme–substrate complex is thus a five-coordinate complex with a chelated catecholate dianion and three remaining endogenous ligands arranged in a facial array.

Exposure of the enzyme–substrate complex to O_2 results in the immediate oxidative cleavage of the substrate. This observation implies that the complex is poised to react with O_2. The nature of this activation has been the subject of some discussion. On the basis of its spectroscopic properties, the enzyme–substrate (ES) complex is best described as an iron(III)–catecholate complex [2]. The ES complex exhibits electron paramagnetic resonance (EPR) and Mössbauer spectra that unequivocally assign the metal center as a high-spin iron(III) ion [14,15]. The complex also has a visible absorption feature that stretches from 500 nm into the near IR region that is associated with a catecholate-to-iron(III) charge transfer transition [16,17]. How does this iron(III)–catecholate complex react with O_2? Since it is highly unlikely that O_2 binds the iron(III) center directly, there are two alternatives to be considered. An O_2 activation mechanism would require the metal center to be reduced by the substrate to an extent that is not detectable by spectroscopy. O_2 binding to this Fe(II) center would then shift the equilibrium to this form and generate the ternary $E \bullet S \bullet O_2$ complex. This mechanism is disfavored by the demonstration that the O_2 analog NO does not react with the enzyme–substrate complex [18]. Alternatively, the reaction may proceed by a substrate activation mechanism [19]. Substrate activation is proposed to occur via a ketonization of the 3-OH moiety that concentrates electron density on the substrate C-4 where O_2 would directly attack (Fig. 3, X = C). This idea has been supported by the fact that substrate analogs that promote this tautomeric form are tight-binding inhibitors of the enzyme (Fig. 3, X = N) [20–23] and the fact that the catecholate is found to be asymmetrically chelated in the crystal structure [11,12]. Indeed, the Fe-O-3 bond is about 0.2 Å longer than the Fe-O-4 bond, a notion corroborated by an 80 cm^{-1} difference observed for the two Fe-O vibrations in the Raman spectrum of the enzyme–substrate complex [12]. The asymmetric chelation probably comes about as a result of differences in the electron donating abilities of the trans ligands, His462 for the substrate O-4 atom and Tyr408

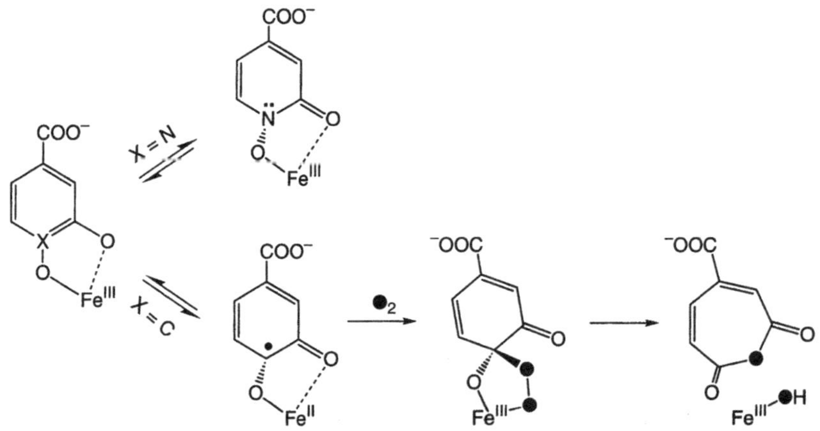

FIG. 3. Postulated mode for substrate activation.

for the O-3 atom. Above the substrate C-4 carbon atom sits a conserved Arg residue that is postulated to stabilize the incipient negative charge that would develop on that carbon atom as the substrate becomes activated.

Attack of O_2 on the substrate C-4 is then postulated to afford the putative ternary $E \bullet S \bullet O_2$ complex shown in Fig. 2d with the dioxygen moiety bridging the substrate C-4 atom and the metal center. This proposed structure derives from altering the coordinates for the "ternary" PCD complex with the analog 3-hydroxyisonicotinic acid N-oxide and cyanide in which the cyanide occupies the vacant sixth coordination site on the metal center [11]. This site is sterically quite restricted and only allows binding of a diatomic species. Decomposition of the ternary complex results in ring cleavage and the expected intradiol product via an anhydride intermediate (Fig. 3).

Model complexes support the substrate activation mechanism. A number of iron(III) catecholate complexes have been shown to undergo the desired intradiol cleavage [24–30]. The rate of cleavage is strongly dependent on the nature of the other ligands bound to the metal center. Ancillary ligands that favor catecholate-to-iron(III) charge transfer transitions in the near-IR region give rise to complexes with the fastest rates of cleavage. The low energy of the LMCT band has been interpreted to reflect the extent of covalency of the metal catecholate bonding [24,26]. On the basis of the observed paramagnetic shifts of the catecholate protons, the covalency is proposed to enhance the Fe(II)-semi-quinone character of the Fe(III)-catecholate moiety (Fig. 3), which in turn would facilitate the direct attack of O_2 on the substrate.

3. Fe(II)-DEPENDENT EXTRADIOL-CLEAVING DIOXYGENASES

Most of the extradiol-cleaving catechol dioxygenases reported thus far require Fe(II). Due to the spectroscopic inaccessibility of Fe(II), these enzymes are not as well understood as their intradiol counterparts, but recent developments have significantly improved the state of our understanding. Notably, the crystal structures of two enzymes are now available: 2,3-dihydroxybiphenyl 1,2-dioxygenase from *Pseudomonas* sp. strain LB400 (BphC) [31,32] and catechol 2,3-dioxygenase (2,3-CTD) from *Pseudomonas putida* mt-2 [33]. As exemplified by the structure of BphC shown in Fig. 4 [31], the metal environment consists of a square-

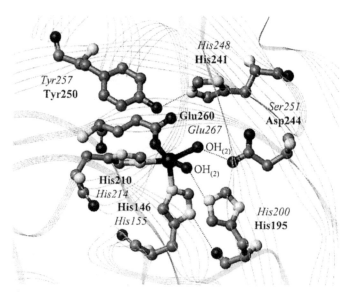

FIG. 4.   Active site structure of BphC based on the coordinates from Han et al. [31]. The Fe(II)-dependent BphC residues are shown in bold while the Mn(II)-dependent MndD residues are shown in italics. The revised sequence of MndD [36] was used for numbering the active site residues.

pyramidal Fe(II) center that is coordinated by three endogenous protein ligands, two His residues and a glutamate, and two solvent molecules. An analogous coordination sphere is also found for the iron(II) center in 2,3-CTD [33]. The three protein ligands are arranged on one face of the square pyramid to form what has been recognized as a 2-His–1-carboxylate facial triad motif common to a diverse array of Fe(II)-dependent oxygen-activating enzymes [34,35].

The structure of the corresponding BphC–substrate complex shows a bidentate catechol substrate that displaces the two solvent ligands and coordinates trans to His210 and the vacant site trans to His146 [32,37]. The site trans to Glu260 is vacant and thus available for O_2 binding. This geometry is consistent with results from previous spectroscopic studies of 2,3-CTD supporting a five-coordinate iron(II) environment for the enzyme–substrate complex [38,39].

Like that of the intradiol-cleaving PCD–substrate complex, the crystal structure of the BphC–substrate complex suggests that the catecholate is unsymmetrically chelated [32,37]. EXAFS analysis of the 2,3-CTD–substrate complex supports this binding mode and reveals Fe-O bond lengths that differ by at least 0.2 Å [39]. Since the crystal structure of the BphC–substrate complex shows that the ligands trans to the catecholate oxygens are both His residues, the unsymmetric chelation mode must have a different chemical basis. We have proposed that the bidentate substrate is a monoanion [39], not a dianion as found for the intradiol-cleaving enzymes. This notion is supported by the crystal structure of an iron(II)–catecholate complex, $[Fe(6-Me_3-TPA)DBC-H]^+$ (Fig. 5), which shows a chelated but monoanionic catecholate where the Fe-O bond is 0.3 Å shorter than the Fe-OH bond [40]. The affinity of catecholate for Fe(III) is quite high [41], sufficiently so to cause ionization of both catechol protons; because its affinity for Fe(II) is significantly lower, only the pK_a of the first catechol proton is decreased enough and a monoanionic complex is formed [41]. The idea of a monanionic substrate moiety in the enzyme active site is supported by the complex of 2,3-CTD with the chromophoric 4-nitrocatechol substrate which exhibits a UV-Vis spectrum characteristic of the 4-nitrocatecholate monoanion [42]. Thus the enzyme–substrate complex of the extradiol-cleaving enzymes is best described as an iron(II)–catecholate monoanion complex.

In contrast to the intradiol-cleaving enzymes, the enzyme–substrate complexes of the extradiol-cleaving enzymes readily bind the O_2

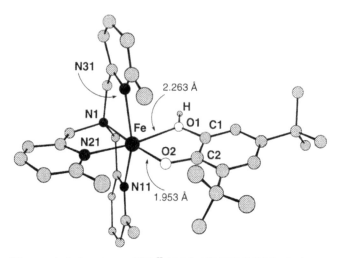

FIG. 5.   The crystal structure of [Fe^{II}-(6-Me$_3$TPA)(DBC-H)$^+$ [39]. (Reproduced with permission from the American Chemical Society.)

analog NO to form ternary E•S•NO complexes [43,44]. This reactivity supports an O$_2$ activation mechanism for these enzymes (Fig. 6). In the proposed mechanism, O$_2$ binding to the iron(II) center generates an iron(III)-superoxo species. Electron transfer from the substrate to the iron(III) center generates an iron(II)-semiquinone species. Indeed Bugg and co-workers [45,46] have demonstrated that radical character is introduced into the substrate aromatic ring during turnover by using substrate analogs that have cyclopropane substituents. The nucleophilic superoxide can then attack the aromatic ring to initiate ring cleavage. Bugg et al. [46] favor the attack of superoxide on one of the enediol carbon atoms to form a peroxo species very similar to that proposed for the intradiol cleavage mechanism. Lipscomb, Que, and co-workers have proposed an alternative mechanism in which the superoxide attacks the carbon atom adjacent to the enediol unit [39] . The crystal structure of the BphC ES complex appears to favor the attack of an enediol carbon atom, since it requires much less dramatic atom motions within the active site to form the peroxo intermediate. This intermediate would then have two options for ring cleavage, intradiol or extradiol, so there must be some mechanism to ensure extradiol cleavage. Attack of the carbon atom adjacent to the enediol unit would have the advantage that the regiospecificity of cleavage would already be built into the mechanism. Further work is needed to clarify the mechanism for extradiol cleavage.

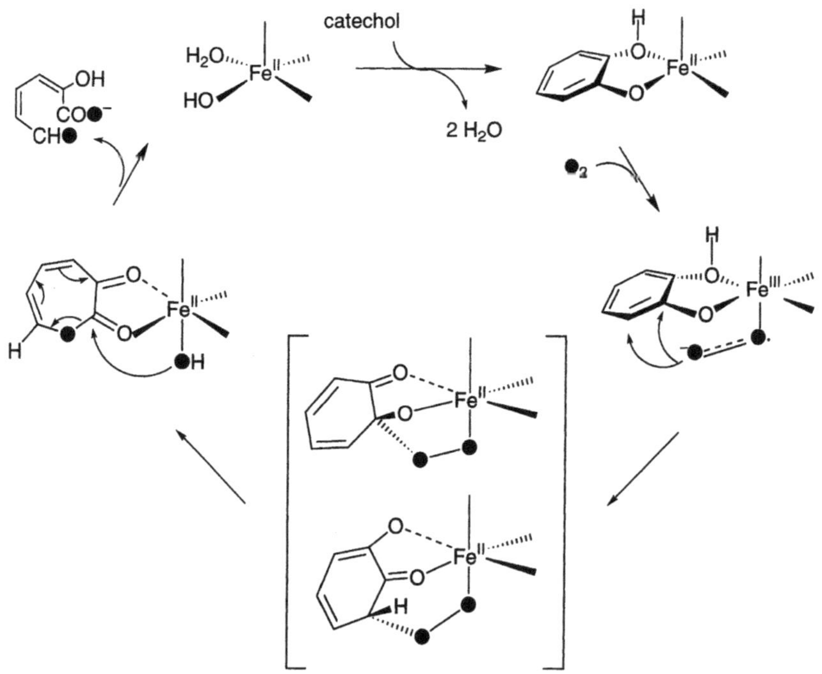

FIG. 6. Proposed mechanism for the extradiol cleavage of catechol.

4. Mn(II)-DEPENDENT DIOXYGENASES

In the course of investigating extradiol-cleaving catechol dioxygenases in general, we discovered that some of these enzymes are actually Mn(II)-dependent. Mn(II)-dependent dioxygenases have now been found in a number of organisms and purified from *Bacillus brevis* [4], *Arthrobacter* sp. strain Mn-1 [47], and *Arthrobacter globiformis* strain CM-2 [5,6]. The involvement of Mn(II) was first indicated by the presence of an intense EPR signal in the $g = 2$ region that exhibited characteristic features of [55]Mn hyperfine splitting [4,6]. Although Mn contamination of metalloenzymes is not uncommon, attempts to remove the Mn "impurity" in the course of purifying the enzyme were unsuccessful, and it was eventually concluded that the Mn center was the key to catalysis.

The best analytical data currently available is for MndD, the 3,4-dihydroxyphenylacetate 2,3-dioxygenase from *A. globiformis* strain

CM-2, whose *mndD* gene has been cloned, sequenced, and then expressed in *E. coli* [5]. Metal analyses by ICP of several preparations of as isolated MndD of comparable specific activity showed an average Mn content of 3.0 ± 0.2 *g*-atoms per homotetramer and an Fe content of 0.7 ± 0.2 *g*-atoms per homotetramer [6]. The importance of the Mn center was established by partial-apo and apo-MndD preparations whose specific activities correlated well with their respective Mn contents and not with their Fe contents [6]. This notion was further supported by the observation that H_2O_2, CN^-, and $K_3Fe(CN)_6$, reagents that all rapidly inactivated the Fe(II)-dependent extradiol dioxygenases, had little effect on the Mn-dependent dioxygenases [6]. These results thus establish a new class of Mn(II)-dependent extradiol cleaving catechol dioxygenases.

4.1. Sequence Information

The cloning and sequencing of the *mndD* gene afforded a wealth of information with which to compare this Mn(II)-dependent enzyme and its many Fe(II)-dependent counterparts [5]. Sequence comparisons of the Fe(II)-dependent extradiol-cleaving dioxygenases reveal that the majority of these enzymes belong to a superfamily with a consensus pattern of 18 residues that uniquely identify this group among the 67 000-member PIR 40 database or the 36 000-member Swiss-Prot 28 database [5,48]. This pattern is located in a region of the enzyme sequences that contain a high concentration of completely conserved residues and minimal gaps or insertions. MndD appears to fit into this superfamily, as it shares 14 of 18 residues in the consensus pattern [5]. When the consensus pattern is relaxed to accommodate the *mndD* sequence, the less restrictive consensus pattern maintains its stringency in identifying only members of the extradiol dioxygenase superfamily.

Three residues in the MndD sequence—H155, H214, and E267—correspond to the three ligand residues in the crystallographically characterized BphC structure (Fig. 4) and are most likely the ligands to the Mn(II) center. This hypothesis has been tested by site-directed mutagenesis [49]. When the His residues were mutated to alanine, the mutant proteins exhibited <0.1% of the specific activity and <2% of the Mn content of the wild-type enzyme. The E267Q mutant protein similarly showed <0.1% of the specific activity of the wild-type enzyme but contained about 1 Mn per homotetramer. These results suggest that the

Gln residue may allow the active site to retain some affinity for Mn(II) but none of the catalytic activity. More interestingly, the replacement of the native Glu ligand with an Asp residue afforded a mutant protein with 12% of the specific activity of the wild-type enzyme. Unfortunately the measurements could only be carried out in crude extracts, as the mutant protein was too unstable to be purified [49]. Taken together, the sequence comparisons with the Fe(II) extradiol dioxygenases and the site-directed mutagenesis experiments provide strong evidence for the presence of a 2-His–1-carboxylate facial triad [34,35] that binds the Mn(II) center in MndD. Thus MndD belongs to this expanding new subclass of metalloenzymes.

4.2. EPR Properties of the as Isolated MndD

As isolated MndD is distinguished from its iron-requiring analogs by the EPR properties of its metal center [6]. Unlike high-spin Fe(II) centers, which have an $S = 2$ spin state that is typically EPR-silent, MndD is EPR-active. Its high-spin Mn(II) center has an $S = 5/2$ spin state with six degenerate spin levels. Its EPR properties are governed by the spin Hamiltonian:

$$\mathbf{H} = g\beta\mathbf{B}\cdot\mathbf{S} + D(\mathbf{S}_z^2 - 35/12) + E(\mathbf{S}_x^2 - \mathbf{S}_y^2) + \mathbf{AI}\cdot\mathbf{S}$$

where D and E quantify the distortion of the ligand field from cubic and axial symmetry, respectively [50]. In a ligand field of cubic symmetry, the ^{6}A state will be split into six equally spaced levels upon the application of a magnetic field. The five allowed $\Delta M_s = 1$ transitions between pairs of levels occur at the same field, and one set of signals is observed at $g = 2.0$, split by the nuclear spin of ^{55}Mn ($I = 5/2$, 100% natural abundance) into six equally spaced peaks. Such a signal is observed for $[\mathrm{Mn(H_2O)_6}]^{2+}$. The presence of a ligand field of less than cubic symmetry partially lifts the sixfold degeneracy and creates a zero field splitting (zfs) that divides the six states into three Kramers doublets ($M_s = \pm1/2, \pm3/2, \pm5/2$). Application of a magnetic field lifts the remaining degeneracies and five sets of signals from the allowed ($\Delta M_s = \pm1$) transitions can in principle be observed in an EPR spectrum. With the inclusion of g anisotropy and ^{55}Mn hyperfine splitting, many more features can be expected, creating a distinct signature for Mn(II) EPR signals.

However, the expected complexity is often not fully resolved in the highly anisotropic outer fine-structure transitions ($\pm 5/2 \rightarrow \pm 3/2$, $\pm 3/2 \rightarrow \pm 1/2$) when Mn(II) is bound to a protein [51]. Fortunately, the central fine structure transition ($+1/2 \rightarrow -1/2$) is nearly isotropic and typically gives rise to an intense signal at $g = 2$ with resolved sixfold hyperfine splitting.

The X-band (9.23 GHz) EPR spectrum of MndD at 2.5 K (Fig. 7A) is typical of a biological Mn(II) center with weak zfs [6]. The spectrum features a strong signal centered at $g = 2.00$ with well-resolved sixfold

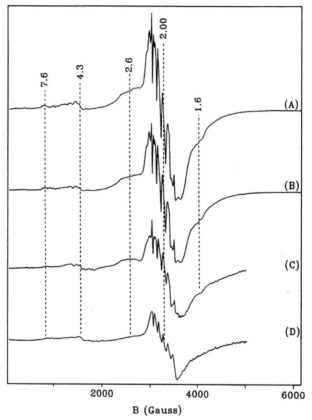

FIG. 7. EPR spectra of as isolated MndD (A) and its complexes with 4-methyl-catechol (B), p-hydroxyphenylacetate (C), and m-hydroxyphenylacetate (D). (From Whiting et al. [6]. Reprinted with permission from the American Chemical Society.)

hyperfine splitting characteristic of the central fine-structure transition ($+1/2 \rightarrow -1/2$). There are also two weaker shoulder-shaped signals at g = 2.6 and g = 1.6 that arise from zfs interactions. All of these features are absent from the spectrum of apo-MndD, thereby supporting their assignment to the catalytically essential Mn(II) site [6]. Interestingly the MndD EPR spectrum is nearly indistinguishable from that of the *B. brevis* enzyme [4]. This level of identity extends to the distribution of linewidths and the intensities of the hyperfine lines (including the intensities of the forbidden hyperfine signals) across the whole g = 2.00 envelope, strongly suggesting that the Mn(II) centers of these two enzymes exist in identical coordination environments.

The region around the g = 2.0 signal of as isolated MndD shows that the hyperfine structure of this signal is more complicated than the typical six-line derivative signal observed for $[Mn(H_2O)_6]^{2+}$. The hyperfine coupling constant, A, which can be measured directly from the spacing of the most intense derivative troughs, is approximately 95 G, a value consistent with a five- or six-coordinate Mn(II) center with oxygen or nitrogen ligands [51]. For comparison, the trigonal bipyramidal Mn(II) center of manganese superoxide dismutase has an A value of 85 G [52], while the distorted octahedral Mn(II) center of concanavalin A has an A value of 93 G [51,53,54].

Figure 8A shows the EPR spectrum of as isolated MndD acquired in parallel mode, where the probing microwave magnetic field ($\mathbf{B_1}$) is rotated from the standard configuration perpendicular to the main magnetic field ($\mathbf{B}$) to a parallel orientation [6]. Under these conditions, the selection rules are different; allowed transitions are ΔM_s = 0. MndD displays a sixfold hyperfine pattern at g = 4.8 and 9.3 with A values of 95 G. These transitions have virtually no intensity for $\mathbf{B_1} \perp \mathbf{B}$ but have a modest intensity for $\mathbf{B_1} \parallel \mathbf{B}$. This spectrum is the first observed for a biological Mn(II) center in parallel mode and demonstrates the potential utility of parallel mode EPR not only for probing integer spin systems [55] but also for studying half-integer spin systems with weak zfs.

4.3. Mode of Substrate Binding

The binding of substrates and inhibitors to MndD affects the EPR spectrum of as isolated MndD [6]. Small perturbations are observed upon the addition of the substrate analog 4-methylcatechol and the inhibitors

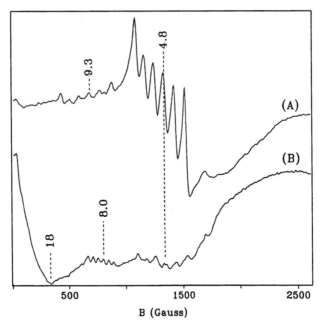

FIG. 8.   Parallel mode EPR spectra of (A) as isolated MndD and (B) its complex with 3,4-dihydroxyphenylacetate. (From Whiting et al. [6]. Reprinted with permission from the American Chemical Society.)

p-hydroxyphenylacetate and m-hydroxyphenylacetate (Fig. 7B–D), but more dramatic changes are observed upon the anaerobic addition of the natural substrate 3,4-dihydroxyphenylacetate (3,4-DHPA), the substrate analog D,L-3,4-dihydroxymandelate, and the tight-binding inhibitor p-nitrocatechol (Fig. 9). The intense [55]Mn-hyperfine split signal at g = 2 found in the as isolated enzyme is reduced significantly in intensity, and new features at g = 1.2, 2.9, 4.3, and 16 are observed. Interestingly, the signal at g = 4.3 displays sixfold hyperfine splitting (A = 95 G) that unambiguously assigns it to a Mn(II) center. These features disappear when the anaerobic MndD–3,4-DHPA complex is exposed to air, allowed to turn over, and then washed of product. The EPR spectrum of the resulting substrate-free sample is identical to that of the as isolated enzyme (as in Fig. 7A), demonstrating that the spectral changes that occur upon substrate binding are reversible [6].

The dramatic changes in the EPR spectrum observed upon substrate binding to MndD suggest that the substrate coordinates to the

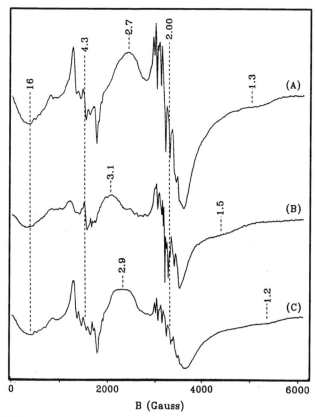

FIG. 9. EPR spectra of MndD with substrates. (A) MndD + D,L-3,4-dihydroxy-mandelic acid, anaerobic; (B) MndD + p-nitrocatechol; and (C) MndD + 3,4-DHPA, anaerobic. (From Whiting et al. [6]. Reprinted with permission from the American Chemical Society.)

metal center (Fig. 9). Similar EPR signals near g = 4.3 with sixfold hyperfine structure have been observed for the Mn(II)-containing proteins phosphoglucomutase [56] and pyruvate kinase [57,58] upon complexation with various strong binding substrates and inhibitors. In these latter cases the appearance of these lower field signals has been attributed to large (5- to 10-fold) increases in zfs caused by coordination of substrates or inhibitors to the Mn(II) center. For BphC, the iron-containing extradiol-cleaving dioxygenase, substrate binds to the Fe(II) center in a bidentate fashion displacing the two bound solvent molecules of the five-coordinate active site [37,59]. By analogy to BphC, it seems likely that the substrate also coordinates directly to the Mn(II) center of MndD. As with 2,3-CTD, the use of the chromophoric 4-nitrocatechol as a probe shows that MndD forms a monoanionic substrate complex [60]. It would appear that the MndD-catalyzed extradiol catechol cleavage mechanism may be analogous to that of iron dioxygenases (Fig. 6), but further work is needed to determine the mechanism.

4.4. Fe versus Mn-Dependent Dioxygenases

Sequence comparisons and site-directed mutagenesis experiments strongly suggest that the Fe- and Mn-dependent extradiol-cleaving dioxygenases represent yet another pair of enzymes that utilize Fe or Mn centers in very similar coordination environments to catalyze a common reaction [5,6,48]. Indeed, the sequence similarity between Fe(II)-dependent 3,4-dihydroxyphenylacetate 2,3-dioxygenase and Mn(II)-dependent MndD is approximately 80% [36,48]. The first examples of metalloenzyme active sites that use Fe or Mn are the Fe- and Mn-dependent superoxide dismutases (SODs). Both FeSOD and MnSOD have been crystallographically characterized and are found to have nearly identical first coordination spheres [61]. Despite this strong similarity, the enzymes are in many cases inactive when substituted with the other metal ion [62–65]. Vance and Miller [66] have recently proposed a simple model to explain the loss of activity when the other metal ion is exchanged into the SOD. They hypothesize that the second coordination sphere modulates the redox potential of the metal ion in the active site so that it can catalyze superoxide dismutation. The enzyme environment poises the reduction potential of the metal ion (Fe or Mn) to within a certain potential window so that superoxide can be oxidized to O_2 and reduced to form peroxide. Since the $Mn^{III/II}$ potential is higher than the $Fe^{III/II}$ potential, the MnSOD protein environment must depress the Mn potential more than is required for the FeSOD protein environment to bring the Fe potential to the correct range. Redox potential measurements indeed show that the $Fe^{III/II}$ potential in Fe-substituted MnSOD is 0.5 V lower than in FeSOD [66]. Thus the metal ion potential of Fe-substituted MnSOD is too low for superoxide to be able to reduce the oxidized Fe^{III}, although the reduced ion can carry out the other half-reaction, the conversion of superoxide to peroxide. Conversely, the Mn-substituted FeSOD should have a metal ion potential that is too high; this upshift appears to be borne out in preliminary experiments [66].

When compared to the Fe- and MnSODs, our understanding of the Fe- and Mn-dependent extradiol-cleaving dioxygenases is at a more rudimentary stage. Thus it is yet unclear what role the redox potential of the metal center plays in the mechanism of oxygen activation for extradiol cleavage. More work needs to be done to determine whether the hypothesis of Vance and Miller [66] applies to the dioxygenases. It is clearly an attractive model to understand metal ion specificity in enzymes.

ACKNOWLEDGMENT

We thank Dr. Steven J. Lange for his help in preparing this manuscript. This work was supported by the National Institutes of Health (GM33162).

ABBREVIATIONS

BphC	2,3-dihydroxybiphenyl 1,2-dioxygenase
2,3-CTD	catechol 2,3-dioxygenase
$DBCH_2$	3,5-di-*tert*-butylcatechol
DHPA	3,4-dihydroxyphenylacetate
EPR	electron paramagnetic resonance
ES	enzyme–substrate complex
EXAFS	extended X-ray absorption fine structure
ICP	inductively coupled plasma
LMCT	ligand-to-metal charge transfer
$6\text{-Me}_3\text{-TPA}$	tris(6-methyl-2-pyridylmethyl)amine
MndD	3,4-dihydroxyphenylacetate dioxygenase
PCD	protocatechuate 3,4-dioxygenase

PIR   Protein Information Resource
SOD   superoxide dismutase
zfs   zero field splitting

REFERENCES

1. D. T. Gibson, *Microbial Degradation of Organic Molecules*, Marcel Dekker, New York, 1984.

2. L. Que, Jr. and R. Y. N. Ho, *Chem. Rev.*, *96*, 2607–2624 (1996).

3. J. D. Lipscomb and A. M. Orville, *Metal Ions Biol. Syst.*, *28*, 243–298 (1992).

4. L. Que, Jr., J. Widom, and R. L. Crawford, *J. Biol. Chem.*, *256*, 10941–10944 (1981).

5. Y. R. Boldt, M. J. Sadowsky, L. B. M. Ellis, L. Que, Jr., and L. P. Wackett, *J. Bacteriol.*, *177*, 1225–1232 (1995).

6. A. K. Whiting, Y. R. Boldt, M. P. Hendrich, L. P. Wackett, and L. Que, Jr., *Biochemistry*, *35*, 160–170 (1996).

7. A. Gibello, E. Ferrer, M. Martin, and A. Garrido-Pertierra, *Biochem. J.*, *301*, 145–150 (1994).

8. D. H. Ohlendorf, P. C. Weber, and J. D. Lipscomb, *J. Mol. Biol.*, *195*, 225–227 (1987).

9. D. H. Ohlendorf, A. M. Orville, and J. D. Lipscomb, *J. Mol. Biol.*, *244*, 586–608 (1994).

10. A. M. Orville, N. Elango, J. D. Lipscomb, and D. H. Ohlendorf, *Biochemistry*, *36*, 10039–10051 (1997).

11. A. M. Orville, J. D. Lipscomb, and D. H. Ohlendorf, *Biochemistry*, *36*, 10052–10066 (1997).

12. T. E. Elgren, A. M. Orville, K. A. Kelly, J. D. Lipscomb, D. H. Ohlendorf, and L. Que, Jr., *Biochemistry*, *36*, 11504–11513 (1997).

13. A. E. True, A. M. Orville, L. L. Pearce, J. D. Lipscomb, and L. Que, Jr., *Biochemistry*, *29*, 10847–10854 (1990).

14. J. W. Whittaker, J. D. Lipscomb, T. A. Kent, and E. Münck, *J. Biol. Chem.*, *259*, 4466–4475 (1984).

15. L. Que, Jr., J. D. Lipscomb, R. Zimmermann, E. Münck, N. R. Orme-Johnson, and W. H. Orme-Johnson, *Biochim. Biophys. Acta*, *452*, 320–334 (1976).

16. L. Que, Jr. and R. H. Heistand, II., *J. Am. Chem. Soc.*, *101*, 2219–2221 (1979).

17. R. H. Felton, L. D. Cheung, R. S. Phillips, and S. W. May, *Biochem. Biophys. Res. Commun.*, *85*, 844–850 (1978).

18. A. M. Orville and J. D. Lipscomb, *J. Biol. Chem.*, *268*, 8596–8607 (1993).

19. L. Que, Jr., J. D. Lipscomb, R. Zimmermann, E. Münck, N. R. Orme-Johnson, and W. H. Orme-Johnson, *Biochim. Biophys. Acta*, *452*, 320–334 (1976).

20. J. W. Whittaker and J. D. Lipscomb, *J. Biol. Chem.*, *259*, 4476–4486 (1984).

21. S. W. May, C. D. Oldham, P. W. Mueller, S. R. Padgette, and A. L. Sowell, *J. Biol. Chem.*, *257*, 12746–12751 (1982).

22. S. W. May, P. W. Mueller, C. D. Oldham, C. K. Williamson, and A. L. Sowell, *Biochemistry*, *22*, 5331–5340 (1983).

23. J. W. Whittaker and J. D. Lipscomb, *J. Biol. Chem.*, *259*, 4487–4495 (1984).

24. H. G. Jang, D. D. Cox, and L. Que, Jr., *J. Am. Chem. Soc.*, *113*, 9200–9204 (1991).

25. L. Que, Jr., R. C. Kolanczyk, and L. S. White, *J. Am. Chem. Soc.*, *109*, 5373–5380 (1987).

26. D. D. Cox and L. Que, Jr., *J. Am. Chem. Soc.*, *110*, 8085–8092 (1988).

27. W. O. Koch and H.-J. Krüger, *Angew. Chem. Int. Ed. Engl.*, *34*, 2671–2674 (1995).

28. R. Viswanathan, M. Palaniandavar, and T. Balasubramanian, *Inorg. Chem.*, *37*, 2943–2951 (1998).

29. M. Duda, M. Pascaly, and B. Krebs, *Chem. Comm.*, 835–836 (1997).

30. T. Funabiki, T. Yamazaki, A. Fukui, T. Tanaka, and S. Yoshida, *Angew. Chem. Int. Ed.*, *37*, 513–515 (1998).

31. S. Han, L. D. Eltis, K. N. Timmis, S. W. Muchmore, and J. T. Bolin, *Science*, *270*, 976–980 (1995).

32. T. Senda, K. Sugiyama, H. Narita, T. Yamamoto, K. Kimbara, M. Fukuda, M. Sato, K. Yano, and Y. Mitsui, *J. Mol. Biol.*, *255*, 735–752 (1996).

33. A. Kita, S.-I. Kita, I. Fujisawa, K. Inaka, T. Ishida, K. Horiike, M. Nozaki, and K. Miki, *Structure*, *7*, 25–34 (1999).

34. E. L. Hegg and L. Que, Jr., *Eur. J. Biochem.*, *250*, 625–629 (1997).

35. S. J. Lange and L. Que, Jr., *Curr. Op. Chem. Biol.*, *2*, 159–172 (1998).

36. M. Wagner and L. Wackett, unpublished results.

37. J. T. Bolin, personal communication.

38. P. A. Mabrouk, A. M. Orville, J. D. Lipscomb, and E. I. Solomon, *J. Am. Chem. Soc.*, *113*, 4053–4061 (1991).

39. L. Shu, Y.-M. Chiou, A. M. Orville, M. A. Miller, J. D. Lipscomb, and L. Que, Jr., *Biochemistry*, *34*, 6649–6659 (1995).

40. Y.-M. Chiou and L. Que, Jr., *Inorg. Chem.*, *34*, 3577–3578 (1995).

41. R. M. Smith and A. E. Martell, *Critical Stability Constants*, Vol. 6, Plenum Press, New York, 1989.

42. C. A. Tyson, *J. Biol. Chem.*, *250*, 1765–1770 (1975).

43. D. M. Arciero, A. M. Orville, and J. D. Lipscomb, *J. Biol. Chem.*, *260*, 14035–14044 (1985).

44. D. M. Arciero and J. D. Lipscomb, *J. Biol. Chem.*, *261*, 2170–2178 (1986).

45. E. L. Spence, G. J. Langley, and T. D. H. Bugg, *J. Am. Chem. Soc.*, *118*, 8336–8343 (1996).

46. T. D. Bugg, J. S. Voisin, and E. L. Spence, *Biochem. Soc. Trans.*, *25*, 81–85 (1997).

47. B. Qi, Masters thesis, University of Minnesota, 1991.

48. Y. Z. Wang and J. D. Lipsomb, *Prot. Expression*, *10*, 1–9 (1997).

49. Y. R. Boldt, A. K. Whiting, M. L. Wagner, M. J. Sadowsky, L. Que, Jr., and L. P. Wackett, *Biochemistry*, *36*, 2147–2153 (1997).

50. A. Abragam and B. Bleaney, *Electron Paramagnetic Resonance of Transition Ions*, Oxford University Press, London, 1970.

51. G. H. Reed and G. D. Markham, *Biol. Magn. Reson.*, *6*, 73–142 (1984).

52. J. W. Whittaker and M. M. Whittaker, *J. Am. Chem. Soc.*, *113*, 5528–5540 (1991).

53. E. Meirovitch and R. Poupko, *J. Phys. Chem.*, *82*, 1920 (1978).

54. G. H. Reed and M. Cohn, *J. Biol. Chem.*, *245*, 662–667 (1970).

55. M. P. Hendrich and P. Debrunner, *Biophys. J.*, *56*, 489–506 (1989).

56. G. H. Reed and W. J. Ray, Jr., *Biochemistry*, *10*, 3190–3197 (1971).

57. D. E. Ash, Ph.D. thesis, University of Pennsylvania, 1982.

58. G. H. Reed and S. D. Morgan, *Biochemistry*, *13*, 3537–3541 (1974).

59. K. Sugiyama, T. Senda, H. Narita, T. Yamamoto, K. Kimbara, M. Fukuda, K. Yano, and Y. Mitsui, *Proc. Jpn. Acad., Ser. B, 71*, 32–35 (1995).

60. A. K. Whiting and L. Que, Jr., unpublished results.

61. M. S. Lah, M. M. Dixon, K. A. Pattridge, W. C. Stallings, J. A. Fee, and M. L. Ludwig, *Biochemistry, 34*, 1646–1660 (1995).

62. J. M. McCord and I. Fridovich, *J. Biol. Chem., 244*, 6049–6055 (1969).

63. F. Yamakura, *J. Biochem., 83*, 849–857 (1978).

64. D. E. Ose and I. Fridovich, *Arch. Biochem. Biophys., 194*, 360–364 (1979).

65. C. J. Brock and J. I. Harris, *Biochem. Soc. Trans., 5*, 1537–1539 (1977).

66. C. K. Vance and A.-F. Miller, *J. Am. Chem. Soc., 120*, 461–467 (1998).

16

Manganese Catalases

Derek W. Yoder,[1] Jungwon Hwang,[1]
and James E. Penner-Hahn[1,2]*

[1]Department of Chemistry, University of Michigan,
930 North University Avenue, Ann Arbor, MI 48109-1055, USA

[2]Section de Bioénergétique, CNRS URA 2096, DBCM CEA Saclay,
F-91191 Gif-sur-Yvette Cedex, France

*Address correspondence to this author at the University of Michigan.

1. INTRODUCTION

1.1. Discovery of Manganese Catalases

Hydrogen peroxide is a toxic molecule, able to both oxidize and reduce organic substrates. Unfortunately, hydrogen peroxide is produced in biological systems, both through the partial reduction of dioxygen by oxidases and by the disproportionation of superoxide by superoxide dismutases. Consequently, aerobic organisms have needed to evolve mechanisms for hydrogen peroxide detoxification. This is most often accomplished by the disproportionation of H_2O_2 to H_2O and O_2, the so-called catalase reaction [Eq. (1)].

$$2H_2O_2 \rightarrow 2H_2O + O_2 \tag{1}$$

Most catalases contain the heme group at their active sites and, like most heme enzymes, are sensitive to inhibition by low concentrations of azide or cyanide. However, it has been known since the 1960s that some catalases are not sensitive to azide and cyanide, suggesting that these might be nonheme catalases [1–3]. In 1983, Kono and Fridovich confirmed the presence of Mn with the isolation and purification of the nonheme catalase from *Lactobacillus plantarum* ATCC 14431 [4]. Although the nonheme catalases have frequently been referred to as "pseudocatalase," this description is inappropriate [2], because there is nothing "false" about the catalase activity of the Mn-containing enzymes. We will describe these as manganese catalase (MnCat).

In addition to the *L. plantarum* enzyme, MnCat has been purified and characterized from *Thermus thermophilus* HB-8 [5] and *Thermoleophilum album* NM [6]. All three enzymes appear to be very similar in their structures and reactivities [7]. The enzymes exist as homohexamers for *L. plantarum* and *T. thermophilus* and as a homotetramer for *T. album*, each containing two manganese atoms per subunit. Electron paramagnetic resonance (EPR) spectra of *T. thermophilus* and *L. plantarum* and a low-resolution crystal structure of *T. thermophilus* confirmed the existence of a binuclear Mn site in both enzymes [8–10]. Recently, another thermostable MnCat was isolated from *Thermus* sp. YS 8-13. This enzyme has a significant homology with *L. plantarum* MnCat [11], but has not as yet been characterized in detail.

1.2. Properties of Manganese Catalases

While heme catalases are found in almost all aerobic organisms, the known Mn catalases have been isolated only from bacteria. All of the Mn catalases have a subunit molecular weight of approximately 30–35 kDa and are believed to fold as a bundle of four antiparallel α helices. Of the Mn catalases, the *L. plantarum* and *T. thermophilus* enzymes are the best characterized. The optical spectrum of the resting enzyme [4,12] is similar to that of oxidized manganese superoxide dismutase, suggesting the presence of Mn(III) in MnCat. This, together with the fact that the metal stoichiometry and the protein folding pattern is similar to that seen in binuclear Fe enzymes (e.g., hemerythrin), led to early speculation that MnCat might contain an oxo-, carboxylato-bridged di-Mn(III) core [13–15].

The MnCat from *T. thermophilus* shows outstanding thermal stability, retaining 85% of activity after heating for 10 min at 95°C [16]. The MnCat from *T. album* also shows good thermal stability, although significant activity is lost on freezing and thawing [6]. Thermostability for the *L. plantarum* enzyme is lower than that found for the thermophilic organisms, losing 40% of its activity after incubation at 80°C for 5 min. However, the *L. plantarum* enzyme is stable to thawing and freezing.

An early experiment showed that the synthesis of MnCat by *T. album* was induced by methyl viologen (paraquat), presumably in response to the oxidative stress that paraquat creates by generating superoxide [6]. This suggests a physiologically important role for MnCat in peroxide detoxification. This was confirmed for *L. plantarum*, where it was shown that an MnCat-deficient strain had reduced viability under stationary growth conditions [17]. Similarly, inactivation of MnCat in an MnCat-sufficient strain resulted in greatly enhanced sensitivity to H_2O_2.

2.   REACTIVITY

2.1.   Comparison with Other Catalase Systems

The disproportionation of hydrogen peroxide is a thermodynamically easy reaction. However, it requires two-electron transfer and is thus kinetically slow in the absence of a catalyst. Although this chapter focuses mainly on manganese catalases, it is useful to review the mechanism of heme catalases as a starting point for understanding the manganese enzyme. The turnover number for heme catalases is extremely high, approximately $1.0 \times 10^7 \ s^{-1}$ [18,19], and close to the diffusion-limited rate. The manganese catalases have a turnover number of about $2.0 \times 10^5 \ s^{-1}$ [5–7], which, while significantly slower, is still quite fast. Heme catalases are also more efficient, as measured by k_{cat}/K_M. The k_{cat}/K_M ratio is $4.0 \times 10^8 \ M^{-1} \ s^{-1}$ for the heme enzymes vs. $5.7 \times 10^5 \ M^{-1} \ s^{-1}$ for MnCat. Heme catalases follow a ping-pong mechanism for hydrogen peroxide disproportionation, as shown in Eqs. (2) and (3) [18–20]. In these equations, "Catalase" and "Compound I" represent the ferric enzyme and an oxo-Fe(IV) porphyrin π-cation intermediate, respectively. The two electrons required for peroxide disproportionation are thus provided by the Fe and by the porphyrin prosthetic group.

$$\text{Catalase} + H_2O_2 \rightarrow \text{Compound I} + H_2O \qquad (2)$$

$$\text{Compound I} + H_2O_2 \rightarrow \text{Catalase} + O_2 + H_2O \qquad (3)$$

Although MnCat does not have a redox-active organic cofactor, it does have two Mn ions, each of which can conceivably adopt one of three oxidation states Mn(II), Mn(III), or Mn(IV). There are thus a variety of ways in which MnCat could provide the two electrons required for peroxide disproportionation. A variety of spectroscopic studies (see Sec. 3) have identified four different oxidation states for MnCat: the reduced

$Mn(II)_2$ state, the mixed-valence $Mn(II)Mn(III)$ state, the oxidized $Mn(III)_2$ state, and the superoxidized $Mn(III)Mn(IV)$ state. There is, to date, no evidence for a $Mn(IV)_2$ state, although the possibility that such a species may form, at least under some conditions, is difficult to rule out.

Compound I for the heme catalases is a highly reactive species and can oxidize other substrates in place of H_2O_2 (e.g., can function as a peroxidase). Alcohol oxidation [Eq. (4)] is particularly important [21], and it has been suggested that heme catalase may provide the dominant pathway for biological ethanol oxidation [22]. There have been only limited investigations of alternate substrates for MnCat. The *L. plantarum* MnCat was found to have no superoxide dismutase activity [4,23]. However, the *T. album* MnCat showed substantial peroxidase activity with *p*-phenylenediamine but not with other substrates [6].

$$\text{Compound I} + RCH_2OH \rightarrow \text{Catalase} + RCHO + H_2O \qquad (4)$$

In recent years, a great deal of effort has been devoted to the synthesis of Mn inorganic complexes that mimic MnCat activity. Even the simplest possible compound, solvated manganese ion $[Mn(H_2O)_6]^{2+}$, shows a low level of catalase activity, with a turnover number of 6.3 $\times 10^{-3}\,s^{-1}$ [24]. By comparison, the most rapid disproportionation of peroxide by a catalase mimic is a million fold faster at $250\,s^{-1}$, although still substantially slower than the enzyme. The most efficient catalase mimic to date is $[Mn^{IV}(\text{salpn})O]_2$, which cycles between $Mn(III)_2$ and $Mn(IV)_2$ [25,26]. Most of the MnCat mimics have been constructed to have some type of bridged manganese dimer at their core in order to be consistent with what is known of the enzymatic active site. However, other models have included manganese tetramers [24,27,28] and a manganese-bound porphyrin system [29]. A variety of redox cycles have been proposed to account for the observed model chemistry, including $Mn(III)_2 \leftrightarrow Mn(IV)_2$ [25,26,29,30], $Mn(II)_2 \leftrightarrow Mn(III)_2$ [24,31–33], $Mn(II)Mn(III) \leftrightarrow Mn(III)Mn(IV)$ [34,35], and $Mn(III) \leftrightarrow Mn(V)$ [29]. These systems are discussed in detail in Chap. 14 of this volume and will not be considered further here.

2.2. Chemical Perturbations of MnCat

A key question for any enzyme is the nature of the substrate–enzyme interaction. Since it has not been possible to trap an intermediate in which H_2O_2 is bound to MnCat, much of the work on MnCat has focused on anion binding as a surrogate for substrate binding. Several anions have been shown to bind to MnCat. Of these, azide is of particular interest because of the similarity of the highest occupied molecular orbitals of peroxide and azide [36]. It is thus likely that information obtained from studies of azide binding will provide direct insight into the interaction of peroxide with the enzyme. This section discusses the evidence that anions bind to and inhibit MnCat. The detailed spectroscopic interpretation of the anion-bound complexes is discussed in Sec. 3. In considering the interactions of anions with MnCat, it is important to remember that while inhibition requires binding, anion binding need not be inhibitory. In addition, it is important to note that anion binding sites can be, but need not be, on the Mn ions.

2.2.1. Anion Binding

Anion binding has been investigated by a variety of probes. For the reduced enzyme, EPR has proven to be very useful, as the EPR spectrum is extremely sensitive to minor perturbations in structure. Thus, as discussed in Sec. 3, the EPR spectrum for anion-free reduced MnCat has a broad, weakly structured signal, while the anion-bound forms show well-resolved hyperfine structure. Based on EPR perturbations, it is clear that halides, oxyanions (e.g., phosphate, sulfate, etc.), and azide all perturb the reduced Mn site [37]. Although these perturbations are likely to involve anion binding to one or both of the Mn ions, this has not been directly proven.

A weakness of EPR as a probe of binding is that it is difficult to determine anion binding constants by EPR (and impossible to determine room temperature binding constants, since cryogenic temperatures are required to observe the EPR spectra). To address this, Whittaker and co-workers used a fluoride-specific electrode to measure the free fluoride concentration as a function of the F^-/MnCat ratio [38]. They found that two fluoride ions bind per active site in reduced $L.$ $plantarum$ MnCat (K_d = 12 μM and 140 μM, pH = 5.5). In addition, by measuring the change in pH when fluoride bound, they determined that approximately one H^+ is taken up per F^- bound. The observation of proton-coupled fluoride binding suggests a possible thermodynamic rationale for the observation that fluoride and other anions bind more tightly at low pH. The structural feature responsible for proton-coupled anion binding could be either simultaneous binding of a proton and an anion [Eq. (5), which would be equivalent to binding of HF] or displacement of a stronger base (e.g., OH^-) when F^- binds [Eq. (6)]. Whittaker et al. favor the latter possibility [38].

$$\text{Enzyme} + 2H^+ + 2F^- \rightarrow \text{enzyme}/2H^+/2F \qquad (5)$$

$$\text{Enzyme} + 2F^- \rightarrow \text{enzyme-2F} + 2OH^- \qquad (6)$$

In contrast to the reduced enzyme, which lacks significant UV-visible absorption, both the oxidized and superoxidized enzyme have electronic absorption bands that can be used to monitor ligand binding directly at room temperature. For the oxidized enzyme, both fluoride and azide have been shown to perturb the electronic structure. For fluoride, only a single binding constant was observed, in contrast with the two binding constants found for the reduced enzyme [38]. Intriguingly, the fluoride binding constant for the oxidized enzyme ($K_d = 0.5$ mM, pH = 5.5) was weaker than either of the binding constants for the reduced enzyme. This is the opposite of expectations, since normally F^-, as a hard anion, would be expected to bind more strongly to Mn(III) than to Mn(II). This may reflect a structural change in the Mn site on oxidation such that tight anion binding is blocked.

Addition of N_3^- perturbs both the absorption and the magnetic circular dichroism (MCD) spectra for oxidized MnCat [39]. An intense new feature, assigned as an $N_3^- \rightarrow$ Mn charge-transfer band, appears providing direct evidence for N_3^- binding to Mn. This is the only case in which there is direct evidence for anion binding to the Mn. All of the other spectral changes, while consistent with direct binding to Mn, could also be caused by indirect effects of ligand binding at a site close to, but not on, the Mn.

Although there have been fewer studies of anion binding to the superoxidized enzyme, both azide and cyanide have been shown to perturb this oxidation state [8,40,41]. Titration of N_3^-, as detected by perturbations in the UV-visible spectrum, indicated positive cooperativity for both azide and cyanide binding. The concentration that gave half-maximal binding, $[N_3^-]_{1/2}$, was 20–40 mM at pH 7.0. As in the reduced enzyme, azide binding was pH-dependent with $[N_3^-]_{1/2} \approx 500$ mM at pH 8.5 and 5 mM at pH 5.5. At pH 5.5, $[CN^-]_{1/2}$ was 28 mM. The $[CN^-]_{1/2}$ values at higher pH were too large to be determined accurately, in part because the protein precipitated from solution at high $[CN^-]$.

2.2.2. Inhibition

Although the Mn catalases were originally identified on the basis of their insensitivity to azide and cyanide, more recent work has shown that they are in fact inhibited by both azide and cyanide, albeit at much higher concentrations than are the heme catalases [6,7,37,42]. The *T. thermophilus* enzyme shows pH-dependent azide inhibition [37]. For a 5.0 mM solution at pH 9.4 in 5 mM borate buffer, only about 7% inhibition was observed. However, this increased to 78% when the pH was lowered to 6.0. The *L. plantarum* enzyme also shows azide inhibition, and in this case azide has been shown to be competitive with peroxide, implying that azide and peroxide share a common binding site [7,42]. At neutral pH, the apparent K_i for azide is 80 ± 4 mM. The apparent inhibition constant falls to around 5 mM at pH 5.5. A variety of models could explain this pH dependence. It may be that the binding site must be protonated before azide will bind or that the actual inhibitory species is HN_3 (the pK_a for azide is 4.72). If the latter were correct, the true K_i for azide would be about 300 μM. Inhibition by HN_3 but not by N_3^- might occur if there were a hydrophobic or an anionic channel leading to the active site such that anions could not enter. Alternatively, it may be that OH^- and N_3^- compete for the same binding site, in analogy with the model proposed above for F^- binding to reduced MnCat [Eq. (6)].

A variety of oxyanions have been shown to inhibit the *T. thermophilus* MnCat. These include phosphate, nitrite, nitrate, acetate, and oxalate [37]. They range in strength from relatively weak inhibitors such as nitrate (50% inhibition by 100 mM nitrate) and oxalate (67% inhibition by 60 mM oxalate) to relatively potent inhibitors such as phosphate and nitrite. Thus, phosphate inhibits by 50% at 20 mM and 90% at 50 mM (pH 6.7), while 5.0 mM nitrite causes 90% inhibition at pH 6.0. Acetate concentrations as high as 100 mM produced no inhibition in pH 7.0 samples, although inhibition was observed at lower pH. No inhibition was observed for sulfate. Oxyanion inhibitors have not been studied in as much detail for the *L. plantarum* enzyme, although phosphate has been reported to give no detectable inhibition for concentrations up to 500 mM between pH 6.5 and 8.0 [42].

Halides are also effective inhibitors of MnCat. Like azide, fluoride and chloride are better inhibitors at lower pH. For *T. thermophilus*, fluoride was not found to be as good an inhibitor as azide, chloride, or phosphate [37]. In contrast, for the *L. plantarum* enzyme fluoride appears to be a better inhibitor than either chloride or phosphate [43,44]. It was found [44] that turnover in the presence of either fluoride or chloride trapped the enzyme in the reduced state. This is in contrast to the behavior in the absence of fluoride, where 30% of the active enzyme remains as Mn(III) following turnover with H_2O_2. The somewhat surprising result that fluoride traps the reduced rather than the oxidized form of MnCat fits nicely with the finding (above) that F^- binds more tightly to the reduced enzyme.

2.2.3. Effect of pH on Activity

The catalase activity of both the *L. plantarum* and the *T. thermophilus* enzymes is independent of pH from 7 to 10 [7,37], although it falls to zero at more extreme pH values. In contrast, the MnCat from *T. album* shows a narrower activity profile, with greatest activity between pH 8.0 and 9.0 [6]. It is interesting that the activity is pH-independent for pH values between 7 and 10 for *L. plantarum* and *T. thermophilus* while anion inhibition depends dramatically on pH. This implies that the factor or factors responsible for the pH dependence of anion inhibition, e.g., obligate protonation of either the anion or the enzyme, or competition with OH^-, do not affect the rate-limiting step in enzyme turnover. Thus, for example, it may be that Mn oxidation (H_2O_2 reduction) becomes rate limiting in the presence of halide, while a different, pH-independent step is rate limiting in the absence of halide.

In addition to the direct effect of pH on activity, there are also indirect effects. For *T. thermophilus*, the rate of air oxidation of the reduced enzyme to give the oxidized state increases as the pH is raised, with oxidation proceeding three to four times faster at pH 9.0 than at pH 7 [8].

2.3. Available Oxidation States

When MnCat is isolated from *L. plantarum* it exists as a mixture of reduced, $Mn(II)_2$, oxidized, $Mn(III)_2$, and superoxidized, $Mn(III)Mn(IV)$, oxidation states, in the approximate ratio of 45%:35%:20% [44]. For the *T. thermophilus* enzyme, the EPR spectrum shows that the mixed-valence, Mn(II)Mn(III) derivative is also present in the as-isolated enzyme [8].

The as-isolated enzyme can be reduced to a homogeneous reduced state by anaerobic incubation with NH_2OH [45]. For *T. thermophilus*, air oxidation of the reduced enzyme appears to give predominantly (about 97%) oxidized enzyme with the remaining 3% present in the mixed-valence oxidation state [8]. A potential weakness of this study is that the presence of the oxidized enzyme was inferred from the absence of an EPR signal (the oxidized enzyme being EPR-silent). A more direct approach to oxidation state determination is to use X-ray absorption spectroscopy (XAS, see Sec. 4), since this is sensitive to all of the Mn in a system, regardless of spin state. For the *L. plantarum*, air oxidation gave a 2:1 mixture of Mn(II) and Mn(III) as determined by X-ray absorption near-edge structure (XANES) [46]. Since the EPR signals characteristic of mixed-valence and superoxidized MnCat were not seen, this mixture was attributed to a 2:1 ratio of reduced/oxidized enzyme. It is not clear as to why the two enzymes are oxidized to a different extent.

Addition of peroxide to the autooxidized enzyme regenerates the EPR signal for the reduced enzyme [12], thus demonstrating that peroxide can reduce the enzyme from $Mn(III)_2$ to $Mn(II)_2$ [Eq. (7)] and suggesting that these are the catalytically relevant oxidation states. It was not possible to test the other half-reaction [Eq. (8)] by EPR since the EPR signal for the reduced enzyme is only readily detectable in the presence of anionic inhibitors, which block the reaction. The oxidative half-reaction *could* be observed by X-ray absorption. Addition of H_2O_2 to reduced *L. plantarum* MnCat gave a 2:1 ratio of Mn(II)/Mn(III), demonstrating that H_2O_2 was able to oxidize reduced MnCat [44], and supporting the assignment of reduced and oxidized MnCat as the active oxidation states.

$$Mn(III)_2 + H_2O_2 \rightarrow Mn(II)_2 + O_2 + 2H^+ \tag{7}$$

$$Mn(II)_2 + H_2O_2 + 2H^+ \rightarrow (Mn(III)_2 + 2H_2O \tag{8}$$

It has been suggested that oxidation of reduced MnCat by peroxide is the rate-limiting step [47]. This is difficult to reconcile with the observed autooxidation of the *T. thermophilus* enzyme, since the autooxidation reaction, the reverse of Eq. (7), should produce H_2O_2 as the O_2 reduction product. If H_2O_2 reacts most rapidly with oxidized MnCat, the peroxide produced during autooxidation should react preferentially by Eq. (7) rather than Eq. (8), thus regenerating the reduced enzyme, resulting in little net autooxidation.

Simultaneous addition of micromolar concentrations of NH_2OH and H_2O_2 converts the enzyme to the catalytically inactive superoxidized state [37,46]. It was originally suggested that this inactivation was irreversible [48], but subsequent work showed that long-term (>1 h) anaerobic incubation with NH_2OH alone was able to restore full activity [46]. These reactions, together with the proposed catalytic cycle, are shown in Fig. 1A. This scheme explains the initial failure to observe reactivation by NH_2OH. Aerobic incubation with NH_2OH does *not* reactivate the enzyme because reinactivation (from NH_2OH + the H_2O_2 produced by autooxidation of either NH_2OH or reduced catalase) competes with reactivation.

The mixed-valence oxidation state is the least well characterized. Although one could imagine a catalytic cycle between the mixed-valence and the superoxidized oxidation states, the mixed-valence enzyme does not appear to be catalytically active. Given the fact ([46], above) that NH_2OH reduction of superoxidized MnCat is slow while NH_2OH reduction of oxidized MnCat is fast, the inactivity of the mixed-valence enzyme may simply be due to the fact that the superoxidized enzyme is not catalytically competent to oxidize H_2O_2. Pecoraro and co-workers have suggested [24] that production of the mixed-valence derivative, perhaps by one-electron reduction of the oxidized enzyme, may be a critical step in the inactivation of the enzyme by H_2O_2 + NH_2OH. This could occur as shown in Eqs. (9) and (10), where the product of the one-electron oxidation of NH_2OH is indicated as "NHOH." This mechanistic possibility is shown in Fig. 1B. Although this reaction sequence takes place in model compounds, it has not yet been demonstrated for the protein.

$$Mn(III)_2 + NH_2OH \rightarrow Mn(II)Mn(III) + \text{"NHOH"} + H^+ \qquad (9)$$

$$Mn(II)Mn(III) + H_2O_2 + 2H^+ \rightarrow Mn(III)Mn(IV) + 2H_2O \qquad (10)$$

For *T. thermophilus* the mixed-valence derivative can be prepared either through the reduction of superoxidized state using I^- or by autooxidation of reduced state [8], although in neither case is homogeneous mixed-valence enzyme produced. There are no reports of chemical production of mixed-valence *L. plantarum* MnCat, although this form was produced by X-ray photoreduction of the oxidized enzyme [44]. The mixed-valence enzyme that was produced by X-ray photoreduction

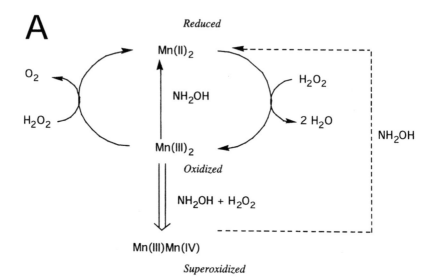

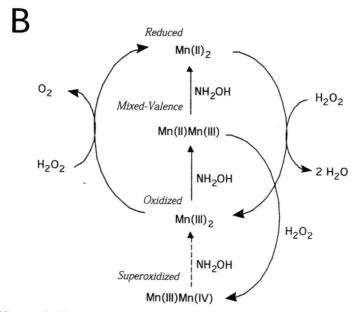

FIG. 1. Oxidation state interconversions of MnCat. The catalytic cycle is shown as solid, curved arrows. (A) Inactivation and reactivation by NH_2OH + H_2O_2 are shown by a double arrow and a dashed arrow, respectively, to indicate the lack of mechanistic detail for these steps. (B) A possible mechanism for inactivation (and subsequent reactivation) is included.

was not stable on thawing to room temperature. This may indicate that the mixed-valence derivative of *L. plantarum* MnCat is unstable with respect to disproportionation [Eq. (11)], although further study is required to confirm this. An analogous disproportionation has been found for the mixed-valence di-iron site in methane monooxygenase [49,50].

$$Mn(II)Mn(III) + Mn(II)Mn(III) \rightarrow Mn(II)_2 + Mn(III)_2 \qquad (11)$$

3. SPECTROSCOPY

3.1. EPR, ENDOR, and ESEEM Studies

3.1.1. Reduced MnCat

The EPR spectra for $Mn(II)_2$ dimers are generally quite complex, typically consisting of four broad transitions each with about 11 hyperfine lines. In the absence of added anions, the EPR signal of reduced MnCat is extremely broad and essentially undetectable [37]. The intensity of the signal increases as the temperature increases, with a maximum at around 50 K, indicating that this signal arises from an excited spin state of an antiferromagnetically coupled $Mn(II)_2$ dimer. Assuming that the EPR signal arises solely from an $S = 1$ state, the exchange coupling, J, for the reduced *T. thermophilus* enzyme was estimated [37] to be 29 cm^{-1} (for this and subsequent discussions, the JS_1S_2 exchange Hamiltonian is used). A revised estimate of $J = 11.2$ cm^{-1} was obtained by including contributions of the $S = 2$ state to the spectrum [51]. Analogous measurements have been reported for the *L. plantarum* enzyme, including spectra measured in both parallel and perpendicular polarization [38]. The dimanganese site was again found to be antiferromagnetically coupled, but with a much stronger exchange interaction ($J = 40$ cm^{-1}).

In addition to the Heisenberg exchange interaction (J), the EPR spectra for $Mn(II)_2$ dimers are also affected by the magnetic dipole interaction between the Mn. This term, $D_{dip} = -g^2\beta^2/r^3$, depends on the distance between the Mn ions and thus can, at least in principle, be used to estimate the Mn-Mn separation. Since the distances estimated from D_{dip} did not agree well with crystallographically determined distances, an empirical correlation was used to estimate the Mn-Mn separation [51]. This gave Mn-Mn distances of 3.31, 3.51, 3.59 Å, and 3.63–3.70 Å, respectively, for the fluoride-, chloride-, phosphate-, and cyanide-bound derivatives of reduced MnCat [51,52]. The aqua (i.e., anion-free) enzyme has the smallest $|D_{dip}|$ and thus the longest Mn-Mn distance (≥ 3.7 Å). These distances are in reasonable agreement with the low-resolution crystal structure but do not appear to be consistent with the distances found by extended X-ray absorption fine-structure (EXAFS) spectroscopy, as described in Sec. 4. Whittaker and co-workers have suggested [38] that the need for an empirical calibration curve (above) resulted from neglect of the single-ion zero field splitting (zfs) terms, which can have a magnitude comparable to D_{dip} for distorted Mn(II) ions. If single-ion zfs is included, the EPR spectrum of the phosphate derivative of reduced *L. plantarum* MnCat gives an apparent Mn-Mn distance of 3.4 Å, i.e., 0.2 Å shorter than that estimated for the *T. thermophilus* enzyme. It is not clear as to whether this difference reflects differences in data analysis or differences between the different MnCat proteins.

Dismukes has suggested [52] that the systematic increase in Mn-Mn distance as the size of the anion is increased (e.g., from 3.3 Å for fluoride to 3.6 Å for phosphate) may indicate that the anions form a bridge between the two Mn. Since the anion-free enzyme has the longest Mn-Mn distance, longer even than chloride, this model would imply that there is no exogenous bridge between the Mn in this form of the enzyme. That is, the reduced enzyme was proposed to have an Mn(II)(μ-carboxylato)$_{1-2}$Mn(II) core, with the carboxylate bridges serving to hold the Mn ions in proximity, as is seen for di-iron proteins [50]. However, in light of the proposal that zfs may affect the apparent Mn-Mn distance [38], the existence of a correlation between anion size and Mn-Mn distance, and the resulting structural interpretations, may need to be re-examined.

The binding of fluoride to reduced *L. plantarum* MnCat gave a fourfold decrease in exchange coupling, to approximately 11 cm^{-1} [38]. This decrease, together with the stoichiometry of fluoride binding [Eq. (6)], led to the proposal that resting MnCat has a di-μ-OH$^-$ bridged structure and that the hydroxide bridges are released when fluoride binds [Eq. (12)]. The decrease in the exchange interaction would thus be a consequence of less effective coupling through the fluoride bridge. Although this model explains the stoichiometry and pH dependence of fluoride binding, it is not clear that an Mn-Mn separation of 3.4 Å is small enough to accommodate the di-μ-OH$^-$ geometry. In addition, this structural picture does not provide a ready explanation for the pronounced sensitivity of the reduced MnCat EPR spectrum to the presence of anions such as phosphate or sulfate.

$$Mn(II)(\mu\text{-}OH)_2Mn(II) + 2F^- \rightarrow Mn(II)(\mu\text{-}F)_2Mn(II) + 2OH^- \quad (12)$$

3.1.2. Mixed-Valence MnCat

As noted above, characterization of the mixed-valence oxidation state is relatively limited, due in part to difficulty in preparing homogeneous samples. This state is characterized by an approximately 18-line EPR signal attributed to an antiferromagnetically coupled $S = 1/2$ ground state [37]. Based on the temperature dependence of the EPR signal amplitude [8,45], the exchange coupling appears to be relatively weak ($J < 40$ cm^{-1}) [53]. Based on the sign of the hyperfine anisotropy ($|A_x|$, $|A_y| > |A_z|$) for Mn(III), the Mn(III) ion was predicted [54] to have the $(d_\pi)^3(d_{z^2})^1$ electronic structure that is expected for an axially elongated site. The hyperfine anisotropy in mixed-valence MnCat was nearly 40% larger than that in superoxidized MnCat. Based on comparison with model compounds, this was correlated with a decrease in the number of oxo bridges. Since superoxidized MnCat is believed to have two oxo bridges (see below), this was interpreted as evidence for a Mn(II)(μ-OH)(μ-carboxylato)$_{1-2}$Mn(III) structure [53]. It is not clear, however, that these data would exclude other structures, e.g., those having a bridging water, or perhaps a single bridging oxo.

3.1.3. Superoxidized MnCat

Superoxidized MnCat has a 16-line EPR signal that is typical of strongly antiferromagnetically coupled Mn(III)Mn(IV) dimers (see Chap. 14 of this volume). There has been a great deal of interest in this signal due to its similarity to the multiline EPR signal that is seen for the photosynthetic oxygen evolving complex. Although a variety of bridging ligands can give rise to a 16-line EPR spectrum, EXAFS data indicate a di-μ-oxo bridging geometry for superoxidized MnCat (see Sec. 4). Detailed investigations of both the *L. plantarum* [55] and the *T. thermophilus* enzyme [53], including measurements at X, P, and S bands, give very similar results. In both cases, the spectra could be simulated using similar axial **g** and **A** tensors. There is substantial hyperfine anisotropy for the Mn(III), but much less anisotropy for the Mn(IV). From the sign of the Mn(III) hyperfine anisotropy, the Mn(III) was again found to have the normal, axially elongated $(d_\pi)^3(d_{z^2})^1$ electronic structure. This places the antibonding d_{z^2} electron in an orbital orthogonal to the $Mn(\mu\text{-}O)_2Mn$ core, giving elongated axial bond lengths and strong Mn-μ-oxo bonds. It was suggested [53] that this may explain the lack of catalase activity for superoxidized MnCat, since such a structure might be expected to have slow ligand exchange rates. This is difficult to reconcile, however, with the observation of facile peroxide disproportionation by structurally similar $Mn(III)_2(\mu\text{-}O)_2$ model compounds [26] (see Chap. 14). An alternative explanation for the lack of catalase activity by superoxidized MnCat is that the two oxo bridges stabilize the Mn against reduction by H_2O_2 [56].

Six resolved pairs of lines were seen in the ^{1}H ENDOR (electron nuclear double resonance) spectra for superoxidized *T. thermophilus* MnCat [57]. All of these are exchangeable in D_2O. These were attributed to two classes of protons and, based on line narrowing in D_2O, it was suggested that there is only a single proton per class. These were attributed to a water (or possibly a hydroxide) that is hydrogen-bonded to an oxygen ligand on the Mn(IV).

Electron spin-echo envelope modulation (ESEEM) spectra for superoxidized *T. thermophilus* MnCat show modulations from ^{14}N that were originally attributed to the remote (nonligated) N of a coordinated histidine imidazole [58]. This assignment was based in part on analogy to ESEEM spectra for Cu(II) [59]. In the Cu case, the hyperfine coupling of the coordinated N is sufficiently large that this nitrogen is not detectable by ESEEM, although it is detectable by ENDOR. If the same situation existed for MnCat, i.e., if the ^{14}N ESEEM signal was due to the remote N of a coordinated histidine, then there should be a second, strongly coupled N that is detectable by ENDOR. However, a subsequent ENDOR study of superoxidized MnCat did not show any ^{14}N lines, despite the fact that four different transitions were detected for model complexes with MnN_4O_2 ligation [57]. The ENDOR results suggested that there are no coordinated histidines in superoxidized MnCat, and the ^{14}N ESEEM signals were attributed to a nitrogen that is close to, but not ligated to, the Mn.

More recent work has suggested a different interpretation of these results [60,61]. It is now known that the nitrogens that are coordinated to Mn often give strong ESEEM signals. The difference relative to Cu reflects the generally lower covalency of Mn-N bonds. The ^{14}N ESEEM parameters for superoxidized MnCat are, in fact, completely consistent with those expected for coordinated nitrogens. However, this leaves open the question of the identity (what amino acid) and the coordination (terminal or bridging) of the N that gives rise to the ESEEM signal.

Reductive methylation of superoxidized *T. thermophilus* MnCat causes significant changes in the EPR and ESEEM spectra [61]. The only amino acid that was methylated to any significant extent was lysine, and these results thus suggested that the ESEEM-detected N might come from a lysine. The ESEEM parameters for native MnCat [61] are similar to those seen for ammonia-inhibited Photosystem II [62]. The latter have been interpreted as arising from a bridging NH_2, thus leading to the suggestion that the N that is seen by ESEEM is a bridging lysine amide [61]. The ^{14}N ESEEM signal is altered but not lost on methylation, as would be expected if methylation converted a bridging ligand into a terminal ligand. Alternatively, the ESEEM signals may arise from the coordinated nitrogen, most likely from a histidine ligand. This is the interpretation that was given for the ESEEM spectra for superoxidized *L. plantarum* MnCat [41], based in part on comparison with ESEEM spectra of model compounds. The ESEEM spectra for *T. thermophilus* and *L. plantarum* MnCat are very similar. Thus it is likely that they arise from a similar structure. Until ESEEM measurements are made on MnCat in which the histidines and/or lysines have been isotopically labeled, it will be difficult to distinguish spectroscopically between lysine and histidine as the origin of this signal.

Crystallographic and EXAFS data (see Sec. 4) suggest that there are two histidine ligands to Mn. It is thus intriguing that at most one, and perhaps neither, of these is seen in the ESEEM (depending on whether the ESEEM signal is attributed to a histidine or a lysine nitrogen). Since there are no ^{14}N ENDOR signals, it is unlikely that the histidines are rendered ESEEM-undetectable as a consequence of being too strongly coupled to the Mn spin [this could happen, for example, if a histidine were axially coordinated to Mn(III)]. In model compounds, nitrogens that are equatorially bound to Mn(III) have highly anisotropic hyperfine tensors [63] that are difficult to detect by both ESEEM and

ENDOR. We therefore favor [41] this as an explanation for the "missing" histidine, or potentially for two missing histidines if the ^{14}N ESEEM signal is due to lysine. In the latter case, this would require either that both histidines be equatorially coordinated to Mn(III) or that another mechanism be found for making a histidine invisible to ESEEM. Since crystallographic data (Sec. 4) suggest that each histidine is close to a different Mn, we provisionally favor assignment of the ^{14}N ESEEM signal to a histidine coordinated to Mn(IV), with the second histidine coordinated to Mn(III), and thus being ESEEM-undetectable.

Addition of either N_3^- or CN^- to superoxidized *L. plantarum* MnCat results in a slight decrease in the Mn hyperfine coupling [41], with almost no change in the **g** tensor. Both anions give similar effects, and both cause modest changes in the ^{14}N ESEEM parameters. Identical spectra are seen for unlabeled and ^{15}N-labeled anions, suggesting that neither anion is coordinated directly to Mn. However, given the changes in the EPR, ESEEM, and UV-visible spectra (see Sec. 3.3), both anions must bind at a site that can perturb the Mn structure.

3.2. Magnetic Susceptibility

Magnetic susceptibility measurements have been used as a direct probe of the exchange coupling in MnCat. An attraction of these measurements is that they can be used to study samples that are not EPR-active. For reduced *T. thermophilus* MnCat, magnetic susceptibility gave $J = 4.8$ cm^{-1}, with this decreasing to 3.4 cm^{-1} when phosphate was added [64]. These couplings are somewhat smaller than those deduced from the EPR for *T. thermophilus* MnCat and significantly smaller than those deduced for *L. plantarum* MnCat. Based on the weak coupling, an Mn(II)(μ-OH$_2$)(μ-carboxylato)$_1$Mn(II) core was proposed for the phosphate-free enzyme, going to a Mn(II)(μ-OH$_2$)(μ-phospato)(μ-carboxylato)Mn(II) structure when phosphate is bound [64].

Magnetic susceptibility data for oxidized *T. thermophilus* MnCat showed evidence for two different species, one weakly coupled ($J \approx 4$ cm^{-1}) and one strongly coupled ($J \approx 200$ cm^{-1}) [65]. These were seen at neutral and basic pH values (6.5 and 9.5), and were attributed to μ-oxo, μ-carboxylato, and di-μ-oxo, μ-carboxylato bridges, respectively. It is not clear, however, how this dramatic pH-dependent change in structure can be reconciled with the lack of pH-dependence to the activity over this pH range. In addition, the pH-dependent doubling of the strongly coupled form (from 42% strongly coupled at pH 6.5 to 80% strongly coupled at pH 9.5) does not match that expected for a 1000-fold change in proton concentration. One potential weakness of magnetic susceptibility is that it is a bulk measurement and thus critically sensitive to sample heterogeneity. Since reduced MnCat is not readily detected by EPR in the absence of added anions, it is difficult to rule out the possibility of minor contamination by this form. A pH-dependent change in the ratio of reduced to oxidized MnCat would account for the pH-dependent bleaching that was observed in the 450- to 500-nm peaks [65]. Additional work will be required to explain the pH dependence of the magnetic susceptibility and to reconcile this with other studies of the oxidized enzyme (below).

3.3. Optical Studies

3.3.1. Oxidized MnCat

Although air oxidized *L. plantarum* MnCat contains both oxidized and reduced enzyme [44], only the oxidized enzyme has significant features in the UV-visible and MCD spectra. This fact has allowed a detailed characterization of the electronic structure of oxidized MnCat [39]. The absorption spectrum of oxidized MnCat is distinct from that of most binuclear Mn(III) models in that it lacks low energy (5000–10 000 cm^{-1}) absorption bands. This difference was attributed to the presence of five-coordinate Mn in oxidized MnCat, probably in a trigonal bipyramidal geometry. There are additional differences between the higher energy features in the absorption and MCD spectra of oxidized MnCat and oxo-bridged Mn(III) models. These suggest that the Mn ions in MnCat may be bridged by a hydroxo or perhaps an aqua group rather than by an oxo group. This is supported by MCD saturation magnetization measurements which suggest that the Mn ions are weakly coupled, since hydroxo bridges should give weaker exchange coupling than oxo bridges. However, it is noteworthy that the MCD data suggest weak *ferro*magnetic coupling for oxidized *L. plantarum* MnCat, while magnetic susceptibility indicates a mixture of weakly and strongly *antiferro*magnetically coupled sites for *T. thermophilus* MnCat. It is not clear whether this is due to genuine differences between the proteins or to limitations in one or both of the determinations of *J*.

When azide is added to oxidized *L. plantarum* MnCat, an intense new transition is seen at 370 nm (27 000 cm^{-1}). This is assigned as an azide → Mn charge-transfer transition [39]. As noted above, this provides the first direct evidence for ligand binding to the Mn, since all of the other anion-induced changes could arise from indirect perturbations in the Mn-dimer structure when anions bind at a distant site. There are only minor changes in the ligand field bands below 25 000 cm^{-1} when azide binds to oxidized MnCat, suggesting that both Mn remain five-coordinate in the azide complex. Based on the pattern of band shifts when N_3^- binds, it appears that N_3^- binding involves primarily N_3^- π overlap with the Mn xy and xz orbitals (z defined as the Mn-bridge direction). This would be consistent either with an end-on nonbridging geometry or with a μ-1,3 bridging geometry for N_3^- (and presumably also for H_2O_2).

3.3.2.   Superoxidized MnCat

The MCD spectrum for superoxidized *L. plantarum* MnCat is similar to that found for di-μ-oxo bridged Mn(III)Mn(IV) binuclear models [40]. However, the MCD transitions attributed to oxo → Mn charge transfer are significantly weaker for MnCat than for the model compounds. This was interpreted as evidence for a bent $Mn_2(μ-O)_2$ core in MnCat. The intensities of the MCD features increase, without a significant change in energy, when azide is bound. This suggests that azide binding causes a slight flattening of the $Mn_2(μ-O)_2$ core. Such a flattening would account for the decrease in Mn hyperfine coupling when azide is added (Sec. 3.1.3), since a flatter core would lead to greater spin delocalization onto the oxo bridges. Taken together, these results and the ESEEM evidence that azide does not bind directly to the Mn lead to a model in which azide and cyanide bind at a protein-derived site, causing a perturbation in the Mn core structure. This is shown schematically in Fig. 2.

It is not clear as to what, if any, role this binding site may play in catalysis. However, it is intriguing that there exists an anion binding site, at least for superoxidized MnCat, that has anion affinity comparable to the anion binding that leads to inhibition of the oxidized and reduced enzyme. It is possible that a nonmanganese binding site accounts for some, or perhaps most, of the anion inhibition of MnCat. This could occur if anion binding occurred at a site (perhaps similar to that in Fig. 2) that blocks a protein channel that peroxide must traverse in order to reach the Mn site.

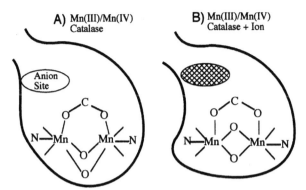

FIG. 2. Schematic illustration of the effect of azide or cyanide binding on the structure of superoxidized MnCat, as deduced from EPR, ESEEM, UV-visible, MCD, and XAS data (see text). The anion binding site (ellipse) is close to, but not on, the Mn. Binding of N_3^- or CN^- at this site (filled ellipse in B) causes a flattening of the $Mn_2(\mu\text{-O})_2$ core, shown in an exaggerated form. An additional carboxylate bridge is shown for consistency with the proposed structures for reduced and oxidized MnCat, but is not required by the data. (Redrawn with permission from [41].)

4. STRUCTURAL CHARACTERIZATION

4.1. XAS Studies

The EXAFS data for reduced *L. plantarum* MnCat show two resolvable shells of nearest-neighbor N/O ligands at 2.11 and 2.27 Å [66]. In addition, there is outer shell carbon scattering at 3.09 Å and 4.41 Å, and an Mn•••Mn feature at 3.54 Å. The 3- to 4-Å Mn-C scattering is assigned to outer shell scattering from coordinated imidazoles. The amplitude was consistent with one histidine per Mn leading to the suggestion [66], subsequently confirmed crystallographically [67], that there are two histidine ligands bound to reduced MnCat. On the basis of comparison with model complexes, the 3.54-Å Mn-Mn distance suggests that there must be at least one single-atom (e.g., aqua or hydroxo) bridge between the Mn, since unbridged structures are unlikely to give detectable Mn•••Mn EXAFS [66]. This distance is probably too long to be consistent with the $Mn_2(\mu\text{-OH})_2$ core structure that was proposed based on the EPR results [38]. An $Mn_2(\mu\text{-OH})_2$ structure would be expected to have an Mn-Mn distance of around 3.3 Å [68]. The XANES spectra for reduced MnCat show a relatively large 1s → 3d transition, suggesting either that the Mn are five-coordinate or the Mn have a very distorted six-coordinate geometry. A five-coordinate structure would be consistent with the structure proposed for oxidized MnCat based on optical spectroscopy (Sec. 3.3.2).

EXAFS data for superoxidized MnCat also show two resolvable shells of nearest-neighbor scattering, in this case at 1.82 and 2.08 Å, together with an intense Mn-Mn feature at 2.70 Å [41]. The combined observation of a 1.82 Å shell (characteristic of Mn-oxo distances) and a 2.7-Å Mn-Mn distance indicate that superoxidized MnCat has an Mn(III)(μ-oxo)$_2$Mn(IV) core structure. The Mn-Mn distance is somewhat longer than expected for a di-μ-oxo-, μ-carboxylato-bridged site [69], but not enough longer to permit this structure to be conclusively excluded. Although these data were compatible with outer shell scattering from coordinated imidazoles, interference from the intense 2.7-Å Mn-Mn shell prevented reliable quantitation of the number of histidine ligands.

Addition of N_3^- to superoxidized MnCat did not cause any significant change in the EXAFS or XANES spectra [41], suggesting, in agreement with the UV-visible, MCD, and EPR data, that azide binding causes only minor changes in the Mn coordination. There was a slight lengthening of the Mn-Mn distance (from 2.70 Å to 2.73 Å) when azide bound, as expected if the Mn_2O_2 core is slightly flattened when N_3^- binds (e.g., Fig. 2).

4.2. Crystallography

Low-resolution crystal structures have been described for both *T. thermophilus* and *L. plantarum* MnCat [9,70]. Both appear to be homohexamers, with subunits consisting of an antiparallel bundle of four α helices. This is the same folding pattern that is found for binuclear iron proteins such as hemerythrin, apoferritin, and ribonucleotide reductase [50]. However, the amino acid sequence deduced from the *L. plantarum* MnCat gene [71] does not show any obvious homologies to the sequences of the known di-iron proteins. It is thus difficult to predict likely Mn ligands from the sequence alone.

The low-resolution *T. thermophilus* structure has two regions of enhanced electron density that can be modeled as two metal ions separated by 3.6 ± 0.3 Å. Unfortunately, a detailed high-resolution structure has not yet been published. A conference abstract [67] cites Mn-Mn distances of 3.18 Å and 3.14 Å for the reduced and oxidized forms, respectively. As the uncertainty in these distances is likely to be fairly large [72], perhaps as large as 0.2 Å, these distances are consistent with most of the structural models that have been proposed for both oxidized and reduced MnCat. Based on this preliminary report, the Mn ions are coordinated to two imidazoles and three carboxylates, as shown in Fig. 3. There are in addition two solvent molecules, which may be water or hydroxide, and which very likely change protonation state depending on the oxidation state of the Mn. Interestingly, the crystal structure shows a lysine and a tyrosine group that are close to, and perhaps within hydrogen bonding distance of, the Mn ligands. It is possible that this is the lysine that is responsible for the change in the ESEEM spectrum on methylation. However, this does not resolve the question of whether this lysine is present as a bridging lysine, since the lysine bridge was proposed [61] for superoxidized MnCat while the available crystal structures are for the reduced and oxidized enzyme.

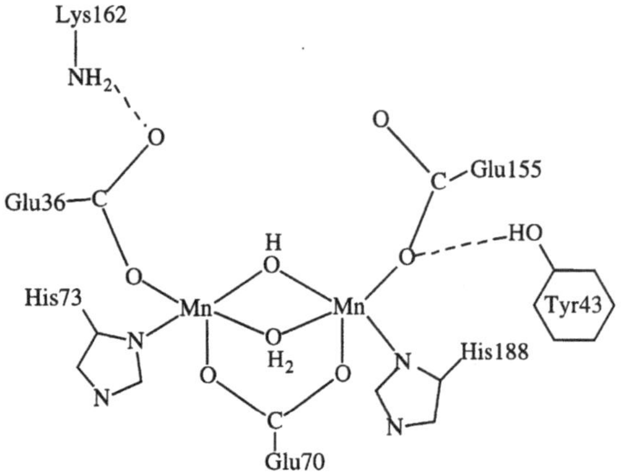

FIG. 3.   Schematic illustration of the Mn core structure for reduced and oxidized MnCat as reported in [67]. The Mn ions are coordinated to two histidine imidazoles, two monodentate glutamate carboxylates, and one bridging glutamate carboxylate. There are, in addition, two solvent molecules. These are shown as a hydroxide and a water, and both are shown to be bridging. However, neither their protonation state nor their geometry (bridging vs. terminal) is well defined at present. Possible hydrogen bonds are suggested by dashed lines but are not required crystallographically.

5.   MECHANISM

From the preceding discussion, it is apparent that while much has been learned, several important questions remain regarding the structure of the different oxidation states of MnCat. A key question is the number and identity of the bridging ligands. Based on the preliminary crystal structure, there appears to be a single bridging carboxylate ligand. However, crystallography, particularly at the present resolution, is not able to decide between oxo, hydroxo, or aqua bridges. Depending on the experimental method used, the proposals for bridging solvent molecules range, in order of increasing bridge strength, from nonbridged [52] to di-μ-hydroxo bridged [38] for reduced MnCat, and from a single hydroxo (or even aqua) bridge [39] to di-μ-oxo bridged [65] for oxidized MnCat. Until these are resolved, it is probably not possible to define a unique catalase mechanism. The combination of additional spectroscopic study with the anticipated solution of the high-resolution structure should answer many of these structural questions. In the meantime, however, it is possible to make some informed mechanistic proposals.

Numerous mechanisms have been suggested for MnCat [7,38,42, 43,52]. Our current preferred mechanism is shown in Fig. 4. In constructing this, we have relied on the general (albeit not universal) consensus that the coupling between the Mn is weak and on the need to accommodate the protons that are produced and consumed during the reaction [see Eqs. (7) and (8)]. For oxidized MnCat, we have interpreted the weak coupling as evidence for either a bridging hydroxide or a bridging water [39]. In Fig. 4, we show a bridging hydroxide. The choice of hydroxide rather than water is based in part on the expectation that coordination to two Mn(III) ions is likely to lower the pK_a of the water below 7, and in part on the need to accommodate protons as the enzyme cycles between oxidized and reduced forms. When Mn is reduced from Mn(III) to Mn(II), the basicity of coordinated solvent molecules increases. A bridging hydroxide in oxidized MnCat would be likely to be protonated in reduced MnCat, thus providing a binding site for one proton. If the bridging ligand was water in oxidized enzyme, then this proton site would not be available. We favor a bridging water molecule in the reduced enzyme as this should give weak enough coupling to be consistent with the EPR, but should also give a rigid enough Mn•••Mn interaction to account for its detectability by EXAFS.

We show only a single solvent bridge in Fig. 4, compared to the two

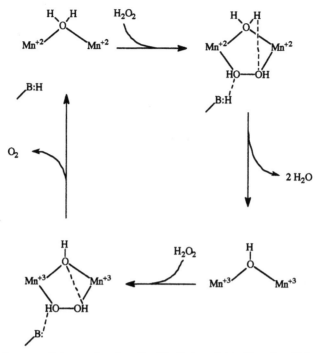

FIG. 4.   One possible mechanism for MnCat activity. For simplicity, only the manganese and a bridging water (hydroxide) are shown as ligands to the Mn. In this scheme, the bridging solvent molecule and a base "B" provides the proton balance that is necessary for the catalase reaction (see text for discussion).

bridging solvents that are suggested in Fig. 3. However, the preliminary crystallography suggests that one of the solvent molecules is disordered [67]; thus the crystallographic data available to date would appear to be consistent with this structure. From the available data, it seems most likely that the Mn ions are five-coordinate in both oxidized and reduced MnCat. However, we do not show either the bridging carboxylate or the terminal Mn ligands in Fig. 4. These are not required for our mechanism and are not, in our opinion, sufficiently well defined for the different oxidation states to warrant their inclusion.

In addition to the proton that is taken up by the bridging solvent, a second proton is released when peroxide is oxidized (i.e., when Mn is reduced). In Fig. 4, this proton is accommodated by an endogenous protein base, "B." We show the peroxide binding in a cis-μ-1,2 fashion. This would facilitate electron transfer from each of the Mn. However, there is to date no data that requires a bridging peroxide, and the mechanism could readily be modified to accommodate terminal peroxide coordination to a single Mn. We show the peroxide as remaining protonated when bound to both the oxidized and reduced enzyme. For the reduced enzyme, this is consistent with the proposed bridging water (i.e., if the local environment were sufficiently polar to cause deprotonation of the peroxide, it is likely that the bridging water would also be deprotonated). For the oxidized enzyme, binding of H_2O_2 rather than HO_2^- is more problematic, and it is possible that proton transfer takes place when H_2O_2 binds. In general, we have simply indicated the proposed pathways of proton transfer by dashed lines, without any indication of the relative timing of proton and electron transfer.

The mechanism shown in Fig. 4 accommodates most of the data available to date and provides testable proposals for the mechanism of MnCat. Future studies in our laboratory and others will be aimed at testing and refining this mechanism.

ACKNOWLEDGMENTS

We gratefully acknowledge support of our studies of Mn redox enzymes by the National Institutes of Health (GM-45205 to J.E.P.H.). D.W.Y. was supported in part by an NIH Molecular Biophysics Training Grant (GM-08270). J.E.P.H. thanks the NIH for support through a Fogarty Senior International Fellowship, Bill Rutherford and his group for support and hospitality during a sabbatical visit in Saclay, and Anabella Ivancich for helpful discussions.

ABBREVIATIONS AND DEFINITIONS

EPR	electron paramagnetic resonance
ENDOR	electron nuclear double resonance
ESEEM	electron spin-echo envelope modulation
EXAFS	extended X-ray absorption fine structure
MCD	magnetic circular dichroism
MnCat	manganese catalase

oxidation state   MnCat can exist in a variety of oxidation states. We refer to these as reduced, $Mn(II)_2$; mixed-valence, $Mn(II)Mn(III)$; oxidized, $Mn(III)_2$; and superoxidized, $Mn(III)Mn(IV)$.

salpn   1,3-bis(salicylideneamino)-2-propane

XAS   X-ray absorption spectroscopy

XANES   X-ray absorption near-edge spectroscopy

zfs   zero field splitting

REFERENCES

1. M. A. Johnston and E. A. Delwiche, *J. Bacteriol*, *83*, 936–938 (1962).

2. M. A. Johnston and E. A. Delwiche, *J. Bacteriol*, *90*, 352–356 (1965).

3. E. A. Delwiche, *J. Bacteriol*, *81*, 416–418 (1961).

4. Y. Kono and I. Fridovich, *J. Biol. Chem.*, *258*, 6015–6059 (1983).

5. V. V. Barynin and A. I. Grebenko, *Dokl. Akad. Nauk SSSR*, *286*, 461–464 (1986).

6. G. S. Allgood and J. J. Perry, *J. Bacteriol*, *168*, 563–567 (1986).

7. J. E. Penner-Hahn, in *Manganese Redox Enzymes* (V. L. Pecoraro, ed.), VCH, New York, 1992, pp. 29–45.

8. S. V. Khangulov, V. V. Barynin, N. V. Voevodskaya, and A. I. Grebenko, *Biochim. Biophys. Acta*, *1020*, 305–310 (1990).

9. B. K. Vainshtein, W. R. Melik-Adamyan, V. V. Barynin, and A. A. Vagin, in *Progress in Bioorganic Chemistry and Molecular Biology* (Y. A. Ovchinnikov, ed.), Elsevier, New York, 1984, pp. 117–126.

10. R. M. Fronko, J. E. Penner-Hahn, and C. J. Bender, *J. Am. Chem. Soc.*, *110*, 7554–7555 (1988).

11. M. Kagawa, N. Murakoshi, T. Mizobata, Y. Kawata, and J. Nagai, *FASEB J.*, *11*, A1138 (1997).

12. S. V. Khangulov, V. V. Barynin, and S. V. Antonyuk-Barynina, *Biochim. Biophys. Acta*, *1020*, 25–33 (1990).

13. J. B. Vincent and G. Christou, *Advances in Chemistry*, *33*, 197–257 (1989).

14. K. Wieghardt, *Angew. Chem. Int. Ed. Engl.*, *28*, 1153–1172 (1989).

15. J. E. Sheats, R. S. Czernuszewicz, G. C. Dismukes, A. L. Rhei

ngold, V. Petrouleas, J. Stubbe, W. H. Armstrong, R. H. Beer, and S. J. Lippard, *J. Am. Chem. Soc.*, *109*, 1435–1444 (1987).

16. V. V. Barynin, *J. Inorg. Biochem.*, *43*, 362 (1991).

17. Y. Kono and I. Fridovich, *J. Bacteriol.*, *155*, 742–746 (1983).

18. A. Deisseroth and A. L. Dounce, *Physiol. Rev.*, *50*, 319–375 (1970).

19. D. Voet and J. G. Voet, *Biochemistry*, 2 ed., John Wiley and Sons, New York, 1995.

20. G. R. Schoenbaum and B. Chance, in *The Enzymes* (P. Boyer, ed.), Academic Press, New York, 1976, pp. 363–408.

21. M. E. Percy, *Can. J. Biochem. Cell. Biol.*, *62*, 1006–1014 (1984).

22. R. G. Thurman and J. A. Handler, *Drug Metab. Rev.*, *20*, 679–688 (1989).

23. W. F. J. Beyer and I. Fridovich, in *Manganese in Metabolism and Enzyme Function* (V. L. Schramm and F. C. Wedler, eds.), Academic Press, Orlando, 1986, pp. 193–219.

24. A. Gelasco, S. Bensiek, and V. L. Pecoraro, *Inorg. Chem.*, *37*, 3301–3309 (1998).

25. A. C. Rosenzweig, C. A. Frederick, S. J. Lippard, and P. Nordlund, *Nature*, *366*, 537–543 (1993).

26. E. J. Larson and V. L. Pecoraro, *J. Am. Chem. Soc.*, *113*, 7809–7810 (1991).

27. Y. Nishida, T. Akamatsu, K. Tsuchiya, and M. Sakamoto, *Polyhedron*, *13*, 2251–2254 (1994).

28. C. P. Horwitz, P. J. Winslow, J. T. Warden, and C. A. Lisek, *Inorg. Chem.*, *32*, 82–88 (1993).

29. Y. Naruta and K. Maruyama, *J. Am. Chem. Soc.*, *113*, 3595–3596 (1991).

30. H. Sakiyama, H. Okawa, and R. Isobe, *J. Chem. Soc. Chem. Commun.*, 882–884 (1993).

31. A. Gelasco and V. L. Pecoraro, *J. Am. Chem. Soc.*, *115*, 7928–7929 (1993).

32. P. Mathur, M. Crowder, and G. C. Dismukes, *J. Am. Chem. Soc.*, *109*, 5227–5233 (1987).

33. P. J. Pessiki and G. C. Dismukes, *J. Am. Chem. Soc.*, *116*, 898–903 (1994).

34. R. T. Stibrany and S. M. Gorun, *Angew. Chem., Int. Ed. Engl.*, *29*, 1156–1158 (1990).

35. U. Bossek, M. Saher, T. Weyhermüller, and K. Wieghardt, *J. Chem. Soc. Chem. Commun.*, 1780–1782 (1992).

36. J. E. Pate, P. K. Ross, T. J. Thamann, C. A. Reed, K. D. Karlin, T. N. Sorrell, and E. I. Solomon, *J. Am. Chem. Soc.*, *111*, 5198–5209 (1989).

37. S. V. Khangulov, M. G. Goldfeld, V. V. Gerasimenko, N. E. Andreeva, V. V. Barynin, and A. I. Grebenko, *J. Inorg. Biochem.*, *40*, 279–292 (1990).

38. A. E. Meier, M. M. Whittaker, and J. W. Whittaker, *Biochemistry*, *35*, 348–360 (1996).

39. T. C. Brunold, D. R. Gamelin, T. L. Stemmler, S. K. Mandal, W. H. Armstrong, J. E. Penner-Hahn, and E. I. Solomon, *J. Am. Chem. Soc.*, *120*, 8724–8738 (1998).

40. D. R. Gamelin, M. L. Kirk, T. L. Stemmler, S. Pal, W. H. Armstrong, J. E. Penner-Hahn, and E. I. Solomon, *J. Am. Chem. Soc.*, *116*, 2392–2399 (1994).

41. T. L. Stemmler, B. E. Sturgeon, D. W. Randall, R. D. Britt, and J. E. Penner-Hahn, *J. Am. Chem. Soc.*, *119*, 9215–9225 (1997).

42. G. S. Waldo, Ph.D. thesis, University of Michigan, Ann Arbor, 1991.

43. T. L. Stemmler, Ph.D. thesis, University of Michigan, Ann Arbor, 1996.

44. G. S. Waldo and J. E. Penner-Hahn, *Biochemistry*, *34*, 1507–1512 (1995).

45. S. V. Khangulov, N. V. Voevodskaya, V. V. Barynin, A. I. Grebenko, and V. R. Melikadamian, *Biofizika*, *32*, 960–966 (1987).

46. G. S. Waldo, R. M. Fronko, and J. E. Penner-Hahn, *Biochemistry*, *30*, 10486–10490 (1991).

47. P. J. Pessiki, S. V. Khangulov, G. C. Dismukes, and V. V. Barynin, in *Macromolecular Host–Guest Complexes: Optical, Optoelectronic, and Photorefractive Properties and Applications* (S. A. Jenekhe, ed.), Materials Research Society, Pittsburgh, 1992, pp. 75–86.

48. Y. Kono and I. Fridovich, *J. Biol. Chem.*, *258*, 13646–13648 (1983).

49. K. E. Paulsen, Y. Liu, B. G. Fox, J. D. Lipscomb, E. Münck, and M. T. Stankovich, *Biochemistry*, *33*, 713–722 (1994).

50. B. J. Wallar and J. D. Lipscomb, *Chem. Rev.*, *96*, 2625–2657 (1996).

51. S. V. Khangulov, P. J. Pessiki, V. V. Barynin, D. E. Ash, and G. C. Dismukes, *Biochemistry*, *34*, 2015–2025 (1995).

52. G. C. Dismukes, *Chem. Rev.*, *96*, 2909–2926 (1996).
53. M. Zheng, S. V. Khangulov, G. C. Dismukes, and V. V. Barynin, *Inorg. Chem.*, *33*, 382–387 (1994).
54. P. J. Pessiki, S. V. Khangulov, D. M. Ho, and G. C. Dismukes, *J. Am. Chem. Soc.*, *116*, 891–897 (1994).
55. A. Haddy, G. S. Waldo, R. H. Sands, and J. E. Penner-Hahn, *Inorg. Chem.*, *33*, 2677–2682 (1994).
56. G. S. Waldo, S. Y. Yu, and J. E. Penner-Hahn, *J. Am. Chem. Soc.*, *114*, 5869–5870 (1992).
57. S. Khangulov, M. Sivaraja, V. V. Barynin, and G. C. Dismukes, *Biochemistry*, *32*, 4912–4924 (1993).
58. S. A. Dikanov, I. D. Tsvetkov, S. V. Khangulov, and M. G. Goldfeld, *Dokl. Akad. Nauk SSSR*, *302*, 1255–1257 (1988).
59. W. B. Mims and J. Peisach, in *Biological Magnetic Resonance*, Vol. 3 (L. J. Berliner and J. Reuben, eds.), Plenum Press, New York, 1981.
60. R. D. Britt and M. P. Klein, in *Pulsed Magnetic Resonance: NMR, ESR, and Optics, a recognition of E. L. Hahn* (D. M. S. Bagguley ed.) Clarendon Press, Oxford, 1992, pp. 361–376.
61. A. Ivancich, V. V. Barynin, and J. L. Zimmermann, *Biochemistry*, *34*, 6628–6639 (1995).
62. R. D. Britt, J. L. Zimmerman, K. Sauer, and M. P. Klein, *J. Am. Chem. Soc.*, *111*, 3522–3532 (1989).
63. D. W. Randall, Ph.D. thesis, The University of California, Davis (1997).
64. L. Jacquamet, I. Michaud-Soret, N. Debaecker-Petit, V. V. Barynin, J. L. Zimmermann, and J. M. Latour, *Angew. Chem., Int. Ed. Engl.*, *36*, 1626–1628 (1997).
65. I. Michaud-Soret, L. Jacquamet, N. Debaecker-Petit, L. Le Pape, V. V. Barynin, and J. M. Latour, *Inorg. Chem.*, *37*, 3874–3876 (1998).
66. T. L. Stemmler, T. M. Sossong, J. I. Goldstein, D. E. Ash, T. E. Elgren, D. M. Kurtz, and J. E. Penner-Hahn, *Biochemistry*, *36*, 9847–9858 (1997).
67. V. V. Barynin, P. D. Hempstead, A. A. Vagin, S. V. Antonyuk, W. R. Melik-Adamyan, V. S. Lamzin, P. M. Harrison, and P. J. Artymiuk, *J. Inorg. Biochem.*, *67*, 196 (1997).
68. N. Kitajima, U. P. Sihgh, H. Amagai, M. Osawa, and Y. Moro-oka, *J. Am. Chem. Soc.*, *113*, 7757–7758 (1991).

69. E. Larson, M. S. Lah, X. H. Li, J. A. Bonadies, and V. L. Pecoraro, *Inorg. Chem.*, *31*, 373–378 (1992).

70. E. Baldwin, Ph.D. thesis, University of North Carolina, Chapel Hill (1990).

71. T. Igarashi, Y. Kono, and K. Tanaka, *J. Biol. Chem.*, *271*, 29521–29524 (1996).

72. J. M. Guss, H. D. Bartunik, and H. C. Freeman, *Acta Crystallogr. B*, *48*, 790–811 (1992).

17

Manganese Peroxidase

Michael H. Gold, Heather L. Youngs,
and Maarten D. Sollewijn Gelpke

Department of Biochemistry and Molecular Biology,
Oregon Graduate Institute of Science and Technology,
Beaverton, OR 97006-8921, USA

1.   INTRODUCTION

Lignin is a plant cell wall, phenylpropanoid polymer synthesized by the free radical condensation of phenolic precursors, resulting in a heterogeneous, random, and highly branched structure [1,2]. The unique structure of lignin requires depolymerization by extracellular, oxidative mechanisms, explaining its recalcitrance to degradation by most microorganisms [3–5]. Indeed, white-rot basidiomycetous fungi are the only known organisms that are capable of degrading lignin extensively to CO_2 and H_2O in axenic culture [4,5]. Early work indicated that lignin degradation by the best studied lignin-degrading fungus, *Phanerochaete chrysosporium*, is both oxidative and nonspecific [4–6]. Lignin degradation by several white-rot fungi is strongly dependent on the presence of Mn in culture [7,8] and MnO_2 precipitates accumulate in wood during decay by many white-rot fungi [9].

In the early 1980s, two extracellular enzymes, lignin peroxidase (LiP) [10,11] and manganese peroxidase (MnP) [12], were discovered in *P. chrysosporium*. These enzymes are major components of the extracellular lignin and aromatic pollutant degradation system of this organism [4,5,13]. This chapter focuses on MnP, a unique heme peroxidase that uses Mn^{II} as its primary substrate. Since its discovery in *P. chrysosporium* [12], MnP has been identified as an extracellular enzyme in all of the lignin-degrading fungi that have been examined to date [7,14–18].

2. GENERAL PROPERTIES OF Mn PEROXIDASE

MnP has been purified from the extracellular medium of *P. chrysosporium* cultures using several combinations of column chromatographies and gel filtration [19–22]. The enzyme exists as a series of glycosylated isoenzymes with pIs ranging from 4.2 to 4.9 and with molecular masses ranging from 45 to 47 kDa [19,20,23–25]. The cDNA sequence of MnP isozyme 1 indicates that the mature protein is composed of 357 amino acids. MnP contains one iron protoporphyrin IX prosthetic group [19,26] and two Ca atoms per molecule of protein [26].

Mn peroxidase activity has been assayed in the extracellular medium of a wide variety of white-rot fungal species [14]. Fungal species from which Mn peroxidases have been purified include *Dichomitus squalens* [27], *Ceriporiopsis subvermispora* [28], *Lentinus edodes* [29,30], *Trametes versicolor* [31], *Phlebia radiata* [32], *Pleurotus ostreatus* [33,34], and *Panus tigrinus* [35,36]. All of these MnPs have molecular masses in the range of 45–55 kDa and are glycoproteins. Where examined, they contain one heme prosthetic group per protein molecule. Furthermore, in the presence of H_2O_2 and a dicarboxylic acid chelator, these MnPs oxidize Mn^{II} to Mn^{III}. A separate group of unusual enzymes apparently capable of oxidizing nonphenolic aromatic compounds, such as veratryl alcohol, as well as Mn^{II}, has been isolated from *Bjerkandera adusta* [37,38] and *Pleurotus eryngii* [37,39].

3. REACTIONS CATALYZED BY Mn PEROXIDASE

In the presence of dicarboxylic acid chelators, such as malonate and oxalate, or α-hydroxy acids, such as lactate and tartrate, the oxidation of Mn^{II} to Mn^{III} by MnP can be monitored at 270–290 nm [40,41]. Mn^{III}-malonate formation is used routinely as a quantitative MnP assay [41]. For the dicarboxylic acid chelators malonate and oxalate, the stoichiometry between the Mn^{III}–chelator complex formed and H_2O_2 consumed is 2:1 [41]. Mn^{III}–chelator complexes are efficient oxidants [41,42] and MnP oxidizes a wide variety of phenols, amines, and dyes in the presence of Mn^{II} [19,20,40]. MnP assays based on 2,6-dimethoxyphenol, vanillyl acetone, ABTS, and phenol red oxidation also have been reported [19,20,41]. In addition, the oxidation of o-dianisidine and guaiacol by Mn^{III} complexes and the reduction of Mn^{III} complexes by vanillyl alcohol [41,42], demonstrate that the Mn^{III}–chelator complex is acting as a mediator in the reaction. Mn^{III}–chelator complexes are stable enough to diffuse through a semipermeable membrane to oxidize a polymeric substrate at a distance [40]. This confirms cytochemical studies showing that MnP is too bulky to diffuse into the wood matrix [43,44], suggesting that the enzyme does not bind directly to lignin in wood but rather oxidizes the substrate via a diffusible Mn^{III}–chelator complex.

The mechanisms proposed for the MnP-catalyzed oxidation of several free phenolic lignin model dimers suggest that the initial one-electron oxidation of the substrate by enzyme-generated Mn^{III} produces a phenoxy radical intermediate [45,46]. This intermediate is further oxidized by Mn^{III} to form a carbon-centered cation. Subsequent loss of a proton yields the ketone dimer II (Fig. 1). Attack of water at the cation followed by alkylphenyl cleavage yields products III–V, and C-C bond cleavage of the arylglycerol-β-aryl ether phenoxy radical intermediate yields products VI-VIII (Fig. 1). Similar cleavage products have been identified when chemically synthesized lignins are oxidized by MnP [47], suggesting that these proposed mechanisms accurately represent processes involved in the oxidation of polymeric lignin.

Nonphenolic substructures are not susceptible to oxidation via mechanisms involving a phenoxy radical intermediate. Therefore, mechanisms whereby MnP could oxidize nonphenolic substructures have been sought. In particular, radical mediator mechanisms have been invoked to explain the oxidation of nonphenolic substructures by MnP. In the presence of Mn^{II}, H_2O_2, and thiols such as glutathione, MnP oxidizes nonphenolic benzyl alcohols and cleaves a nonphenolic β-aryl ether dilignol [48]. This mechanism can account for the degradation of synthetic lignin by MnP in the presence of thiols [49] and suggests that relatively long-lived radicals could mediate the oxidation of nonphenolic lignin substructures by MnP. The slow oxidation of nonphenolic lignin substructures by MnP in the presence of unsaturated fatty acids suggests that these or similar compounds may act as mediators [50]. Whether radical mediator mechanisms can explain the degradation of nonphenolic lignin substructures requires further clarification.

MnP is also able to generate H_2O_2 from NADPH and thiols in the presence of Mn^{II} [20,40]. In the absence of added H_2O_2, MnP oxidizes oxalate, glyoxalate, and malonate to generate H_2O_2 [51–54]. Since these

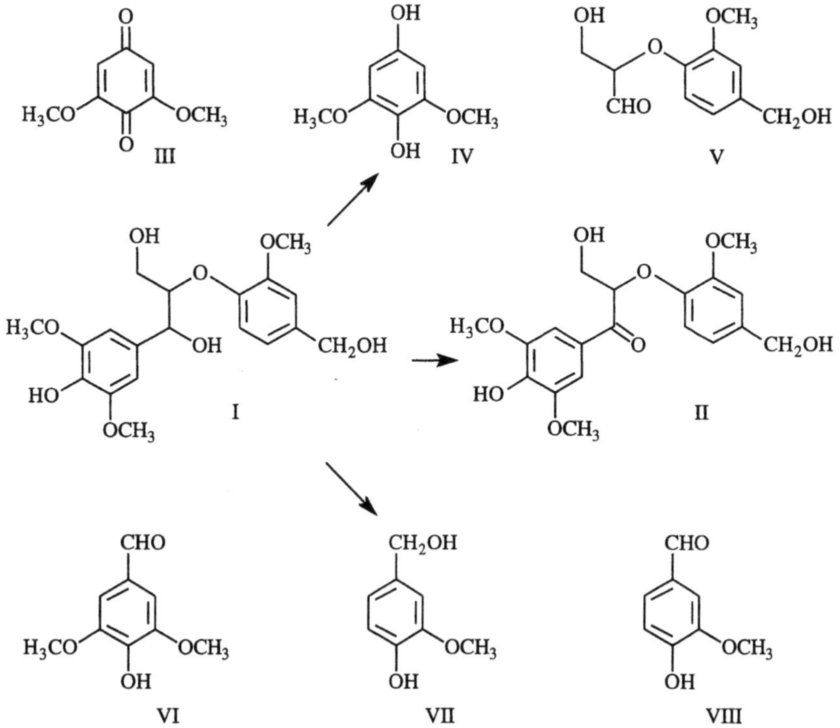

FIG. 1.   Products obtained from the oxidation of a phenolic arylglycerol β-aryl ether lignin substructure (I) by MnP. Reactions are described in the text [45]. (Reprinted with permission from [45]. Copyright 1992, American Chemical Society.

carboxylic acids are produced by white-rot fungi [41,52], these reactions may play an important role in the generation of H_2O_2 by some white-rot fungi [53,55]. Finally, as with LiP [56], MnP can oxidize Br^- and I^- at low pH, resulting in the halogenation of a variety of aromatic substrates [57].

4.   BIOPHYSICAL STUDIES OF Mn PEROXIDASE

4.1.   Spectroscopic Studies

Electronic absorption maxima for native, oxidized, and various ligated forms of MnP have been reported (Table 1) [4,19] and are similar to those of both horseradish peroxidase (HRP) and LiP [19,42,58–61],

TABLE 1

Spectroscopic Characteristics of MnP,[a] LiP,[a] and HRP

	Electronic absorption maxima (nm)[b]		
	MnP	LiP	HRP
Ferric	406, 502, 632	407, 500, 632	403, 498, 640
Ferric-N$_3^-$	417, 542, 580	418, 540, 575	416, 534, 565, 635
Ferric-CN$^-$	421, 542, 580, 640	423, 540, 580	422, 439, 580
Ferrous	433, 544, 585	435, 556, 580	440, 510, 557, 580
Ferrous-CO	423, 541, 570	420, 535, 568	423, 542, 572
Compound I	407, 558, 605, 650	408, 550, 608, 650	400, 557, 622, 650
Compound II	420, 528, 555	420, 525, 556	420, 527, 554
Compound III	417, 545, 579	419, 543, 578	413, 546, 583

[a]From *P. chrysosporium*.
[b]References are cited in the text.

which indicates that the heme iron is high-spin, ferric, and pentacoordinate, with a histidine acting as the fifth ligand. Detailed electron paramagnetic resonance (EPR) and resonance Raman studies of various forms of MnP confirm that the native enzyme exists as a high-spin, ferric, heme protein [62]. Resonance Raman and nuclear magnetic resonance (NMR) studies show that the native enzyme forms low-spin complexes with CN$^-$ and N$_3^-$ [62–64] and a high-spin complex with F$^-$ [62] and that the heme environment of MnP is similar to those of HRP and LiP [62–64]. NMR studies of native, ferric, MnP confirm that the fifth ligand to the heme iron is a histidine moiety [63,64]. Spectra of the reduced enzyme are typical of high-spin, pentacoordinate, ferrous heme with the heme iron ligated to the protein through a proximal His [62]. The ferrous enzyme forms a complex with CO which has a spectrum typical of other peroxidases [19,60]. Finally, EPR of the ferrous heme-^{14}NO and -^{15}NO adducts of MnP confirms that the fifth ligand is the N-imidazole of a histidine residue as in LiP and HRP [62].

4.2. Catalytic Cycle and Kinetic Mechanism

The catalytic cycle of MnP is shown in Fig. 2. Optical absorption maxima for the oxidized intermediates of MnP also are compared with those

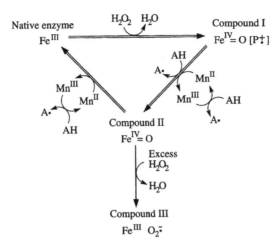

FIG. 2.   Catalytic cycle of MnP. AH is a phenolic or aromatic amine substrate and A• is the radical produced upon one-electron oxidation. [P⁺] is a porphyrin π-cation radical. (Reprinted with permission from [4]. Copyright 1989, American Chemical Society.)

of LiP and HRP in Table 1 [42,60,61]. The two-electron oxidation of ferric MnP by H_2O_2 yields the oxyferryl, porphyrin cation radical intermediate, Compound I [42]. Reduction of Compound I by one electron, using one equivalent of ferrocyanide or Mn^{II}, yields Compound II [42]. Compound II is then reduced back to the ferric enzyme by a single electron step in the presence of the substrate, Mn^{II}. The addition of excess H_2O_2 to the native enzyme yields Compound III [42]. While Mn^{II} and a variety of phenols or aromatic amines reduce Compound I to Compound II, only Mn^{II} efficiently reduces Compound II to native enzyme (Fig. 2) [42,65]. This indicates that Mn^{II} serves as an obligatory substrate for MnP Compound II, enabling the enzyme to complete its catalytic cycle [42,65].

Steady-state kinetic analysis of Mn^{II} oxidation suggests a peroxidase-type ping-pong kinetic mechanism [41]. The k_{cat}/K_m for Mn^{II} and H_2O_2 (in the presence of malonate) are 3.94×10^6 and 8.34×10^6 M^{-1} s^{-1}, respectively [21,66].

Transient state kinetic results support the mechanism described above. The reduction rate of compound I by Mn^{II} in malonate buffer is too fast to measure ($>10^7$ M^{-1} s^{-1}) at the pH optimum, 4.5. However, at pH 3.0 the second-order rate constant for Compound I reduction by Mn^{II} is 4×10^4 M^{-1} s^{-1} in malonate buffer. At pH 4.5, the second-order rate constant for reduction of Compound I by dimethoxyphenol (DMP) is ~5.0 $\times$ 10^3 M^{-1} s^{-1} [65,67,68], which is ~10^4-fold slower than that for Mn^{II} at this pH. In malonate buffer, the first-order rate constant for reduction of Compound II by Mn^{II} is about 5.48 $\times$ 10^2 s^{-1}, while the rate constant for reduction of Compound II by DMP is >650-fold lower [65,67–69]. Indeed, the rate constant for reduction of Compound II by DMP is too slow to support efficient enzyme turnover. Likewise, while the dissociation constant for Mn^{II} is around 1.66 x 10^{-4} M, the dissociation constant for DMP suggests that the binding of DMP is 100-fold weaker [67].

4.3. Role of Chelators

To date, MnP appears to be the only enzyme that uses Mn as a diffusible substrate rather than a permanent enzyme-bound cofactor. Therefore, the binding site must be able to bind Mn^{II} and release Mn^{III}. The role of chelators in this process has been studied; however, it is still not well understood. As previously mentioned, a dicarboxylic acid or α-hydroxy acid chelator is required for complete turnover of the enzyme by Mn^{II} [41,66,69]. Although *P. chrysosporium* secretes several organic acids such as oxalate, malonate, citrate, and glyoxalate during idiophasic metabolism [41,52,70,71], only oxalate is produced at concentrations sufficient to stimulate MnP activity [52,69].

The formation and reduction of Compound I do not appear to be affected by the presence or type of chelator in reaction mixtures at pH 4.5 [66,67,69]. In contrast, the reduction of Compound II is greatly affected by chelators [66,69]. Maximum rates for the reduction of Compound II are observed when the Mn^{II} in solution is stoichiometrically chelated by oxalate [66,69]. Based on this, the formation of an enzyme–Mn^{II}–oxalate ternary complex during the reaction cycle has been postulated [66]. However, recent NMR [72] and crystal structure [26] studies show that Mn^{II}, rather than an Mn^{II}–chelator complex, binds to the native ferric enzyme as proposed earlier by Gold and co-workers [41]. The binding of Mn^{III} to MnP is difficult to study due to the instability of Mn^{III} complexes [41]. Trivalent lanthanides (Ln^{III}), which also bind at the Mn binding site [73], have been proposed to mimic the behavior of Mn^{III} [72]. Although the binding site is on the surface of the enzyme [26], bound Mn^{II} is difficult to remove completely from the native ferric enzyme [72,74,75]. In contrast, lanthanide ions are easily removed by oxalate [72,73,75]. These results support the proposal that MnP has a strong affinity for free Mn^{II}, $K_D \simeq 10$ µM, while a chelator facilitates the removal of Mn^{III} from the enzyme [41].

5. Mn PEROXIDASE cDNA AND GENOMIC SEQUENCES

In *P. chrysosporium*, MnP occurs as a series of isozymes encoded by a family of genes [76]. The sequences of cDNA [25,77–79] and genomic clones encoding three alleles of MnP isozymes from this species [77,80,81] have been determined. *mnp1* and *mnp3* each contain six introns, whereas *mnp2* contains seven [77,80,81]. Although the introns differ in size and sequence, the positions of five of the introns (1,3,4,5,6 of *mnp1* and *mnp3* and 1,4,5,6,7 of *mnp2*) align precisely in all three genomic sequences [81]. Intron 2 of *mnp2* aligns with intron 2 of *mnp1* while intron 3 of *mnp2* aligns with intron 2 of *mnp3* [81]. Sequences from the three genes share 66–70% nucleotide identity within the protein coding regions and several short regions of sequence identity in their promoters, including a TATAAA element, inverted CCAAT elements, and several putative AP-2 binding sites [77,80,81]. All three genes contain putative heat-shock elements [76,81]. Finally, all three *mnp* genes contain putative metal response elements [77,80–84].

cDNA sequences of the three *mnp* genes encode precursor enzymes that contain 21–24 amino acid signal peptides and mature proteins consisting of 357–358 amino acids [77–81]. The deduced amino acid sequences show that 10 Cys residues known to be involved in disulfide bond formation [26], two putative N-glycosylation sites [76,81], and sequences flanking catalytic amino acids (see Sec. 6.2) are conserved among the three genes and are similar to those in other peroxidases [25,76,78,81]. Finally, sequences surrounding and including the residues which constitute the functional Mn binding site (see Sec. 6.2) share amino acid identity [25,77–81].

Genes apparently encoding MnPs have been sequenced from several white-rot fungi in addition to *P. chrysosporium*. These gene sequences appear to form two distinct groups. The first group includes genes from *D. squalens* [18], *C. subvermispora* [85,86], and *P. chrysosporium* [77,80,81], which encode proteins containing at least 350 amino acid residues and 5 disulfide linkages, one of which is found in a long

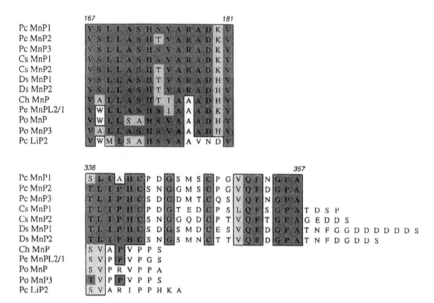

FIG. 3. Alignments of the deduced amino acid sequences from several *mnp* genes in the region of the proximal His and C-terminal regions. Pc, *Phanerochaete chrysosporium*; CS, *Ceriporiopsis subvermispora*; DS, *Dichomitus squalens*; Ch, *Coriolus hirsutus*; Pe, *Pleurotus eryngii*; Po, *Pleurotus ostreatus*. The amino acid numbering refers to the Pc MnP sequences. References are cited in the text.

carboxy terminal tail (Fig. 3). These *mnp* genes also encode a signal peptide, suggesting that they are produced as a precursor protein [18,76,78,81,85]. The deduced amino acid sequences of these genes appear to contain the three acidic amino acid residues found in the Mn binding site (see Sec. 6.2), although this has been experimentally tested only for *mnp* genes from *P. chrysosporium* [22,68,74]. They also contain a loop comprising residues 229–235 which is not found in LiP. Finally, all of these MnPs [18,76,81,85] contain a Ser at the site occupied by the critical Trp171 residue in LiP [87,88] (Fig. 3).

The second group of genes from *P. ostreatus* [89,90], *P. eryngii* [91], *Coriolus hirsutus* [92], and *T. versicolor* [93,94] encode peroxidases with characteristics of both MnP and LiP. While these sequences appear to contain the acidic amino acid residues involved in the Mn binding site of MnP, they all encode proteins, which, like LiP, contain a shorter carboxy terminal tail [87,89,91,94] and lack Arg177 (Fig. 3), a residue essential for the activity of the *P. chrysosporium* enzyme [67]. Furthermore, like LiP, the proteins in this group contain only four of the five disulfide bonds found in MnP [26] and contain both a signal peptide and a short propeptide, suggesting that, like LiP [95], members of this group are synthesized as preproenzymes [89,91,94]. Members of this group also contain a Trp or an Ala [89,91,93,94] at the position equivalent to the important Trp171 in LiP [88]. Thus, these enzymes have characteristics of both MnP and LiP and more work is required to determine how these enzymes and their genes should be classified.

6.   CRYSTAL STRUCTURE OF Mn PEROXIDASE

The crystal structure of MnP from *P. chrysosporium* has been solved [26,74]. Previous studies indicated that MnP is a glycosylated peroxidase containing one iron protoporphyrin IX [19,20,25]. Detailed spectroscopic studies show that the heme iron is ferric, high-spin, pentacoordinate, and ligated to a histidine residue, as in other plant and fungal peroxidases [19,42,62,63]. The crystal structure confirms these observations and further shows that the overall polypeptide fold is similar to that of other plant and fungal peroxidases (see Ref. 26 and references therein) [96–99].

The crystal structure shows that MnP contains 1 minor and 10 major helices arranged in two approximately equal-sized domains, proximal and distal to the heme, each containing one calcium atom (Fig. 4) [26]. The positions of the calcium sites are homologous to those in LiP, *Arthromyces ramosus* peroxidase (ArP), and *Coprinus cinereus* peroxidase (CiP), although the exact ligands are not conserved [26,96,100]. In MnP, each calcium is septacoordinate. The distal calcium is bound by the side chains of Asp47, Ser66, and Asp64, the backbone carbonyls of Gly62 and Asp47, as well as two water molecules. Recent studies show that the distal calcium provides thermal stability to the enzyme [101,102]. One of the water ligands to the calcium is bound to Glu74 which forms an H-bond network through Gln80 with the distal His46 [26]. In MnP and LiP, the distal calcium is coordinated to Asp47 on helix B which forms part of the active site [26,100]. Indeed, this Asp residue is conserved in many peroxidases [103]. The proximal calcium is bound by the backbone carbonyls of Thr196, Ser174, and Thr193 and the side chains of Asp191, Thr193, Asp198, and Ser174, which is adjacent to the proximal His173 [26].

MnP contains five disulfide linkages, four of which are identical to those in LiP, ArP, and CiP [26,96,97,99,100,104]. The disulfide linkage

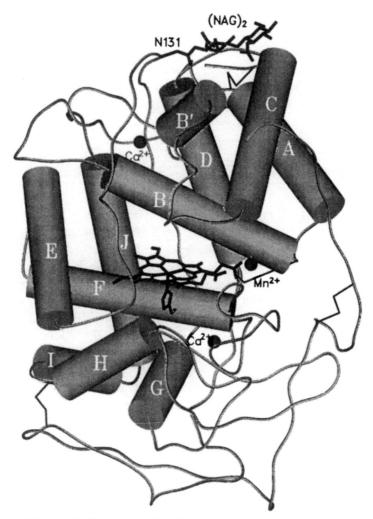

FIG 4.   Schematic diagram of the *P. chrysosporium* MnP crystal structure.
(Kindly provided by M. Sundaramoorthy and reprinted with permission granted
by the American Society for Biochemistry and Molecular Biology [26].)

pattern of these first four bridges in MnP, 1–3, 2–7, 4–5, 6–8, is identical to that found in other fungal peroxidases and differs from the linkage pattern of homologous plant peroxidases [98,105]. It has been proposed that the fifth linkage, Cys341–Cys348, which is unique to MnP,
not only stabilizes the enzyme's carboxy terminal tail, which is longer

than that of LiP (see Sec. 6.1), but may also participate in stabilization of the Mn binding site [26].

The MnP crystal structure exhibits N-glycosylation at Asn131 [26], one of the putative sites predicted by the cDNA sequence [25] and O-mannosylation has been observed at Ser336 [73]. This is consistent with glycosylation patterns observed in other extracellular fungal peroxidases [105].

6.1. The Heme Environment and Peroxide Binding Site

Amino acid residues in the distal domain are involved in the heterolytic cleavage of peroxide and in heme stabilization, including His46, Arg42, Asn80, Glu74, and Phe45 (Fig. 5). As in all peroxidases, His46 acts as an acid-base catalyst, accepting a proton from peroxide, facilitating cleavage [106,107]. Arg42, the distal Arg, appears to stabilize Compound I and may facilitate heterolytic cleavage of the peroxide anion [108]. Mutation studies of the homologous residue Arg51 in CiP suggest that the distal Arg may also influence the occupancy of the H_2O_2-binding pocket [109]. The distal Arg in many other peroxidases interacts directly, or through a bridging water molecule, with one of the heme propionates, whereas in MnP this propionate is rotated such that it cannot interact with Arg42 [26]. Asn80, Glu74, and His46 form a hydrogen bonding network believed to participate in modulation of the acid-base character and positioning of the distal histidine for peroxide cleavage (Fig. 5). Finally, extracellular plant and fungal peroxidases contain a Phe residue adjacent to the heme in the position of Phe45 [26,103,110], which is involved in stabilizing Compound I [111].

In the proximal domain, His173, Asp242, and Phe190 are important conserved residues (Fig. 5). His173, the proximal histidine, is the fifth ligand to the heme iron, thereby tethering the heme to the protein [26]. Asp242 forms a hydrogen bond with His173 and thus may render more anionic character to His173, which would, in turn, lower the redox potential of the heme iron, enabling the formation of the oxyferryl intermediates [106]. Phe190 is conserved in LiP [100], peanut peroxidase [98], and HRP [112] but is replaced by Trp in cytochrome c peroxidase and ascorbate peroxidase [103] and Leu in ArP and CiP [96,97]. The orientations of Phe190 in MnP and LiP differ considerably [26,100]. This difference in orientation may influence the redox potential of the two enzymes [63,64].

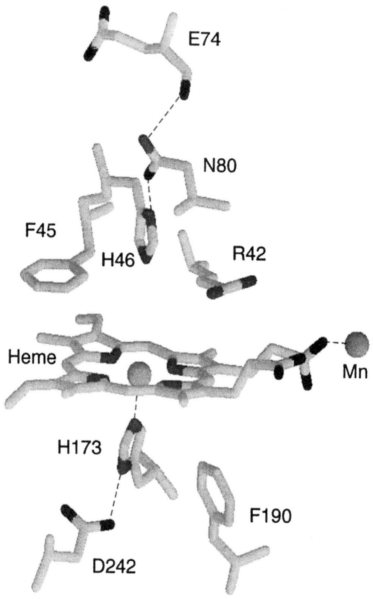

FIG. 5.   Heme environment of MnP. D = Asp; E = Glu; F = Phe; H = His; N = Asn; R = Arg. (Reprinted with permission from [113]. Copyright 1997, American Chemical Society.)

6.2. Manganese Binding Site

Prior to the elucidation of the crystal structure of MnP, several Mn binding sites were proposed on the basis of heme modification experiments
and homology-based molecular modeling [115,116]. The addition of
azides to the δ-meso carbon of the heme in MnP and LiP has been used
to assess the availability of the heme to substrates [115,117]. While Co^{II}
competitively inhibits Mn^{II} oxidation by the enzyme, it does not inhibit
inactivation by azides, suggesting that Mn^{II} binds at some distance from
the δ-meso carbon [115]. NMR studies indicate that the upper limit for
this distance is around 11 Å [118]. Three different Mn binding sites were
proposed by homology model comparisons of two MnP isozymes [116].
The most favorable binding site proposed in that study was the only apparent Mn^{II} binding site in the crystal structure [26]. Recent pH titration studies suggest that there may be a second low-affinity Mn^{II} binding site not apparent in the crystal structure [119].

The enzyme-bound Mn at the functional site (Fig. 6) is hexacoordinate, with two water ligands and four carboxylate ligands from three
acidic amino acids, Glu35, Glu39, and Asp179, and heme propionate 6.
One water ligand is hydrogen-bonded to heme propionate 7 (Fig. 6) and
all ligand-metal bond distances range from 2.34 to 2.82 Å [26], typical
of coordinated Mn^{II} [120]. Electron transfer is presumed to occur via a
direct pathway through the heme propionate 6 ligand. Of the amino
acids forming the Mn binding site, only Glu39 is present in LiP and none
of the residues are present in ArP or CiP [26,96,97]. Arg177 forms a salt
bridge with Glu35 (Fig. 6) thereby orienting this ligand, which is at the
surface of the protein, and perhaps neutralizing the charge at the Mn
binding site [26]. Arg177 is not conserved in LiP nor, it has been argued,
can the LiP structure accommodate this residue [26].

Other metals such as Co^{II}, Cd^{II}, Sm^{III}, Eu^{III}, Gd^{III}, and Ce^{III} can
bind at the Mn binding site as shown by competitive inhibition kinet-
ics and binding experiments [72,75,115]. The crystal structure of the
Cd-substituted enzyme reveals that this metal binds at the Mn binding
site with the same geometry as Mn^{II}. In contrast, Sm^{III} binds at the Mn
binding site with a slightly different geometry, presumably due to the
ability of Sm^{III} to accept additional ligands [73]. It has been suggested
that lanthanide ions may act as models for Mn^{III} binding [72]. Slight

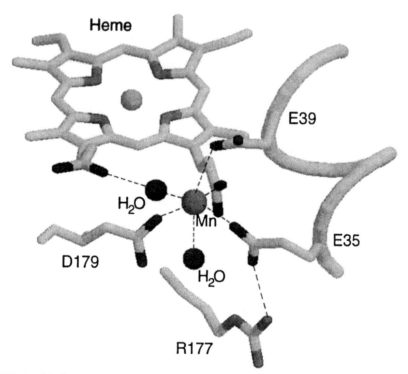

FIG. 6. Mn binding site of MnP [26]. For the one-letter code, see legend of Fig. 5. (Reprinted with permission from [67]. Copyright 1999, American Chemical Society.)

changes in geometry, coupled with the fairly large size difference between Mn^{II}, 0.80 Å, and Mn^{III}, 0.66 Å, [121], as well as differing affinities for dicarboxylic acid chelators may explain the difference in the enzyme affinities for Mn^{II} and Mn^{III}, thus facilitating binding of Mn^{II} and release of Mn^{III} (see Sec. 4.3).

7.   STRUCTURE–FUNCTION STUDIES OF Mn PEROXIDASE

7.1.   Homologous and Heterologous Expression of Mn Peroxidase

An efficient system for the expression of recombinant enzyme is required for structure and function studies of MnP. Heterologous expression of *mnp* from *P. chrysosporium* has been achieved in *Escherichia coli* [122] and *Aspergillus oryzae* [123]. Enzyme expressed in *E. coli* is not glycosylated and is produced as inclusion bodies requiring reconstitution with heme and the two structural calciums under anaerobic conditions [122]. rMnP expressed in *E. coli* exhibits many kinetic features similar to wild-type MnP (wtMnP) [68,122]. However, neither detailed spectroscopic nor crystallographic studies of this enzyme have been reported; therefore, the degree of similarity of this enzyme to the wild-type (wt) enzyme is not known. Expression of rMnP in *A. oryzae* produces active, glycosylated protein in yields comparable to the homologous system (see below) [123]. However, addition of heme to cultures is required which may lead to adventitiously bound heme. Furthermore, the only rMnP produced in this system to date has Mn^{II} oxidation kinetics significantly lower than the wt enzyme [123].

Homologous expression of rMnP in *P. chrysosporium* results in the secretion of active enzyme with kinetic properties similar to wtMnP [21]. Homologous expression in *P. chrysosporium* is possible because the wt enzyme is only expressed during secondary (idiophasic) metabolism triggered by nutrient nitrogen depletion [5,76]. Placing the *mnp* gene under the control of a primary metabolic promoter results in expression of the recombinant protein during primary metabolic growth in the presence of high nitrogen levels [21]. This system yields sufficient enzyme for biochemical and spectroscopic studies which show that the rMnP produced is similar to the wtMnP, suggesting proper heme insertion and essentially identical posttranslational modification and secretion [21,22, 74,113].

7.2.   Site-Directed Mutations at the Mn Binding Site

The putative Mn^{II} binding site (Fig. 6) and heme environment (Fig. 5) have been identified by X-ray crystallographic analysis. In the first site-directed mutagenesis studies on MnP [22,124] each of the three amino acid ligands in the Mn binding site was changed to its respective amide to obtain Asp179Asn, Glu35Gln, and Glu39Gln. In addition, one double mutant, Asp179Asn-Glu35Gln, was constructed. These mutant MnPs, homologously expressed in *P. chrysosporium*, are essentially identical to wtMnP in chromatographic properties, molecular weight, and spectral characteristics of the ferric enzymes and oxidized intermediates [22,124]. Resonance Raman spectra of these mutants show that the coordination and spin states of the heme irons are identical to wtMnP, indicating that the heme environment is apparently not affected by the mutations at the Mn binding site [22]. Indeed, preservation of the heme environment geometry was confirmed by crystallographic analysis of several mutants [74]. Furthermore, mutations at the Mn binding site do not affect kinetic constants for binding and reactivity toward peroxide, ferrocyanide, and small phenolic compounds such as p-cresol [22,124]. However, steady-state kinetic analyses of all the mutants show significant increases in K_m and decreases in k_{cat} for Mn^{II} compared to wtMnP [22,124]. The catalytic efficiency of the enzyme for Mn^{II}, k_{cat}/K_m, is approximately 10^4-fold lower for the single mutants and 10^5-fold lower for the double mutant [22,124].

Transient-state kinetic analysis of Compound II reduction of MnP variants by Mn^{II} shows first-order kinetics. The K_D values are around 100-fold higher for the single mutants and 200-fold higher for the double mutant compared to wtMnP. The first-order rate constants for the single and double mutants are around 200-fold and 4000-fold less, respectively, than that of wtMnP [22,124]. Crystal structures of the mutants show dramatically decreased electron density at the Mn binding site compared to wtMnP, indicating much weaker binding of Mn at the altered sites [26,74]. The orientation of the Mn binding site ligands in the mutant MnPs also are considerably altered [74]. All of the mutations result in increased exposure of the binding site to solvent, primarily by rotation of residues 35 and 39, at the surface of the enzyme, to a more open configuration [74].

More recently, a different set of Mn^{II} binding site mutations, Asp179Ala, Glu35Asp, and Glu39Asp, was constructed and expressed as apoenzyme in $E.$ $coli$ and reconstituted with heme [68]. However, no detailed spectroscopic analysis of these mutants has been published. The binding and reactivity toward ferrocyanide and small phenols are not altered by mutations of the Mn binding ligands [68], confirming previous results [22,124]. Steady-state kinetic analyses of Asp179Ala and Glu35Asp show decreases in k_{cat} and increases in K_m, and approximately 10^4-fold decreases in catalytic efficiency (k_{cat}/K_m) for Mn^{II} when compared to unaltered rMnP [68], similar to results with the Mn binding mutants described above [22]. Transient-state kinetics reveal that Compound I reduction by Mn^{II} is reduced 63- and 220-fold for Glu35Asp and Asp179Ala, respectively. Compound II reduction by Mn^{II} shows first-order kinetics with K_D values 42- and 240-fold higher for Glu35Asp and Asp179Ala, respectively, and the first-order rate constants decreased about 110-fold compared to unaltered rMnP [68]. In contrast, the kinetic analysis of Glu39Asp suggested that this mutation has little effect on the catalytic properties of the rMnP [68]. The researchers concluded [68], that Glu39 is not a ligand to the Mn. However, Glu39 is a ligand in the crystal structure [26] and is conserved in all *mnp* genes examined to date [77–81]. Furthermore, the Glu39Asp mutation [68] does not change the functional carboxylate moiety of the ligand. Studies of mutations such as Glu39Gln [22,74] and Glu39Ala [75], which eliminate the functional carboxylate, clearly demonstrate that Glu39 is a ligand.

Arg177 is believed to form a salt bridge with the Mn binding ligand, Glu35 (Fig. 6). Steady-state kinetic analysis of two Arg177 mutants, Arg177Lys and Arg177Ala [67], show increases in the K_m for Mn^{II}, confirming involvement of this residue in Mn binding. No decrease in k_{cat} is observed in these mutants. Transient-state kinetic analysis indicates a decrease in the second-order rate constant for the reduction of Compound I in these variants. The reduction of Compound II shows an increase in the K_D for Mn^{II}, indicating a decrease in the binding affinity for Mn^{II}. No change in the first-order rate constant is observed, consistent with the steady-state data, suggesting that the electron transfer rate for the oxidation of Mn^{II} is not affected by the mutations [67]. These results suggest that Mn^{II} oxidation by MnP can be separated into two events: binding of Mn^{II}, which is facilitated by Arg177; and electron transfer from Mn^{II} to the enzyme, where Arg177 is apparently not directly involved [67].

7.3.   Site-Directed Mutations of the Proximal Residue, Phe190

Phe190 is located on the proximal side of the heme cavity in MnP (Fig. 5) and is equivalent to Trp191 in yeast CcP [125]. In most plant and fungal peroxidases, Trp191 is replaced by either a Phe [26,100,103,104] or a Leu [96,97]. A series of homologously expressed site-directed mutants, Phe190Tyr, Phe190Leu, Phe190Ile, and Phe190Ala, were constructed to investigate the role of this amino acid residue in MnP [113]. The variant proteins exhibit spectral and steady-state characteristics similar to those of wtMnP for both Mn^{II} and peroxide [113], indicating that Phe190 is not directly involved in binding or reactivity with these substrates [113].

The stabilities of the native and oxidized states of the enzyme are affected in several of the Phe190 variant MnPs. Replacement of Phe190 with either Ile or Ala significantly enhances the rate of thermal denaturation of the protein [113]. Moreover, the rates of spontaneous reduction of the oxidized intermediates, MnP Compounds I and II, are dramatically increased for the Phe190Ala mutant [113]. At pH 9.0, the absorption spectra of the wt and Phe190 variant MnP proteins exhibit a ferric high- to low-spin transition which apparently involves direct coordination of the distal His residue to the heme iron to form a bis-His structure [113,114]. When this low-spin, bis-His form of the enzyme is reduced, it exhibits a UV-visible spectrum similar to that of cytochrome b_{558}, which contains a bis-His structure [114]. This transition is reversible, but only in the presence of calcium, suggesting that one or both of the two structural calciums are lost at high pH [114]. Thus, the presence of the calcium may help to maintain the pentacoordination of the heme iron by keeping the distal His apart from the heme iron. Loss of calcium may result in movement of His46 closer to the heme, allowing formation of a bis-His–iron complex. The pH at which this transition occurs is considerably lower for the Phe190Ala and Phe190Ile mutant proteins compared to the wtMnP [113,114]. These results suggest that Phe190 plays several important roles. First, it may act as a wall to protect the oxidized heme from spontaneous reduction by amino acid residues in the protein. Second, it appears to help dock and stabilize the heme in its binding cavity, providing thermal stability. Finally, Phe190 helps stabilize the pentacoordinate heme iron, possibly preventing the loss of calcium at neutral pH.

8.   REGULATION OF Mn PEROXIDASE GENE EXPRESSION

The regulation of *mnp* expression has been the subject of an extensive review [76]. In *P. chrysosporium*, MnP is expressed only under secondary metabolic conditions that are triggered by nutrient nitrogen depletion in culture [25,78]. However, in several other lignin-degrading fungi *mnp* gene expression occurs under high organic nitrogen conditions [7,39]. In *P. chrysosporium*, *mnp* gene transcription also is regulated by the levels of Mn in the medium. Addition of 180 µM Mn to nitrogen-depleted cells, grown in the absence of Mn, results in the rapid appearance of *mnp* mRNA [76,82,83]. *mnp* promoter/gene reporter studies have demonstrated that this regulation of *mnp* transcription by nitrogen and Mn is dependent on cis-acting sequences found in the promoter region of the *mnp* gene, within about 1 kb upstream of the translation start site [126]. This has been confirmed for the *mnp1* and *mnp2* genes of *P. chrysosporium* by reverse transcriptase–polymerase chain reaction, using specific primers [84].

MnP gene transcription is also regulated by heat shock and by peroxide concentrations in culture [127,128]. If nitrogen-depleted cultures, grown in the absence of Mn, are exposed to a 15-min heat shock at 45°C or to exogenous H_2O_2, the rapid appearance of the *mnp* mRNA is observed [127,128]. However, no MnP protein is expressed under these conditions [127,128]. The heat- shock regulation of *mnp* gene transcription correlates with the occurrence of putative heat shock elements in the promoters of the *P. chrysosporium mnp* genes [77,80,81].

ACKNOWLEDGMENTS

We thank our collaborators, T. Poulos and M. Sundaramoorthy, University of California, Irvine; T. M. Loehr and P. Moënne-Loccoz, Oregon Graduate Institute; and A. G. Mauk, University of British Columbia, for their excellent contributions. Research in M.H.G.'s laboratory on aspects of MnP biochemistry and molecular biology has been funded by National Science Foundation grants MCB-9723725 and MCB-9506338 and grant DE-FG03-96ER20235, U.S. Dept. of Energy, Division of Energy Biosciences.

ABBREVIATIONS

ABTS	2,2′-azinobis(3-ethylbenzthiazoline-6-sulfonic acid)
ArP	*Arthromyces ramosus* peroxidase
CcP	cytochrome *c* peroxidase
CiP	*Coprinus cinereus* peroxidase
DMP	2,6-dimethoxyphenol
EPR	electron paramagnetic resonance
GSH	reduced glutathione
HRP	horseradish peroxidase

LiP	lignin peroxidase
MnP	manganese peroxidase protein
mnp	manganese peroxidase gene
NADPH	nicotinamide adenine dinucleotide phosphate (reduced)
NMR	nuclear magnetic resonance
pI	negative logarithm of the isoelectric point
rMnP	recombinant MnP
wtMnP	wild-type MnP

REFERENCES

1. K. V. Sarkanen and C. H. Ludwig, *Lignins. Occurrence, Formation, Structure and Reactions*, Wiley-Interscience, New York, 1971.

2. K. Freudenberg, in *Constitution and Biosynthesis of Lignin* (A. C. Neish and K. Freudenberg, eds.), Springer-Verlag, New York, 1968, pp. 47–122.

3. K.-E. Eriksson, R. A. Blanchette and P. Ander, in *Microbial and Enzymatic Degradation of Wood and Wood Components*, Springer-Verlag KG, Berlin, 1990, pp. 225–333.

4. M. H. Gold, H. Wariishi, and K. Valli, *ACS Symp. Ser.*, *389*, 127–140 (1989).

5. T. K. Kirk and R. L. Farrell, *Annu. Rev. Microbiol.*, *41*, 465–505 (1987).

6. J. K. Glenn and M. H. Gold, *Appl. Environ. Microbiol.*, *45*, 1741–1747 (1983).

7. F. H. Périé and M. H. Gold, *Appl. Environ. Microbiol.*, *57*, 2240–2245 (1991).

8. G. F. Leatham, *Appl. Environ. Microbiol.*, *24*, 51–58 (1986).

9. R. A. Blanchette, *Phytopathology*, *74*, 725–730 (1984).

10. J. K. Glenn, M. A. Morgan, M. B. Mayfield, M. Kuwahara, and M. H. Gold, *Biochem. Biophys. Res. Commun.*, *114*, 1077–1083 (1983).

11. M. Tien and T. K. Kirk, *Science*, *221*, 661–663 (1983).

12. M. Kuwahara, J. K. Glenn, M. A. Morgan, and M. H. Gold, *FEBS Lett.*, *169*, 247–250 (1984).

13. K. E. Hammel, *Enzyme Microb. Technol.*, *11*, 776–777 (1989).

14. A. Hatakka, *FEMS Microbiol. Rev.*, *13*, 125–135 (1994).

15. A. B. Orth, D. J. Royse, and M. Tien, *Appl. Environ. Microbiol.*, *59*, 4017–4023 (1993).

16. L. Homolka, F. Nerud, O. Kofronová, E. Novotná, and V. Machurová, *Folia Microbiol.* (Praha), *39*, 37–43 (1994).

17. F. Pelaez, M. J. Martinez, and A. T. Martinez, *Mycol. Res.*, *99*, 37–42 (1995).

18. D.-M. Li, N. Li, M. B. Mayfield, and M. H. Gold, *Biochim. Biophys. Acta*, in press (1999).

19. J. K. Glenn and M. H. Gold, *Arch. Biochem. Biophys.*, *242*, 329–341 (1985).

20. A. Paszczyński, V. B. Huynh, and R. Crawford, *Arch. Biochem. Biophys.*, *244*, 750–765 (1986).

21. M. B. Mayfield, K. Kishi, M. Alic, and M. H. Gold, *Appl. Environ. Microbiol.*, *60*, 4303–4309 (1994).

22. K. Kishi, M. Kusters-van Someren, M. B. Mayfield, J. Sun, T. M. Loehr, and M. H. Gold, *Biochemistry*, *35*, 8986–8994 (1996).

23. M. S. A. Leisola, B. Kozulic, F. Meussdoerffer, and A. Fiechter, *J. Biol. Chem.*, *262*, 419–424 (1987).

24. E. A. Pease and M. Tien, *J. Bacteriol.*, *174*, 3532–3540 (1992).

25. D. Pribnow, M. B. Mayfield, V. J. Nipper, J. A. Brown, and M. H. Gold, *J. Biol. Chem.*, *264*, 5036–5040 (1989).

26. M. Sundaramoorthy, K. Kishi, M. H. Gold, and T. L. Poulos, *J. Biol. Chem.*, *269*, 32759–32767 (1994).

27. F. H. Périé, D. Sheng, and M. H. Gold, *Biochim. Biophys. Acta*, *1297*, 139–148 (1996).

28. S. Lobos, J. Larrain, L. Salas, D. Cullen, and R. Vicuna, *Microbiology*, *140*, 2691–2698 (1994).

29. I. T. Forrester, A. C. Grabski, C. Mishra, B. D. Kelley, W. N. Strickland, G. F. Leatham, and R. R. Burgess, *Appl. Microbiol. Biotechnol.*, *33*, 359–365 (1990).

30. H. Kofujita, T. Ohta, Y. Asada, and M. Kuwahara, *Mokuzai Gakkaishi*, *37*, 562–569 (1991).

31. T. Johansson, K. G. Welinder, and P. O. Nyman, *Arch. Biochem. Biophys.*, *300*, 57–62 (1993).

32. E. Karhunen, A. Kantelinen, and M.-L. Niku-Paavola, *Arch. Biochem. Biophys.*, *279*, 1, 25–31 (1990).

33. H. Kofujita, Y. Asada, and M. Kuwahara, *Mokuzai Gakkaishi*, *37*, 555–561 (1991).

34. S. Sarkar, A. T. Martinez, and M. J. Martinez, *Biochim. Biophys. Acta, 1339*, 23–30 (1997).

35. O. V. Maltseva, M.-L. Niku-Paavola, A. A. Leontievsky, N. M. Myasoedova, and L. A. Golovleva, *Biotechnol. Appl. Biochem.*, *13*, 291–302 (1991).

36. L. A. Golovleva, A. A. Leontievsky, O. V. Maltseva, and N. M. Mya-soedova, *J. Biotechnol.*, *30*, 71–77 (1993).

37. A. Heinfling, F. J. Ruiz-Duenas, M. J. Martinez, M. Bergbauer, U. Szewzyk, and A. T. Martinez, *FEBS Lett.*, *428*, 141–146 (1998).

38. T. Mester and J. A. Field, *J. Biol. Chem.*, *273*, 15412–15417 (1998).

39. M. J. Martinez, F. J. Ruiz Duenas, F. Guillen, and A. T. Martinez, *Eur. J. Biochem.*, *237*, 424–432 (1996).

40. J. K. Glenn, L. Akileswaran, and M. H. Gold, *Arch. Biochem. Biophys.*, *251*, 688–696 (1986).

41. H. Wariishi, K. Valli, and M. H. Gold, *J. Biol. Chem.*, *267*, 23688–23695 (1992).

42. H. Wariishi, L. Akileswaran, and M. H. Gold, *Biochemistry*, *27*, 5365–5370 (1988).

43. R. A. Blanchette, E. W. Krueger, J. E. Haight, M. Akhtar, and D. E. Akin, *J. Biotechnol.*, *53*, 203–213 (1997).

44. G. Daniel, B. Pettersson, T. Nilsson, and J. Volc, *Can. J. Bot.*, *68*, 920–933 (1990).

45. U. Tuor, H. Wariishi, H. E. Schoemaker, and M. H. Gold, *Biochemistry*, *31*, 4986–4995 (1992).

46. H. Wariishi, K. Valli, and M. H. Gold, *Biochemistry*, *28*, 6017–6023 (1989).

47. H. Wariishi, K. Valli, and M. H. Gold, *Biochem. Biophys. Res. Commun.*, *176*, 269–275 (1991).

48. H. Wariishi, K. Valli, V. Renganathan, and M. H. Gold, *J. Biol. Chem.*, *264*, 14185–14191 (1989).

49. I. T. Forrester, A. C. Grabski, R. R. Burgess, and G. F. Leatham, *Biochem. Biophys. Res. Commun.*, *157*, 992–999 (1988).

50. W. Bao, Y. Fukushima, K. A. Jensen, Jr., M. A. Moen, and K. E. Hammel, *FEBS Lett.*, *354*, 297–300 (1994).

51. I. C. Kuan and M. Tien, *Arch. Biochem. Biophys.*, *302*, 447–454 (1993).

52. I. C. Kuan and M. Tien, *Proc. Natl. Acad. Sci. USA*, *90*, 1242–1246 (1993).

53. U. Urzua, P. J. Kersten, and R. Vicuna, *Arch. Biochem. Biophys.*, *360*, 215–222 (1998).

54. M. Hofrichter, D. Ziegenhagen, T. Vares, M. Friedich, M. G. Jager, W. Fritsche, and A. Hatakka, *FEBS Lett.*, *434*, 362–366 (1998).

55. M. H. Gold (unpublished observations).

56. V. Renganathan, K. Miki, and M. H. Gold, *Biochemistry*, *26*, 5127–5132 (1987).

57. D. Sheng and M. H. Gold, *Arch. Biochem. Biophys.*, *345*, 126–134 (1997).

58. W. E. Blumberg, J. Peisach, B. A. Wittenberg, and J. B. Wittenberg, *J. Biol. Chem.*, *243*, 1854–1862 (1968).

59. M. Tamura, T. Asakura, and T. Yonetani, *Biochim. Biophys. Acta*, *268*, 292–304 (1972).

60. H. B. Dunford and J. S. Stillman, *Coord. Chem. Rev.*, *19*, 187–251 (1976).

61. V. Renganathan and M. H. Gold, *Biochemistry*, *25*, 1626–1631 (1986).

62. Y. Mino, H. Wariishi, N. J. Blackburn, T. M. Loehr, and M. H. Gold, *J. Biol. Chem.*, *263*, 7029–7036 (1988).

63. L. Banci, I. Bertini, E. A. Pease, M. Tien, and P. Turano, *Biochemistry*, *31*, 10009–10017 (1992).

64. L. Banci, I. Bertini, I. C. Kuan, M. Tien, P. Turano, and A. J. Vila, *Biochemistry*, *32*, 13483–13489 (1993).

65. H. Wariishi, H. B. Dunford, I. D. MacDonald, and M. H. Gold, *J. Biol. Chem.*, *264*, 3335–3340 (1989).

66. I. C. Kuan, K. A. Johnson, and M. Tien, *J. Biol. Chem.*, *268*, 20064–20070 (1993).

67. M. D. Sollewijn Gelpke, P. Moënne-Loccoz, and M. H. Gold, *Biochemistry*, *38*, 11481–11489 (1999).

68. R. E. Whitwam, K. R. Brown, M. Musick, M. J. Natan, and M. Tien, *Biochemistry*, *36*, 9766–9773 (1997).

69. K. Kishi, H. Wariishi, L. Marquez, H. B. Dunford, and M. H. Gold, *Biochemistry*, *33*, 8694–8701 (1994).

70. D. P. Barr, M. M. Shah, T. A. Grover, and S. D. Aust, *Arch. Biochem. Biophys.*, *298*, 480–485 (1992).

71. M. V. Dutton, C. S. Evans, P. T. Atkey, and D. A. Wood, *Appl. Microbiol. Biotechnol.*, *39*, 5–10 (1992).

72. L. Banci, I. Bertini, L. Dal Pozzo, R. Del Conte, and M. Tien, *Biochemistry*, *37*, 9009–9015 (1998).

73. M. Sundaramoorthy, H. L. Youngs, M. H. Gold, and T. Poulos (in preparation).

74. M. Sundaramoorthy, K. Kishi, M. H. Gold, and T. L. Poulos, *J. Biol. Chem.*, *272*, 17574–17580 (1997).

75. H. L. Youngs, M. D. Sollewijn-Gelpke, M. Sundaramoorthy, and M. H. Gold (in preparation).

76. M. H. Gold and M. Alic, *Microbiol. Rev.*, *57*, 605–622 (1993).

77. M. B. Mayfield, B. J. Godfrey, and M. H. Gold, *Gene*, *142*, 231–235 (1994).

78. E. A. Pease, A. Andrawis, and M. Tien, *J. Biol. Chem.*, *264*, 13531–13535 (1989).

79. A. B. Orth, M. Rzhetskaya, D. Cullen, and M. Tien, *Gene*, *148*, 161–165 (1994).

80. B. J. Godfrey, M. B. Mayfield, J. A. Brown, and M. H. Gold, *Gene*, *93*, 119–124 (1990).

81. M. Alic, L. Akileswaran, and M. H. Gold, *Biochim. Biophys. Acta*, *1338*, 1–7 (1997).

82. J. A. Brown, J. K. Glenn, and M. H. Gold, *J. Bacteriol.*, *172*, 3125–3130 (1990).

83. J. A. Brown, M. Alic, and M. H. Gold, *J. Bacteriol.*, *173*, 4101–4106 (1991).

84. J. M. Gettemy, B. Ma, M. Alic, and M. H. Gold, *Appl. Environ. Microbiol.*, *64*, 569–574 (1998).

85. S. Lobos, L. Larrondo, L. Salas, E. Karahanian, and R. Vicuna, *Gene*, *206*, 185–193 (1998).

86. G. R. Corsini, S. Lobos, and R. Vicuna, Genbank Accession No. AF036254.

87. T. G. Ritch, Jr. and M. H. Gold, *Gene*, *118*, 73–80 (1992).

88. W. A. Doyle, W. Blodig, N. C. Veitch, K. Piontek, and A. T. Smith, *Biochemistry*, *37*, 15097–15105 (1998).

89. Y. Asada, A. Watanabe, T. Irie, T. Nakayama, and M. Kuwahara, *Biochim. Biophys. Acta*, *1251*, 205–209 (1995).

90. T. Irie, Y. Honda, Y. Matsuyama, T. Watanabe, and M. Kuwahara, GenBank Accession No. AB016519,

91. F. J. Ruiz-Duenas, M. J. Martinez, and A. T. Martinez, *Mol. Microbiol.*, *31*, 223–235 (1999).

92. Y. Kawai, J. Sugiura, and Y. Kita, GenBank Accession No. E12284.

93. L. Jonsson, H. G. Becker, and P. O. Nyman, *Biochim. Biophys. Acta*, *1207*, 255–259 (1994).

94. T. Johansson and P. O. Nyman, *Gene*, *170*, 31–38 (1996).

95. T. G. Ritch, Jr., V. J. Nipper, L. Akileswaran, A. J. Smith, D. G. Pribnow, and M. H. Gold, *Gene*, *107*, 119–126 (1991).

96. N. Kunishima, K. Fukuyama, H. Matsubara, H. Hatanaka, Y. Shibano, and T. Amachi, *J. Mol. Biol.*, *235*, 331–344 (1994).

97. J. F. Petersen, J. W. Tams, J. Vind, A. Svensson, H. Dalboge, K. G. Welinder, and S. Larsen, *J. Mol. Biol.*, *232*, 989–991 (1993).

98. D. J. Schuller, N. Ban, R. B. Huystee, A. McPherson, and T. L. Poulos, *Structure*, *4*, 311–321 (1996).

99. S. L. Edwards, R. Raag, H. Wariishi, M. H. Gold, and T. L. Poulos, *Proc. Natl. Acad. Sci. USA*, *90*, 750–754 (1993).

100. T. L. Poulos, S. L. Edwards, H. Wariishi, and M. H. Gold, *J. Biol. Chem.*, *268*, 4429–4440 (1993).

101. G. Sutherland, L. Zapanta, M. Tien, and S. Aust, *Biochemistry*, *36*, 3654–3662 (1997).

102. G. R. Sutherland and S. D. Aust, *Arch. Biochem. Biophys.*, *332*, 128–134 (1996).

103. K. G. Welinder, *Curr. Opin. Struct. Biol.*, *2*, 388–393 (1992).

104. K. Piontek, T. Glumoff, and K. Winterhalter, *FEBS Lett.*, *315*, 119–124 (1993).

105. P. Limongi, M. Kjalke, J. Vind, J. W. Tams, T. Johansson, and K. G. Welinder, *Eur. J. Biochem.*, *227*, 270–276 (1995).

106. T. L. Poulos and B. C. Finzel, in *Peptide and Protein Reviews*, Vol. 4, Marcel Dekker, New York, 1984, pp. 115–171.

107. B. D. Howes, J. N. Rodriguez-Lopez, A. T. Smith, and G. Smulevich, *Biochemistry*, *36*, 1532–1543 (1997).

108. T. L. Poulos and J. Kraut, *J. Biol. Chem.*, *255*, 8199–8205 (1980).

109. F. Neri, C. Indiani, K. G. Welinder, and G. Smulevich, *Eur. J. Biochem.*, *251*, 830–838 (1998).

110. K. G. Welinder, in *Biochemical, Molecular and Physiological Aspects of Plant Peroxidases* (J. Lobarzewski, H. Greppin, C. Penel, and T. Gaspar, eds.), University of Geneva, Geneva, 1991, pp. 3–14.

111. A. T. Smith, S. A. Sanders, R. N. Thorneley, J. F. Burke, and R. R. Bray, *Eur. J. Biochem.*, *207*, 507–519 (1992).

112. M. Gajhede, D. J. Schuller, A. Henriksen, A. T. Smith, and T. L. Poulos, *Nature Struct. Biol.*, *4*, 1032–1038 (1997).

113. K. Kishi, D. P. Hildebrand, M. Kusters-van Someren, J. Gettemy, A. G. Mauk, and M. H. Gold, *Biochemistry*, *36*, 4268–4277 (1997).

114. P. Moenne-Loccoz, H. L. Youngs, and M. H. Gold (in preparation).

115. R. Z. Harris, H. Wariishi, M. H. Gold, and P. R. Ortiz de Montellano, *J. Biol. Chem.*, *266*, 8751–8758 (1991).

116. F. Johnson, G. H. Loew, and P. Du, *Proteins*, *20*, 312–319 (1994).

117. G. D. DePillis, H. Wariishi, M. H. Gold, and P. R. Ortiz de Montellano, *Arch. Biochem. Biophys.*, *280*, 217–223 (1990).

118. L. Banci, I. Bertini, T. Bini, M. Tien, and P. Turano, *Biochemistry*, *32*, 5825–5831 (1993).

119. M. R. Mauk, K. Kishi, M. H. Gold, and A. G. Mauk, *Biochemistry*, *37*, 6767–6771 (1998).

120. H. Demmer, I. Hinz, H. Keller-Rudex, K. Koeber, H. Kottelwesch, and D. Schneider, in *Coordination Compounds of Manganese*, Vol. 56, (E. Schleitzer-Rust, ed.), 8th ed., Springer-Verlag, New York, 1980, pp. 1–185.

121. F. A. Cotton and G. Wilkinson, *Advanced Inorganic Chemistry: A Comprehensive Text*, 4th ed., Wiley Interscience, New York, 1980, p. 14.

122. R. Whitwam and M. Tien, *Arch. Biochem. Biophys.*, *333*, 439–446 (1996).

123. P. Stewart, R. E. Whitwam, P. J. Kersten, D. Cullen, and M. Tien, *Appl. Environ. Microbiol.*, *62*, 860–864 (1996).

124. M. Kusters-van Someren, K. Kishi, T. Lundell, and M. H. Gold, *Biochemistry*, *34*, 10620–10627 (1995).

125. J. M. Mauro, L. A. Fishel, J. T. Hazzard, T. E. Meyer, G. Tollin, M. A. Cusanovich, and J. Kraut, *Biochemistry*, *27*, 6243–6256 (1988).

126. B. J. Godfrey, L. Akileswaran, and M. H. Gold, *Appl. Environ. Microbiol.*, *60*, 1353–1358 (1994).

127. J. A. Brown, D. Li, M. Alic, and M. H. Gold, *Appl. Environ. Microbiol.*, *59*, 4295–4299 (1993).

128. D. Li, M. Alic, J. A. Brown, and M. H. Gold, *Appl. Environ. Microbiol.*, *61*, 341–345 (1995).

18

Manganese Superoxide Dismutase

James W. Whittaker

Department of Biochemistry and Molecular Biology,
Oregon Graduate Institute of Science and Technology,
Beaverton, OR 97006-8921, USA

1. INTRODUCTION

1.1. Role of Manganese in Biological Antioxidant Defense

Among the biologically important transition ions (V, Mn, Fe, Co, Ni, Cu, Mo, and W), manganese plays a special role in the redox buffering of living cells, a result of the unique stability of the reduced Mn(II) ion in the cellular environment. In aqueous solution, manganous ion resists oxidation beyond 1 V ($E^0_{Mn(II)/Mn(III)}$ = +1.51 V vs. NHE), leaving the reduced ion available to meet extreme oxidative challenges that arise as a consequence of aerobic lifestyles. This redox buffering action is expressed by manganese ions both as inorganic complexes and in enzyme active sites [1], including manganese superoxide dismutase (MnSOD) [2] and manganese catalase [3]. Some aerotolerant fermentative organisms, including certain lactobacilli, appear to accumulate mineralized Mn(II) phosphate intracellularly [4,5] and thereby avoid the need to genetically template an antioxidant defense protein. However, many organisms have evolved specialized enzyme systems that allow the cell to mount an effective defense against the oxidative challenges. Superoxide dismutase [6–9], one of the most important of these antioxidant enzymes, serves as the front line molecular defense against superoxide, $O_2^{-\bullet}$, a reactive free radical oxygen metabolite that is thought to be responsible (directly or indirectly) for the oxidative damage to living cells underlying aging, cancer, and neurodegenerative disease [10].

1.2. Superoxide and Oxidative Stress

Superoxide is formed in a variety of processes through reaction of molecular oxygen (O_2) with reductants such as organic free radicals (1a) or reduced metal ions (1b):

$$O_2 + R\bullet \rightarrow O_2^{-\bullet} + R \tag{1a}$$

$$O_2 + M^{n+} \rightarrow O_2^{-\bullet} + M^{(n+1)+} \tag{1b}$$

The respiratory chain of aerobic organisms is particularly susceptible to these reactions, since reduced electron transfer cofactors (quinones, flavins, iron-sulfur clusters, and cytochromes) lie exposed to dioxygen in these redox systems. In mitochondria, the cytochrome bc_1 complex has been identified as the primary source of superoxide formation [11], a leak that allows approximately 5% of electrons in the respiratory chain to be diverted to one-electron reduction of O_2 [12].

The toxic effects of reactive oxygen species, including superoxide, are a consequence of reactions with cellular components as shown in Fig. 1. Superoxide can damage iron-sulfur clusters in enzymes and electron transfer proteins [13], releasing iron that may contribute to formation of additional superoxide via equation (1b), or react with hydrogen peroxide (H_2O_2) via Fenton chemistry [14]:

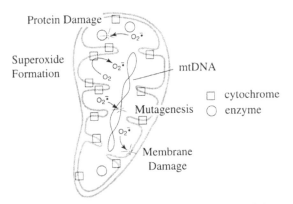

FIG. 1. Schematic of superoxide reactions in the mitochondrial matrix. Superoxide formed by autooxidation of respiratory chain cofactors is implicated in oxidative damage to proteins, membranes, and mitochondrial DNA.

$$Fe(II) + H_2O_2 \rightarrow Fe(III) + HO^{\bullet} + H_2O \tag{2}$$

The hydroxyl radical ($HO^{\bullet}$) produced in this process is an exceptionally aggressive oxidant capable of inserting indiscriminantly into any covalent bond in proteins, membrane lipids, or DNA, effectively burning the cell from within. Enzymes inactivated by damage from superoxide or its reactive byproducts block biosynthetic pathways and homeostatic control circuits, bringing metabolism to a grinding halt. Peroxidation of membrane lipids by oxidative reactions interferes with membrane permeability and the stability of the lipid bilayer, further compromising the essential structure of the living cell. Oxidative damage to DNA has particularly pervasive effects, threatening the viability and fate of the genome itself [15]. Extranuclear organelle genomes (like mitochondrial DNA, mtDNA) are vulnerable to oxidative damage. Mutagenesis of mtDNA can profoundly alter the function of mitochondria, producing disease states that are the focus of an emerging new field of mitochondrial medicine [12].

The superoxide radical is fundamentally unstable, as illustrated in Fig. 2, a volt-equivalent or Frost diagram for dioxygen species where relative stability (in units of volts) is plotted vs. the average oxidation number, the element oxidation number being taken as 0. The observation that both O_2 and H_2O_2 lie below superoxide on this plot implies that the oxy radical can react with itself, spontaneously disproportionating

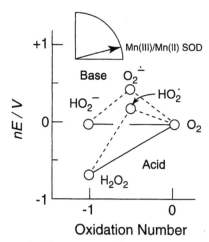

FIG. 2.   Frost diagram for dioxygen species.

(dismutating) into the more stable products, hydrogen peroxide and dioxygen:

$$2O_2^{-\bullet} + 2H^+ \rightarrow H_2O_2 + O_2 \tag{3}$$

Although superoxide is thermodynamically unstable, at physiological pH the radical is fairly long-lived because of unfavorable disproportionation kinetics. At low pH, superoxide anion radical is protonated and the neutral hydroperoxyl radical ($HO_2^{\bullet}$, pK_a = 4.9) disproportionates with a bimolecular rate constant that approaches the diffusion limit, obviating any need for dismutation catalysis. However, at neutral pH, electrostatic repulsion between superoxide anions dramatically lowers the reaction rate, and superoxide dismutases have evolved to function under these conditions to remove toxic oxygen radicals. Because oxygen radicals equilibrate efficiently with a variety of other radical species [Eqs. (1) and (2)], superoxide dismutation can also contribute to cellular defense against other radical processes. Free radical storms initiated by ionizing radiation or oxidative challenges can ravage cells, propagating as free radical chain reactions that knock out essential metabolic pathways and leave the cell dying. SOD can intercept the superoxide radicals formed in connection with these reactions and efficiently terminate the radical chain process.

In order to serve as a superoxide dismutase, a redox catalyst must have an electrochemical potential (E^0) lying between the potentials for $O_2^{-\bullet}/O_2$ and $O_2^{-\bullet}/H_2O_2$ redox couples, allowing it to perform each reaction efficiently. The slope of a line segment connecting two species in Fig. 2 is proportional to the standard potential for the corresponding redox couple, and the observation that the slope of the redox vector for the Mn(II)/Mn(III) couple in MnSOD (E^0 = +0.31 V vs. NHE) [16] (Fig. 2, *insert*) lies midway between the slopes for superoxide reactions indicates that this metal center is well suited to an antioxidant function catalyzing superoxide dismutation chemistry.

2. MANGANESE SUPEROXIDE DISMUTASE

2.1. Phylogenetic Distribution

Superoxide dismutases are ubiquitous metalloenzymes found in virtually all aerobic organisms from bacteria to humans and, more surprisingly, have also been detected in strict anaerobes [17]. However, not all organisms contain the manganese-cofactored dismutase [2]. Other forms of superoxide dismutase are known to contain Fe [18], binuclear Cu/Zn [19]/[20], or even Ni [20] active sites. Based on sequence analysis the Fe and Mn enzymes form a distinct family and the diversity of superoxide dismutases appears to be an example of convergent evolution to this antioxidant defense function [21,22]. While a small fraction of (Mn,Fe)SODs are able to function with either metal [23,24], most are specialized to function with only one or the other of these two metal ions. Phylogenetic arguments suggest that the FeSOD branch of the family may be evolutionarily older, with the Mn enzyme branch emerging relatively recently. Manganese superoxide dismutases have been isolated from thermophilic eubacteria (e.g., *Thermus thermophilus*) [25] and are common constituents of mesophilic bacteria and higher eukaryotes.

2.2. Subcellular Localization

When several distinct superoxide dismutase isozymes (Mn, Fe, Cu/Zn or Ni) are present in a single cell (whether prokaryotic or eukaryotic), each form appears to be targeted to a specific subcelluar site. For example, in *E. coli*, a Cu/Zn enzyme is translocated to the periplasmic space [19], while Fe and Mn forms occur cytoplasmically in that organism [26,27]. Within the cytoplasmic compartment, the latter two enzymes appear to have distinct distributions. Immunohistochemical studies indicate that FeSOD is associated with the bounding membranes while the MnSOD is more uniformly distributed throughout the cytoplasm [28].

For eukaryotes, the situation is distinct but equally predictable. Within the compartments (nuclear, mitochondrial, peroxisomal, etc.) of the highly partitioned eukaryotic cell, the MnSOD appears to be exclusively associated with mitochondria, while the cytoplasmic/peroxisomal SOD is in the Cu/Zn form [29,30]. The mitochondrial enzyme is encoded by a nuclear gene and must be transported across two mitochondrial membranes to the matrix space where it functions. This process involves translation of a proenzyme that in the case of the human MnSOD includes a 24-amino-acid N-terminal leader peptide targeting the protein to the mitochondrion. The delivery of the enzyme to the mitochondrial matrix is essential for organelle function, and defects in MnSOD or its expression have been linked to certain cancers. Other evidence for the importance of this enzyme comes from genetically engineered organisms: homozygous knockout mice lacking a functional MnSOD gene die shortly after birth and exhibit a number of severe neurological abnormalities [31,32].

2.3. Kinetics and Mechanism

The elementary mechanism of MnSOD catalysis has emerged from elegant kinetic studies [33] that have led to the overall reaction scheme shown in Fig. 3. The enzymatic reaction replaces the bimolecular reaction (3) with a catalytic cycle involving two distinct half-reactions, an oxidative reaction (4) in which the substrate, superoxide, is oxidized to dioxygen and a reductive half-reaction (5) in which superoxide is converted to hydrogen peroxide:

$$O_2^{-\bullet} + Mn(III)SOD \rightarrow O_2 + Mn(II)SOD \tag{4}$$

$$O_2^{-\bullet} + 2H^+ + Mn(II)SOD \rightarrow H_2O_2 + Mn(III)SOD \tag{5}$$

These two reactions differ in the oxidation state of the metal ion and the involvement of protons in the reductive half-reaction. The bimolecular rate constants for reaction of oxidized (4) and reduced (5) *T. thermophilus* MnSOD with superoxide, measured by pulse radiolysis, are near the diffusion limit $(2.0 \times 10^9 \, M^{-1} s^{-1}, 2.2 \times 10^9 \, M^{-1} s^{-1})$ [33], making MnSOD among the fastest of all enzymes, consistent with the simplicity of the catalyzed reaction, which is essentially electron transfer

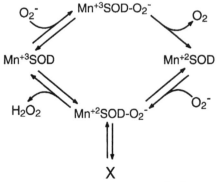

FIG. 3.   Kinetic scheme for manganese superoxide dismutase catalysis.

between a protein-bound metal ion and a diatomic redox partner. Under the conditions of stopped-flow kinetic measurements, a dead-end peroxide complex forms (X, Fig. 3) that effectively inactivates approximately 95% of the enzyme in the steady state. This peroxide complex appears to be an isomer of the peroxy intermediate formed during turnover, and conversion to the dead-end complex exhibits a solvent isotope effect less than unity, suggesting that proton transfer to the productive peroxyanion complex prevents formation of the dead-end complex. The close balance between oxidative and reductive rates is expected to be important for efficient cycling of the enzyme during turnover. Recent kinetic studies have demonstrated similar behavior for the recombinant human MnSOD [34].

3.   MOLECULAR STRUCTURES

3.1.   Overview of the Structures

Crystal structures have now been solved at high resolution for MnSODs isolated from *T. thermophilus* (PDB ID code 1MNG) [35], *E. coli* (PDB ID code 1VEW) [36], and for the recombinant human mitochondrial enzyme (PDB ID code 1ABM) [37–40]. These enzymes share a high degree of structural homology, but differ in quaternary organization, the *E. coli* enzyme being a homodimer, while both human and *T. thermophilus* MnSODs are homotetramers (more precisely, dimers of dimers). In each case, the subunits are composed of two domains, an all-α N-terminal domain and an α/β C-terminal domain (Fig. 4). The overall similarity to the homologous FeSOD structures is remarkable [41,42], and a subunit superposition between MnSOD and FeSOD from *E. coli* yields an rms difference of only 0.6 Å over 388 main chain atoms [36].

This structural homology is mirrored in significant sequence similarities within the family of Mn/Fe superoxide dismutases [43–45] (e.g., 45% sequence identity between the Fe and Mn enzymes from *E. coli*) [36], indicating that the differences between these enzymes are the result of divergent evolution from a common ancestor. Sequence alignments between Fe and Mn enzymes have been used to identify residues that appear to be conserved within a subfamily but differ between Fe

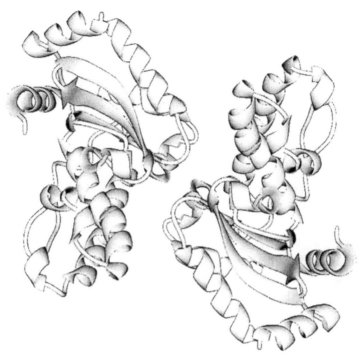

FIG. 4.   Structural elements of the dimeric *E. coli* manganese superoxide dismutase.

and Mn proteins and thus may relate to metal specificity [43,44], and work is in progress in a number of laboratories targeting these residues for protein engineering experiments attempting to interconvert Mn and Fe enzymes. In addition, there are a number of residues that appear to be strictly conserved over both subfamilies that are expected to represent groups essential for catalytic function [45]. Four of these (H26, H81, D167, and D171 in *E. coli* MnSOD sequence numbering) are metal ligands, two more (H30 and Y34) form the gateway to the active site (Fig. 5), and another (E170) lies in the outer sphere of the metal binding site. The latter residue is part of a pattern that is highly conserved over all Fe/Mn SOD protein sequences ($D_{167}XWE_{170}H_{171}XXY_{174}$) including two metal ligands (D167 and H171) that form a DX_3H metal-binding motif, and two residues (E170, Y174) that span the dimer interface, bridging between active sites in opposite halves of the dimer (Fig. 6). Thus, the

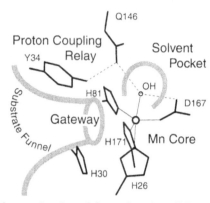

FIG. 5.   Functional organization of the active site of Mn superoxide dismutase.

glutamate residue lying in the outer sphere of the Mn complex in one subunit arises from the polypeptide chain of the other subunit [36]. As a result of the twofold symmetry of the dimeric protein, corresponding glutamates in the two subunits form a double bridge between the active sites whose role has been investigated by mutagenesis (see below).

The dimeric protein has a somewhat irregular form that leaves a hemicylindrical groove between the subunits as a conserved feature of MnSOD structure [36]. The diameter of the cleft, approximately 22 Å, is close to the diameter of B-form DNA, suggesting that this feature may be involved in the nonspecific association with DNA that has been ob-

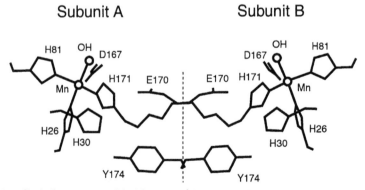

FIG. 6.   Strictly conserved bridges crossing the subunit interface connect active sites in the MnSOD dimer.

served for *E. coli* MnSOD [28]. Potato mitochondrial MnSOD, which was originally isolated as an RNA-binding protein and only identified as superoxide dismutase following N-terminal sequence analysis, also appears to bind nucleic acids [46]. The intersubunit cleft is lined with polar residues and bears a slight net positive charge, but lacks features characteristic of sequence-specific DNA-binding proteins, and more closely resembles the clamp structures associated with nonspecific DNA interactions. Molecular dynamics modeling allows B-form DNA to be docked within the cleft with only minor rearrangement of amino acid side chains [36] (Fig. 7). In FeSOD, the corresponding cleft region contains protruding loops preventing this type of interaction, and there is no evidence for FeSOD–DNA interactions [36,47]. These considerations suggest a unique role for MnSOD in protecting DNA from reactive oxygen species.

3.2. Focus on the Active Sites

The active site metal complex in MnSOD is formed from four protein side chains (three histidine imidazoles in $N\pi$ coordination and a monodentate aspartic carboxylate) and a molecule of coordinated solvent (water or hydroxide, depending on metal oxidation state) for overall five-coordination at the metal center (Fig. 5). The ligands forms a nearly perfect trigonal bipyramidal coordination polyhedron for the bound metal ion, with the carboxylate and two imidazoles comprising the equatorial ligand set and the remaining imidazole and solvent aligned axially. The complex has approximate C_S site symmetry with the mirror plane bisecting the equatorial pair of histidines. In the outer sphere of the complex, the E170 glutamate residue (Fig. 6) is hydrogen-bonded to the noncoordinating $N\tau$ nitrogen of the H171 ligand and contributes to charge compensation for the buried metal ion, effectively neutralizing the single unit of residual charge unbalanced by anionic ligands in the inner sphere [36,48–50].

The only nonprotein ligand for the active site Mn ion is the coordinated solvent, which, unlike solvent associated with other catalytic metalloenzyme complexes, is not the substrate binding site. X-ray crystallography shows that this solvent is buried inside the protein, sequestered from bulk water in a discrete binding pocket (Fig. 5), and is

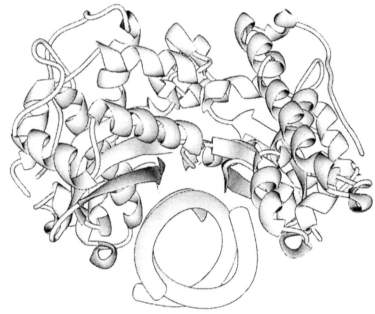

FIG. 7.   Molecular dynamics adapted structure of *E. coli* Mn superoxide dismutase DNA complex.

hydrogen-bonded to the noncoordinated oxygen of the carboxylate ligand, forming a six-atom ring including the metal ion. Other important outer sphere interactions radiate from the solvent pocket, including a conserved interaction with a glutamine residue (Q146 in *E. coli* MnSOD) which arises from a different region of the polypeptide chain in Mn and Fe proteins. This hydrogen bonding interaction extends to a conserved tyrosine (Y34) which, together with a histidine residue (H30), forms the gateway to the active site metal complex (see Fig. 5). The hydrogen bonding chain Y34-Q146-OH has been identified as a relay pathway for proton transfer in and out of the solvent pocket [50]. The gateway formed by Y34 and H30 controls the coordination chemistry of the metal complex. These residues lie at the base of a substrate funnel that extends out to the surface of the globular protein that restricts access to the active site to small molecules.

The structure of the thermophilic *Thermus thermophilus* MnSOD, the first MnSOD structure to be solved [35], is virtually identical in many respects to the mesophilic *E. coli* enzyme, and the active sites of both prokaryotic enzymes can be aligned with the human enzyme to give atomic superposition extending into the outer sphere of the metal complexes. The structure of the azide complex of the *Thermus* enzyme has also been solved [35], providing a model for anion interactions with the active site. In this complex, the azide binds directly to the Mn ion, expanding the inner sphere and increasing the coordination number to six. The complex adopts a roughly octahedral geometry, with the angle between the equatorial histidine rings opening from 131° to 148° and the Mn-O(carboxylate) distance stretching from 1.8 Å to 2.25 Å.

3.3. Mechanistic Implications of Structural Studies

The combination of X-ray crystallographic studies with sequence correlations over all known Mn and Fe superoxide dismutases allows certain elements of the enzyme structures to be recognized as key features essential for biological function. These conserved structural features include the inner sphere ligand set (including the sequestered solvent and the carboxylate opposite to the gateway) and the hydrogen bonding pathways from the active site out through the gateway. Based on the crystallographic evidence for an increase in coordination number in the *Thermus* MnSOD azide complex, an expansion of the coordination sphere has been incorporated into a "5-6-5" mechanism for SOD [42] involving alternate formation of five-coordinate ligand-free and six-coordinate ligand-bound complexes during turnover.

4. LIGAND INTERACTIONS

4.1. Coordination Chemistry

Spectroscopic studies on MnSOD provide additional information on ligand interactions [51,52] directly probing the electronic structure of the active site metal complex. The optical absorption spectrum of the oxidized enzyme arises from the four spin-allowed ligand field ($d \rightarrow d$) excitations of the d^4 Mn(III) metal ion. Titration of the Mn(III) form of the enzyme with small anions (azide, fluoride) results in characteristic changes in the absorption spectra reflecting changes in coordination number or geometry of the metal complex [51]. A change in coordination number is ruled out by the similarity of ligand field spectra for *E. coli* MnSOD native and anion complexes at ambient temperatures.

These spectra demand five coordination for both forms, which implies displacement of one of the endogenous ligands on anion binding [52]. Low-temperature magnetic circular dichroism (MCD) spectroscopy provides higher resolution information on the ground state electronic structure complementing the information available from optical absorption experiments. MCD spectra for the ligand-free enzyme are characteristic of a high-spin ($S = 2$) Mn(III) ion in a rhombically distorted trigonal environment. Anion binding perturbs this complex and low-temperature MCD spectra indicate a tetragonal Mn(III) site in both azide and fluoride adducts [52]. Thus, an apparent discrepancy has arisen between spectroscopic and crystallographic characterization of these complexes, the ambient temperature spectra requiring a five-coordinate azide complex for *E. coli* MnSOD [52], while X-ray crystallography defines a six-coordinate Mn(III) in the corresponding azide complex of *T. thermophilus* MnSOD [35].

4.2. Temperature-Dependent Structures

A more detailed investigation of the temperature dependence of the optical spectra of *E. coli* MnSOD complexes has resolved this apparent discrepancy and revealed an unexpected subtlety in the behavior of the protein [53,54]. While spectra of the ligand-free enzyme are essentially the same at ambient and cryogenic temperatures, the spectra of anion adducts (including the azide adduct, Fig. 8) change dramatically as the temperature is lowered, converting from a spectrum characteristic of a five-coordinate Mn(III) ion (all ligand field transitions > 15000 cm^{-1}) at ambient temperature to one characteristic of six-coordinate Mn(III) (with the lowest energy ligand field band near 10000 cm^{-1}) at cryogenic temperature (below 150 K). This structural transition between six- and five-coordinate complexes behaves like a simple two-state process with a midpoint for the conversion T_m = 220 K and has been analyzed in terms of thermochemical parameters (ΔH_{vH} = 4.97 kcal/mol, ΔS_{vH} = 22 cal/mol·K) in the range characteristic of ligand dissociation processes. The observation that this process approaches completion at the physiological temperature for *E. coli* MnSOD function suggests that this thermally activated transition in active site structure may relate to enzyme function. In particular, it emphasizes that structural patterns revealed by crystallography imply dynamic motifs in protein motion that

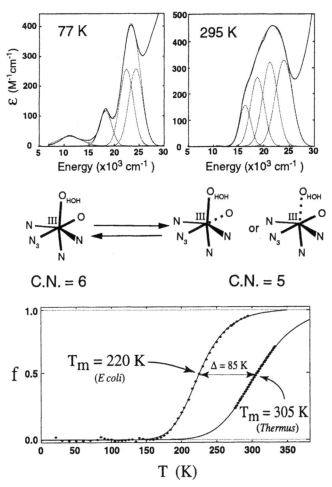

FIG. 8.   Temperature-dependent spectra for MnSOD azide complexes imply temperature-dependent structures. (top) Optical absorption spectra for Mn(III)SOD in 25 mM potassium phosphate buffer, pH 7, in 50% glycerol with 100 mM sodium azide at 77 K (left) and 295 K (right). (middle) Active site complexes stabilized at low temperature (left) and ambient temperature (right) differ in coordination number and geometry. (bottom) Thermal interconversion between low- and high-temperature active site azide complexes of *Escherichia coli* and *Thermus thermophilus* MnSOD illustrating a thermophilic shift in active site properties.

are tuned to a specific temperature range [54]. In MnSOD, these dynamical motifs may be important in (de)stabilizing certain exogenous ligand interactions in the path for catalysis, replacing the 5-6-5 mechanism with a 5-5-5 process.

Based on this hypothesis, one might predict that a thermophilic MnSOD will exhibit analogous behavior but over a higher temperature range. In fact, the corresponding transition for the *Thermus* MnSOD azide complex has been observed, and occurs at a higher temperature (T_m = 305 K), nearly 85 K above that found for the mesophilic *E. coli* MnSOD [55]. This represents a thermophilic shift in the anion interactions for the *Thermus* enzyme. The apparent discrepancy between the crystallographic and spectroscopic characterization of the MnSOD azide complex is thus resolved: an ambient temperature crystal structure for the *Thermus* MnSOD represents cryogenic conditions for that enzyme and only the six-coordinate azide complex is observed. On the other hand, the five-coordinate azide complex characterized by the ambient temperature spectra for *E. coli* MnSOD reflects an enzyme studied under more physiological conditions.

4.3. Role of Covalency in Redox Catalysis

Electronic structure calculations complement spectroscopic and crystallographic studies of the Mn active site and give a detailed analysis of metal–ligand interactions extending beyond the atomic level of resolution [48,56]. Density functional theory ab initio calculations of the ground state based on the crystallographic ligand coordinates results in a computed redox potential of −1.2 V [56] compared to an experimental value of +0.31 V [16]. The discrepancy may be a result of protein environmental effects or may be a consequence of errors in the crystallographic model. Metric features of protein–metal complexes are particularly susceptible to errors since they cannot be included in the refinement cycles that are applied to the organic portion of the protein because universal models for metal–ligand potentials do not exist. For redox-active metal ions, oxidation state heterogeneity may also contribute to structural averaging. The complexity of metal–ligand interactions requires that calculations must construct ligand potentials ab initio to solve for the energy-minimized ground state geometry [48].

Once an optimized geometry is reached, it is possible to solve for a reliable ground state electronic structure.

Geometry optimization on a model for the MnSOD active site leaves the essential trigonal bipyramidal coordination unchanged but results in a significant shortening in the Mn-OH bond distance, from the crystallographic value of 2.08 Å to 1.77 Å [48]. Adding one electron to the model and repeating the energy minimization procedure yields an optimized geometry for the reduced Mn(II)-OH complex in which this distance is stretched to 1.98 Å, increasing further (to 2.14 Å) on protonation of the solvent site. In these calculations, the bond distance to the axial imidazole also increases on reduction, from 2.07 Å to 2.28 Å. This behavior can be understood in terms of an orbital picture of the redox process. The LUMO for the Mn(III) active site model, represented in Fig. 9, is the redox orbital in the complex. This MO clearly has a large contribution from Mn d_{z^2} valence orbital as previously predicted from analysis of the low-temperature MCD spectra, but the coordinated solvent oxygen valence shell also makes a significant contribution, reflecting the covalency of ligand interactions in this complex. The Mn-O interactions are antibonding in character (indicated by the change in phase of the LUMO between Mn and O) accounting for the dramatic stretching along the Mn-O vector in the Mn(II) complex, when this orbital becomes occupied. These considerations show that the axial directions in MnSOD represent an important electron transfer coordinate. In particular, changes in oxidation state of the metal center are expected to affect the chemistry of the solvent site [48].

4.4. Role of the Bound Solvent in Proton Coupling

The sequestered solvent is known to play a special role in SOD catalysis [42]. Reduction of the metal center in FeSOD results in uptake of a proton, attributed to protonation of the coordinated solvent [57]. Calculations (see above) support this picture of coupling between redox and ligand protonation, which is also firmly based in the chemistry of manganese aqua ions. While water coordinated to Mn(II) ion is relatively basic (pK_a = 9.82) oxidation of the metal ion (to Mn(III)) converts the coordinated solvent to the equivalent of a mineral acid (pK_a = 0.2) [58]. This strong coupling between metal oxidation state and ligand acidity

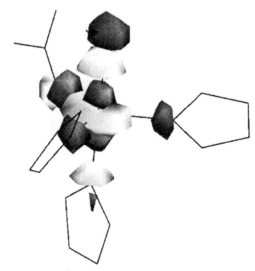

FIG. 9.   Ground state redox orbital calculated for a MnSOD-optimized model using nonlocal density functional theory methods.

accounts for the delivery of at least one of the protons required in the reductive half-reaction of MnSOD in Eq. (5). Transfer of this proton between the solvent pocket and the substrate funnel may be facilitated by the relay pathway involving Q146 glutamine and Y34 tyrosine side chains as shown in Fig. 5.

5.   MUTAGENIC DISSECTION OF THE ACTIVE SITE

Mutagenesis allows the functional role of individual protein residues to be investigated experimentally through site-specific amino acid substitutions. One of the first residues in MnSOD to be targeted for mutagenesis was the strictly conserved gateway tyrosine residue, Y34, that has been proposed to participate as a proton donor in catalysis. Substitution by phenylalanine (Y34F mutagenesis) conserves most of the interactions of the amino acid side chain but eliminates the phenolic hydroxyl. *Escherichia coli* MnSOD(Y34F) [50] retains approximately 80% of the wild-type enzyme activity under normal assay conditions (low superoxide flux). However, the coordination chemistry of the Mn center is perturbed indirectly and a six-coordinate azide complex is stabilized at ambient temperatures. Binding of hydroxide at high pH is also eliminated. This altered chemistry of the active site has been interpreted in terms of interruption of a proton linkage pathway involving Y34 and Q146 that would have a function analogous to the proton relay chains of peroxidases. The corresponding Y34F mutant of recombinant human MnSOD has also been prepared [59], and a detailed kinetic analysis of the mutant enzyme indicates that the most dramatic effects of this mutation are revealed at high superoxide flux, conditions that inactivate the mutant enzyme by conversion to the dead-end species "X" (Fig. 3) leaving only about 1% of the wild-type activity. This has led to a proposal that the strict requirement for the gateway tyrosine is based on the behavior of the enzyme under extreme conditions [59], and that MnSOD has been selected to perform well under (oxidative) stress.

The role of the conserved glutamate bridge (Fig. 6) has also been investigated by mutagenesis [49]. The *E. coli* MnSOD(E170A) mutant, in which the bridging glutamate is replaced by alanine, is isolated as an Fe-containing protein even when the culture is supplemented with manganese salts, indicating that in vivo the mutant protein preferentially binds Fe rather than the native metal ion, Mn. Size exclusion chromatography shows that the stability of the dimeric protein is severely affected by loss of the bridge, dissociating into monomers under mild conditions. Physiological studies on this expression of this mutant in *sodA*-deficient and *sodA*-proficient *E. coli* strains (with and without a functional MnSOD gene, respectively) has demonstrated that it is toxic to the cells and that its toxicity is a dominant trait. Since the isolated enzyme does not appear to exhibit unusual peroxidative activity, it appears that the toxic gain of function may result from the instability of the dimer, which exposes the hydrophobic dimer interface and allows it to engage in nonspecific protein interactions.

6. METAL SPECIFICITY: THE IRONY OF Mn SUPEROXIDE DISMUTASE

In general, Mn and Fe SODs form discrete classes, and although metal binding selectivity may be low (as evidenced by the isolation of all combinations of Mn_2-MnSOD, (Fe,Mn)-MnSOD hybrid, and Fe_2-MnSOD from *E. coli*) [60], the catalytic specificity for the metal is high, and in general the activity is associated almost exclusively with the preferentially bound metal ion. There are exceptions to this general rule, and a class of "cambialistic" superoxide dismutases has been described in which either Fe or Mn equally supports turnover [23,24]. Thus, one of the perplexing questions regarding the Fe/Mn superoxide dismutase family is the structural basis for metal specificity.

Crystal structures for iron and manganese superoxide dismutases have confirmed the high degree of structural homology that was anticipated based on the strong sequence similarities between these two classes of enzyme. In addition to the structural alignments that can be made over the homologous folds (see above), atomic alignment is possible for all metal ligands (Fig. 10) and a close superposition extends even to the outer sphere of the metal complexes. It would seem likely that substitution of Fe for Mn in MnSOD would lead to essentially identical coordination in the protein containing the "wrong" metal ion. It is therefore ironic that Fe_2-MnSOD, containing iron in place of manganese, has a distinct metal geometry relative to the native Mn_2-MnSOD [61] (Fig. 10). The Fe complex is six-coordinate, with a ligating solvent (interpreted as hydroxide) leading to a roughly octahedral metal environment. This observation provides a structural explanation for metal specificity of MnSOD, as the hydroxide ion fills the substrate access funnel and blocks access to the active site metal ion [61]. Potentiometric studies have shown that this complex has a perturbed redox potential,

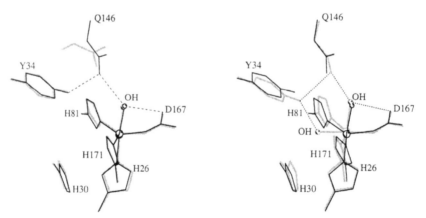

FIG. 10.   Comparison of Fe and Mn superoxide dismutase structures. (left) Superposition of structures for active site complexes of *E. coli* MnSOD (black) and FeSOD (gray). (right) Superposition of structures for active site complexes of *E. coli* Mn_2-MnSOD (black) and the iron-substituted derivative Fe_2-MnSOD (gray).

consistent with the decreased catalytic efficiency [62]. However, the decreased activity is a direct consequence of hydroxide binding and below the pK_a for hydrolysis (= 6.5 for the iron-substituted enzyme) [50,63,64] the activity of Fe_2-MnSOD increases nearly eightfold. Metal specificity is thus related to the tuning of the coordination chemistry of the active site that prevents rusting of the native iron enzyme. Part of this tuning is likely to relate to outer sphere interactions of the metal centers. The effect of E170A mutagenesis on metal binding selectivity (the relative affinity for Mn and Fe) has been described above. In addition, the iron-substituted Y34F mutant has been found to be active (as an FeSOD) through the physiological pH range as a result of destabilization of the hydroxide adduct [50].

7. SUPEROXIDE DISMUTASE AS A ONE-ELECTRON REDOX ENGINE

The active site manganese complex in MnSOD is an efficient redox catalyst that performs two distinct reactions: the one-electron oxidation and reduction of superoxide. In the oxidative half-reaction, as the Mn(III) ion removes an electron from the first molecule of superoxide forming dioxygen, the coordinated solvent is protonated as a result of the increased basicity of that ligand in the Mn(II) complex. The reaction with a second molecule of superoxide in the reductive cycle requires two protonation steps to release the peroxy dianion product from the complex. One of the protons may derive from bulk water, but the other will be delivered from the coordinated solvent in a step that might represent the power stroke displacing the product from the metal ion. The tight coupling between redox and protonation processes is a key feature of this active site that involves a water ligand serving as an inorganic cofactor for storage and delivery of protons during the reaction cycle.

ACKNOWLEDGMENTS

Support from the National Institutes of Health (GM 42680) and the M. J. Murdock Charitable Trust is gratefully acknowledged. I would also like to take this opportunity to express my appreciation to the talented co-workers who have made our research on Mn superoxide dismutase possible, including Dr. Mei M. Whittaker (Oregon Graduate Institute, Portland) and Dr. Edward N. Baker and colleagues in the Structural Biology Laboratory, University of Auckland, New Zealand.

ABBREVIATIONS

LUMO   lowest unoccupied molecular orbital
MCD   magnetic circular dichroism
mt-DNA   mitochondrial DNA
NHE   normal hydrogen electrode
SOD   superoxide dismutase
rms   root mean square

REFERENCES

1. P. L. Cheton and F. S. Archibald, *Free Radic. Biol. Med.*, *5*, 325–333 (1988).

2. B. B. Keele, Jr., J. M. McCord, and I. Fridovich, *J. Biol. Chem.*, *245*, 6176–6181 (1970).

3. Y. Kono and I. Fridovich, *J. Biol. Chem.*, *258*, 6015–6019 (1983).

4. F. S. Archibald and I. Fridovich, *J. Bacteriol.*, *146*, 928–936 (1981).

5. F. Archibald, *Crit. Rev. Microbiol.*, *13*, 63–109 (1986).

6. J. M. McCord, *New Horiz.*, *1*, 70–76 (1993).

7. I. Fridovich, *J. Biol. Chem.*, *272*, 18515–18517 (1997).

8. I. Fridovich, *Annu. Rev. Biochem.*, *64*, 97–112 (1995).

9. I. Fridovich, *Arch. Biochem. Biophys.*, *247*, 1–11 (1986).

10. E. R. Stadtman, *Science*, *257*, 1220–1224 (1992).

11. L. Zhang, L. Yu, and C. A. Yu, *J. Biol. Chem.*, *273*, 33972–33976 (1998).

12. R. Luft and B. R. Landau, *J. Int. Med.*, *238*, 405–421 (1995).

13. D. H. Flint, J. F. Tuminello, and M. H. Emptage, *J. Biol. Chem.*, *268*, 22369–22376 (1993).

14. P. Wardman and L. P. Candeias, *Radiat. Res.*, *145*, 523–531 (1996).

15. J. A. Imlay and S. Linn, *Science*, *240*, 1302–1309 (1988).

16. G. D. Lawrence and D. T. Sawyer, *Biochemistry*, *18*, 3045–3050 (1979).

17. J. M. McCord, *Adv. Exp. Med. Biol.*, *74*, 540–550 (1976).

18. F. J. Yost and I. Fridovich, *J. Biol. Chem.*, *248*, 4905–4908 (1973).

19. L. Benov, L. Y. Chang, and I. Fridovich, *Arch. Biochem. Biophys.*, *319*, 508–511 (1995).

20. H. D. Youn, H. Youn, J. W. Lee, Y. I. Yim, J. K. Lee, Y. C. Hah, and S. O. Kang, *Arch. Biochem. Biophys.*, *334*, 341–348 (1996).

21. S. C. Grace, *Life Sci.*, *47*, 1875–1886 (1990).

22. W. C. Stallings, A. L. Metzger, K. A. Pattridge, J. A. Fee, and M. L. Ludwig, *Free Radic. Res. Commun.*, *12–13*, 259–268 (1991).

23. M. E. Martin, B. R. Byers, M. O. Olson, M. L. Salin, J. E. Arceneaux, and C. Tolbert, *J. Biol. Chem.*, *261*, 9361–9367 (1986).

24. R. Gabbianelli, A. Battistoni, F. Polizio, M. T. Carri, A. De Martino, B. Meier, A. Desideri, and G. Rotilio, *Biochem. Biophys. Res. Commun.*, *216*, 841–847 (1995).

25. S. Sato and K. Nakazawa, *J. Biochem. (Tokyo)*, *83*, 1165–1171 (1978).

26. S. D. Ravindranath and I. Fridovich, *J. Biol. Chem.*, *250*, 6107–6112 (1975).

27. E. M. Gregory, F. J. Yost, Jr., and I. Fridovich, *J. Bacteriol.*, *115*, 987–991 (1973).

28. H. M. Steinman, L. Weinstein, and M. Brenowitz, *J. Biol. Chem.*, *269*, 28629–28634 (1994).

29. R. A. Weisiger and I. Fridovich, *J. Biol. Chem.*, *248*, 3582–3592 (1973).

30. R. A. Weisiger and I. Fridovich, *J. Biol. Chem.*, *248*, 4793–4776 (1973).

31. R. M. Lebowitz, H. Zhang, H. Vogel, J. Cartwright, Jr., L. Dionne, N. Lu, S. Huang, and M. M. Matzuk, *Proc. Natl. Acad. Sci. USA*, *93*, 9782–9787 (1996).

32. S. Melov, J. A. Schneider, B. J. Day, D. Hinerfeld, P. Coskun, S. S. Mirra, J. D. Crapo, and D. C. Wallace, *Nature Genet.*, *18*, 159–163 (1998).

33. C. Bull, E. C. Niederhoffer, T. Yoshida, and J. A. Fee, *J. Am. Chem. Soc.*, *113*, 4069–4076 (1991).

34. J. L. Hsu, Y. Hsieh, C. Tu, D. O'Connor, H. S. Nick, and D. N. Silverman, *J. Biol. Chem.*, *271*, 17687–17691 (1996).

35. M. L. Ludwig, A. L. Metzger, K. A. Pattridge, and W. C. Stallings, *J. Mol. Biol.*, *219*, 335–358 (1991).

36. R. A. Edwards, H. M. Baker, M. M. Whittaker, J. W. Whittaker, G. B. Jameson, and E. N. Baker, *J. Biol. Inorg. Chem.*, *3*, 161–171 (1998).

37. U. G. Wagner, M. M. Werber, Y. Beck, J. R. Hartman, F. Frolow, and J. L. Sussman, *J. Mol. Biol.*, *206*, 787–788 (1989).

38. U. G. Wagner, K. A. Pattridge, M. L. Ludwig, W. C. Stallings, M. M. Werber, C. Oefner, F. Frolow, and J. L. Sussman, *Protein Sci.*, *2*, 814–825 (1993).

39. G. E. Borgstahl, H. E. Parge, M. J. Hickey, W. F. Beyer, Jr., R. A. Hallewell, and J. A. Tainer, *Cell*, *71*, 107–118 (1992).

40. G. E. Borgstahl, H. E. Parge, M. J. Hickey, M. J. Johnson, M. Boissinot, R. A. Hallewell, J. R. Lepock, D. E. Cabbelli, and J. A. Tainer, *Biochemistry*, *35*, 4287–4297 (1996).

41. W. C. Stallings, K. A. Pattridge, R. K. Strong, and M. L. Ludwig, *J. Biol. Chem.*, *259*, 10695–10699 (1984).

42. M. S. Lah, M. M. Dixon, K. A. Pattridge, W. C. Stallings, J. A. Fee, and M. L. Ludwig, *Biochemistry*, *34*, 1646–1660 (1995).

43. M. W. Parker, C. C. F. Blake, D. Barra, F. Bossa, M. E. Schinina, W. H. Bannister, and J. V. Bannister, *Protein Eng.*, *1*, 393–397 (1987).

44. M. W. Parker and C. C. F. Blake, *FEBS Lett.*, *229*, 377–382 (1988).

45. T. Hunter, K. Ikeburkuro, W. H. Bannister, J. V. Bannister, and G. J. Hunter, *Biochemistry*, *36*, 4925–4933 (1997).

46. T. Fester and W. Schuster, *Biochem. Mol. Biol. Int.*, *36*, 67–75 (1995).

47. K. A. Hopkin, M. A. Papazian, and H. M. Steinman, *J. Biol. Chem.*, *267*, 24253–24258 (1992).

48. M. M. Whittaker, C. A. Ekberg, R. A. Edwards, E. N. Baker, G. B. Jameson, and J. W. Whittaker, *J. Phys. Chem. B*, *102*, 4668–4677 (1998).

49. M. M. Whittaker and J. W. Whittaker, *J. Biol. Chem.*, *273*, 22188–22193 (1998).

50. M. M. Whittaker and J. W. Whittaker, *Biochemistry*, *36*, 8923–8931 (1997).

51. B. B. Keele, Jr., J. M. McCord, and J. A. Fee, *J. Biol. Chem.*, *245*, 6176–6181 (1970).

52. J. W. Whittaker and M. M. Whittaker, *J. Am. Chem. Soc.*, *113*, 5528–5540 (1991).

53. M. M. Whittaker and J. W. Whittaker, *Biochemistry*, *35*, 6762–6770 (1996).

54. J. W. Whittaker, *J. Phys. Chem. B*, *101*, 674–677 (1997).

55. M. M. Whittaker and J. W. Whittaker, *J. Biol. Inorg. Chem.*, *2*, 667–671 (1997).

56. C. L. Fisher, J.-L. Chen, J. Li, D. Bashford, and L. Noodleman, *J. Phys. Chem. B*, *100*, 13498–13505 (1996).

57. C. Bull and J. A. Fee, *J. Am. Chem. Soc.*, *107*, 3295–3304 (1985).

58. C. F. Baes, Jr. and R. E. Messmer, *The Hydrolysis of Metal Cations*, R. E. Krieger, Malabar, FL, 1986.

59. Y. Guan, M. J. Hickey, G. E. Borgstahl, R. A. Hallewell, J. R. Lepock, D. O'Connor, Y. Hsieh, H. S. Nick, D. N. Silverman, and J. A. Tainer, *Biochemistry*, *37*, 4722–4730 (1998).

60. W. F. Beyer, Jr. and I. Fridovich, *J. Biol. Chem.*, *266*, 303–308 (1991).

61. R. A. Edwards, M. M. Whittaker, J. W. Whittaker, G. B. Jameson, and E. N. Baker, *J. Am. Chem. Soc.*, *120*, 9684–9685 (1998).

62. C. K. Vance and A.-F. Miller, *J. Am. Chem. Soc.*, *120*, 461–467 (1998).

63. F. Yamakura, K. Kobayashi, H. Ue, and M. Konno, *Eur. J. Biochem.*, *227*, 700–706 (1995).

64. F. Yamakura, H. Taka, T. Fujimora and K. Murayama, *J. Biol. Chem.*, *273*, 14085–14089 (1998).

19

Mechanistic Aspects of the Tyrosyl Radical–Manganese Complex in Photosynthetic Water Oxidation

Curtis W. Hoganson and Gerald T. Babcock

Department of Chemistry, Michigan State University,
East Lansing, MI 48824-1322, USA

1. INTRODUCTION

The photosynthetic oxidation of water to molecular oxygen by Photo-system II is an example of a splendidly effective catalyst. Duplication of that catalytic ability in industrial settings would have considerable economic benefit but will require a solid understanding of the mechanism of the biological catalyst. We will describe the most pertinent experimental results, discuss current models for the chemical mechanism by which plants and algae oxidize water, and relate the results to these models. We will also incorporate insights from recent theoretical work related to oxygen evolution. Although the subject is still controversial, the chemistry underlying oxygen evolution is becoming much clearer.

1.1. Composition and Organization of Photosystem II

Photosystem II (PS II) is found in most higher plants, algae, and cyano-bacteria and is highly similar among these groups of organisms. It is a complex of membrane proteins composed of a reaction center that carries out the conversion of light energy to stable chemical energy and an antenna rich with chlorophylls and carotenoids that harvests light and transfers the energy to the reaction center. The reaction center is composed mainly of two intrinsic membrane proteins, called D1 and D2, and its bound cofactors. PS II comprises, also, several water-soluble extrinsic polypeptides that shield the water oxidizing site from too intimate contact with solutes present in the aqueous phase. For a detailed examination of the polypeptides in PS II, see the chapter by Debus in this volume [1].

Reaction-center cores are the smallest particles active in oxygen production and contain, in addition to D1 and D2, several other polypeptides, including the chlorophyll-binding proteins CP47 and CP43. Particles much larger than these have been frequently used for studies. PS II membrane fragments containing additional chlorophyll-binding antenna proteins can be isolated from plant chloroplasts by detergent solubilization of most of the Photosystem I, cytochrome b_6f, and ATP synthase. The relative simplicity of the preparation, its stability, and the small amount of PS I present have made these particles very useful [2].

Photosystem II contains a number of cofactors involved in charge separation, including chlorophyll, pheophytin, and plastoquinone. Reduction of the mobile plastoquinone pool is facilitated by a nonheme iron atom, one of whose ligands is a bicarbonate ion. Water binding and oxidation occur at a tetra-manganese cluster that requires one calcium and one chloride ion for activity. One or two copies of cytochrome b_{559} are also present, but its function is not yet well understood.

Electron paramagnetic resonance (EPR) has been very useful in studying the electron transfer reactions of PS II. EPR signals are associated with chlorophyll P_{680}, with tyrosine residues Y_Z and Y_D, with the manganese complex, and with plastoquinone radicals and the nonheme iron [3].

1.2. Electron-Transfer Sequence

P_{680} is a dimer or higher multimer of chlorophyll that receives excitation energy from the antenna chlorophyll molecules. Upon excitation, P_{680} loses an electron that first moves to a pheophytin, then to a bound plastoquinone, Q_A, and finally to an exchangeable plastoquinone, Q_B. On losing an electron, P_{680} becomes a radical cation, P_{680}^+. It receives an electron from a tyrosine residue Y_Z of the D1 polypeptide, and the tyrosyl radical, $Y_Z^\bullet$, thus formed is reduced by the manganese cluster. The manganese cluster not only binds the substrate but also serves to accumulate and store the oxidizing power necessary for the four-electron oxidation of two water molecules to give O_2.

1.3. The S-State Cycle

When exposed to flashes of light that are sufficiently short and bright, nearly all of the reaction centers in a sample undergo one photochemical charge-separation event. Short flashes take advantage of the fact that a second charge separation is limited by the rates by which P_{680}^+ can be reduced and Q_A^- oxidized [4].

When PS II is allowed to rest for several minutes in darkness and then subjected to a sequence of short, intense flashes, oxygen release is detected in amounts that oscillate with a period of four, with maximal amplitudes following the third and seventh flash, and the oscillation is progressively damped with increasing number of flashes. These findings imply that each photochemical reaction center is coupled to only one oxidant storage center, which we now know to be the manganese complex. Furthermore, some of the oxidation states of the manganese cluster are reactive enough to undergo reduction in the dark.

This pattern of oxygen release indicates that the manganese complex cycles through four stable oxidation states, called S_0, S_1, S_2, and S_3, where the index denotes the number of electrons removed from the metal centers [5]. Oxidation of S_3 leads to the release of O_2 and regeneration of S_0, possibly by way of an unstable S_4. States S_2 and S_3 undergo reduction to S_1 during lengthy dark adaptation, accounting for the maximal yield of O_2 on the third flash. Perfect synchronization is not possible, however, as both misses and double hits occur, and these account for the damping of the oscillation of oxygen release. This damping complicates the analysis of many experiments.

Besides oxygen release, a number of other S-state-dependent phenomena have been observed. EPR signals from the S_2 state of the manganese cluster have been detected since 1981 [6]. A $g = 2$ multiline spectrum indicates that S_2 has an odd number of electrons. This and other spectroscopic measurements will be discussed in more detail below. The kinetics of redox reactions also depend on S state. In S_0 and S_1, P_{680}^+ is reduced monophasically in about 20 ns, while in S_2 and S_3, P_{680}^+ reduction is multiphasic with half-times of about 50 and 200 ns and 35 μs [7]. Reduction of $Y_Z^\bullet$ occurs in about 50, 100, 300, and 1300 μs, from S_0 to S_3, respectively, but structural perturbations can slow these rates quite markedly. A detailed discussion of electron and proton flow through $Y_Z^\bullet$ is provided in [8].

1.4. Inhibitions of the S-State Cycle Due to Loss of Cofactors

Loss of manganese from PS II inhibits oxygen evolution and alters some of the electron-transfer kinetics. Manganese depletion by heating, by washing with 0.8 M Tris at pH 8, or by incubation with reductants, especially hydroxylamine, has been much used in the study of PS II. These treatments usually release extrinsic polypeptides from PS II [9].

The optimum range of pH for oxygen evolution is between 5.5 and 7.5, with a maximum at about 6.5. The maximum can be shifted to higher pH with increased chloride ion concentration [10], and kinetic studies show an apparent competition between activating Cl^- and inhibiting OH^- [11]. This suggests either that OH^- and Cl^- compete for the same binding site or that chloride binding requires binding of a proton, perhaps to maintain charge neutrality. Chloride depletion by alkaline treatment causes the S-state cycle to stop at S_2 [12], but no EPR signals are detected from this state. Studies with essentially intact PS II show that there is one tightly bound, slowly exchanging chloride ion per manganese complex [13].

Calcium is also thought to be required for oxygen evolution [9,14]. Calcium depletion, like chloride depletion, causes the S-state cycle to stop at S_2, and a multiline spectrum is observed. A second EPR signal is observed by freezing calcium-depleted PS II under illumination [15]. This signal has a linewidth of about 160 G and is attributed to an interaction of the manganese complex in the S_2 state with $Y_Z^{\bullet}$ [16,17].

1.5. Similarities and Differences Relative to Bacterial Photoreaction Centers

The reaction centers (RC) of PS II resemble those of purple photosynthetic bacteria, in that they perform similar charge-separation reactions using similar cofactors; their polypeptides share strong amino acid sequence similarities and tertiary structure [18]. These facts suggest that the bacterial RC, whose geometry has been determined by X-ray crystallography [19], can serve as a model for the RC of PS II (Fig. 1). The bacterial RC is composed of a heterodimer with approximate twofold rotation symmetry, where each polypeptide spans the membrane five times. The bacteriochlorophylls and bacteriopheophytins are bound in symmetry-related positions, and the nonheme iron lies on the rotation axis. The approximate rotation symmetry was one clue that led to identification of the specific tyrosine residues on the D1 and D2 polypeptides responsible for the $Y_Z^{\bullet}$ and $Y_D^{\bullet}$ EPR signals in PS II. Thus, the C2 symmetry extends beyond the primary charge-separation cofactors to the redox-active tyrosines and the histidine bases that form hydrogen bonds with them [20].

There are significant differences, as well, between the reaction centers of purple bacteria and PS II. Purple bacteria do not generate tyrosyl radicals and are unable to oxidize water. Their photochemistry is

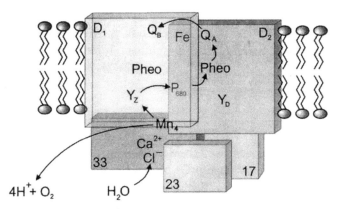

FIG. 1.   Cartoon structure of the Photosystem II reaction center, showing the electron-transfer cofactors.

aimed at generating a cyclic electron flow to be used to generate the electrochemical proton gradient that drives ATP synthesis.

2.   STRUCTURE OF THE CATALYTIC SITE

Because high-resolution structural information is not yet available for PS II, our knowledge of the active site structure comes from less direct observations. For recent reviews on this subject, see [21–24].

2.1.   Electron Magnetic Resonance

The S_2 multiline EPR spectrum has a large number of lines, due to hyperfine interactions between the unpaired electrons and the manganese nuclei. The hyperfine couplings cannot be extracted directly from the spectra, however, and relatively successful spectral simulations have been performed by assuming either a binuclear or a tetranuclear cluster. The manganese hyperfine couplings have been estimated through an electron spin echo-detected ENDOR experiment [25]. With these values and the overall width of the EPR spectrum, it was shown that all four manganese contribute to that spectrum, consistent only with a tetranuclear complex. A second EPR signal from an S_2 state has been observed at $g = 4.1$ and is due to a high-spin, ground state of the manganese cluster [26]. The implications that this high-spin species has for recent structural models of the manganese cluster are considered below.

2.2.   Manganese XAFS

X-ray absorption fine-structure spectra (XAFS) of PS II in the S_1 state indicate the presence of two Mn-Mn vectors of about 2.7 Å, generally interpreted as due to two $Mn(\mu\text{-}O)_2Mn$ dimers. A third distance of 3.3 Å is also detected and may reflect another Mn-Mn distance or an Mn-Ca distance. The Mn-Mn distances depend somewhat on S state and electron spin state. From samples in which the PS II membrane fragments are partially oriented, an angle between the Mn-Mn vectors of about 60° has been deduced. This fact allows further distinction of the Mn-Mn separations: in S_1, 2.71 Å and 2.74 Å; in S_2 multiline, 2.72 Å and 2.72 Å; in S_2 $g = 4.1$, 2.72 Å and 2.85 Å; and in S_3, 2.8 Å and 3.0 Å [21,22].

The Mn XAFS spectra also exhibit features due to the ligand atoms. An average distance of 1.9 Å is indicated, which is typical for oxygen or nitrogen donor atoms. Mn-O distances are expected to range from 1.75 Å for the bridging oxo atoms to 2.1 Å for water ligands. This spread of expected distances precludes an accurate measurement of the coordination numbers of the Mn atoms.

The determination of the angle between the two Mn-Mn vectors has led to proposals of possible arrangements of the four manganese atoms. One of these structures (see Fig. 2) in particular has caught the eye of many investigators and has been incorporated into models for the mechanism of oxygen production. In this model, the two manganese dimers are connected to each other, Mn to Mn, by one oxo and one or two carboxylate ligands to give the 3.3-Å distance mentioned above. The other two Mn are not joined directly, but the angle of about 60° and the assumption of coplanarity of the two Mn_2O_2 units puts their separation at about 5.5 Å.

There is, however, some uncertainty as to whether this dimer-of-dimers structure can account for the S_2 $g = 4.1$ EPR signal. From work with model compounds, one expects strong antiferromagnetic coupling within each dimer and weak coupling between the dimers [27]. For the set of manganese valence states determined for S_2, a low-spin ground state is, therefore, to be expected, consistent with the S_2 multiline sig-

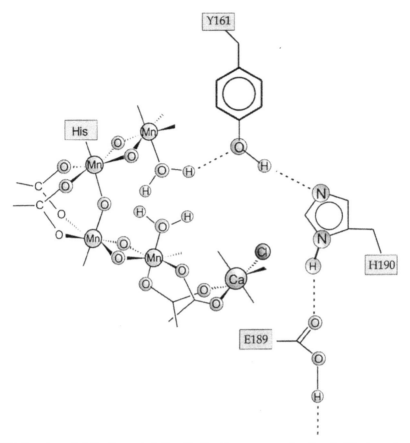

FIG. 2. A model for the catalytic site for dioxygen production in Photosystem II. The site includes the manganese cluster as a dimer of dimers, tyrosine Y_Z, and its hydrogen-bonded partner, histidine-190.

nal at $g = 2$, but varying from the $g = 4.1$ signal. To accommodate the results of XAFS experiments on strontium-substituted PS II, a new structural proposal includes a three-atom bridge (O-Ca-O) connecting the two manganese at the "open" end of the cluster [28].

2.3. Manganese Ligands

Electron spin-echo envelope modulation spectroscopy has been applied to the S_2 multiline spectra. This technique is very sensitive for nuclei having a nuclear spin of 1, such as ^2H and ^{14}N. The spectra show the presence of a histidine ligand, and this was confirmed by isotopic labeling of histidine added to the growth medium of a histidine-tolerant strain of *Synechocystis* [29]. No evidence for more than one histidine ligand was obtained. The majority of the manganese ligands must, therefore, contain oxygen atoms.

Site-directed mutagenesis has been applied in order to identify the protein-derived ligands to the essential metal atoms. Attention has focused mainly on carboxylic acid residues. The most likely candidates for these ligands all lie on the D1 polypeptide: D170, E333, E342, and the carboxy terminus, A344 [1]. Additional evidence for carboxylate ligands to manganese or calcium comes from Fourier transform infrared (FTIR) measurements before and after the S_1-to-S_2 transition [30,31].

2.4.   Chloride Is a Likely Ligand to Manganese

A number of aliphatic amines inhibit oxygen evolution. Kinetic studies show competition between chloride and the amine inhibitors, whose inhibition constants parallel their pK_a values [32]. The fact that these amines are competitive, with respect to chloride, suggests that both the amines and chloride bind to the same Lewis acid, most likely the manganese. (The inhibition due to ammonia is more complex, due to binding at a second site on the manganese cluster, possibly a substrate binding site.) Chloride is required to promote the S_2-to-S_3 and S_3-to-S_0 transitions, but not those from S_0 to S_1 and S_1 to S_2 [12]. The S_2 state formed in the absence of chloride does not exhibit either of the usual S_2 EPR signals, but dark addition of chloride to such samples causes the multiline signal to form. The affinity of the oxygen-evolving complex (OEC) for chloride is also modulated by the S state [33]. Although chloride binding to the manganese complex has not yet been demonstrated by spectroscopic measurements, it is reasonable to conclude that chloride is a ligand to manganese in the higher S states.

2.5.   Properties of Tyrosyl Radical, $Y_Z^{\bullet}$

The EPR spectrum of $Y_Z^{\bullet}$ in manganese-depleted PS II has a g value that indicates that the radical is deprotonated. With an oxygen-evolving preparation, the EPR spectrum is similar [34], indicating that $Y_Z^\bullet$ is deprotonated in active PS II as well. These results are consistent with the fact that phenoxyl radicals have pK_a values of -2.

Mutagenesis experiments established that Y161 of D1 is Y_Z and that the symmetry related Y160 is Y_D (*Synechocystis* numbering [20]). Symmetry-related histidines, H189 of D2 and H190 of D1, strongly influence the properties of Y_D and Y_Z, respectively, and are believed to form hydrogen bonds to the redox-active tyrosines. H190-D1 is required for rapid reduction of P_{680}^+ by Y_Z [35–39], presumably because it accepts the proton from Y_Z upon its oxidation. H190 is also required for reduction of $Y_Z^\bullet$ by electron-transfer reagents [37,38]. The UV absorbance spectrum of Y_Z exhibits some phenolate character [40,41], which suggests that the hydrogen bond to H190 is quite strong. Density functional calculations show that a suitable proton acceptor is needed for oxidation of a phenol by a chlorophyll radical [42] and that, when the phenol is hydrogen-bonded to a histidine, there is no barrier for proton transfer during oxidation of the phenol [43].

The 160-G-wide EPR spectrum, observed after illumination of calcium-depleted PS II, is due to a magnetic interaction between $Y_Z^\bullet$ and the manganese complex in an S_2 state. Spin-echo detected ENDOR of this signal established that $Y_Z^\bullet$ is the radical responsible for the EPR signal [16]. A similar but narrower signal is observed in acetate-treated PS II. Simulation analysis of these signals in three different labs [17,44,45] indicates that both exchange and dipolar coupling are significant and that the center-to-center distance between $Y_Z^\bullet$ and the manganese complex is about 8.5 Å (Fig. 2).

2.6.   Chemical Nature of the Oxidations

During the S-state cycle, PS II must accumulate and stabilize three oxidizing equivalents to be used when Y_Z is oxidized a fourth time and dioxygen can be made. It is of great interest to know what molecular species store the oxidizing power. It may seem obvious that the manganese atoms should perform this function, and experimental evidence largely supports that idea. However, some evidence has been interpreted as indicating that a species other than manganese is oxidized on the S_2-to-S_3 transition.

Ultraviolet difference spectra obtained for the various S-state transitions show a peak at 300 nm and have been interpreted in terms of manganese-centered oxidations [46]. The spectral changes on the S_1-to-S_2 and the S_2-to-S_3 transitions are essentially identical to each other, and those on the S_0-to-S_1 transition are somewhat less intense. All three transitions were interpreted as oxidation of Mn(III) to Mn(IV).

The observation of a multiline EPR signal from S_2 implies that that state has an odd number of electrons. A recent study used partially oriented PS II membranes to examine the orientation dependence of the multiline signal and came to the conclusion that the spectra were probably due to an Mn(III)Mn(IV)$_3$ cluster [47]. Because the hyperfine anisotropy of Mn(III) is much larger than that of Mn(IV), the rather small orientation dependence of the multiline spectrum suggests that Mn(IV) is the more prevalent oxidation state. An earlier study came to a different conclusion [48], however.

X-ray absorbance near-edge spectroscopy (XANES) has been used to study oxidation state changes of many transition-metal compounds, because the position of the onset of absorbance reflects the electronic structure of the molecule and, in particular, the oxidation state of the metal atom. XANES studies of PS II show significant shifts in the edge positions on the S_0-to-S_1 and S_1-to-S_2 transitions [49–51]. Together with model-compound studies, these results indicate that these oxidations are manganese-centered oxidations. The S_2-to-S_3 transition has been more controversial, with two groups [49,51] reporting a significant advance of the edge and one group finding a minimal edge shift [50]. The task of defining the edge position is complicated by the presence of fine structure in the X-ray spectra, and to some extent the discrepancy may be due to differing methods for extracting the edge position. The bulk of the evidence from XANES favors the interpretation that the S_2-to-S_3 transition is manganese-centered.

The XANES spectra of the S_0 state contains a shoulder [51] that appears in many model compounds containing Mn(II). Thus, the oxidation states of the four manganese atoms deduced from the XANES of PS II and of model compounds are these: S_0, II, III, IV, IV; S_1, III, III, IV, IV; S_2, III, IV, IV, IV; S_3, IV, IV, IV, IV.

2.7.   Reduction Potentials

The reduction potentials of the various S-state transitions are not all the same (Table 1), but they differ much less than do the four one-elec-

TABLE 1

Reduction Potentials of
Photosystem II Components

$P_{680} \rightarrow P_{680}^+ + e^-$	1120 mV
$Y_Z \rightarrow Y_Z^{\cdot} + H^+ + e^-$	970 mV
$S_0 \rightarrow S_1 + e^-$	<700 mV
$S_1 \rightarrow S_2 + e^-$	925 mV
$S_2 \rightarrow S_3 + e^-$	925 mV
$Y_D \rightarrow Y_D^{\cdot} + H^+ + e^-$	740 mV

tron reduction potentials for the uncatalyzed oxidation of water. S_3 and S_2 are stronger oxidants than S_1, and, during dark incubation, they are reduced in a few seconds to S_1 by endogenous or exogenous reductants, while S_1 and S_0 are stable. During prolonged dark incubation, S_0 is advanced to S_1 at the expense of $Y_D^{\cdot}$, the stable tyrosine radical of PS II.

3. WATER BINDING AND EXCHANGE

3.1. Mass Spectrometry

The binding of substrate water to the OEC can be studied by mass spectrometry of the O_2 produced. Starting with dark-adapted PS II in water containing either ^{16}O or ^{18}O, one or more flashes of light are given; then the isotopic composition of the water is very rapidly altered, and one or more additional flashes of light are given. The exchange of ^{16}O for ^{18}O water, or vice versa, can be done on the millisecond time scale, and the isotopic composition of the O_2 subsequently produced indicates the rate of substrate exchange.

These experiments provide evidence for the binding of two substrate molecules in S_3 [52]. Two exchange rates, 4.9 s^{-1} and 56 s^{-1}, were measured at 20°C, having activation energies of 19 and 9 kcal/mol, respectively. These rates were compared with those of model inorganic complexes and one enzyme. It was noted that bridging oxo ligands in the models exchange more slowly than does the substrate in S_3 by factors of 10^4 or greater.

Preliminary reports of substrate exchange from the other S states by the same group show that the exchange rates vary with S state [53]. If the substrate binding sites are on manganese, the S-state dependence would be a natural consequence of the changing manganese-oxidation states during the catalytic cycle. In general, the exchange rates slow as the manganese oxidation state increases. Interpretation of these data is complicated, because the exchange rates should depend also on the number and type of other ligands to the metal.

3.2.   Electron Magnetic Resonance

The S_2 state has been studied after incubation with water labeled with either ^2H or ^{17}O, in the expectation that alterations of the multiline EPR spectrum from these magnetic nuclei might indicate the presence of bound substrate. Although the EPR spectra are little affected, the related ENDOR and ESEEM spectra show more significant effects [23]. Deuterons, in particular, are detected. This suggests that manganese-bound water or hydroxide ions are present in S_2.

4.   PROTON RELEASE

Protons are the most numerous product of the OEC and have sparked considerable interest and debate (for reviews, see [8,54]). Measuring the number of protons released on each step of the S-state cycle might be interpretable in terms of the chemical changes occurring at the OEC. At the very least, one would like to know how the overall charge of the cluster changes on each S-state advancement.

Protons released to the thylakoid lumen can be detected optically as they react with acid–base indicator dyes [54]. Such measurements show that the protons are not released all four at once, together with the oxygen molecule. Instead, the release of protons is spread over the four S-state transitions. A uniform pattern of one proton released per transition is sometimes, but not usually, observed. These observations raise the possibility that charge accumulates in or near the manganese cluster, and charge accumulation is often cited as one of its functions.

The protons released may originate from several possible sources (Fig. 3). Ligands to manganese, including water, hydroxide, and the im-

$$P^+ \,[MnLH] \longrightarrow P\,[MnL]\,H_3O^+$$

$$P^+ \,[MnL]\,HB_{int}\,H_2O \longrightarrow P\,[MnL]^+\,B_{int}^-\,H_3O^+$$

$$P^+ \,MnL \longrightarrow P\,[MnL]^+$$

$$P^+ \,MnL\text{-}H\cdots B\text{-}H\cdots B_{int}^- \longrightarrow P\,MnL\cdots H\text{-}B\cdots H\text{-}B_{int}$$

FIG. 3.   OEC oxidation accompanied (top two reactions) or not (bottom two reactions) by proton release may in either case be either electroneutral or charge the manganese cluster. Here, P represents P_{680}, [MnL] and [MnLH] describe the manganese cluster with a ligand in two different protonation states, B and B_{int} represent protein acid–base groups, and H_3O^+ indicates proton release to bulk solution.

idazole of histidine, may deprotonate as the metal is oxidized. Amino acid residues or other molecules not bound to manganese may respond to a changing charge on the manganese complex or to reorientations of electric dipoles or hydrogen bonds. The chemical changes at the manganese complex may be communicated either through-space or through-bond to the deprotonating group, which may even be on the surface of the protein. Unfortunately, the multitude of potential sources of protons makes it impossible to unambiguously determine the chemical changes occurring at the manganese cluster from observations of proton release.

For example, the manganese cluster may acquire a positive charge during oxidation (Fig. 3). No proton is released to the aqueous phase, then, unless a nearby base, perhaps at the protein surface, deprotonates due to an electrostatic interaction with the newly charged manganese cluster. For a second example, the manganese cluster may acquire no charge if a ligand deprotonates during oxidation. A proton would then be detectable in the aqueous phase, unless a base at the protein surface takes up the proton. This could result from a reorientation of hydrogen bonds within a hydrogen-bonded chain connecting the manganese cluster with the protein surface. Such hydrogen-bonded chains are likely to exist in all of the S states, as indicated by the generally rapid exchange of substrate molecules. A third possibility is that a rearrangement within the cluster might change its electric dipole whose electrostatic interaction with residues on the protein surface could lead to their protonation or deprotonation.

The position of the manganese complex will tend to suppress excess proton uptake or release because to bury uncompensated charges in a low dielectric environment is energetically costly. On the other hand, oxidation of the manganese cluster without its deprotonation might be electrically compensated by reorientation of a hydrogen-bonded chain connecting the cluster with the protein surface, where a higher dielectric constant exists. Such a hydrogen-bonded chain would, however, provide a conduit for protons to move from the cluster to the protein surface.

4.1. Pigment Bandshifts

Before considering the proton release measurements in detail, it is useful to introduce another sort of measurement that may be relevant to the question of charge accumulation. Changes in the absorption spectrum of PS II in the visible and UV regions occur simultaneously with the chemical changes initiated by light. These are bandshifts in regions where chlorophyll absorbs strongly. These bandshifts have been widely interpreted as due to a changing electrostatic environment at the chromophore, and the effect is often termed "local electrochromism." Here, we will use the term "pigment bandshift," to avoid prejudicing the discussion. One such bandshift, occurs between 424 and 440 nm, in response to the presence of $Y_Z^{\bullet}$. Another is a persistent bandshift at 695 nm that occurs on S_1 to S_2 and is reversed on S_3 to S_0. Neither the transient signal [55] nor the persistent signal [56,57] is much influenced by pH, even when proton release depends on pH. From the latter signal, it has been widely concluded that a positive charge develops on the manganese cluster on S_1 to S_2 that is neutralized during S_3 to S_0. From the former signal, it has been concluded that a positive charge remains near $Y_Z^{\bullet}$. Alternate explanations for these phenomena have been proposed recently that preserve the cluster's electroneutrality and allow for deprotonation of $Y_Z^{\bullet}$ to the bulk phase [58].

4.2. Patterns of H+ Release and Their pH Dependencies

Early measurements of proton release from PS II in thylakoids were interpreted in terms of a 1:0:1:2 proton release pattern (i. e., 1 proton on S_0 to S_1, none on S_1 to S_2, and so on). This pattern leads to the prediction that one positive charge is stored on S_1 to S_2 and is discharged on S_3 to S_0, and this would nicely account for the S-state dependence of P_{680}^{+} reduction and certain pigment bandshifts. Later measurements, however, found proton release to be noninteger and strongly pH-dependent [54]. Although nearly the above pattern was obtained recently from thylakoid membranes at pH 7.3, the pattern reversed at pH 6.2 to become 1:1.7:1:0.3 [59]. Furthermore, the proton-release patterns differ widely among different PS II preparations [54], even though the pigment bandshifts and P_{680}^+ reduction kinetics do not. These facts underscore the difficulty of interpreting the proton-release data.

Reaction-center cores, to take another example, have a flat proton-release pattern of 1:1:1:1, independent of pH; this has been taken as evidence for an electroneutral S-state cycle [60]. An alternate interpretation is that residues exposed on the surface of the protein, after release of extrinsic polypeptides, buffer and smooth an intrinsic, non-uniform release pattern [54,57,61].

If the intrinsic pattern of proton release from the manganese cluster itself is 1:1:1:1, how are the actual patterns to be interpreted? The noninteger patterns may arise from changes in electric dipoles or hydrogen bonds during the cycle that interact with the acid–base residues exposed on the protein surface. Questions for future research are to discover how large the dipoles would need to be and to identify the putative hydrogen-bonding networks that connect the manganese complex with the protein surface.

4.3.   Kinetics of H⁺ Release

With pH-indicating dyes present, proton release in as little as 10 μs is observed [54,59]. By this time, P_{680}^+ has oxidized Y_Z to $Y_Z^{\bullet}$ and H190-D1 has been protonated. Although proton release is measured in 10 μs, it is not likely that the proton released to H190 is so rapidly transported to the pH-indicating dye. Two explanations seem possible. The proton released from Y_Z may remain in the protein on H190, and, via a purely electrostatic effect, cause the release of a proton from an amino acid residue at the protein surface. Alternately, the proton released from Y_Z may enter a hydrogen-bonded chain running between Y_Z and the protein surface, forcing the hydrogen bonds within the chain to reorient and release a proton at the protein surface.

Substantial evidence indicates that a charge migration follows the oxidation of Y_Z. Chlorophyll fluorescence and P_{680}^+ reduction both exhibit 30- to-50-μs kinetic-decay components on the $S_2 \rightarrow S_3$ and $S_3 \rightarrow S_0$ transitions, which may be due to the migration of a proton away from

Y_Z toward the protein surface [62–64]. These observations may reflect the fact that $Y_Z^\bullet$ becomes a stronger reductant as the proton moves away from it [8,42], and the reaction $Y_Z\,P_{680}^+ \rightarrow Y_Z^\bullet\,P_{680}$ can then go to completion. The decay of the $Y_Z^\bullet$-related bandshift has a similar fast phase on $S_3 \rightarrow S_0$ [55] (see also [65]) and was interpreted in the same way. A 30-μs lag phase also occurs in the $Y_Z^\bullet\,S_3 \rightarrow Y_Z\,S_0$ reaction [65,66], even though $Y_Z^\bullet$ is presumably becoming a weaker oxidant. This observation is consistent with the notion that this reaction is not an electron-transfer reaction but a hydrogen-atom-transfer reaction that is impeded until H190 can deprotonate. An alternate explanation is that the proton is released not from H190 but from the manganese cluster, making it a stronger reductant [65].

The fast release of one full proton is not observed on each S-state transition, however. In particular, on the S_1-to-S_2 transition of thylakoids at pH 7.4, only about half of a proton is released with 10-μs kinetics [59]. This is also the transition in which many measurements have found little proton release to occur. On this transition, in particular, it appears that the usual pattern of proton release upon Y_Z oxidation is not followed. This observation disfavors the idea that the proton released upon Y_Z oxidation remains trapped on His 190 and returns to $Y_Z^\bullet$ during its reduction. Instead, a fraction of the protons released by Y_Z may bind to a basic ligand of the manganese cluster in the S_1 state rather than acidifying the aqueous phase. This hypothesis is consistent with the proximity of Y_Z to the manganese cluster that is required for $Y_Z^\bullet$ to function as an H-atom abstractor. On this transition, P_{680}^+ is reduced in the nanosecond regime, with no 35-μs kinetic phase [67]. The idea that S_1 especially contains a basic site is supported by the fact that, at lower pH where this basic site might be protonated, more than one proton is released during the S_1-to-S_2 transition. The proton remaining bound in the newly formed S_2 state might be the trigger for the chloride migration suggested by Tommos and Babcock [68]. It would be useful to know how many fast protons are released on this transition at lower pH.

Proton release (at high pH) or uptake (at low pH) on a slower time scale can be observed on the S_3-to-S_0 transition with kinetics corresponding to that of $Y_Z^\bullet$ reduction and O_2 release. These slow phases follow the rapid proton release mentioned above. During this transition, manganese is reduced, one or two water molecules may bind to the cluster, and a chloride ion may migrate. These structural changes may cause proton release or uptake from the cluster or from the protein surface by mechanisms set forth above.

5.   MECHANISMS FOR OXYGEN PRODUCTION

Many mechanisms for oxygen production have been proposed. The mechanisms we discuss here either have received wide attention or are recent proposals. We first consider the problem of water oxidation with regard to thermodynamic and kinetic issues and then describe several proposed mechanisms.

5.1.   General Considerations

5.1.1.   Krishtalik Analysis

The primary oxidant of PS II, P_{680}^+, has a reduction potential of about +1.12 V, which limits the driving force available for water oxidation. The reduction potential of $O_2 + 4H^+ + 4e^- \rightarrow 2H_2O$ is 0.93 V at pH = 5. At this pH, the average volume that contains exactly one H^+ ion is a cube with 55-nm sides, so there can be on average no H^+ ions present in the small volume of the enzyme active site, and certainly no OH^- ions to substitute for water as reactant. The presence of any H^+ ions after the reaction that produces O_2 would lower the effective pH so far as to render the reaction thermodynamically unfavorable. This is the essence of Krishtalik's analysis, which he put on a rigorous, quantitative basis by introducing the configurational potential, a thermodynamic quantity that is independent of concentration [69].

The analysis suggests that formation and release of O_2 can be made thermodynamically favorable only by providing bases in the active site to bind protons or by the prior transfer of the protons to the bulk medium. The first possibility, i.e., providing bases in the active site, introduces conceptual difficulties relating to both pK_a considerations for the base and electrostatics associated with generating (or neutralizing) charge in the active site. Accordingly, several mechanisms outlined below describe most or all of the S-state transitions as being electrically neutral losses of an electron and a proton from a manganese atom and its ligand, respectively.

5.1.2. Water as a Ligand to Manganese

Water molecules ligated to a metal ion experience large changes in their pK_a upon oxidation or reduction of the metal. One-electron oxidation coupled with deprotonation occurs frequently and is equivalent to loss of a hydrogen atom from the complex. From the acid dissociation constant and the reduction potential measured electrochemically, an O-H bond strength can be calculated. Model manganese dimer complexes containing aquo or hydroxo ligands are found to have O-H bond strengths between 76 and 94 kcal/mol [70,71]. Density-functional calculations on manganese complexes predict similar values [72]. These bond strengths are considerably lower than that of H_2O, 119 kcal/mol, and more in line with that of tyrosine, about 86 kcal/mol.

The model-compound studies show that the second oxidation of a complex can have a similar potential to the first oxidation, if the first oxidation includes a deprotonation so that the charge of the complex is not changed by that oxidation [24,71,73] (see also [74,75]). Thus, the studies on inorganic manganese dimer complexes imply that electrically neutral oxidations of the manganese complex can form the basis for the S-state cycle. The loss of a proton on each step of the cycle allows consecutive oxidations by $Y_Z^\bullet$ to proceed with similar driving force.

5.1.3. H-Atom Transfers

A key feature of several mechanisms below is that the tyrosyl radical functions not simply as a cofactor for electron transfer. Instead, it performs the critical functions of extracting both the protons and electrons from the substrate water molecules. Because of the large change in the pK_a of the phenolic proton upon oxidation, tyrosine Y_Z is perfectly suited to perform this function, which it may do by abstracting neutral hydrogen atoms from water bound to the manganese cluster. For tyrosine Y_Z to transfer electrons only would require that the protein actively suppress its natural reactivity. Furthermore, compared with the much larger chlorophyll molecules that do transfer only electrons, tyrosine is an unlikely electron-transfer cofactor because the Franck-Condon factors that govern the electron-transfer rate are not nearly so favorable for tyrosine as for the chlorophylls. In PS II and bacterial reaction centers, pure electron transfers utilize macrocyclic compounds, but when proton uptake or release is to be coupled with electron transfer, smaller, single-ring molecules such as quinones are used.

Additional support for the idea that $Y_Z^\bullet$ functions to remove both protons and electrons from substrate water in PS II comes from the kinetic data on proton release described above, from the O-H bond strengths of tyrosine and model-manganese complexes, and from the proximity of $Y_Z^\bullet$ to the manganese cluster. Furthermore, this proposal recognizes the hydrogen-atom-transfer role that tyrosyl radicals play in other enzymes [76–78].

5.2.   Cubane-Adamantane Rearrangement

The first chemically explicit molecular model for oxygen evolution proposed that oxygen was formed during a rearrangement of a cluster of manganese and oxygen atoms [79]. In this mechanism, the S_3 and the metastable S_4 states were proposed to be adamantane-like Mn_4O_6 clusters in which each pair of manganese atoms is bridged by one η_2 oxo ligand. The S_4 structure is proposed to release oxygen as it rearranges to an Mn_4O_4 cluster in which each η_3 oxo ligand bridges between three manganese atoms. This cubane structure would exist in S_0, S_1, and S_2. However, XAFS data that were obtained subsequent to this proposed mechanism did not support the presence of such highly symmetric clusters in PS II, and this model has been superseded.

5.3.   Bridging Oxo Fusion

The possibility that two bridging oxo ligands might come together to form O_2 is the idea that underlies a recent proposal [21] based on XAFS, XANES, and EPR data that indicate manganese oxidation-state changes and variations in Mn-Mn distances, as the sample is stepped through the S-state cycle. It suggests that the manganese cluster takes the form of a C-shaped dimer of dimers. Only one of the two di-μ-oxo dimers is proposed to be involved in the redox activity, and oxygen is formed from the two bridging oxo atoms in this dimer. The other dimer remains in the IV/IV oxidation state throughout the S-state cycle and no role for it is suggested. The active dimer is suggested to progress through the following oxidation states: S_0, II/III; S_1, III/III; S_2, III/IV; S_3, III/IV/bridging oxyl; S_4, III/IV/(bridging oxyl)$_2$ ↔ III/IV/peroxo. Only in the S_0 structure are the oxo ligands protonated, resulting in a proton-release pattern from the cluster of 2,0,0,2, but interactions between the manganese cluster and the protein side chains could result in a smoothing of this intrinsic pattern to yield the observed proton-release patterns.

Formation of dioxygen from two bridging oxo ligands is an attractive possibility, because of their proximity in such a structure-2.3–2.4 Å apart. However, whether exchange of substrate water into the bridging oxo positions can occur in the millisecond time regime that the mass spectroscopic experiments indicate is yet to be determined. The particular formulation of S_3 as containing a bridging oxyl ligand adjacent to an Mn(III) is surprising and is not supported by recent calculations [72]. The involvement of bridging oxyl radicals [21] seems unlikely, owing to the lack of precedent for oxidations in model di-μ-oxo manganese dimer complexes to oxidation states higher than Mn(IV)$_2$ [27].

5.4. Metalloradical Mechanism

The novel features of the metalloradical mechanism when it was proposed [60,76] were as follows: (1) $Y_Z^\bullet$ functions as a hydrogen-atom abstractor, (2) oxygen is formed from water bound to manganese as terminal rather than bridging ligands, and (3) the manganese cluster stays electrically neutral through the S-state cycle rather than acquire increasing positive charge as a charge accumulator. The C-shaped cluster proposed by the Berkeley group was used to illustrate the mechanism, although the mechanistic features above are not specifically dependent on this structure, and the two manganese atoms at the open end of the cluster were proposed as the catalytic manganese, which bind substrate and undergo the redox chemistry (Fig. 4). The two structural manganese atoms anchor the catalytic Mn to the protein in a geometry appropriate to template and catalyze O-O bond formation. Two additional features of the model, as it has developed, are the participation of $Y_Z^\bullet$ in the oxygen-oxygen bond forming chemistry [80] and a role for chloride ion and its migration on the S_1-to-S_2 and S_3-to-S_0 transitions [68].

The function of chloride is proposed to be to ensure that an abstractable hydrogen atom is present near $Y_Z^\bullet$ in the higher S states. In the absence of chloride, a substrate water in S_0 might be converted to a terminal oxo ligand in S_2, which, having no abstractable proton, would not allow further S-state advancement. Chloride binding to the Mn(IV)=O in S_2 brings with it a proton, giving Cl-Mn(IV)-OH. Oxidation to S_3 yields not an Mn(V)=O but, rather, an Mn(IV)=O from the one remaining Mn(III). Upon release of O_2 and formation of S_0, chloride dissociates from the manganese atom. Calcium is proposed to be a binding site for the chloride ion in S_0 and S_1. One possible scheme [68] embodying these suggestions is shown in Fig. 4.

Oxygen-oxygen bond formation is proposed to occur in a radical reaction initiated by and with the direct participation of $Y_Z^{\bullet}$ [80]. A concerted reaction that breaks two bonds and makes two bonds by transferring a hydrogen atom to $Y_Z^{\bullet}$ while the O-O σ bond forms is proposed (Fig. 5). In this process, both $Y_Z^{\bullet}$ and the manganyl manganese atom would be reduced.

5.5.   Monomanganese Mechanism

This proposal is based on density-functional calculations [81] and also adopts the C-shaped dimer of dimers. It invokes Y_Z as an abstractor of hydrogen atoms and O-O bond formation from a terminal, rather than bridging, manganese ligand. Only one manganese atom is included in most of the calculations, and it is proposed that only one manganese atom of the cluster is redox-active. It changes oxidation state and its key terminal ligand evolves through the cycle: S_0, II/aquo; S_1, III/hydroxo; S_2, IV/oxo; S_3, IV/oxyl $\leftrightarrow$ III/hydroperoxo; S_4, III/superoxy. The other three manganese have III/IV/IV oxidation states; no explicit role is proposed for them.

The density-functional calculations indicate that O-O bond formation by a radical mechanism can have an acceptably low activation barrier of only 10 kcal/mol. This barrier is obtained for the 1,3 reductive addition of a water molecule to two oxygen ligands of an Mn(IV)–oxyl radical complex (Fig. 5). The O-O distance in the cyclic transition structure is 1.90 Å. The reactive manganese complex is six-coordinate with primarily oxygen ligands, which give the Mn(IV)-oxyl state a lower energy than the related Mn(V)-oxo excited state.

The reactive manganese-oxyl state cannot be generated simply by transferring a hydrogen atom to a tyrosyl radical, however. When the O-H bond is weak enough for the H-atom transfer to occur, the ground state is always the unreactive, double-bonded Mn(V)-oxo, and the Mn(IV)-oxyl excited state is 20 kcal/mol or more higher in energy. Forming the six-coordinate Mn(IV)-oxyl species by hydrogen-atom transfer to the tyrosyl radical is typically 20 kcal/mol endothermic.

To overcome this difficulty, it was proposed that additional stabilization is gained by relegation of both the calcium and manganese

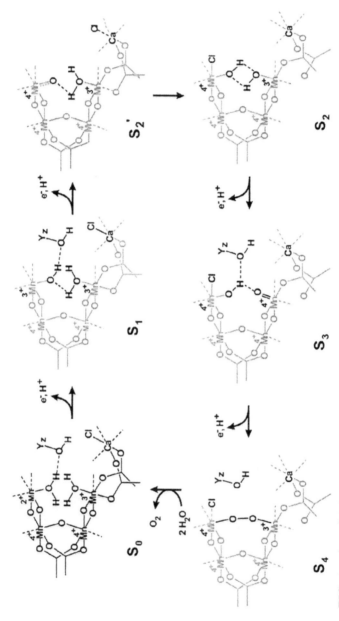

FIG. 4. A model for the S-state cycle of Photosystem II (Reproduced with permission from [68]. Copyright 1998 American Chemical Society.)

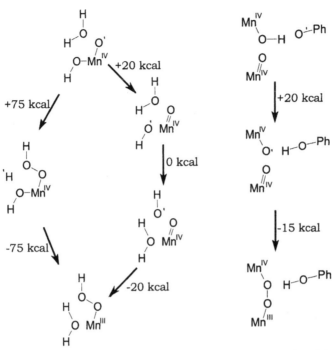

FIG. 5.   Two proposed radical mechanisms for oxygen-oxygen bond formation. For purposes of analysis, the concerted reactions are here decomposed into the corresponding stepwise reactions and estimated energies are given. The cyclic proposal on the left [81] has two branches in principle, but the hydrogen-atom branch on the far left is so high in energy that it is probably irrelevant. The remaining branch strongly resembles the tyrosyl-based mechanism on the right [80]; therefore, the activation energies of the two concerted mechanisms are probably similar.

atoms. Thus, S_2 contains a Ca and an Mn(IV), both six-coordinate, weakly bridged by aquo and oxo ligands. After hydrogen-atom transfer to $Y_Z^{\bullet}$ and several other steps, the Mn(IV)oxyl state of S_3, with Mn and Ca bridged by two hydroxo ligands, is formed. The scheme derives its functionality from the calculated result that the μ-oxo, μ-aquo S_2 state is higher in energy than the corresponding bis-μ-hydroxo structure.

There is, however, no obvious way to obligatorily couple the metal ion relegations with oxidation of the manganese. After the oxyl is formed, it is likely to reoxidize Y_Z, and the energy associated with the changes in calcium and manganese ligation will be lost. Even formation of a peroxide bond in S_3 cannot prevent the exothermic reoxidation of

Y_Z, because the Mn(III)peroxide, Mn(IV)oxyl, and Mn(V)oxo structures have similar energies. These difficulties are due to the weakness of the O-O single bond and affect all mechanisms that propose O-O bond formation prior to S_4.

5.6. Dual-Dimer Mechanism

Several manganese enzymes, including manganese catalase, contain binuclear active sites [24,82]. PS II contains two manganese dimers that might function independently, one to oxidize water to peroxide and the other to oxidize peroxide to O_2 [73]. This proposal also suggests a role for calcium in O-O bond formation and it includes the hypothesis of Y_Z as a hydrogen-atom abstractor, although not on each S-state advancement. In particular, on S_0 to S_1, a pure electron-transfer function for Y_Z is suggested. This would lead to an intrinsic proton release pattern of 0:1:1:2. The transition between S_0 and S_1 operates at a lower reduction potential than the others, so there is less need for a strict coupling between the electron and proton reaction coordinates during the reduction of $Y_Z^{\bullet}$. The other transitions are described as proton-coupled electron transfers, which can also be described formally as hydrogen-atom transfers. The S_2-to-S_3 transition is unique, in that the proton is proposed to originate from a water bound to the calcium ion, which, in turn, is bridged by a ligand to the manganese cluster. These oxidations result in an Mn(V)=O in S_4. This species is thought to be strongly electrophilic, rendering it susceptible to nucleophilic attack by a hydroxo ligand of the calcium ion, with resulting O-O bond formation. The transiently formed peroxide at one manganese dimer is then oxidized by the second dimer.

Although Mn=O species may react as electrophiles, oxo ligands retain a considerable negative charge [72]. The reaction between the oxo and a nucleophilic hydroxide will be disfavored by the electrical repulsion between the two negatively charged oxygen atoms and lead to high activation energies [81].

5.7. Chloride-Switched Nucleophilic Hydroxide

Another suggested mechanism [83] proposes a largely electroneutral cycle of hydrogen-atom transfers. In this mechanism, only one dimer is redox active, one substrate water binds terminally to manganese, and another binds as a hydroxide to the calcium ion. As above, the O-O bond is to be formed by the nucleophilic attack by the calcium-bound hydroxide on an electrophilic Mn(V)-oxo. In this variation, a chloride ion bridging between the calcium and a manganese controls the nucleophilicity of the hydroxide. As manganese is oxidized to Mn(V), it becomes a stronger Lewis acid and draws the chloride to it, and this increases the Lewis acidity of the calcium also. It was suggested that this would make the hydroxide more nucleophilic, favoring reaction with the oxo.

5.8.   Other Possibilities

Studies on inorganic complexes suggest some other possibilities. Oxomanganese porphyrins have been synthesized and are strong oxidants. The condensation of two terminal oxos may form the basis for the report that manganese porphyrin dimers catalyze the electrochemical oxidation of water to O_2 [84]. Manganyl oxo species have been suggested in the reactions of nonporphyrin manganese complexes, very few of which produce O_2. One such compound that does produce O_2 is a di-μ-oxo bridged manganese dimer with one open coordination site on each manganese [85]. Oxygen-atom transfer from hypochlorite may produce a manganyl oxo species that yields O_2 on further reaction. Reactions of oxo-containing manganese complexes have been examined by theoretical methods, and high barriers to reaction are found [86], apparently due to the large repulsion between two negatively charged oxo ligands.

6.   THE NATURE OF S-STATE CYCLE INTERMEDIATES

6.1. Mn_2O_2 Diamond Cores

A large number of compounds containing di-μ-oxo-manganese dimers with manganese in the III and IV oxidation states have been prepared in solution and crystallized. Many are quite stable in solution allowing detailed study of their redox and acid–base chemistry. The stability is, in part, due to the planar di-μ-oxo bridges. Most of these model compounds are prepared with ligands that prevent the formation of higher nuclearity clusters.

The chemical bonding within the Mn_2O_2 diamond core is complex

[87,110] and may include contributions from ionic as well as covalent σ and π bonding. A full, accurate, theoretical treatment of these systems is not yet available. The complexes exhibit octahedral coordination and, when Mn(III) is present, the long Jahn-Teller axis lies normal to the plane of the diamond, indicating the presence of an electron in the d_{z^2} orbital [28,110].

From study of the magnetic properties, the ground states are usually found to be low spin, indicating an antiferromagnetic interaction between the two manganese atoms, which individually are expected to be high spin [28,88]. The antiferromagnetic interactions suggest the existence of π bonds involving the bridging oxygen atoms. Three-center π bonds can be formed by overlap of an oxygen $2p_z$ orbital with a d_{xz} and a d_{yz} orbital on different metal atoms. These oxygen atoms, each participating in three covalent bonds (two σ and one π), are formally hypervalent. The strength of these π bonds is unknown.

Strong bonding within the Mn_2O_2 dimers may be mechanistically significant because it will weaken the bonds that other ligands form to the metal. If π bonding within the dimer is significant, then orbital arguments suggest that an axial ligand will not form strong covalent π bonds to the manganese because the relevant manganese d_{xz} and d_{yz} orbitals are already involved in bonds. As discussed below, the manganese-oxygen bonds in the higher S states are likely to be rather weak. The need to keep these bonds weak may be one reason that a tetranuclear cluster containing two Mn_2O_2 units is used in the OEC, when only two manganese atoms are sufficient to accumulate the required four oxidizing equivalents. Thus, the bridging oxos in the OEC may play a role analogous to that proposed for the spectator oxo group in several molybdenum enzymes [89].

An interconversion between di-μ-oxo and peroxy ligation has been suggested for the PS II reaction [21] on the basis of experimental results with Cu_2O_2 dimers where the bridging oxo $\leftrightarrow$ peroxo transformation does occur. In the copper dimers, the bonding within the diamond is weaker than in the manganese dimers. Each of the copper t_{2g} orbitals is doubly occupied and cannot π bond with the bridging oxo ligands. The copper oxidation state is only II, so ionic bonding will also not be as strong. In manganese dimers, the conversion of bridging oxos to a bridging peroxide or oxygen is considerably endothermic, so this process is unlikely to form the basis for photosynthetic oxygen evolution.

In Fe_2O_2 dimers, significant spin density can occur on bridging oxo ligands [72,92] and is likely to be important in the soluble methane mono-oxygenase and in type I ribonucleotide reductase. Neutral Mn dimers, however, have little spin density on the bridging oxo ligands [72].

6.2.   Redox Leveling and Mn-O Bond Strengths

One function of the manganese cluster is to enable the four sequential one-electron processes to be driven by the modest oxidizing power inherent in a phenoxyl radical. By contrast, the uncatalyzed oxidation of water proceeds through intermediates that are strong oxidants, namely, hydrogen peroxide and the hydroxyl radical. In two models of the PS II reaction, one substrate molecule binds, as an aquo ligand, to Mn(II), which then is oxidized to Mn(III)-OH and finally to Mn(IV)=O. What makes the O-H bond energies similar on these two transitions? First, they are both neutral oxidations of manganese. Second, both oxidations remove an electron from an e_g orbital in the octahedral complex. It is not yet clear as to whether binding the substrate to an axial or equatorial position on the Mn_2O_2 unit is important.

It is useful to estimate the strengths of the bonds between manganese and the substrate oxygen atoms, particularly in S_3. Although the possibility that chloride ion and proton migrations occur during the S-state cycle complicates the analysis, it is possible to consider a simplified cycle lacking these migrations. In this cycle, S_0 corresponds to $Mn_A^{III}(Cl)$-OH_2 Mn_B^{II}-OH_2 and S_1 to $Mn_A^{III}(Cl)$-OH_2 Mn_B^{III}-OH, where Mn_A is the upper Mn atom in Fig. 4. This cycle may be relevant at high-turnover rates, whereas chloride migration has been experimentally implicated only at low-turnover rates. The chloride ion and proton migrations must be only weakly driven; therefore the high-turnover S_0 and S_1 structures can be thought of as slightly higher-energy isomers of the structures shown in Fig. 4.

The strength of the Mn_B^{III}-OH bond in S_1 can be estimated from a thermodynamic cycle (Fig. 6). The H-atom transfer reactions to $Y_Z^{\bullet}$ from S_0 or from unligated H_2O are 7 kcal/mol exothermic (from the redox potentials of Table 1) or 33 kcal/mol endothermic, respectively. If the Mn-OH_2 heterolytic bond dissociation energy is taken as 4 kcal/mol (see below), the Mn(III)-OH homolytic BDE is found to be 44 kcal/mol.

The S_1-to-S_2 transition is only 2 kcal/mol exothermic. If we assume that the heterolytic binding energy of water is again 4 kcal/mol, then, by a thermodynamic cycle similar to the one above, the strength of the bond in $Mn_A(IV)$-OH in S_2 is found to be 38 kcal/mol.

To estimate the strength of a possible $Mn(IV)=O$ bond in S_3, we consider the two-step conversion of $Mn_B(II)$-OH_2 to $Mn(III)$-OH and to $Mn(IV)=O$ that may occur during the S_0-to-S_1 and S_2-to-S_3 transitions, which together are exothermic by about 9 kcal/mol. A thermodynamic cycle incorporating these reactions can be evaluated by making the same assumptions as above. Again, the binding energy of water to $Mn(II)$ of 4 kcal/mol enters, as do the O-H bond strengths of Y_Z, H_2O, and $OH^\bullet$, 86, 119, and 102 kcal/mol, respectively. From these values, the BDE of the $Mn(IV)=O$ bond in S_3 is estimated to be 62 kcal/mol.

To check the validity of this estimate, we calculate the energy change of the S_3 $Y_Z^\bullet$ reaction to produce O_2 without rebinding water to S_0. Using $Mn(IV)=O$ and $Mn(IV)$-OH bond energies of 62 and 38 kcal/mol, respectively, this reaction is found to be 3 kcal/mol exother-

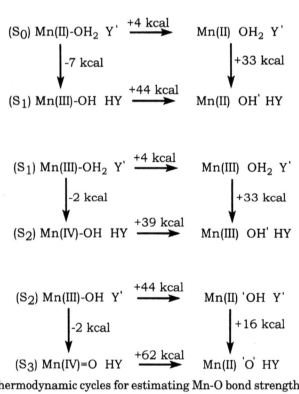

FIG. 6.   Thermodynamic cycles for estimating Mn-O bond strengths (see text).

mic, confirming the reasonableness of the estimates. Consistent with the nature of S_3 as a species about to produce O_2, these Mn-O bonds are quite weak compared to other metal-oxygen bonds [90,91].

The calculations of Mn-O bond strengths illustrate that two separate factors are responsible for the effectiveness of the manganese complex in producing O_2. First, the oxidizing power of $Y_Z^{\bullet}$ is not squandered by allowing the developing Mn-O bonds to become too strong. This is equivalent to saying either that the reduction potential of the manganese must not be too low or that reactive H-OMn bonds must not be too weak. The calculations show that the strengthening of the Mn-O bond resulting from oxidation governs the strength of the H-O bond broken in the reaction with $Y_Z^{\bullet}$. Second, the strength of substrate binding has a direct influence on the strength of product binding. If the substrate were to bind too tightly, the product would be bound too tightly to be released. For that reason, O_2 formation from six-coordinate rather than five-coordinate manganese complexes is likely to be strongly favored.

6.3. The S_0 State

The models of the S-state cycle described above all suppose a substrate molecule to be bound to manganese in S_0. Water binding to Mn(III) complexes has been modeled quantum mechanically, and it is found that a six-coordinate aquo complex is comparable in energy to a five-coordinate complex containing a hydrogen-bonded water molecule in the second coordination sphere [92]. The results suggest the dative H_2O-Mn(III) bond to be worth, at most, 5 kcal/mol. The rapid water-exchange rates observed in S_0 are consistent with weak binding and a rapid conversion between five- and six-coordinate manganese, as is observed for related manganese complexes [93]. The ultimate release of O_2 is likely, also, to involve these two stable coordination geometries. The properties of Mn(II) in an oxo-bridged dimer are not so well understood, and four and five coordination may be competitive, so that the catalytic Mn(II) atom in S_0 may be five coordinate with a water molecule bound that exchanges rapidly. It is also possible that a bridging oxo ligand is protonated in S_0 [21].

An EPR spectrum of the S_0 state has recently been observed, but so far only when methanol has been added to the suspending medium

[94–97]. It is a multiline spectrum with $g = 2$ and an overall width exceeding that of the S_2 spectrum. It is not yet known as to why native S_0 gives no multiline spectrum or how methanol enables the spectrum to be detected. The width of the S_0 EPR spectrum suggests the presence of an Mn(II), in addition to one Mn(III) and two Mn(IV) [94,95]. This assignment is favored over three Mn(III) and one Mn(IV), because Mn(II) has a higher intrinsic hyperfine coupling than do the other two oxidation states.

6.4. The S_1 State

S_1 is the state most stable in the dark, so it is most easily studied, but it has no conventional EPR spectrum. By using parallel-mode EPR, however, two different S_1 spectra have been observed. One, at $g = 4.8$, has no hyperfine structure [98,99], but a second signal with $g = 12$ does have manganese hyperfine structure [100].

Several of the mechanisms proposed above suggest that the S_0-to-S_1 transition corresponds to loss of a hydrogen atom from an Mn(II)-OH_2. As shown in Fig. 4, an Mn(III)-OH would result and could be the species, if five coordinate, that exchanges its substrate oxygen with bulk water very slowly (Table 2).

The S_1-to-S_2 transition corresponds to oxidation of an Mn(III) to Mn(IV). The reaction induced by $Y_Z^{\bullet}$ is only about 2 kcal/mol exothermic. An important question is whether the manganese cluster acquires a positive charge on this transition.

The above arguments rule out the possibility that the OEC functions as charge accumulator on each step but not the possibility that one of the S-state transitions does store a positive charge. An increase of positive charge on the cluster specifically on the $S_1 \rightarrow S_2$ transition has been proposed from proton-release patterns, local electrochromic absorbance measurements, and the kinetics of P_{680}^+ reduction. Such a charge increase would probably cause significant differences between the $S_1 \rightarrow S_2$ and $S_2 \rightarrow S_3$ transitions. The XANES edge shifts and $Y_Z^{\bullet}$ reduction kinetics are quite similar on the two transitions and suggest, instead, that there is no charge increase on $S_1 \rightarrow S_2$. Furthermore, the reduction potentials of the S_3/S_2 and S_2/S_1 couples are quite similar [101], which is hard to explain except by supposing that both transitions are electrically neutral [71,73].

TABLE 2

Substrate Exchange
Rates

State	R_1	R_2
S_0	>100	>100
S_1	0.02	>100
S_2	2	>175
S_3	2	40

[a]Exchange is measured at
10°C. Rates are in units of s^{-1}.

6.5.   The S_2 State

The S_2 state is uniquely sensitive to chloride depletion, calcium depletion, and treatment with amines. These treatments all inhibit the S-
state cycle such that $Y_Z^{\bullet}$ does not efficiently oxidize the S_2 state. It may
be, however, that the S_2-to-S_3 oxidation can occur in the absence of chloride, although at a reduced rate [102].

These observations can be explained by the hypothesis that chlo-
ride is a ligand to the catalytic manganese atom from which $Y_Z^{\bullet}$ abstracts
H atoms. Removal of the chloride ion causes the abstractable proton to
be lost and converts a terminal hydroxo ligand to an oxo. Because of geometrical constraints, H-atom transfer to $Y_Z^{\bullet}$ requires there be a proton
on the closer catalytic manganese atom, and the reaction is frustrated
if the proton is absent. The binding of chloride may be facilitated by an
ionic interaction with the calcium ion, consistent with steady-state kinetics that indicate calcium binding precedes chloride binding [103]. A
small rate of S-state advance would be allowed by a small equilibrium
concentration of a geminal dihydroxo species, in which chloride is replaced by hydroxide.

The S_2-to-S_3 transition has the highest activation energy of all the
$S_i Y_Z^{\bullet}$ reactions [104,105]. A simple explanation is that the more distant
catalytic manganese atom is involved, and its ligand is too far away to
donate a hydrogen atom directly to $Y_Z^{\bullet}$. The hydrogen-atom transfer
might be mediated by the hydroxo ligand bound to the nearer catalytic

manganese atom that is not oxidized on S_2 to S_3. Such mediated H-atom transfers have been studied theoretically [106] and have reasonable activation energies.

6.6. The S_3 State

Several models for the S_3 state include a terminal oxo ligand to one of the catalytic manganese atoms. Here we consider the properties of manganyl bonds and the evidence regarding the presence of a terminal oxo group in the OEC.

Based on the usual valence of oxygen, one expects that a terminal oxo ligand will form two bonds with its metal atom. One of these is a normal covalent σ bond. Augmenting this are two half-bonds derived from the oxygen $2p_x$ and $2p_y$ orbitals and the manganese $3d_{xz}$ and $3d_{yz}$ orbitals, respectively. (We take the z axis along the Mn-O internuclear axis.) Each pair of interacting π orbitals contains three electrons, giving a bond order of 1/2. The unpaired electrons largely belong to the manganese, but the mixing of orbitals puts a spin on the oxygen of about 0.2–0.3 [92], and the oxygen obtains a Mulliken charge of about -0.4 [72]. This type of covalent double bond is clearly different from the double bonds of alkenes and carbonyl compounds but is similar to the double bond in dioxygen itself.

Another useful model for the Mn=O bond is the semipolar N-O bond of amine oxides. Ab initio calculations suggest a covalent N-O bond order close to 1, which is augmented by an ionic attraction between the negatively charged oxygen and the positively charged atoms around the nitrogen. The N-O bonds in amine oxides are weak, probably less than 50 kcal/mol. A number of organic N-oxides where resonance stabilization is possible have dissociation energies between 53 and 83 kcal/mol [88]. These bonds are weak because the nitrogen orbitals required for π bonding to the oxygen are used for bonding to other atoms.

Manganese-oxo compounds become more reactive when a strong base coordinates trans to the oxo (see [83]). In theoretical studies of related compounds, the ligand trans to the oxo tends to come off, and the remaining ligands distort toward a trigonal bipyramidal arrangement [92]. Clearly, one way for the OEC to keep a terminal O=Mn bond weak is to prevent the stabilizing loss of the trans ligand by arranging that ligand to be a strong base, such as the imidazole ring of histidine [83].

One histidine ligand has been identified and may be present in the OEC for this reason.

Vibrational spectroscopy has the potential to provide evidence of a manganese oxo bond [107], but results are not yet available. XAFS measurements may be relevant to this question, because they suggest that one of the Mn-Mn distances increases on the S_2-to-S_3 transition from 2.7 to about 2.9 Å. A similar effect is seen in the g = 4.1 S_2 state. These observations could be due to formation of a terminal oxo ligand perpendicular to the Mn_2O_2 plane. In this position, the $2p_x$ and $2p_y$ orbitals of the oxygen ligand would overlap with the manganese d_{xz} and d_{yz} orbitals involved in intradimer π bonding. Doing so would weaken and lengthen the bonds within the Mn_2O_2 unit and could cause a shift to ferromagnetic coupling within the dimer and produce a high-spin ground state. Protonation of a bridging oxo ligand would also lead to lengthening of the Mn-Mn distance [21], but this is unlikely to occur in S_3 because the bridging oxos become less basic as the manganese oxidation state increases.

Formation of an oxo in S_3 is expected to slow the rate of substrate oxygen exchange with solvent, and this is observed (Table 2), although the exchange rate obtained is faster than that in S_1. It may be that a relatively fast-exchanging oxo in S_3 is bound to a manganese with an additional water ligand, while the slowly exchanging OH in S_1 has no adjacent water ligands.

6.7.   O-O Bond Formation

The S-state cycle models described above include detailed descriptions of how an oxygen-oxygen bond might form. Three of these suggest radical mechanisms and two suggest a nonradical mechanism. Two of them include a peroxo intermediate with a significant lifetime. As described above, the weakness of the O-O bond in peroxides makes these species thermodynamically difficult to form and, as a result, they are kinetically labile. On the other hand, formation of O_2 from water in one step is a four-electron process, and such a redox process may be unfavorable because of the possibility of a high reorganization energy. However, by use of several one-electron acceptors, it is possible for a multielectron process to have an acceptably low reorganization energy [108]. Furthermore, the tendency to describe the chemistry of the OEC, in terms of manganese oxidation states, obscures the strongly covalent character of the Mn-O bonds [87,92], which is an additional mitigating factor that may allow O_2 formation to proceed in a process that is formally four electron.

Regardless of whether a peroxide intermediate occurs, it is important to describe the formation of the O-O σ bond and π bond separately. The σ bond in peroxides is weak and, for energetic reasons, its formation will limit the overall rate of O_2 production. In PS II, where O_2 formation does occur rapidly, there are unlikely to be any additional kinetic impediments to formation of this σ bond. Therefore, we expect the reaction to be spin-allowed, orbital-symmetry-allowed, and adiabatic. The radical mechanisms described above satisfy these expectations. The nonradical reaction of an electrophilic Mn(V)=O with a nucleophilic hydroxide would likely result first in a low-spin manganese product. For a mononuclear Mn(V) complex, the initial low-spin product would be an excited state of Mn(III), and a nucleophilic reaction would be disfavored. For an Mn(IV,V) dimer, however, the product could be a low-spin, ground state of an Mn(III,IV) dimer, making a nucleophilic reaction possible.

The tyrosyl [80] and cyclic [81] radical mechanisms for O-O bond formation are similar in some ways. The reactions are built from atom or group transfer and addition reactions, familiar in radical organic chemistry, and, in particular, they both involve a hydrogen-atom transfer. Both involve concerted reactions in which two covalent bonds are formed and two are consumed, although, in the cyclic mechanism, one of the consumed bonds does persist as a dative Mn-O bond. The transition states show delocalization of the spin density. In the cyclic reaction, all five atoms in the cycle have some spin, and this may help give this reaction a relatively low activation energy. In the tyrosyl mechanism, the spin density is expected primarily where it is most stable: on the tyrosine, on the manganyl manganese, and to a lesser extent on the oxygen of a hydroxo ligand.

The two radical mechanisms differ in that one proposes a manganese(III) hydroperoxide intermediate. As noted above, such a species is expected to be reactive. The homolytic cleavage of the O-O bonds of alkyl hydroperoxides by Mn(III) compounds with production of alkoxy radicals has been reported [109]. The proposed PS II intermediate would also react homolytically by abstracting hydrogen atoms from the surrounding protein.

The tyrosyl mechanism avoids this problem by delaying O-O bond formation until the S_3-to-S_0 transition. We envision a concerted reaction composed of the two radical reactions that separately are described as, first, the H-atom transfer to $Y_Z^\bullet$ from Mn-O-H to give an oxyl radical (Mn-O$^\bullet$), and, second, the addition of that oxyl radical to the O=Mn bond (Fig. 5). In the concerted reaction, the oxyl radical is not a discrete intermediate, but the transition state would have some spin density on that particular oxygen atom, giving it partial radical character. The energy of the product state, Mn(III)-O-O-Mn(IV), can be estimated as the sum of the excitation energy of Mn(IV)=O (20 kcal/mol [92]) and the energy to produce Mn(IV)-O$^\bullet$ (20 kcal/mol [81]) minus the O-O bond energy. If the last quantity is about 35 kcal/mol, as in organic peroxides, then the concerted reaction to produce the peroxide is about 5 kcal/mol endothermic. This is less than the actual activation energy of 9 kcal/mol for the S_3 $Y_Z^\bullet$ reaction and lends support to this proposed mechanism.

7. CONCLUSIONS

Beginning with the recognition of the S-state cycle and the first true molecular mechanisms for water oxidation in PS II [5,23,79], research on the chemistry of the oxygen-evolving process has progressed significantly. Molecular structures for the Mn_4 cluster, although still a matter of considerable discussion and debate, have emerged, and a fundamental role of the tyrosyl radical in the overall process has been recognized. Small-molecule, model-compound studies and, more recently, sophisticated quantum-chemical calculations have been invaluable in propelling progress in deciphering how plants produce O_2 with remarkably small overall driving forces. Progress continues to accelerate, as the principal factors that control tyrosyl radical, manganese, and ligand energetics and reactivity are being elucidated. This chapter has aimed at documenting this progress and at illuminating promising directions for future work.

ACKNOWLEDGMENTS

NIH GM37300 and the USDA Office of Competitive Research Grants supported the work that was performed at Michigan State and described above. We thank Drs. Margareta Blomberg, Dave Britt, Gary

Brudvig, Rick Debus, Bruce Diner, Wolfgang Junge, Jim Mayer, Vince Pecoraro, Fabrice Rapapport, Gernot Renger, Per Siegbahn, Cecilia Tommos, and Charlie Yocum for illuminating discussions on the mechanism of water oxidation in photosynthesis.

ABBREVIATIONS

ATP	adenosine 5'-triphosphate
BDE	bond dissociation energy
D1, D2	polypeptides of the PS II reaction center
ENDOR	electron nuclear double resonance
EPR	electron paramagnetic resonance
ESEEM	electron spin-echo envelope modulation
FTIR	Fourier transform infrared
OEC	oxygen-evolving complex
PS II	Photosystem II
P_{680}	primary electron donor of PS II; its absorbance maximum is at 680 nm
RC	photochemical reaction center
Tris	tris(hydroxymethyl)methylamine
XAFS	X-ray absorbance fine-structure spectroscopy
XANES	X-ray absorbance near-edge spectroscopy

REFERENCES

1. R. J. Debus, this volume, Chapter 20.

2. D. F. Ghanotakis and C. F. Yocum, *Annu. Rev. Plant Phys. Plant Mol. Biol.*, *41*, 255–276 (1990).

3. A.-F. Miller and G. W. Brudvig, *Biochim. Biophys. Act*, *1056*, 1–18 (1991).

4. J. H. A. Nugent, *Eur. J. Biochem.*, *237*, 519–531 (1996).

5. B. Kok, B. Forbush, M. McGloin, *Photochem. Photobiol.*, *11*, 457–475 (1970).

6. G. C. Dismukes and Y. Siderer, *Proc. Natl. Acad. Sci. USA*, *78*, 274–278 (1981).

7. B. A. Diner and G. T. Babcock, in *Advances in Photosynthesis Oxygenic Photosynthesis: The Light Reactions* (D. R. Ort and C. F. Yocum, eds.), Kluwer Academics, Dordrecht, 1996, pp. 213–247.

8. C. Tommos and G. T. Babcock, *Biochim. Biophys. Act*, submitted.

9. R. J. Debus, *Biochim. Biophys. Act, 1102*, 269–352 (1992).

10. P. R. Gorham and K. A. Clendenning, *Arch. Biochem. Biophys., 37*, 199–223 (1952).

11. P. H. Homann, *Biochim. Biophys. Act, 809*, 311–319 (1985).

12. H. Wincencjusz, H. J. van Gorkom, and C. F. Yocum, *Biochemistry, 36*, 3663–3670 (1997).

13. K. Lindberg, T. Vänngård, and L. E. Andréasson, *Photosyn. Res., 38*, 410–408 (1993).

14. C. F. Yocum, *Biochim. Biophys. Act, 1059*, 1–15 (1991).

15. A. Boussac, J.-L. Zimmermann, A. W. Rutherford, and J. Lavergne, *Nature, 347*, 303–306 (1990).

16. M. L. Gilchrist, J. A. Ball, D. W. Randall, and R. D. Britt, *Proc. Natl. Acad. Sci. USA, 92*, 9545–9549 (1995).

17. J. M. Peloquin, K. A. Campbell, and R. D. Britt, *J. Am. Chem. Soc., 120* 6840–6841 (1998).

18. K. H. Rhee, E. P. Morris, J. Barber, and W. Kühlbrandt, *Nature, 396* 283–286 (1998).

19. J. Deisenhofer, O. Epp, K. Miki, R. Huber, and H. Michel, *Nature, 318* 618–624 (1985).

20. G. T. Babcock, B. A. Barry, R. J. Debus, C. W. Hoganson, M. Atamian, L. McIntosh, I. Sithole, and C. F. Yocum, *Biochemistry, 28*, 9557–9565 (1989).

21. V. K. Yachandra, K. Sauer, and M. P. Klein, *Chem. Rev., 96*, 2927–2950 (1996).

22. J. E. Penner-Hahn, in *Structure and Bonding*, Vol. 90 (H. A. O. Hill, P. J. Sadler, and A. J. Thomson, eds.), Springer-Verlag, Berlin, 1998, pp. 1–36.

23. R. D. Britt, in *Advances in Photosynthesis Oxygenic Photosynthesis: The Light Reactions* (D. R. Ort and C. F. Yocum, eds.), Kluwer Academics, Dordrecht, 1996, pp. 137–164.

24. N. A. Law, M. T. Caudle, and V. L. Pecoraro, *Adv. Inorg. Chem., 46*, 305–440 (1999).

25. D. W. Randall, B. E. Sturgeon, J. A. Ball, G. A. Lorigan, M. K.

Chan, M. P. Klein, W. H. Armstrong, and R. D. Britt, *J. Am. Chem. Soc.*, *117*, 11780–11789 (1995).

26. A. Haddy, W. R. Dunham, R. H. Sands, and R. Aasa, *Biochim. Biophys. Act*, *1099*, 25–34 (1992).

27. R. Manchanda, G. W. Brudvig, and R. H. Crabtree, *Coord. Chem. Rev.*, *144*, 1–38 (1995).

28. R. M. Cinco, J. H. Robblee, A. Rompel, C. Fernandez, V. K. Yachandra, K. Sauer, and M. P. Klein, *J. Phys. Chem. B*, *102*, 8248–8256 (1998).

29. X.-S. Tang, B. A. Diner, B. S. Larsen, M. L. Gilchrist, and R. D. Britt, *Proc. Natl. Acad. Sci. USA*, *91*, 704–708 (1994).

30. T. Noguchi, T. Ono, and Y. Inoue, *Biochim. Biophys. Act*, *1228*, 189–200 (1995).

31. T. Noguchi, T. Ono, and Y. Inoue, *Biochim. Biophys. Act*, *1232*, 56–66 (1995).

32. P. O. Sandusky and C. F. Yocum, *Biochim. Biophys. Act*, *849*, 85–93 (1986).

33. H. Wincencjusz, C. F. Yocum, and H. J. van Gorkom, *Biochemistry*, *37*, 8595–8604 (1998).

34. C. W. Hoganson and G. T. Babcock, *Biochemistry*, *27*, 5848–5855 (1988).

35. R. A. Roffey, D. M. Kramer, Govindjee, and R. T. Sayre, *Biochim. Biophys. Act*, *1185*, 257–270 (1994).

36. H.-A. Chu, A. P. Nguyen, and R. J. Debus, *Biochemistry*, *34*, 5839–5858 (1995).

37. A.-M. A. Hays, I. R. Vassiliev, J. H. Golbeck, and R. J. Debus, *Biochemistry*, *37*, 11352–11365 (1998).

38. F. Mamedov, R. T. Sayre, and S. Styring, *Biochemistry*, *37*, 14245–14256 (1998).

39. B. A. Diner, D. A. Force, D. W. Randall, and R. D. Britt, *Biochemistry*, *37*, 17931–17943 (1998).

40. M. Haumann, A. Mulkidjanian, and W. Junge, *Biochemistry*, *38*, 1258–1267 (1999).

41. L. P. Candeias, S. Turconi, and J. H. A. Nugent, *Biochim. Biophys. Act*, *1363*, 1–5 (1998).

42. M. R. A. Blomberg, P. E. M. Siegbahn, and G. T. Babcock, *J. Am. Chem. Soc.*, *120*, 8812–8824 (1998).

43. P. J. O'Malley, *J. Am. Chem. Soc.*, *120*, 11732–11738 (1998).

44. P. Dorlet, M. Di Valentin, G. T. Babcock, and J. McCracken, *J. Phys. Chem. B*, *102*, 8239–8249 (1998).

45. V. A. Szalai, H. Kühne, K. V. Lakshmi, and G. W. Brudvig, *Biochemistry*, *37*, 13594–13603 (1998).

46. P. J. Van Leeuwen, C. Heimann, P. Gast, J. P. Dekker, H. J. Van Gorkom, *Photosynthesis Research*, *34*, 145–145 (1992).

47. K. Hasegawa, M. Kusunoki, Y. Inoue, and T. Ono, *Biochemistry*, *37*, 9457–9465 (1998).

48. M. Zheng and G. C. Dismukes, *Inorg. Chem.*, *35*, 3307–3319 (1996).

49. T. Ono, T. Noguchi, Y. Inoue, M. Kusunoki, T. Matsushita, and H. Oyanagi, *Science*, *258*, 1335–1337 (1992).

50. T. A. Roelofs, W. Liang, M. J. Latimer, R. M. Cinco, A. Rompel, J. C. Andrews, K. Sauer, V. K. Yachandra, and M. P. Klein, *Proc. Natl. Acad. Sci. USA*, *93*, 3335–3340 (1996).

51. L. Iuzzolini, J. Dittmer, W. Dörner, W. Meyer-Klaucke, and H. Dau, *Biochemistry*, *37*, 17112–17119 (1998).

52. W. Hillier, J. Messinger, and T. Wydrzynski, *Biochemistry*, *37*, 16908–16914 (1998).

53. W. Hillier and T. Wydrzynski, personal communication.

54. J. Lavergne and W. Junge, *Photosyn. Res.*, *38*, 279–296 (1993).

55. F. Rappaport, M. Blanchard-Desce, and J. Lavergne, *Biochim. Biophys. Act*, *1184*, 178–192 (1994).

56. M. Haumann, O. Bogershausen, and W. Junge, *FEBS Lett.*, *355*, 101 (1994).

57. H. Kretschmann, E. Schlodder, and H. T. Witt, *Biochim. Biophys. Act*, *1274*, 1–8 (1996).

58. C. Tommos, C. W. Hoganson, M. Di Valentin, N. Lydakis-Simantiris, P. Dorlet, K. Westphal, H.-A. Chu, J. McCracken, and G. T. Babcock, *Curr. Opin. Chem. Biol.*, *2*, 244–252 (1998).

59. M. Haumann and W. Junge, *Biochemistry*, *33*, 864–872 (1994).

60. C. W. Hoganson, N. Lydakis-Simantiris, X.-S. Tang, C. Tommos, K. Warncke, G. T. Babcock, B. A. Diner, J. McCracken, and S. Styring, *Photosyn. Res.*, *46*, 177–184 (1995).

61. H. T. Witt, *Ber. Bunsenges.*, *100*, 1923–1942 (1996).

62. G. Christen, F. Reifarth, and G. Renger, *FEBS Lett.*, *429*, 49–52 (1998).

63. G. Christen and G. Renger, *Biochemistry*, *38*, 2068–2077 (1999).

64. M. J. Schilstra, F. Rappaport, J. H. A. Nugent, C. J. Barnett, and D. R. Klug, *Biochemistry, 37,* 3974–3981 (1998).

65. G. Christen, A. Seeliger, and G. Renger, *Biochemistry,* in press.

66. M. R. Razeghifard and R. J. Pace, *Biochemistry, 38,* 1252–1257 (1999).

67. E. Schlodder, K. Brettel, and H. T. Witt, *Biochim. Biophys. Acta, 808,* 123–131 (1985).

68. C. Tommos and G. T. Babcock, *Acct. Chem. Res., 31,* 18–25 (1998).

69. L. I. Krishtalik, *Biochim. Biophys. Act, 849,* 162–171 (1986).

70. M. J. Baldwin and V. L. Pecoraro, *J. Am. Chem. Soc., 118,* 11325–11326 (1996).

71. M. T. Caudle and V. L. Pecoraro, *J. Am. Chem. Soc., 119,* 3415–3416 (1997).

72. M. R. A. Blomberg, P. E. M. Siegbahn, S. Styring, G. T. Babcock, B. Åkermark, and P. Korall, *J. Am. Chem. Soc., 119,* 8285–8292 (1997).

73. V. L. Pecoraro, M. J. Baldwin, M. T. Caudle, W.-Y. Hsieh, and N. A. Law, *Pure Appl. Chem., 70,* 925–929 (1998).

74. H. H. Thorp, J. E. Sarneski, G. W. Brudvig, and R. H. Crabtree, *J. Am. Chem. Soc., 111,* 9249–9250 (1989).

75. O. Horner, E. Anxolabehere-Mallart, M.-F. Charlot, L. Tchertanov, J. Guilhem, T.A. Mattioli, A. Boussac, and J.-J. Girerd, *Inorg. Chem., 38,* 1222–1232 (1999).

76. G. T. Babcock, in *Photosynthesis: from Light to Biosphere,* Vol. 2, (P. Mathis, ed.), Kluwer Academic, Dordrecht, 1995, pp. 209–215.

77. G. T. Babcock, M. Espe, C. W. Hoganson, N. Lydakis-Simantiris, J. McCracken, W. Shi, S. Styring, C. Tommos, and K. Warncke, *Acta Chem. Scand., 51,* 533–540 (1997).

78. J. Stubbe and W. A. van der Donk, *Chem. Rev., 98,* 705–762 (1998).

79. G. W. Brudvig and R. H. Crabtree, *Proc. Natl. Acad. Sci. USA, 83,* 4586–4588 (1985).

80. C. W. Hoganson and G. T. Babcock, *Science, 253,* 1953–1956 (1997).

81. P. E. M. Siegbahn and R. H. Crabtree, *J. Am. Chem. Soc., 121,* 117–127 (1999).

82. G. C. Dismukes, *Chem. Rev., 96,* 2909–2926 (1996).

83. J. Limburg, V. A. Szalai, and G. W. Brudvig, *J. Chem. Soc., Dalton Trans.*, in press.

84. Y. Naruta, M. Sasayama, and T. Sasaki, *Angew. Chem. Int. Ed. Engl.*, *33*, 1839 (1994).

85. J. Limburg, M. S. Vrettos, L. M. Liable-Sands, A. L. Rheingold, R. H. Crabtree, and G. W. Brudvig, *Science*, *283*, 1524–1527 (1999).

86. D. M. Proserpio, R. Hoffman, and G. C. Dismukes, *J. Am. Chem. Soc.*, *114*, 4374–4382 (1992).

87. X. G. Zhao, W. H. Richardson, J.-L. Chen, J. Li, L. Noodleman, H.-L. Tsai, and D. N. Hendrickson, *Inorg. Chem.*, *36*, 1198–1217 (1997).

88. W. Rüttinger and G. C. Dismukes, *Chem. Rev.*, *97*, 1–24 (1997).

89. R. Hille, *Chem. Rev.*, *96*, 2757–2816 (1996).

90. R. H. Holm and J. P. Donahue, *Polyhedron*, *12*, 571–589 (1993).

91. O. González-Blanco, V. Branchadell, K. Monteyne, and T. Ziegler, *Inorg. Chem.*, *37*, 1744–1748 (1998).

92. M. R. A. Blomberg and P. E. M. Siegbahn, *Theor. Chem. Acta*, *97*, 72–80 (1997).

93. V. L. Pecoraro, *Photochem. Photobiol.*, *48*, 249–264 (1988).

94. J. Messinger, J. H. A. Nugent, and M. C. W. Evans, *Biochemistry*, *36*, 11055–11060 (1997).

95. K. A. Åhrling, S. Peterson, and S. Styring, *Biochemistry*, *36*, 13148–13152 (1997).

96. J. Messinger, J. H. Robblee, W. O. Yu, K. Sauer, V. K. Yachandra, and M. P. Klein, *J. Am. Chem. Soc.*, *119*, 11349–11350 (1997).

97. K. A. Åhrling, S. Peterson, and S. Styring, *Biochemistry*, *37*, 8115–8120 (1998).

98. S. L. Dexheimer and M. P. Klein, *J. Am. Chem. Soc.*, *114*, 2821–2826 (1992).

99. T. Yamauchi, H. Mino, T. Matsukawa, A. Kawamori, and T. Ono, *Biochemistry*, *36*, 7520–7526 (1997).

100. K. A. Campbell, W. Gregor, D. P. Pham, J. M. Peloquin, R. J. Debus, and R. D. Britt, *Biochemistry*, *37*, 5039–5045 (1998).

101. I. Vass and S. Styring, *Biochemistry*, *30*, 830–839 (1991).

102. K. Lindberg and L.-E. Andréasson, *Biochemistry*, *35*, 14259 (1996).

103. C. M. Waggoner, V. L. Pecoraro, and C. F. Yocum, *FEBS Lett.*, *244*, 237–240 (1989).

104. G. Renger and B. Hanssum, *FEBS Lett.*, *299*, 28–32 (1992).

105. M. Karge, K.-D. Irrgang, and G. Renger, *Biochemistry*, *36*, 8904–8913 (1997).

106. P. E. M. Siegbahn, M. R. A. Blomberg, and R. H. Crabtree, *Theor. Chem. Acta*, *97*, 289–300 (1997).

107. H.-A. Chu, M. T. Gardner, J. P. O'Brien, and G. T. Babcock, *Biochemistry*, *38*, 4533–4541 (1999).

108. L. I. Krishtalik, *Bioelectrochem. Bioenerg.*, *23*, 249–263 (1990).

109. M. T. Caudle, P. Riggs-Gelasco, A. K. Gelasco, J. E. Penner-Hahn, and V. L. Pecoraro, *Inorg. Chem.*, *35*, 3577–3584 (1996).

110. J. E. McGrady and R. Stranger, *J. Am. Chem. Soc.*, *119*, 8512–8522.

20

The Polypeptides of Photosystem II and Their Influence on Manganotyrosyl-Based Oxygen Evolution

Richard J. Debus

Department of Biochemistry,
University of California at Riverside,
Riverside, CA 92521-0129, USA

1. INTRODUCTION

Photosynthetic water oxidation is the source of nearly all oxygen in the atmosphere and is the indirect source of nearly all biomass on Earth. Photosynthetic water oxidation takes place in Photosystem II (PS II) near the lumenal surface of the thylakoid membranes in plants, algae, and cyanobacteria. Photosystem II is an integral membrane protein complex that utilizes solar energy to reduce plastoquinone and to extract electrons and protons from water. The catalytic site for water oxidation contains four Mn ions that are arranged in a multinuclear cluster. This cluster accumulates oxidizing equivalents in response to photochemical events within PS II, then catalyzes the oxidation of two molecules of water, releasing one molecule of O_2 as a byproduct. During each catalytic cycle, two plastoquinone molecules are reduced and protonated, four protons are removed from the stroma, and four protons are deposited into the lumen. These protons contribute to the transmembrane proton gradient that is utilized for ATP formation. By forming plastoquinol and contributing to the transmembrane proton gradient, PS II provides the reducing equivalents and much of the electrochemical potential that is required for the synthesis of organic compounds from carbon dioxide. For general reviews on water oxidation in PS II, see [1–6] and Chap. 19 of this volume.

1.1. The Cofactors of Photosystem II

The photochemical events that precede water oxidation are initiated by the capture of light by an array of light-harvesting pigments that are located in proteins peripheral to the PS II core. The excitation energy is transferred to the photochemically active chlorophyll species known as P_{680} (Fig. 1). This species may be a weakly coupled multimer of up to four chlorophyll a and two pheophytin a molecules [7], although the $P_{680}^{\bullet+}$ cation is probably localized on two chlorophyll a molecules [8,9]. Excitation of P_{680} results in formation of the charge-separated state, $P_{680}^{\bullet+}Pheo^{\bullet-}$. This separation of charge is stabilized by the rapid oxidation of $Pheo^{\bullet-}$ by a plastoquinone-9 molecule, Q_A, and by the rapid re-

PHOTOSYSTEM II

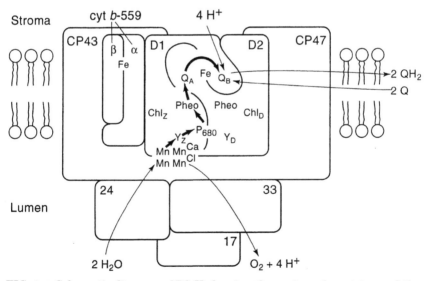

FIG. 1.   Schematic diagram of PS II showing the major *psb* proteins and the electron transfer cofactors. Heavy arrows show the direction of electron flow. (Modified from [1], copyright 1992, by permission of Elsevier Science.)

duction of $P_{680}^{\bullet+}$ by a nearby tyrosine residue, Y_Z [3]. The oxidized form of Y_Z is the neutral tyrosine radical, $Y_Z^\bullet$. Subsequently, $Q_A^{\bullet-}$ reduces a second plastoquinone molecule, Q_B, and $Y_Z^\bullet$ oxidizes the Mn cluster. A second light-induced charge separation results in further oxidation of the Mn cluster and in the reduction and protonation of $Q_B^{\bullet-}$ to form the Q_BH_2 plastoquinol. The latter exchanges out of PS II and is replaced by another molecule of plastoquinone from the membrane-bound plastoquinone pool. Both $Q_A^{\bullet-}$ and $Q_B^{\bullet-}$ are magnetically coupled to an atom of nonheme iron.

The oxidation of two water molecules requires four oxidizing equivalents. Consequently, four light-induced charge separations take place during each catalytic cycle and the Mn cluster cycles through five oxidation states. These states are termed S_n, where n denotes the number of oxidizing equivalents stored by the Mn cluster. The S_1 state predominates in dark-adapted samples and probably consists of two Mn(III) and two Mn(IV) ions [1–6]. The S_3 state may have one oxidizing equivalent localized on an Mn ligand: whether or not an Mn ion is oxidized during the $S_2 \rightarrow S_3$ transition is currently under debate (e.g., see [10] vs. [11]). The S_4 state is a transient intermediate that reverts to the S_0 state with the concomitant release of O_2.

The Mn cluster is a magnetically coupled tetramer [12,13]. On the basis of extended X-ray absorption fine structure (EXAFS) data, the Mn cluster has been proposed to be arranged as a bridged pair of di-μ_2-oxo bridged Mn dimers [4,14]. This structure is compatible with data showing that two of the Mn ions are more labile than the others [15,16] and with data suggesting that exogenous reductants attack different sites in the Mn cluster [17,18]. However, this structure may be incompatible with magnetic resonance studies of the S_2 state [19]. Other structures are compatible with the EXAFS data [4] and may need further consideration [6]. One Ca^{2+} ion [20,21] and one Cl^- ion [22] are required for catalytic activity and are believed to be located in the vicinity of the Mn cluster.

Other electron transfer cofactors in PS II are Chl_Z (a redox-active monomeric chlorophyll a molecule), Chl_D (a redox-inactive monomeric chlorophyll a molecule), tyrosine Y_D, and cytochrome b-559, and one molecule of carotenoid (Car). Tyrosine Y_D and Car are oxidized by $P_{680}^{\bullet+}$ in competition with Y_Z [23–25,334]. The function of Y_D and Chl_D are unknown. Cytochrome b-559 and Chl_Z reduce $Car^{\bullet+}$ [334] and all three species may be involved in protecting PS II against photoinduced damage (for a discussion of $Chl_Z^{\bullet+}$ in this role, see [27–29]; for reviews of cytochrome b-559 in this role, see [28–30]; for the possible participation of $Car^{\bullet+}$ in this role, see [334]).

Recent data show that $Y_Z^\bullet$ is located close to the Mn cluster. Simulations of electron paramagnetic resonance (EPR) and electron nuclear double resonance (ENDOR) data from inhibited samples trapped in the $S_2Y_Z^\bullet$ state has yielded an Mn-$Y_Z^\bullet$ point-dipole distance of ≈ 8 Å [13,31,32]. This distance is consistent with a geometrical center-to-center distance of ≈ 9 Å between Y_Z and the Mn cluster and is consistent with a hydrogen bond existing between Y_Z and an Mn-bound water molecule [33]. These data, plus data showing that $Y_Z^\bullet$ is rotationally mobile [34–36], have led to new models for the mechanism of water oxidation in PS II. These models postulate that Y_Z participates directly in water oxidation by abstracting protons [2,36] or hydrogen atoms [33–35,37–41] from water-derived ligands of the Mn cluster. Whether these abstractions occur during all of the S-state transitions [34,35, 37–40], only the $S_2 \rightarrow S_3$ and $S_3 \rightarrow (S_4) \rightarrow S_0$ transitions [2,33], or only the $S_2 \rightarrow S_3$ transition [41] is currently under debate. These models are described in detail in Chap. 19 of this volume.

2.   THE POLYPEPTIDES OF PHOTOSYSTEM II

The PS II complex in vivo contains nearly 30 different polypeptides, including those involved in light harvesting (for review, see [1,42–44]). About 25 of these polypeptides are the PS II core proteins and are encoded by the psb genes. Most of the psb genes are located on the chloroplast genome. The light-harvesting polypeptides of higher plants are the chlorophyll a/b proteins. These are LHC II and the minor chlorophyll proteins, CP29, CP26, and CP24 (for review, see [45–49]). These are encoded on the nuclear genome by the six $lhcb$ genes. The light-harvesting polypeptides of green algae and most other lower plants are similar to those of higher plants [46,47]. The light-harvesting proteins of cyanobacteria and eukaryotic red algae are the phycobiliproteins. These are water-soluble proteins with covalently attached linear tetrapyrrole pigments known as phycobilins. The phycobiliproteins and associated linker polypeptides form phycobilisomes, complexes that are located on the stromal surface of the thylakoid membrane [50,51]. The phycobili-proteins and linker polypeptides are encoded by the *apc* and *cpc* genes.

2.1. The Antenna Proteins, LHC II, CP29, CP26, and CP24

Single-particle image averaging [44,52–55] and electron crystallogra-phy [56–60] show that PS II in higher plants is dimeric and has twofold rotational symmetry (for review, see [44,59,61]). Biochemical data sup-port this conclusion [53,62,63]. Photosystem II is also dimeric in cyanobacteria [52,64–67], with one phycobilisome associating with each dimer [64]. In higher plants, the *psb*-encoded proteins of the PS II core are surrounded by single copies of CP29, CP26, CP24, and by one to four LHC II trimers. The best characterized dimeric PS II–LHC II complex contains one copy each of CP29 and CP26 and one LHC II trimer per PS II monomeric unit, with CP29 and CP26 interfacing between the LHC II trimer and the PS II core complex in each monomer [44,52,53,55]. This dimeric complex, referred to as the "PS II–LHC II supercomplex," has a total molecular mass of ≈700 kDa and contains ≈100 chlorophyll molecules per monomeric unit. Larger complexes con-taining CP24 and additional LHC II trimers have been isolated [68–70]. The largest of these contain two PS II–LHC II supercomplexes bridged by LHC II trimers and by CP26 and CP24 proteins [70]. These com-plexes have molecular masses of ≈1600 kDa [70]. The multiplicity of these complexes reinforce the belief that the antenna system of PS II in higher plants has a dynamic structure in vivo [71–74].

The LHC II monomer contains three α-helical domains and its structure has been determined by electron crystallography to an in-plane resolution of 3.4 Å [75,76]. Twelve chlorophyll and two carotenoid (xanthophyll) molecules are present in the model, although two addi-tional xanthophyll sites were not identified in the structure, possibly because of their variable occupancy in vivo [49,77–79]. Of the 12 chloro-phyll molecules, 7 are tentatively assigned as being chlorophyll *a* and 5 are tentatively assigned as being chlorophyll *b* [75,76]. The LHC II trimer is made up of varying proportions of the *lhcb1* and *lhcb2* pro-teins. Whether the *lhcb3* protein forms heterodimers with the *lhcb1* and *lhcb2* proteins, forms homotrimers, or exists in monomeric form remains unknown [45,48]. It is absent from the most recent preparations of the

PS II–LHC II supercomplex [80]. The *lhcb1* and *lhcb2* proteins are reversibly phosphorylated near their N termini. This phosphorylation causes lateral movement of LHC II from PS II to PS I, thereby regulating the excitation balance between photosystems as a short-term response to changes in light quality [71,72,74]. This lateral movement may be caused by the dissociation of the LHC II trimer into monomers that diffuse through the thylakoid membrane and have a higher affinity for PS I than PS II [74,81].

The CP29, CP26, and CP24 proteins are evolutionarily related to the LHC II polypeptides and are encoded by the *lhcb4*, *lhcb5*, and *lhcb6* genes, respectively. A stromally exposed residue is reversibly phosphorylated in CP29 independently of the kinase that phosphorylates LHC II and has been proposed to be involved in a signal transduction pathway [82]. Analyses of native and reconstituted proteins have shown that CP29, CP26, and CP24 bind 8, 9, and 10 chlorophyll molecules, respectively, with chlorophyll *a/b* ratios of 6:2 in CP29 [78,83], 6:3 in CP26 [78,84], and 5:5 in CP24 [78,85], compared to 7:5 in the LHC II monomer [75,76].

The molar ratios of xanthophyll to chlorophyll in CP29, CP26, and CP24 are higher than in the LHC II monomer and the xanthophyll compositions of these three proteins are enriched in violaxanthin [79,86,87]. Furthermore, specific carboxylate residues on CP29 and CP26 react with dicyclohexylcarbodiimide (DCCD) [88,89]. Consequently, CP29, CP26, and CP24 have been proposed to play a critical role in the xanthophyll cycle that protects PS II from photodamage by dissipating excess excitation energy as heat (for review, see [49,73,90–92]). This cycle is activated when excess excitation of PS II overacidifies the lumen, increasing the transmembrane pH gradient. This overacidification (possibly sensed by the DCCD-reactive residues in CP29 and CP26) results in the enzymatic deepoxidation of violaxanthin to zeaxanthin, leading to nonradiative dissipation of excess excitation energy by mechanisms that may correlate with changes in the oligomerization state of the PS II antenna complex [93,94] but are not fully understood. Recently, one weakly bound violaxanthin molecule was reported to be present in each LHC II monomer as well as in each CP29 and CP26 protein [79]. These weakly bound violaxanthin molecules are more likely to participate in the xanthophyll cycle than tightly bound violaxanthin [79] because they would be in equilibrium with the lipid phase and, therefore, would have facile access to the violaxanthin deepoxidase enzyme [95] that binds to the lumenal surface of the thylakoid membrane when the lumen becomes acidified [96]. Therefore, the entire PS II antenna system may participate in the xanthophyll cycle of nonradiative photoprotection [79].

The LHC II polypeptides and the CP29, CP26, and CP24 proteins can be removed from higher plant PS II by detergent treatment, yielding a PS II complex that retains O_2-evolving activity [53,97–100]. A similar PS II complex can be isolated from cyanobacteria by similar methods [66,101]. One such complex from spinach was recently studied by electron crystallography and a two-dimensional projection map was obtained with a resolution of 9 Å [60]. Additional polypeptides can be removed from this complex [62,102–104] to yield a preparation containing only CP47, D1, D2, cytochrome b-559, and the smaller PS II polypeptides encoded by the $psbI$, $psbK$, $psbL$, $psbT_C$, and $psbW$ genes [62]. This complex retains the ability to oxidize Y_Z (or Y_D) [63,105,106] and reduce Q_A [63,106], but does not oxidize water. This complex was recently studied by electron crystallography [107–109] and its three-dimensional structure was determined to an in-plane resolution of 8 Å [61,109] (Fig. 2). An even smaller PS II complex has been isolated [110,111] that contains only D1, D2, the α and β polypeptides of cytochrome b-559, and the products of the $psbI$ and $psbW$ genes [110–114]. This complex retains the ability to form the charge-separated state, $P_{680}^{\bullet+}Pheo^{\bullet-}$ [115], but is unable to photooxidize Y_Z or Y_D, or to photoreduce Q_A.

2.2. The D1 and D2 Proteins

At the core of PS II is a heterodimer of two homologous 38- to 39-kDa polypeptides known as D1 and D2. These polypeptides are the products of the $psbA$ and $psbD$ genes and each contains five membrane-spanning helical domains. In higher plants, the N-terminal threonine residues of D1 and D2 are acetylated and reversibly phosphorylated following posttranslational removal of their initiating N-formylmethionine residues [116,117]. The D1 polypeptide is also posttranslationally cleaved after Ala344 [117–119]. The D1 polypeptide turns over more rapidly than any

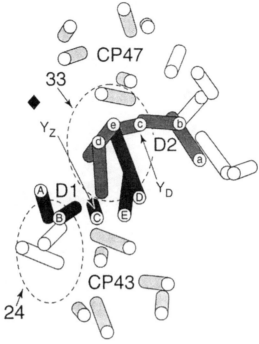

FIG. 2.   Helix organization of the major polypeptides of the PS II core, as viewed from the lumen. All helices expect those of CP43 are present in the 8-Å structure of the CP47/D2/D1 complex [109]. The helices of CP43 are modeled into the 9-Å projection map of an O_2-evolving dimeric PS II complex, assuming that they exhibit twofold symmetry with those of CP47 [60]. Dark-shaded helices denoted A–E are those of the D1 protein. Medium-shaded helices denoted a–e are those of the D2 protein. Light-shaded helices are those of CP47 and CP43. The unidentified nonshaded helices presumably correspond to those of the α and β polypeptides of cytochrome b-559 and the psbI, psbK, psbL, psbT_C, and psbW proteins. The black diamond in the upper left denotes the twofold symmetry axis that relates the two monomeric PS II units in the O_2-evolving dimeric PS II complex [60,61]. Additional protein density, presumably corresponding to one or more additional small intrinsic subunits, is present in this region but not depicted in the figure [60]. The large dashed oval represents the position of the extrinsic 33-kDa polypeptide. The small dashed oval represents the position of the extrinsic 24-kDa polypeptide. The positions of tyrosines Y_Z and Y_D, near the lumenal ends of the C helices of D1 and D2, respectively, are indicated. (Modified from [61], copyright 1999, by permission of Elsevier Science.)

other polypeptide in the thylakoid membrane [120]. This rapid turnover is a response to the photo-induced damage (known as photoinhibition) that is an inevitable byproduct of the highly oxidizing radicals and toxic activated oxygen species that are intermediates in the mechanism of water oxidation (for review of the photo-induced damage and repair cycle of PS II, see [43,121–123]).

The D1/D2 heterodimer contains the cofactors involved in light-induced electron transfer. The heterodimer contains six chlorophyll a, two pheophytin a, and two β-carotene molecules [124–126], plus the plastoquinones Q_A and Q_B, the redox-active tyrosines Y_Z and Y_D, and one atom of nonheme iron. The D1/D2 heterodimer probably also contains most of the residues that ligate the Mn and Ca^{2+} ions that are located at the catalytic site of water oxidation (Sec. 4). The amino acid sequences of the D1 and D2 polypeptides are homologous to those of the L and M polypeptides of reaction centers from purple nonsulfur bacteria. Because of the sequence and functional similarities between the two photosystems [127,128], the bacterial reaction center has long served as a structural model for PS II. Consequently, the electron transfer cofactors of PS II are believed to be arranged in two pseudosymmetric branches that are surrounded and supported by the ten pseudosymmetrically arranged helices of the D1 and D2 polypeptides. In this model, P_{680} is believed to be coordinated by D1-His198 and D2-His198, the pheophytin electron acceptor is believed to interact with D1-Glu130, and the nonheme iron atom is believed to be coordinated by D1-His215, D1-His272, D2-His215, and D2-His269 (Fig. 3A). Recent Fourier transform infrared (FTIR) studies have shown that the fifth and sixth coordination positions of the iron atom in PS II are occupied by bicarbonate [129].

The appropriateness of the bacterial model for the D1/D2 heterodimer has been verified by the 8-Å structure of the CP47/D2/D1 complex [61,109] (Fig. 2). In this structure, the lateral positions of the 10 helices of the D1/D2 heterodimer deviate no more than 3.5 Å from the positions of the 10 helices of the L/M heterodimer of *Rhodopseudomonas viridis*, and most of these differences are confined to only 3 of the 10 helices [109]. The 8-Å structure contains regions of electron density that appear to correspond to the positions of the four bacteriochlorophyll and two bacteriopheophytin molecules in bacterial reaction centers. One difference between the two photosystems is that the distance between the central pair of chlorophyll molecules in PS II is greater than the corresponding distance between the special pair of bacteriochlorophyll molecules in bacterial reaction centers (the center-to-center distance is ≈11 Å in PS II compared to 7.6 Å in bacterial reaction centers) [109]. The greater distance is consistent with the weaker exciton coupling of the pigments comprising P_{680} compared to that in bacterial reaction centers [3,7]. The two extra chlorophyll a molecules in the D1/D2 heterodimer, Chl_Z and Chl_D, are not visible in the 8-Å structure. Nevertheless, these chlorophylls are believed to be located in the heterodimer's periphery, with Chl_Z ligated to D1-His118 and Chl_D ligated to D2-His118 [130–132] (see below).

The original bacterial model for the D1/D2 heterodimer inspired the site-directed mutagenesis studies that identified tyrosine Y_D as Tyr161 of the D2 polypeptide [133,134] and Y_Z as Tyr161 of the D1 polypeptide [135,136]. More refined versions of this model have been developed [137–140] and used as predictive tools for mutagenesis studies of the environments of Y_D and Y_Z (Sec. 3) and other cofactors (for review of earlier site-directed mutagenesis studies, see [139,141,142]). In recent work, mutations at D1-His198 shifted the optical absorption spectrum [143,144] and reduction potential of P_{680} [144] and altered the quantum yield and free energy of the $P_{680}^{\bullet+}$ Pheo$^{\bullet-}$ radical pair [145]. These alterations are consistent with the predicted role of this residue in ligating P_{680}. Similarly, mutations at D1-Glu130 shifted the optical absorption spectrum of Pheo$^{\bullet-}$ [146] and altered the quantum yield and free energy of the $P_{680}^{\bullet+}$ Pheo$^{\bullet-}$ radical pair [145,146]. These alterations are consistent with the predicted interaction of this residue with the pheophytin electron acceptor. Recently, a resonance Raman study of mutations at D1-His118 showed that this residue ligates Chl_Z [132] as predicted [130,131]. Additional studies imply that D2-His118 ligates Chl_D [132,147]. Also, a recent ESEEM study involving a glycine mutation at D2-Ala260 showed that the peptide nitrogen of this residue forms a predicted hydrogen bond to $Q_A^{\bullet-}$ [148].

Despite the successes mentioned in the previous paragraph, the bacterial model for the D1/D2 heterodimer provides limited insight into the nature or location of the catalytic site for water oxidation because bacterial reaction centers do not oxidize water and because the lumenal domains of the D1 and D2 polypeptides are much larger than the corresponding domains of bacterial reaction centers.

D1 PROTEIN

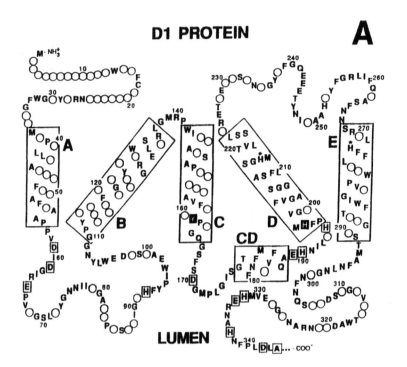

A

LUMEN

D2 PROTEIN

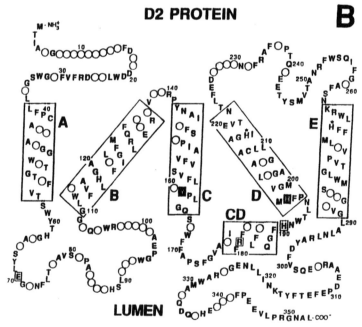

B

LUMEN

2.3. The CP47 and CP43 Proteins

The CP47 and CP43 polypeptides have molecular masses of approximately 56 and 50 kDa, respectively, and are encoded by the *psbB* and *psbC* genes, respectively [1,42,149]. In higher plants, the first two amino acid residues of CP43 are posttranslationally cleaved and the resulting N-terminal threonine residue is acetylated and reversibly phosphorylated [116]. The recent 8-Å structure of the CP47/D1/D2 complex shows that the CP47 polypeptide contains six transmembrane helices that are arranged as a trimer of dimers [61,109]. The CP43 polypeptide is believed to have a similar structure [60,61] (Fig. 2). In both proteins, helices V and VI are linked by a large hydrophilic loop that is located on the lumenal side of the thylakoid membrane (Fig. 4B). This loop contains ≈190 residues in CP47 and ≈130 residues in CP43. These loops are believed to fold over part of the lumenal domains of the D1/D2 heterodimer because amino acid residues in these loops strongly influence water oxidation (Sec. 4) and because in the absence of the extrinsic proteins (Sec. 2.6 and 2.7), Y_D is located ≈27 Å [150] or ≈20 Å [151] from the lumen despite its location near the lumenal terminus of helix C of the D2 polypeptide (Fig. 2).

The recent 9-Å projection map of a dimeric O_2-evolving PS II complex shows that CP47 and CP43 are arranged symmetrically on either side of the D1/D2 heterodimer and appear to be related by the same pseudo-twofold symmetry axis that relates D1 and D2 [60] (Fig. 2). On the basis of crosslinking studies [152,153], it is believed that CP47 is located adjacent to the D2 polypeptide in this structure [60,61,109]. The symmetric structure of the CP47/CP43/D2/D1 complex resembles that of the core of Photosystem I (Fig. 4). The structure of PS I has been de-

---

FIG. 3.   The predicted folding patterns for the D1 protein (A) and the D2 protein (B). Residues conserved in 39 sequences of D1 and 15 sequences of D2 are shown by their one-letter symbols. The circles represent nonconserved residues. The sequence numberings correspond to those of spinach. The Y_Z and Y_D tyrosine residues (D1-Tyr161 and D2-Tyr161, respectively), and the proposed histidine ligands to P_{680} (D1-His198 and D2-His198) are denoted by white letters on black backgrounds. The proposed histidine ligands for the nonheme iron (D1-His215, D1-His272, D2-His215, D2-His269) are marked with asterisks. Residues known to influence the properties of Y_Z, Y_D, or the Mn cluster are enclosed in boxes. (Modified from [137], copyright 1990, by permission of Oxford University Press.)

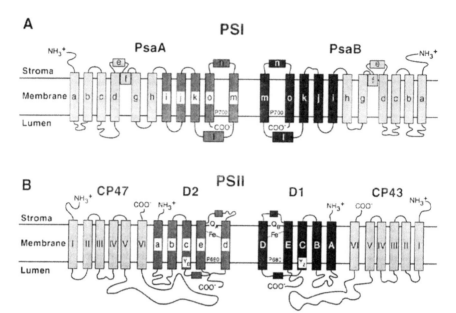

FIG. 4. Comparison of the folding model of the Photosystem I (PS I) *psaA* and *psaB* proteins (A) in comparison with those of CP47/D2 and CP43/D1 (B). Note, the large lumenal loops of CP47 and CP43 are drawn to cover part of the lumenal domains of the D1 and D2 proteins. (Modified from [60], copyright 1999, by permission of Nature America, Inc.)

termined to a resolution of 4 Å [154–157]. At its core is a heterodimer of two ≈83-kDa polypeptides that are the products of the *psaA* and *psaB* genes. The helical domains of the *psaA* and *psaB* polypeptides are arranged around a pseudo-twofold symmetry axis. The five C-terminal helices of each polypeptide are arranged like the helices of the L/M heterodimer in bacterial reaction centers and the D1/D2 heterodimer in higher plants. The six N-terminal helices of each polypeptide each form a trimer of dimers [154,155] and show sequence similarities with the CP47 and CP43 polypeptides of PS II [158]. On the basis of the structural analogies between PS I (a type 1 reaction center, having iron-sulfur clusters as electron acceptors) and bacterial reaction centers (a type 2 reaction center, having quinones as electron acceptors), it was proposed that all oxygenic and anoxygenic photosystems derive from a common ancestor and that CP47 and CP43 in PS II would be located on either side of the D1/D2 heterodimer and share the same pseudo-twofold symmetry axis as D1 and D2 [159,160]. The recent 9-Å projection map [60] confirms this prediction (Fig. 2). In both CP47 and CP43, helices V and VI are believed to correspond to the pair of helices located closest to the D1/D2 heterodimer, so that the large hydrophilic loops that connect these helices fold over the lumenal domains of D1 and D2 [109] (Fig. 2).

Both CP47 and CP43 contain approximately 15 molecules of chlorophyll a and 2–3 molecules of β-carotene [62]. The helices of CP47 and CP43 contain 12 and 8 conserved histidine residues, respectively [42,149]. The possibility that many of these residues serve as axial ligands to chlorophyll molecules has been supported by site-directed mutagenesis studies of CP47 [161–163] and CP43 [164]. Most of these residues are located near the stromal or lumenal ends of their respective helices. In the 8-Å structure of the CP47/D2/D1 complex (Fig. 2), 14 small ellipsoidal densities attributed to chlorophyll molecules were observed in CP47 [61,109]. These densities were distributed in two layers near the stromal and lumenal ends of the six helices. A similar distribution of chlorophyll molecules was found previously in the 3.4-Å structure of the light harvesting LHC-II complex from pea [75,76].

The CP47 polypeptide is required for the stable assembly of PS II [165,166]. The CP43 polypeptide may facilitate the assembly of PS II because PS II accumulates in thylakoid membranes to only ≈10% of wild-type levels when $psbC$ is deleted or inactivated [106,165]. The photooxidation of Y_Z and/or Y_D requires the presence of CP47 but can take place in the absence of CP43 [63,105,106]. Similarly, the photoreduction of Q_A requires the presence of CP47 but can take place in the absence of CP43 [63,106]. The CP43 polypeptide is more weakly associated with the D1/D2 heterodimer than CP47 and can be easily removed with chaotropic salts [103,104] or mild detergents [62,102]. This ease of removal may reflect the position of CP43 at the periphery of the dimeric CP47/CP43/D2/D1 complex [60] (Fig. 2). This ease of removal may also play an important physiological role in the repair processes that replace the D1 polypeptide after photooxidative damage (photoinhibition): disassociation of CP43 may be required for removal of damaged D1 from the PS II core complex [43,167].

The CP47 and CP43 proteins are believed to play a role in transferring energy from the light-harvesting pigments to the D1/D2 heterodimer [42,43,149]. However, the large hydrophilic loops of CP47 and

CP43 appear to bind the 33-kDa protein (Sec. 2.6) and may play direct or indirect roles in water oxidation (Secs. 4.3 and 4.4)

2.4. Cytochrome b-559

Cytochrome b-559 consists of two polypeptides in 1:1 stoichiometry [168]. These polypeptides are known as the α and β polypeptides, are encoded by the $psbE$ and $psbF$ genes, and have molecular masses of 9.3 and 4.4 kDa [169]. Each polypeptide contains one membrane-spanning region and is oriented with its C terminus on the lumenal side of the membrane [170–172]. The N-terminal threonine residue of the β polypeptide is acetylated following posttranslational removal of its initiating N-formylmethionine residue [169]. The heme is coordinated by two histidine residues [173]. Because the α and β polypeptides each contain a single histidine residue, cytochrome b-559 is generally considered to be arranged as an $\alpha\beta$ dimer with its heme group located near the stromal surface of the membrane (Fig. 1; for review, see [28,30,174]). Whether each monomeric unit of PS II contains one (e.g., [175]) or two (e.g., [176]) copies of cytochrome b-559 (with one heme being more labile than the other [176]) remains controversial (see the discussions in [28,175,176]). If there are two copies, then whether the cytochrome is arranged as two $\alpha\beta$ heterodimers or as α_2 and β_2 homodimers remains unresolved, although the $\alpha\beta$ configuration is generally favored (e.g., see the discussion in [177], but also see [178,179]).

The proper coordination of the heme of cytochrome b-559 is required for the stable assembly of PS II. If either the $psbE$ or $psbF$ genes are deleted or truncated in the membrane-spanning hydrophobic domain [177,180–182], or if one of the axial histidine ligands is mutated to Leu [181], then the D2 polypeptide fails to accumulate in the thylakoid membrane.

Cytochrome b-559 is oxidized by $P_{680}^{\bullet+}$ via Chl_Z [26] or Car [334], and reduced by $Q_A^{\bullet-}$ [183], $Q_B^{\bullet-}$ (or Q_BH_2) [25], or $Pheo^{\bullet-}$ [184], depending on conditions. These electron transfer reactions are too slow to be part of the normal electron transfer reactions of water oxidation but are believed to function to protect PS II from photooxidative damage (photoinhibition, see below).

A striking characteristic of cytochrome b-559 is its low and variable midpoint potential compared to other b-type cytochromes [28,30,

174,185]. Cytochrome b-559 can exist in at least three potential forms: high (375–435 mV), intermediate (170–240 mV), and low (5–45 mV) [186–188]. The higher potential forms dominate in intact, O_2-evolving PS II reaction centers, whereas the lower potential forms usually dominate in preparations that have been depleted of the Mn cluster or of their extrinsic 24-and 17-kDa polypeptides (Sec. 2.7) (e.g., [186, 189–191]). However, the high potential form can be stabilized by Ca^{2+} ions if the extrinsic 33-kDa polypeptide remains attached [192,193]. The photooxidation of Mn^{2+} ions, such as occurs during light-driven assembly (photoactivation) of the Mn cluster, results in conversion of the intermediate potential form to the high potential form [183]. This process requires two light-driven steps, with $Q_A^{\bullet-}$ reducing the heme on the first step and with $Q_B^{\bullet-}$ possibly reducing the heme on the second [183]. Restoration of rapid electron transfer from $Q_A^{\bullet-}$ to Q_B appears to accompany the conversion of intermediate to high potential form [183], either by a decrease in the midpoint potential of Q_A [194] or by increased binding of Q_B [195]. Consequently, cytochrome b-559 has been proposed to act as a "molecular switch" to regulate electron transfer on the acceptor side of PS II and, with it, the assembly of the Mn cluster on the donor side of PS II [183].

Cytochrome b-559 has also been proposed to function as a molecular switch in protecting PS II from photooxidative damage (photoinhibition) caused by highly reactive radical species, either to switch between different mechanisms of photoprotection [184,196] or to switch photoprotection "on" [28,29]. These mechanisms involve cytochrome b-559 either accepting electrons from $Pheo^{\bullet-}$ to prevent the formation of $^3P_{680}$ and singlet oxygen [184,196–198], donating electrons to $P_{680}^{\bullet+}$ via Chl_Z or Car to eliminate long-lived oxidizing radicals [26,184,196], or permitting the accumulation of $Chl_Z^{\bullet+}$ or $Car^{\bullet+}$, which would act as fluorescence quenchers to dissipate excess excitation energy, thereby limiting subsequent charge separations [25,27–29,334] (for review, see [28,30]).

2.5. Other Intrinsic Proteins

With the exception of the ≈22-kDa product of the *psbS* gene, all other intrinsic polypeptides in PS II have molecular masses ≤10 kDa and contain a single transmembrane helix. These are the products of the *psbH*,

$psbI, psbJ, psbK, psbL, psbM, psbN, psbR, psbT_N, psbT_C, psbW$, and $psbX$ genes. The functions of most of these polypeptides are unknown.

The $psbH$ protein has a molecular mass of ≈ 8 kDa and is reversibly phosphorylated in higher plants near its N terminus after posttranslational removal of its initiating N-formylmethionine residue [199]. In cyanobacteria, the first 12 amino acids are posttranslationally cleaved and the resulting ≈ 6.5 kDa polypeptide may be phosphorylated near its N terminus [200]. The function of the $psbH$ protein is not known but it is not essential for the stable assembly of PS II complexes: the deletion of $psbH$ does not abolish the photoautotrophic growth of the cyanobacterium $Synechocystis$ sp. PCC 6803, but electron transfer from $Q_A^{\bullet-}$ to Q_B is slowed and the mutant is more sensitive to photooxidative damage (photoinhibition) [201]. The $psbH$ protein is absent from preparations that lack CP43 [62]. Therefore, its transmembrane helix is not in the 8-Å structure of the CP47/D2/D1 complex [61,109]. However, it has been suggested to be located in the central region of the O_2-evolving dimeric PS II complex, between the two monomeric units [60] (Fig. 2).

The $psbI$ protein has a molecular mass of 4.2 kDa and retains the initiating N-formyl group on its N-terminal methionine residue [169]. Crosslinking studies show that the $psbI$ protein is intimately associated with the D1/D2 heterodimer [202] and it is present in all PS II preparations that retain the ability to form the charge-separated state, $P_{680}^{\bullet+}Pheo^{\bullet-}$. Therefore, it may correspond to one of the unidentified helices in the 8-Å structure of the CP47/D2/D1 complex (Fig. 2). The function of the $psbI$ protein remains unknown. Deletion of the $psbI$ gene from $Synechocystis$ sp. PCC 6803 has little effect on photoautotrophic growth or light-saturated rates of O_2 evolution [203]. Consequently, the $psbI$ protein is not essential for the stable assembly or function of PS II. Nevertheless, in the absence of $psbI$, PS II is slightly more sensitive to photooxidative damage (photoinhibition) [203].

The $psbJ$ and $psbK$ proteins have molecular masses of ≈ 4.2 kDa [62,204]. The first eight residues of the $psbK$ protein are posttranslationally cleaved to yield a product that is believed to have its N terminus on the lumenal side of the thylakoid membrane [205]. Neither protein is essential for the assembly or function of PS II because mutants of $Synechocystis$ sp. PCC 6803 that lack $psbJ$ [204] or $psbK$ [205,206] grow photoautotrophically, but at somewhat diminished rates. The $psbJ$ protein may have some influence on the stability or assembly of PS II because in its absence there are ≈50% fewer PS II complexes in the thylakoid membrane [204]. The *psbJ* protein must be located at the periphery of the PS II core complex because it is absent from preparations that lack CP43 [62]. Therefore, its transmembrane helix is not in the 8-Å structure of the CP47/D2/D1 complex (Fig. 2). In contrast, the *psbK* protein is present in these preparations [62], although it is lost when the dimeric complex is converted to monomers [62]. Therefore, it may correspond to one of the unidentified helices in the 8-Å structure (Fig. 2) or be located in the central region of the dimeric PS II complex [60], between the two monomeric units.

The *psbL* protein has a molecular mass of 4.4 kDa [62]. Deletion of *psbL* abolishes photoautotrophic growth of *Synechocystis* sp. PCC 6803 [207] and biochemical reconstitution studies show that the *psbL* protein is required for the oxidation of Y_Z by $P_{680}^{\bullet+}$ [208]. The inability to oxidize Y_Z in the absence of the *psbL* protein prevents the stable formation of $Q_A^{\bullet-}$ because of rapid charge recombination between $Q_A^{\bullet-}$ and $P_{680}^{\bullet+}$ [208]. This lack of stable $Q_A^{\bullet-}$ formation in the absence of the *psbL* protein was previously attributed to an influence of the *psbL* protein on the binding or photoreduction of Q_A [209]. The *psbL* protein is present in the dimeric form of PS II preparations that lack CP43 [62] but is lost when the dimeric complex is converted to monomers [62]. Therefore, like the *psbK* protein, it may correspond to one of the unidentified helices in the 8-Å structure (Fig. 2) or be located in the central region of the dimeric PS II complex [60], between the two monomeric units.

The *psbM* and *psbN* proteins each have molecular masses of ≈4.7 kDa [210]. They have no known functions. Deletion of both *psbN* and *psbH* from *Synechocystis* sp. PCC 6803 caused no effects other than those observed in the absence of *psbH* alone [201]. The *psbM* and *psbN* proteins must be located at the periphery of the PS II core complex because neither is present in preparations that lack CP43 [62]. Consequently, neither the *psbM* nor *psbN* proteins is in the 8-Å structure of the CP47/D2/D1 complex (Fig. 2).

The *psbR* protein is nuclear-encoded and has a molecular mass of ≈10 kDa [211]. It has no known function and is absent from O_2-evolving PS II preparations that lack the LHC II, CP29, CP26, and CP24 antenna proteins [53,97–100]. Its presence is not required to bind the extrinsic 24-and 17-kDa proteins (Sec. 2.7) [100], contrary to earlier reports.

The *psbS* protein is nuclear-encoded and evolutionarily related to the LHC II, CP29, CP26, and CP24 antenna proteins. However, it contains four α-helical domains rather than three and has shorter loops between its helices. It binds ≈5 chlorophyll molecules, has a chlorophyll *a/b* ratio of ≈6, and binds substoichiometric amounts of several xanthophylls [212,213]. However, the exciton coupling between the chlorophyll pigments is believed to be weak [213] and, unlike any other known chlorophyll-binding protein, the *psbS* protein is stable in the thylakoid membrane in the absence of pigments [214]. Furthermore, the developmental regulation of *psbS* differs from that of any other chlorophyll-binding protein [215]. Consequently, rather than serve as a light-harvesting protein, the *psbS* protein is believed to be a chlorophyll storage protein that donates or scavanges pigments during the biosynthesis, degradation, or turnover of PS II antenna or core polypeptides [213,214]. A similar role has been postulated for the ELIPs (early light-inducible proteins), which are also related to the LHC II proteins of PS II [216]. The *psbS* protein is absent from O_2-evolving PS II preparations that lack the LHC II, CP29, CP26, and CP24 antenna proteins [53,97–100] and is not present in cyanobacteria.

The chloroplast-encoded *psbT$_C$* protein has a molecular mass of 3.9 kDa and retains the initiating *N*-formyl group on its N-terminal methionine residue [62]. The function of this protein is unknown, but the deletion of *psbT$_C$* from the green alga *Chlamydomonas reinhardtii* renders PS II more sensitive to photooxidative damage (photoinhibition) [217]. The *psbT$_C$* protein is present in the monomeric CP47/D2/D1 complex [62]. Therefore, it may correspond to one of the unidentified helices in the recent 8-Å structure (Fig. 2).

The nuclear encoded *psbT$_N$* protein has a molecular mass of ≈3 kDa [218]. It is absent from preparations that lack CP43 [62]. Therefore, is not present in the 8-Å structure of the CP47/D2/D1 complex (Fig. 2). It is believed to be an extrinsic protein [218]. Its function is unknown.

The *psbW* protein is nuclear-encoded [114,219], has a molecular mass of 5.9 kDa [62], and is oriented with its N terminus facing the lumen [114,220]. Consequently, the *psbW* protein's orientation in the thylakoid membrane is opposite to that of all other *psb* proteins with the possible exception of the *psbK* protein. The *psbW* protein is intimately associated with the D1/D2 heterodimer in higher plants [114,219,220]. Therefore, it is present in the CP47/D2/D1 complex [62] and may correspond to one of the unidentified helices in the 8-Å structure (Fig. 2). The function of this protein is unknown. It is not present in cyanobacteria.

The *psbX* protein has a molecular mass of ≈4.1 kDa [221]. It is nuclear-encoded in *Arabidopsis thaliana* [221] and chloroplast-encoded in algae [22]. It is also present in cyanobacteria. The *psbX* protein is absent from PS II preparations that lack CP43 [62]. Therefore, it is not present in the 8-Å structure of the CP47/D2/D1 complex (Fig. 2). The function of the *psbX* protein is unknown.

2.6. The Extrinsic 33-kDa Protein

The extrinsic "33-kDa polypeptide" has a molecular mass of ≈26.5 kDa [223] and is encoded by the *psbO* gene. It is nuclear-encoded in plants and algae and is present in cyanobacteria. In solution, it is a "natively unfolded" protein [224] that is conformationally flexible [225]. Its conformation changes when it binds to the intrinsic subunits of PS II [225,226]. It binds more tightly in the presence of the Mn cluster than in the cluster's absence [227–229]. Whether each monomeric unit of PS II contains one [55,61,230] or two [229,231,232] copies of the extrinsic 33-kDa polypeptide (with one copy binding to a structural site and the other to a regulatory site [232]) remains controversial. Nevertheless, single-particle image-averaging studies [52,55], in combination with the 8-Å structure for the CP47/D2/D1 complex [109], show that one extrinsic 33-kDa polypeptide covers the central region of the D1/D2 heterodimer near the putative locations of helices V and VI of CP47 [61] (Fig. 2). Because the large hydrophilic loops of CP47 and CP43 that connect these helices are believed to cover lumenal domains of the D1/D2 heterodimer (Sec. 2.3), this location is consistent with numerous crosslinking, accessibility, deletion mutagenesis, and site-directed mutagenesis studies that show that the large hydrophilic loop of CP47 interacts with the extrinsic 33-kDa polypeptide (for recent reviews of these studies, see [233,234]). Several crosslinking studies used the zero-length crosslinking agent 1-ethyl-3-[3-(dimethylamino)propyl]carbodiimide (EDC). These studies showed that the large hydrophilic loop of CP47 comes within van der Waals contact of the extrinsic 33-kDa polypeptide [230,235,236]. The hydrophilic loop that connects helices I and II of CP47 can also be crosslinked to the extrinsic 33-kDa protein with EDC [237]. Additional studies show that the large hydrophilic loop of CP43 is exposed to the lumen in the absence of the extrinsic 33-kDa polypeptide and may be required for binding this polypeptide [238]. The lumenal domains of the α polypeptide of cytochrome b-559 and the $psbI$ protein have also been crosslinked to the extrinsic 33-kDa polypeptide [239]. However, these proteins may be farther from the extrinsic 33-kDa protein than CP47 because a crosslinking agent with an 11-Å chain length was employed [239].

The extrinsic 33-kDa polypeptide is not required for O_2 evolution in vitro [240] or for photoautotrophic growth of the cyanobacteria *Synechocystis* sp. PCC 6803 [241–243] or *Synechoccocus* sp. PCC 7942 [244]. However, in its absence, the rates of O_2 release [245,246] and $Y_Z^{\bullet}$ reduction [247] during the $S_3 \rightarrow (S_4) \rightarrow S_0$ transition are slowed approximately fivefold, the S_2 state is abnormally stable [245,246,248], and PS II is more susceptible to photooxidative damage (photoinhibition) [242,243]. Furthermore, unless the polypeptide-depleted preparations are maintained in high concentrations of Cl^- [16], two Mn ions are gradually lost from the Mn cluster as Mn^{2+} ions [15,16]. Therefore, the extrinsic 33-kDa polypeptide protects the Mn cluster from endogenous reductants and optimizes its catalytic efficiency. Indeed, reducing the Mn cluster in the presence of the extrinsic 33-kDa polypeptide and Ca^{2+} produces Mn^{2+} ions that are retained in a sequestered environment and can be reoxidized by illumination [17,18]. Therefore, the extrinsic 33-kDa polypeptide appears to serve as a diffusion barrier. As a consequence of this apparent role, the extrinsic 33-kDa polypeptide also impedes the access of Mn^{2+} ions to sites on the apoprotein: when the Mn cluster is absent, the efficiency of Mn^{2+} photooxidation [249] and the quantum yield of the light-driven assembly (photoactivation) of the Mn cluster [250] increase substantially in the absence of this polypeptide.

2.7.   Other Extrinsic Proteins

In higher plants and green algae, two additional extrinsic polypeptides are associated with PS II. These are the 24-kDa and 17-kDa polypeptides, the products of the nuclear-encoded *psbP* and *psbQ* genes [1,42,233]. They are present in a 1:1:1 stoichiometry with the extrinsic 33-kDa polypeptide [251,252]. The 24-kDa polypeptide appears to bind to a site created by the binding of the extrinsic 33-kDa polypeptide [227]. Similarly, the 17-kDa polypeptide appears to bind to a site created by the binding of the 24-kDa polypeptide [227]. Single-particle image-averaging studies [55], in combination with the 8-Å structure for the CP47/D2/D1 complex [109], show that one 24-kDa polypeptide binds next to the extrinsic 33-kDa polypeptide near CP43, covering part of the D1 protein [61] (Fig. 2). Both the 24-kDa and 17-kDa proteins appear to serve as diffusion barriers, with the 24-kDa protein maintaining an optimal concentration of Ca^{2+} ions near the Mn cluster [21] and the 17-kDa polypeptide and/or the 24-kDa polypeptide maintaining an optimal concentration of Cl^- ions near the Mn cluster [253]. In the absence of these polypeptides, high rates of O_2 evolution require elevated concentrations of these ions in solution [21,253]. The magnetic properties of the Mn cluster are altered in the absence of these polypeptides as shown by the appearance of the S_1-state parallel polarization multiline EPR signal in their absence, but not in their presence [254]. An influence of the 24-kDa and 17-kDa polypeptides on the properties of the Mn cluster is also evident from narrowing of the EPR signal of the $S_2Y_Z^\bullet$ state in Ca^{2+}-depleted samples in the absence of these polypeptides [255].

The 24-kDa and 17-kDa polypeptides are not present in cyanobacteria or eukaryotic red algae. Instead, these organisms contain two other extrinsic polypeptides, the products of the *psbU* and *psbV* genes [233]. The *psbU* protein has a molecular mass of ≈10.5 kDa [256] but is generally referred to as the "12-kDa polypeptide." It is nuclear-encoded in red algae. The *psbV* protein is known as cytochrome c-550 and has a molecular mass of ≈17 kDa [257]. It is chloroplast-encoded in red algae. The heme group of this cytochrome has a very low potential (-260 mV). Its function is unknown. In cyanobacteria, cytochrome c-550 can bind to the intrinsic polypeptides in the absence of the extrinsic 33-kDa polypeptide, but the binding of the *psbU* protein requires the prior binding of either the extrinsic 33-kDa polypeptide or cytochrome c-550 [258]. In red algae, neither protein can bind in the absence of an additional extrinsic 20-kDa polypeptide whose function is unknown [259].

In cyanobacterial mutants lacking *psbU*, normal rates of photoautotrophic growth are retained [256], but the rate of O_2 evolution decreases slightly [256] and the S_2 state is more stable [256,260]. In addition, photoautotrophic growth is slowed in the absence of Ca^{2+} and Cl^- ions [256], suggesting that the *psbU* protein helps maintain optimal concentrations of Ca^{2+} and Cl^- ions near the Mn cluster.

In mutants lacking cytochrome c-550, photoautotrophic growth is retained in the presence of Ca^{2+} and Cl^- ions, but not in their absence

[257,260]. Furthermore, $\approx$40% fewer PS II complexes are stably incorporated into the thylakoid membranes [257], the quantum yield for the light-driven assembly (photoactivation) of the Mn cluster increases substantially [260], the rate of O_2 release during the $S_3 \rightarrow (S_4) \rightarrow S_0$ transition is slower [260], and the Mn cluster is as sensitive to exogenous reductants as it is in the absence of the extrinsic 33-kDa polypeptide [260]. These results show that cytochrome c-550 plays a much greater role than the $psbU$ protein in maintaining optimal concentrations of Ca^{2+} and Cl^- ions near the Mn cluster, and that, like the extrinsic 33-kDa protein, it protects the Mn cluster from endogenous reductants and optimizes its catalytic activity. Indeed, although photoautotrophic growth is retained in the absence of either the extrinsic 33-kDa or cytochrome c-550 proteins, such growth is abolished in the absence of *both* proteins [261].

3. THE ENVIRONMENTS OF THE REDOX-ACTIVE TYROSINE RESIDUES

3.1. Tyrosine Y_D

Tyrosines Y_D and Y_Z are D2-Tyr161 [133,134] and D1-Tyr161 [135,136], respectively, and are located symmetrically in the D1/D2 heterodimer [262] near the lumenal ends of the C helices (Figs. 2, 3B, and 4B). Despite its position in the D1/D2 heterodimer, Y_D is located $\approx$27 Å [150] or $\approx$20 Å [151] from the lumen in the absence of the extrinsic polypeptides, perhaps because this region of the heterodimer is covered by the lumenal domains of D1 or D2 or by the large hydrophilic loops of CP47 or CP43. The $Y_D^{\bullet}$ radical is extremely stable under physiological conditions and is well shielded from solvent, as shown by $^2H_2O/^1H_2O$ exchange [263,264] and reductant accessibility [265,266] studies. Modeling studies predict that Y_D is located in a hydrophobic environment, surrounded by the hydrophobic residues D2-Phe170, D2-Phe182, D2-Phe189, D2-Leu290, and D2-Ala291, and by D2-Phe186, which is a Leu residue in cyanobacteria [137–139] (Fig. 5B). Tyrosine Y_D is predicted to form hydrogen bonds with D2-His190 and D2-Gln165, to be spatially positioned by D2-Pro162, and to be in van der Waals contact with D2-Phe186 and D2-Ala291 [139]. The prediction of a hydrogen bond between $Y_D^{\bullet}$ and D2-His190 [133,137–139] has been supported by CW-ENDOR [263] and

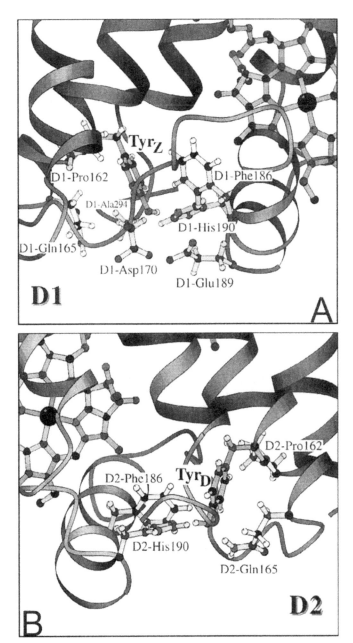

FIG. 5.   The predicted environments of Y_Z (Tyr_Z, A), and Y_D (Tyr_D, B). (Modified from [139], copyright 1996, by permission of the American Chemical Society. Figures kindly provided by B. Svensson.)

high-field EPR [267] studies and shown unambiguously by a pulsed ENDOR study that used ^{15}N-histidine to show that $Y_D^{\bullet}$ accepts a hydrogen bond from the τ-nitrogen of D2-His190 [268]. There may be a second hydrogen bond to $Y_D^{\bullet}$ in *Synechocystis* sp. PCC 6803 [264]. The EPR line shape of $Y_D^{\bullet}$ is altered in all D2-His190 mutants [263,267,269]. Because the spin density distributions of tyrosine radicals in proteins are largely independent of the radical's hydrogen bonding status [34,270,271], these altered line shapes must be caused by perturbations in the environment or orientation of $Y_D^{\bullet}$ in the absence of the hydrogen bond from D2-His190. Perturbations in protein backbone conformation or side chain interactions were invoked to explain the altered $Y_D^{\bullet}$ EPR line shapes observed in mutants of D2-Pro162 and D2-Gln165 [272]. Such perturbations probably also explain the altered $Y_D^{\bullet}$ EPR line shapes recently observed in mutants of D2-Arg181 [273]. Mutations of this residue presumably perturb the structure of the loop connecting helices C and D (Figs. 3B, 5B). These mutations also appear to influence the redox potential of P_{680} [273].

3.2.   Tyrosine Y_Z

As shown by $^2H_2O/^1H_2O$ exchange [264,274] and reductant accessibility [265,266] studies, tyrosine Y_Z is readily accessible to solvent in the absence of the Mn cluster, unlike Y_D. Modeling studies predict that Y_Z is located in a hydrophilic environment, with the polar residues D1-Gln165, D1-Ser169, D1-Asp170, D1-Glu189, and D1-His190 located nearby and D1-Phe186 and D1-Ala294 making van der Waals contact [137–139] (Fig. 5A). A combinatorial mutagenesis study has shown that residues 160, 162, and 163 of the D1 polypeptide are permissive to substitution [275] (Fig. 3A). In O_2-evolving PS II preparations, Y_Z is believed to form a strong hydrogen bond with D1-His190 [2,33,35–41]. In Mn-depleted PS II preparations, $Y_Z^{\bullet}$ forms a strong hydrogen bond that is disordered [267,276,277]. Whether $Y_Z^{\bullet}$ interacts with D1-His190 directly [264,278] or via one or more hydrogen-bonded H_2O molecules [279] in Mn-depleted preparations is under debate.

In both O_2-evolving and Mn-depleted PS II preparations, the oxidation of Y_Z by $P_{680}^{\bullet+}$ is believed to be facilitated by the deprotonation of Y_Z by D1-His190 [2,33,35–41]. This presumption has been supported by site-directed mutagenesis studies showing that electron transfer from

Y_Z to $P_{680}^{\bullet+}$ is severely impaired in D1-His190 mutants [279–285] and by chemical complementation studies [279,284] showing that the electron transfer rate is substantially restored when imidazole or other small organic bases are added to mutant PS II preparations. Several carboxylate residues have been proposed to influence the redox potential of Y_Z by interacting with D1-His190, including D1-Asp170 and D1-Glu189 [279,286–289]. In support of this idea, charge recombination between $Q_A^{\bullet-}$ and $P_{680}^{\bullet+}$ is accelerated in the mutants D1-Asp170Ala [290] and D1-Glu189Asp [286,288]. Because Y_Z is located near the Mn cluster [13,31,32] (Sec. 1.1), one or more of the carboxylate residues proposed to interact with D1-His190 may ligate Mn (Sec. 4). The mutation D1-His195Asp appears to alter the redox potential of Y_Z [280], perhaps by altering the conformation of the loop connecting helices C and D.

4. THE ENVIRONMENT OF THE MANGANESE CLUSTER

If each Mn ion is octahedrally coordinated, the tetranuclear Mn cluster will have 24 ligands. If the cluster is arranged as a bridged pair of di-μ_2-oxo bridged Mn dimers [4,14], 10 ligands will be provided by bridging oxygen atoms, and the rest will be provided by amino acid residues, peptide carbonyl groups, substrate H_2O molecules, and Cl^-. The amino acids that coordinate the Mn cluster are believed to be primarily carboxylate residues plus one or two histidine residues. Coordination by histidine has been demonstrated by electronic spin-echo envelope modulation (ESEEM) studies using ^{15}N-histidine [291]. Coordination by a carboxylate residue that forms a bridge to a Ca^{2+} ion has been proposed on the basis of an FTIR study that compared the S_2-*minus*-S_1 difference spectrum of intact and Ca^{2+}-depleted samples [292]. Coordination by both carboxylate and histidine residues has been supported by chemical modification studies showing that both types of residues are involved in ligating an Mn^{2+} ion that is photooxidized by the apoprotein [293–296].

Most attempts to identify individual ligands of the Mn cluster have focused on the D1, D2, CP47, and CP43 polypeptides. Neither the extrinsic 33-kDa protein nor any of the characterized smaller intrinsic proteins are likely to contribute ligands to the Mn cluster because, except for the *psbL* protein, photoautotrophic growth is retained when the genes encoding these proteins are individually deleted (Secs. 2.5 and 2.6). Also, the helical domains of most of the smaller proteins are located far from Y_Z (Fig. 2). Similarly, cytochrome b-559 is unlikely to contribute ligands because photoautotrophic growth is retained when the lumenal domain of the α polypeptide is truncated by 31 residues [297] and because the β polypeptide lacks a lumenal domain [28,30]. The increased sensitivity to photooxidative damage (photoinhibition) seen in the absence of many of the smaller polypeptides, and in the presence of site-directed mutations in C-terminal domain of the α polypeptide of cytochrome b-559 [30], may be caused by the release of toxic, activated oxygen species from Mn clusters that have been perturbed by long-range changes in protein backbone conformation. The release of activated oxygen species from perturbed Mn clusters has been proposed to explain why mutants containing such clusters are often much more sensitive to photooxidative damage (photoinhibition) than mutants lacking Mn clusters [282,298].

However, a terminal ligand of the Mn cluster might be functionally replaced by an H_2O molecule, a Cl^- ion, or by a repositioned amino acid residue from another protein. Therefore, it is not possible to rigorously exclude the 33-kDa protein as potentially contributing ligands to the Mn cluster and, until the unidentified helices in the structure of the CP47/CP43/D2/D1 complex (Fig. 2) are identified, it will not be possible to rigorously exclude any of the small intrinsic proteins as potentially contributing ligands to the Mn cluster either.

4.1.   The D1 Protein

Because of the proximity of Y_Z to the Mn cluster [13,31,32], most efforts to identify Mn ligands have targeted the D1 protein. Site-directed mutagenesis studies have identified D1-Asp170, D1-His190, D1-His332, D1-Glu333, D1-His337, D1-Asp342, and the C terminus of Ala344 as potential ligands of the Mn cluster.

4.1.1.   D1-Asp170

At least 15 mutations have been constructed at D1-Asp170 [282,290,299–301]. The Glu and His mutants are photoautotrophic, whereas O_2 evolution is abolished in the Ala, Ser, Thr, and Pro mutants, nearly abolished in the Asn mutant, and severely diminished in most others. The Mn content of PS II particles isolated from the Asn mutant is also diminished substantially [300] and a high-affinity Mn binding site on the apoprotein is abolished in the Asn, Ala, and Ser mutants [299,302]. On the basis of these studies, it was concluded that D1-Asp170 forms part of the binding site for the first Mn^{2+} ion that is photooxidized during the light-driven assembly (photoactivation) of the Mn cluster and that D1-Asp170 may be a ligand to the assembled Mn cluster. In apparent contradiction to the latter conclusion, the Val, Leu, and Ile mutants were found to be photoautotrophic [282]. One explanation is that D1-Asp170, although required for efficient photooxidation of the first Mn ion ligated during assembly of the Mn cluster, does not remain as a ligand to the final, *assembled* Mn cluster. However, if D1-Asp170 is not a ligand to the *assembled* Mn cluster, it is difficult to explain why replacement of this residue with Asn is more deleterious to O_2 evolution than replacement with Val, Leu, or Ile. To explain this dilemma, it was proposed that Val, Leu, and Ile, being bulky and hydrophobic, cause structural perturbations that permit the missing carboxylate moiety to be replaced by another residue, a peptide carbonyl group, or a H_2O molecule [282]. Compensatory, mutation-induced structural rearrangements have been observed in ferredoxin I of *Azotobacter vinelandii* [303], ricin A [304], and human alcohol dehydrogenase [305]. Therefore, D1-Asp170 is still considered to be a probable ligand of the assembled Mn cluster, but additional spectroscopic studies are needed.

4.1.2. D1-His190

At least 15 mutations have been constructed at D1-His190 [280–282, 284,285]. All abolish photoautotrophic growth. Because of this, several authors have suggested that D1-His190 may ligate the Mn cluster [2, 280,282,291,306]. Both the Arg and Lys mutants evolve O_2, but at only ≈13% the rate of wild-type cells [282,284]. Because Arg can replace His [307] and Lys can replace Met [308,309] as ligands to Fe in cytochrome *c*, it was proposed that D1-His190 may indeed ligate the Mn cluster [282]. A dual role for D1-His190, interacting with both Y_Z (Sec. 3.2) and the Mn cluster, has been proposed [2]. However, it will be difficult to test whether D1-His190 ligates the Mn cluster because only the Arg and Lys mutants contain photooxidizable Mn ions in vivo and these contain photooxidizable Mn ions in only a minority of PS II reaction centers [282].

4.1.3. D1-His332

At least 10 mutations have been constructed at D1-His332 [298,306]. None are photoautotrophic. Only the Gln and Ser mutants evolve O_2, and at only 10–15% the rate of wild-type cells. In all mutants except Asp and Glu, substantial fractions of PS II complexes lack photooxidizable Mn ions in vivo [298]. These data show that D1-His332 influences the assembly or stability of the Mn cluster. However, the high-affinity Mn site identified in the D1-Asp170 mutants (Sec. 4.1.1) remains intact [306]. Several D1-His332 mutants are extremely sensitive to photooxidative damage (photoinhibition), possibly because toxic, activated oxygen species are released from perturbed Mn clusters [298]. Because Gln and Glu functionally replace His as a ligand to Fe in cytochrome c peroxidase [310], and because Asp and Ser are potential ligands to Mn, it was proposed that D1-His332 may ligate the Mn cluster and that its redox properties are substantially altered in the Asp and Glu mutants [298]. In PS II particles isolated from the His332Glu mutant, the quantum yield for Mn oxidation is very low, the temperature threshold for the $S_1 \rightarrow S_2$ transition is ≈70°C higher than in wild-type, the S_2-state multiline EPR signal is altered exhibiting more lines and narrower spacings than the wild-type signal, and the mutant is unable to advance beyond the $S_2 Y_Z^{\bullet}$ state (R. J. Debus, K. A. Campbell, J. M. Peloquin, D. P. Pham, and R. D. Britt, submitted). Studies are underway to determine if the nitrogen couplings observed in the ESEEM spectrum of the wild-type S_2-type multiline EPR signal [291] are diminished in the Glu mutant, as would be expected if D1-His332 ligates the Mn cluster.

4.1.4. D1-Glu333

At least six mutations have been constructed at D1-Glu333 [298,306]. Only the Gln mutant is photoautotrophic. This mutant evolves O_2 at ≈36% the rate of wild-type cells. In all mutants, substantial fractions of PS II complexes lack photooxidizable Mn ions in vivo [298], showing that D1-Glu333 influences the assembly or stability of the Mn cluster. However, the high-affinity Mn site identified in the D1-Asp170 mutants (Sec. 4.1.1) remains intact [306]. All D1-Glu333 mutants are extremely sensitive to photooxidative damage (photoinhibition), possibly because toxic, activated oxygen species are related from perturbed Mn clusters

[298]. Because the Gln mutant evolves O_2 and because Gln can functionally replace His as a ligand to Fe in cytochrome c peroxidase [310], D1-Glu333 was proposed to be a possible ligand of the Mn cluster. This residue may also ligate a Ca^{2+} ion: electron transfer from Y_Z to $P_{680}^{\bullet+}$ is slowed dramatically when D1-Glu333 mutants are propagated in the absence of Ca^{2+} [298].

4.1.5. D1-His337

At least 10 mutations have been constructed at D1-His337 [298,306]. The Arg, Gln, and Phe mutants are photoautotrophic and the Glu, Asp, Asn, and Leu mutants evolve O_2 [298]. In many mutants, substantial fractions of PS II complexes lack photooxidizable Mn ions in vivo, showing that D1-His337 influences the assembly or stability of the Mn cluster [298]. However, the high-affinity Mn site identified in the D1-Asp170 mutants (Sec. 4.1.1) remains intact [306]. Several D1-His337 mutants are extremely sensitive to photooxidative damage (photoinhibition), possibly because toxic, activated oxygen species are released from perturbed Mn clusters [298]. Because Arg can replace His as a ligand to Fe in cytochrome c [307] and Gln can replace His as a ligand to Fe in cytochrome c peroxidase [310], D1-His337 was proposed to be a possible ligand of the Mn cluster [298]. This had been proposed previously on the basis of chemical modification and proteolysis studies [311]. Whereas the Mn clusters in the Val mutant are severely perturbed, those in the Leu mutant evolve O_2 and those in the Phe mutant support photoautotrophic growth [298]. To explain why progressively larger hydrophobic residues cause progressively fewer perturbations, the bulky Leu and Phe residues were proposed to cause structural perturbations that permit the missing imidazole moiety to be replaced by another residue, a peptide carbonyl group, or an H_2O molecule [298]. As mentioned in Sec. 4.1.1, compensatory, mutation-induced structural rearrangements have been observed in ferredoxin I of *Azotobacter vinelandii* [303], ricin A [304], and human alcohol dehydrogenase [305].

4.1.6. D1-Asp342

At least five mutations have been constructed at D1-Asp342 [298,306]. Only the Glu mutant is photoautotrophic, although the Asn mutant evolves O_2 at $\approx 33\%$ the rate of wild-type cells when propagated in dim light. In all mutants, some fraction of PS II complexes lack photooxidizable Mn ions in vivo, showing that D1-Asp342 influences the assembly or stability of the Mn cluster. However, the high-affinity Mn site identified in the D1-Asp170 mutants (Sec. 4.1.1) remains intact [306]. Most of the D1-Asp342 mutants are extremely sensitive to photooxidative damage (photoinhibition), possibly because toxic, activated oxygen species are released from perturbed Mn clusters [298]. Because Asn can replace Asp as a ligand to Fe in cytochrome *bo* ubiquinol oxidase [312], D1-Asp342 was proposed to be a possible ligand of the Mn cluster. This residue may also ligate a Ca^{2+} ion: electron transfer from Y_Z to $P_{680}^{\bullet+}$ is slowed dramatically when the Glu and Asn mutants are propagated in the absence of Ca^{2+} [298].

4.1.7. The C Terminus of D1-Ala344

The mutations Ala344stop and Ser345Pro abolish photoautotrophic and O_2 evolution [249,313], although the high-affinity Mn site identified in the D1-Asp170 mutants (Sec. 4.1.1) remains intact [313]. Because the D1 polypeptide in the Ala344stop mutant is shortened by one residue and the C-terminal domain is not posttranslationally processed in the Ser345Pro mutant, it was proposed that the C terminus of D1-Ala may be a ligand to the assembled Mn cluster [313].

4.1.8. Other D1 Residues

All mutants constructed at D1-Asp59, D1-Asp61, D1-Glu65, and D1-His92 are photoautotrophic [282,306]. None of these residues appear to be essential for the assembly or stability of the Mn cluster [282]. Therefore, none appears likely to ligate Mn. Nevertheless, the Mn clusters in all of the mutants are perturbed to some degree, particularly in the Asp61Asn, Asp61Ala, Glu65Gln, and Glu65Ala mutants. These mutants evolve O_2 at only $\approx 20\%$ the rate of wild-type cells [282]. In the Asp61Asn and Asp61Ala mutants, O_2 release during the $S_3 \rightarrow (S_4) \rightarrow S_0$ transition is slowed ≈ 10-fold [314]. The $S_3 \rightarrow (S_4) \rightarrow S_0$ transition and O_2 release are also slowed in the Asp49Asn and Asp61Glu mutants, but to lesser extents [315]. Photoautotrophic growth of the Asp59Asn and Asp61Ala mutants is abolished and electron transfer from Y_Z to $P_{680}^{\bullet+}$ is slowed dramatically in the absence of Ca^{2+} [282]. Therefore, it was proposed that

D1-Asp59 and D1-Asp61 may directly coordinate a Ca^{2+} ion [282]. It was subsequently proposed that binding Ca^{2+} to this site promotes repositioning of the C-terminal domain of the D1 polypeptide during the light-driven assembly (photoactivation) of the Mn cluster [316]. Recent data show that intermediates in the assembly and photoactivation of the Mn cluster are greatly destabilized in both the Asp59Asn and Asp61Glu mutants [315].

At least 17 mutations have been constructed at D1-Glu189 [286, 288,289,298]. Only the Gln, Lys, Arg, Leu, and Ile mutants are photoautotrophic. The influence of the D1-Glu189 mutants on the assembly or stability of the complex is minor [282], so this residue is not believed to ligate Mn [282]. Neither the Asp nor Gly mutants appear able to advance beyond the $S_2Y_Z^{\bullet}$ state and neither exhibits an S_2-state multiline EPR signal [288]. The Glu189Asp mutant appears to alter the redox potential of Y_Z: charge recombination between $Q_A^{\bullet-}$ and $P_{680}^{\bullet+}$ is accelerated in this mutant [286,288]. It has been proposed that D1-Glu189 interacts with D1-His190 and that both residues form part of a network of hydrogen bonds involving Y_Z [279,286–289] (Sec. 3.2).

4.2.   The D2 Protein

The mutations D2-Glu70Gln and D2-Glu70Val abolish photoautotrophic growth [317]. The Glu70Gln mutant evolves O_2, but the rate declines rapidly during illumination, presumably because of photooxidative damage (photoinhibition). Because the addition of Mn^{2+} ions stabilized the rate of O_2 evolution in this mutant, D2-Glu70 was proposed to be a ligand of the Mn cluster [317]. However, in the recent structure of the CP47/D2/D1 complex (Fig. 2), D2-Glu70, located in the loop connecting helices A and B of the D2 polypeptide (Fig. 4B), seems far from the Mn cluster, located near Y_Z. Furthermore, exogenous Mn^{2+} ions may protect against light-induced damage by donating electrons to $Y_Z^{\bullet}$, in the same manner that some other electron donors offer protection (see discussion in [1]). Therefore, it seems unlikely that D2-Glu70 is a ligand to the Mn cluster.

None of the other mutations constructed in the lumenal domains of the D2 polypeptide by site-directed [141] or random chemical [318] mutagenesis, including mutations constructed at all conserved carboxylate and histidine residues, abolish photoautotrophic growth, with the exception of the mutation D2-Ser80Phe [318]. Like D2-Glu70Gln, this mutant evolves O_2 but is sensitive to photooxidative damage (photoinhibition) [318]. Several deletion mutants have been constructed in the D2 protein. Photoautotrophic growth is retained in mutants lacking the C-terminal 11 residues or containing 7–8 amino acid deletions within the C-terminal domain [319]. These deletion mutants are also sensitive to photooxidative damage (photoinhibition).

On the basis of the available data and the structure of the CP47/D2/D1 complex (Fig. 2), it seems unlikely that the D2 protein provides any ligands to the Mn cluster. Instead, mutations or deletions in the lumenal domains of the D2 protein probably perturb the Mn cluster by perturbing the backbone conformations of this and other polypeptides. Nevertheless, because a terminal ligand of the Mn cluster might be functionally replaced by an H_2O molecule, a Cl^- ion, or by a repositioned amino acid residue from another protein, it is not possible to rigorously exclude the D2 protein as a potential source of one or more terminal ligands of the Mn cluster.

4.3.   The CP47 Protein

The large hydrophilic loop of CP47 interacts with the extrinsic 33-kDa polypeptide (Sec. 2.6) and is believed to cover part of the lumenal domains of the D1/D2 heterodimer (Sec. 2.3). The importance of specific domains in this loop has been probed by segment deletion [166, 320–323], site-directed [320,323–329], combinatorial [330], and random [163] mutagenesis. Segment deletion mutagenesis identified the regions extending from Ala373 to Asp380 and from Arg384 to Val392 as crucial for tight association of the extrinsic 33-kDa protein and for the stability of a functional Mn cluster [321,322]. Site-directed mutagenesis studies show that Arg384 and Arg385 are required for the proper binding of the extrinsic 33-kDa protein [331]. Therefore, as might be expected (Sec. 2.6), mutations of these residues slow O_2 release during the $S_3 \rightarrow (S_4)$ $\rightarrow S_0$ transition [326], stabilize the S_2 state [326], increase the sensitivity of PS II to photooxidative damage (photoinhibition) [324,326], and increase the quantum yield of light-driven assembly (photoactivation) of the Mn cluster [331]. In other domains of the large hydrophilic loop, the residues Lys321 [328], Phe363 [329], and Arg448 [163,325], plus

residues in the domain extending from Asp440 to Pro447 [330], critically influence the Cl^- requirement for photoautotrophic growth and O_2
evolution. Mutations at these residues increase the sensitivity of PS II
to light-induced damage and abolish photoautotrophic growth and O_2
evolution at low Cl^- concentrations. Other residues of interest are
Gly342 [163] and Glu364 [323]. The mutation Gly342Asp impairs photoautotrophic growth [163], while the mutation Glu364Gln abolishes
photoautotrophic growth in the absence of the *psbV* protein [323]. In addition, mutation of Tyr167, a residue in the smaller hydrophilic loop
connecting helices III and IV of CP47 (Fig. 4B), severely retards photoautotrophic growth, decreases the amount of PS II stability incorporated in the thylakoid membrane, and increases the sensitivity of PS II
to photooxidative damage (photoinhibition) [327].

In contrast to the D1 protein, no individual residues on CP47 have
been identified whose mutation abolishes photoautotrophic growth and
O_2 evolution under normal growth conditions without concurrently preventing the stable assembly of PS II. Therefore, no specific residues on
CP47 have been proposed as potential ligands for Mn. Nevertheless, because a terminal ligand of the Mn cluster might be functionally replaced
by a H_2O molecule, a Cl^- ion, or a repositioned amino acid residue from
another protein, it is not possible to rigorously exclude CP47 as potentially contributing one or more terminal ligands. In any event, the critical influence of specific residues of CP47 on the Cl^- requirement for O_2
evolution shows that the large hydrophilic loop of CP47 strongly influences the environment of the Mn cluster.

4.4. The CP43 Protein

The large hydrophilic loop of CP43 also interacts with the extrinsic 33-
kDa polypeptide (Sec. 2.6) and is believed to cover part of the lumenal
domains of the D1 protein (Sec. 2.3). The importance of specific domains
in this loop has been probed by segment deletion [332] and site-directed
[333] mutagenesis. Photoautotrophic growth and O_2 evolution were
abolished in all of the deletion mutants [332]. In contrast, some of the
deletion mutations in CP47 showed little effect on either photoautotrophic growth or O_2 evolution [166,320]. The mutation Arg305Ser
slightly impairs O_2 evolution, whereas the mutation Arg342Ser com-

pletely abolishes photoautotrophic growth and O_2 evolution under normal growth conditions [333]. The Arg342Ser mutant stably assembles PS II and its PS II content, on a chlorophyll basis, is 60–70% of that in wild-type cells [333]. However, these PS II complexes are extremely sensitive to photooxidative damage (photoinhibition) [333].

The CP43 protein is present in every O_2-evolving PS II complex yet isolated (Sec. 2.1). However, a recent study shows that the light-driven assembly and photoactivation of the Mn cluster can proceed in the absence of CP43 in vitro [335]. Therefore, it seems unlikely that CP43 provides any ligands to the Mn cluster unless such ligands can be functionally replaced by a H_2O molecule, a Cl^- ion, or a repositioned amino acid from another protein.

5.   CONCLUDING REMARKS

Our understanding of photosynthetic water oxidation has increased steadily over the last 5 years. The overall structure of PS II is becoming clearer, as is the role of the antenna proteins of higher plants and green algae in protecting PS II from light-induced damage. New models for water oxidation have been proposed that incorporate proton-coupled electron transfer events, and amino acid residues that interact with tyrosines Y_Z and Y_D have been identified. Although no amino acid ligand of the Mn cluster has been identified unambiguously, many candidates have been identified and spectroscopic characterization of site-directed mutants is being pursued vigorously. The next 5 years should see continued progress in our understanding of the structure and function of the core proteins of PS II and their role in promoting manganotyrosyl-based oxygen evolution.

ACKNOWLEDGMENTS

I am very grateful to J. Barber for providing a preprint of Ref. 60, to B. Svensson for providing Fig. 5A and B, to the NIH for support (Grant GM 43496), and to G.T. Babcock, J.J. Eaton-Rye, and M. Seibert for critical comments on the manuscript.

ABBREVIATIONS

ATP	adenosine triphosphate
Car	carotenoid
Chl	chlorophyll a
Chl_Z	monomeric Chl species coordinated by D1-His118 and oxidized by $P_{680}^{\bullet+}$ via a molecule of carotenoid
Chl_D	monomeric Chl species coordinated by D2-His118
CP	chlorophyll protein
CW	continuous wave
DCCD	dicyclohexylcarbodiimide
EDC	1-ethyl-3-[3-(dimethylamino)propyl]carbodiimide
ENDOR	electron nuclear double resonance
EPR	electron paramagnetic resonance
ESEEM	electron spin-echo envelope modulation
EXAFS	extended X-ray absorption fine structure
FTIR	Fourier transform infrared
LHC	light-harvesting complex
OEC	oxygen evolving complex
PS II	Photosystem II
PS I	Photosystem I
P_{680}	multimeric Chl species that serves as the light-induced electron donor in PS II
Pheo	pheophytin
Q_A	primary plastoquinone electron acceptor
Q_B	secondary plastoquinone electron acceptor
Y_Z	tyrosine residue that mediates electron transfer between the Mn cluster and $P_{680}^{\bullet+}$
Y_D	tyrosine residue that acts as an alternate electron donor to $P_{680}^{\bullet+}$

REFERENCES

1. R. J. Debus, *Biochim. Biophys. Acta*, *1102*, 269–352 (1992).

2. R. D. Britt, in *Oxygenic Photosynthesis: The Light Reactions* (D. R. Ort and C. F. Yocum, eds.), Kluwer Academic, Dordrecht, 1996, pp. 137–164.

3. B. A. Diner and G. T. Babcock, in *Oxygenic Photosynthesis: The Light Reactions* (D. R. Ort and C. F. Yocum, eds.), Kluwer Academic, Dordrecht, 1996, pp. 213–247.

4. V. K. Yachandra, K. Sauer, and M. P. Klein, *Chem. Rev.*, *96*, 2927–2950 (1996).

5. G. Renger, *Physiol. Plant.*, *100*, 828–841 (1997).

6. J. E. Penner-Hahn, *Structure and Bonding*, *90*, 1–36 (1998).

7. J. R. Durrant, D. R. Klug, S. L. Kwa, R. van Grondelle, G. Porter, and J. P. Dekker, *Proc. Natl. Acad. Sci. USA*, *92*, 4798–4802 (1995).

8. S. E. J. Rigby, J. H. A. Nugent, and P. J. O'Malley, *Biochemistry*, *33*, 10043–10050 (1994).

9. T. Noguchi, T. Tomo, and Y. Inoue, *Biochemistry*, *37*, 13614–13625 (1998).

10. L. Iuzzolino, J. Dittmer, W. Dörner, W. Meyer-Klaucke, and H. Dau, *Biochemistry*, *37*, 17112–17119 (1998).

11. T. A. Roelofs, W. Liang, M. J. Latimer, R. M. Cinco, A. Rompel, J. C. Andrews, K. Sauer, V. K. Yachandra, and M. P. Klein, *Proc. Natl. Acad. Sci. USA*, *93*, 3335–3340 (1996).

12. D. W. Randall, B. E. Sturgeon, J. A. Ball, G. A. Lorigan, M. K. Chan, M. P. Klein, W. H. Armstrong, and R. D. Britt, *J. Am. Chem. Soc.*, *117*, 11780–11789 (1995).

13. J. M. Peloquin, K. A. Campbell, and R. D. Britt, *J. Am. Chem. Soc.*, *120*, 6840–6841 (1998).

14. V. K. Yachandra, V. J. DeRose, M. J. Latimer, I. Mukerji, K. Sauer, and M. P. Klein, *Science*, *260*, 675–679 (1993).

15. T.-A. Ono and Y. Inoue, *FEBS Lett.*, *168*, 281–286 (1984).

16. M. Miyao and N. Murata, *FEBS Lett.*, *170*, 350–354 (1984).

17. R. Mei and C. F. Yocum, *Biochemistry*, *31*, 8449–8454 (1992).

18. P. J. Riggs-Gelasco, R. Mei, C. F. Yocum, and J. E. Penner-Hahn, *J. Am. Chem. Soc.*, *118*, 2387–2399 (1996).

19. M. Zheng and G. C. Dismukes, *Inorg. Chem.*, *35*, 3307–3319 (1996).

20. K.-C. Han and S. Katoh, *Plant Cell Physiol.*, *34*, 585–593 (1993).

21. P. Ädelroth, K. Lindberg, and L.-E. Andréasson, *Biochemistry*, *34*, 9021–9027 (1995).

22. K. Lindberg, T. Vänngård, and L.-E. Andréasson, *Photosynth. Res.*, *38*, 401–408 (1993).

23. C. A. Buser, L. K. Thompson, B. A. Diner, and G. W. Brudvig, *Biochemistry*, *29*, 8977–8985 (1990).

24. I. Vass and S. Styring, *Biochemistry*, *30*, 830–839 (1991).

25. C. A. Buser, B. A. Diner, and G. W. Brudvig, *Biochemistry*, *31*, 11449–11459 (1992).

26. L. K. Thompson and G. W. Brudvig, *Biochemistry*, *27*, 6653–6658 (1988).

27. R. H. Schweitzer and G. W. Brudvig, *Biochemistry*, *36*, 11351–11359 (1997).

28. D. H. Stewart and G. W. Brudvig, *Biochim. Biophys. Acta*, *1367*, 63–87 (1998).

29. D. H. Stewart and G. W. Brudvig, in *Photosynthesis: Mechanism and Effects*, Vol. 2 (G. Garab, ed.), Kluwer Academic, Dordrecht, 1999, pp. 1113–1116.

30. J. Whitmarsh and H. B. Pakrasi, in *Oxygenic Photosynthesis: The Light Reactions* (D. R. Ort and C. F. Yocum, eds.), Kluwer Academic, 1996, pp. 249–264.

31. P. Dorlet, M. Di Valentin, G. T. Babcock, and J. L. McCracken, *J. Phys. Chem. B*, *102*, 8239–8247 (1998).

32. K. V. Lakshmi, S. S. Eaton, G. R. Eaton, H. A. Frank, and G. W. Brudvig, *J. Phys. Chem. B*, *102*, 8327–8335 (1998).

33. J. Limburg, V. A. Szalai, and G. W. Brudvig, *J. Chem. Soc., Dalton Trans.*, 1353–1361 (1999).

34. C. Tommos, X.-S. Tang, K. Warncke, C. W. Hoganson, S. Styring, J. McCracken, B. A. Diner, and G. T. Babcock, *J. Am. Chem. Soc.*, *117*, 10325–10335 (1995).

35. C. W. Hoganson, N. Lydakis-Simantiris, X.-S. Tang, C. Tommos, K. Warncke, G. T. Babcock, B. A. Diner, J. McCracken, and S. Styring, *Photosynth. Res.*, *46*, 177–184 (1995).

36. M. L. Gilchrist, Jr., J. A. Ball, D. W. Randall, and R. D. Britt, *Proc. Natl. Acad. Sci. USA*, *92*, 9545–9549 (1995).

37. G. T. Babcock, in *Photosynthesis: From Light to Biosphere*, Vol. 2 (P. Mathis, ed.), Kluwer Academic, Dordrecht, 1995, pp. 209–215.

38. C. W. Hoganson and G. T. Babcock, *Science*, *277*, 1953–1956 (1997).

39. C. Tommos and G. T. Babcock, *Acc. Chem. Res.*, *31*, 18–25 (1998).

40. C. Tommos, C. W. Hoganson, M. Di Valentin, N. Lydakis-Sima-

tiris, P. Dorlet, K. Westphal, H.-A. Chu, J. McCracken, and G. T. Babcock, *Curr. Opin. Chem. Biol.*, *2*, 244–252 (1998).

41. M. Haumann and W. Junge, *Biochim. Biophys. Acta*, *1411*, 86–91 (1999).

42. T. M. Bricker and D. F. Ghanotakis, in *Oxygenic Photosynthesis: The Light Reactions* (D. R. Ort and C. F. Yocum, eds.), Kluwer Academic, Dordrecht, 1996, pp. 113–136.

43. J. Barber, J. Nield, E. P. Morris, D. Zheleva, and B. Hankamer, *Physiol. Plant.*, *100*, 817–827 (1997).

44. B. Hankamer, J. Barber, and E. J. Boekema, *Annu. Rev. Plant Physiol. Plant Mol. Biol.*, *48*, 641–671 (1997).

45. S. Jansson, *Biochim. Biophys. Acta*, *1184*, 1–19 (1994).

46. B. R. Green and D. G. Durnford, *Annu. Rev. Plant Physiol. Plant Mol. Biol.*, *47*, 685–714 (1996).

47. D. J. Simpson and J. Knoetzel, in *Oxygenic Photosynthesis: The Light Reactions* (D. R. Ort and C. F. Yocum, eds.), Kluwer Academic, Dordrecht, 1996, pp. 493–506.

48. E. Pichersky and S. Jansson, in *Oxygenic Photosynthesis: The Light Reactions* (D. R. Ort and C. F. Yocum, eds.), Kluwer Academic, Dordrecht, 1996, pp. 507–521.

49. R. Bassi, D. Sandonà, and R. Croce, *Physiol. Plant.*, *100*, 769–779 (1997).

50. W. A. Sidler, in *The Molecular Biology of Cyanobacteria* (D. A. Bryant, ed.), Kluwer Academic, Dordrecht, 1994, pp. 139–216.

51. R. MacColl, *J. Struct. Biol.*, *124*, 311–334 (1998).

52. E. J. Boekema, B. Hankamer, D. Bald, J. Kruip, J. Nield, A. F. Boonstra, J. Barber, and M. Rögner, *Proc. Natl. Acad. Sci. USA*, *92*, 175–179 (1995).

53. B. Hankamer, J. Nield, D. Zheleva, E. Boekema, S. Jansson, and J. Barber, *Eur. J. Biochem.*, *243*, 422–429 (1997).

54. C. Eijckelhoff, J. P. Dekker, and E. J. Boekema, *Biochim. Biophys. Acta*, *1321*, 10–20 (1997).

55. E. J. Boekema, J. Nield, B. Hankamer, and J. Barber, *Eur. J. Biochem.*, *252*, 268–276 (1998).

56. K. M. Marr, D. N. Mastronarde, and M. K. Lyon, *J. Cell Biol.*, *132*, 823–833 (1996).

57. K. M. Marr, R. L. McFeeters, and M. K. Lyon, *J. Struct. Biol.*, *117*, 86–98 (1996).

58. E. P. Morris, B. Hankamer, D. Zheleva, G. Friso, and J. Barber, *Structure*, *5*, 837–849 (1997).

59. M. K. Lyon, *Biochim. Biophys. Acta*, *1364*, 403–419 (1998).

60. B. Hankamer, E. P. Morris, and J. Barber, *Nature Struct. Biol.*, 6, 560–564 (1999).

61. J. Barber, J. Nield, E. P. Morris, and B. Hankamer, *Trends Biochem. Sci.*, *24*, 43–45 (1999).

62. D. Zheleva, J. Sharma, M. Panico, H. R. Morris, and J. Barber, *J. Biol. Chem.*, *273*, 16122–16127 (1998).

63. M. Bianchetti, D. Zheleva, Z. Deak, S. Zharmuhamedov, V. Klimov, J. H. A. Nugent, I. Vass, and J. Barber, *J. Biol. Chem.*, *273*, 16128–16133 (1998).

64. E. Mörschel and G. H. Schatz, *Planta*, *172*, 145–154 (1987).

65. M. Rögner, J. P. Dekker, E. J. Boekema, and H. T. Witt, *FEBS Lett.*, *219*, 207–211 (1987).

66. J. P. Dekker, E. J. Boekema, H. T. Witt, and M. Rögner, *Biochim. Biophys. Acta*, *936*, 307–318 (1988).

67. E. J. Boekema, A. F. Boonstra, J. P. Dekker, and M. Rögner, *J. Bioenerg. Biomemb.*, *26*, 17–29 (1994).

68. E. Boekema, H. Van Roon, and J. P. Dekker, *FEBS Lett.*, *424*, 95–99 (1998).

69. R. Harrer, R. Bassi, M. G. Testi, and C. Schäfer, *Eur. J. Biochem.*, *255*, 196–205 (1998).

70. E. J. Boekema, H. Van Roon, F. Calkoen, R. Bassi, and J. P. Dekker, *Biochemistry*, *38*, 2233–2239 (1999).

71. J. F. Allen, *Biochim. Biophys. Acta*, *1098*, 275–335 (1992).

72. J. F. Allen, *Physiol. Plant.*, *93*, 196–205 (1995).

73. P. Horton, A. V. Ruban, and R. G. Walters, *Annu. Rev. Plant Physiol. Plant Mol. Biol.*, *47*, 655–684 (1996).

74. J. F. Allen and A. Nilsson, *Physiol. Plant.*, *100*, 863–868 (1997).

75. W. Kühlbrandt, D. N. Wang, and Y. Fujiyoshi, *Nature*, *367*, 614–621 (1994).

76. W. Kühlbrandt, *Curr. Opin. Struct. Biol.*, *4*, 519–528 (1994).

77. J. P. Connelly, M. G. Müller, R. Bassi, R. Croce, and A. R. Holzwarth, *Biochemistry*, *36*, 281–287 (1997).

78. D. Sandonà, R. Croce, A. Pagano, M. Crimi, and R. Bassi, *Biochim. Biophys. Acta*, *1365*, 207–214 (1998).

79. A. V. Ruban, P. J. Lee, M. Wentworth, A. J. Young, and P. Horton, *J. Biol. Chem.*, *274*, 10458–10465 (1999).

80. S. Eshaghi, B. Andersson, and J. Barber, *FEBS Lett.*, *446*, 23–26 (1999).

81. A. Nilsson, D. Stys, T. Drakenberg, M. Spangfort, S. Forsén, and J. F. Allen, *J. Biol. Chem.*, *272*, 18350–18357 (1997).

82. M. G. Testi, R. Croce, P. Polverino-De Laureto, and R. Bassi, *FEBS Lett.*, *399*, 245–250 (1996).

83. E. Giuffra, D. Cugini, R. Croce, and R. Bassi, *Eur. J. Biochem.*, *238*, 112–120 (1996).

84. F. Ros, R. Bassi, and H. Paulsen, *Eur. J. Biochem.*, *253*, 653–658 (1998).

85. A. Pagano, G. Cinque, and R. Bassi, *J. Biol. Chem.*, *273*, 17154–17165 (1998).

86. R. Bassi, B. Pineau, P. Dainese, and J. Marquardt, *Eur. J. Biochem.*, *212*, 297–303 (1993).

87. A. V. Ruban, A. J. Young, A. A. Pascal, and P. Horton, *Plant Physiol.*, *104*, 227–234 (1994).

88. R. G. Walters, A. V. Ruban, and P. Horton, *Proc. Natl. Acad. Sci. USA*, *93*, 14204–14209 (1996).

89. P. Pesaresi, D. Sandonà, E. Giuffra, and R. Bassi, *FEBS Lett.*, *402*, 151–156 (1997).

90. H. Y. Yamamoto and R. Bassi, in *Oxygenic Photosynthesis: The Light Reactions* (D. R. Ort and C. F. Yocum, eds.), Kluwer Academic, Dordrecht, 1996, pp. 539–563.

91. A. M. Gilmore, *Physiol. Plant.*, *99*, 197–209 (1997).

92. M. Eskling, P.-O. Arvidsson, and H.-E. Åkerlund, *Physiol. Plant.*, *100*, 806–816 (1997).

93. A. V. Ruban, D. Phillip, A. J. Young, and P. Horton, *Biochemistry*, *36*, 7855–7859 (1997).

94. A. V. Ruban, D. Phillip, A. J. Young, and P. Horton, *Photochem. Photobiol.*, *68*, 829–834 (1998).

95. R. C. Bugos, A. D. Hieber, and H. Y. Yamamoto, *J. Biol. Chem.*, *273*, 15321–15324 (1998).

96. A. Hager and K. Holocher, *Planta*, *192*, 581–589 (1994).

97. M. Ikeuchi and Y. Inoue, *Arch. Biochem. Biophys.*, *247*, 97–107 (1986).

98. D. F. Ghanotakis, D. M. Demetriou, and C. F. Yocum, *Biochim. Biophys. Acta*, *891*, 15–21 (1987).

99. E. Haag, K.-D. Irrgang, E. J. Boekema, and G. Renger, *Eur. J. Biochem.*, *189*, 47–53 (1990).

100. R. K. Mishra and D. F. Ghanotakis, *Photosynth. Res.*, *42*, 37–42 (1994).

101. X.-S. Tang and B. A. Diner, *Biochemistry*, *33*, 4594–4603 (1994).

102. K. Akabori, H. Tsukamoto, J. Tsukihara, T. Nagatsuka, O. Motokawa, and Y. Toyoshima, *Biochim. Biophys. Acta*, *932*, 345–357 (1988).

103. D. F. Ghanotakis, J. C. de Paula, D. M. Demetriou, N. R. Bowlby, J. Petersen, G. T. Babcock, and C. F. Yocum, *Biochim. Biophys. Acta*, *974*, 44–53 (1989).

104. J. P. Dekker, N. R. Bowlby, and C. F. Yocum, *FEBS Lett.*, *254*, 150–154 (1989).

105. J. Petersen, J. P. Dekker, N. R. Bowlby, D. F. Ghanotakis, C. F. Yocum, and G. T. Babcock, *Biochemistry*, *29*, 3226–3231 (1990).

106. M. Rögner, D. A. Chisholm, and B. A. Diner, *Biochemistry*, *30*, 5387–5395 (1991).

107. K. H. Rhee, E. P. Morris, D. Zheleva, B. Hankamer, W. Kühlbrandt, and J. Barber, *Nature*, *389*, 522–526 (1997).

108. K. Mayanagi, T. Ishikawa, C. Toyoshima, Y. Inoue, and K. Nakazato, *J. Struct. Biol.*, *123*, 211–224 (1998).

109. K. H. Rhee, E. P. Morris, J. Barber, and W. Kühlbrandt, *Nature*, *396*, 283–286 (1998).

110. O. Nanba and Ki. Satoh, *Proc. Natl. Acad. Sci. USA*, 84, 109–112 (1987).

111. J. Barber, D. J. Chapman, and A. Telfer, *FEBS Lett.*, 220, 67–73 (1987).

112. M. Ikeuchi and Y. Inoue, *FEBS Lett.*, *241*, 99–104 (1988).

113. A. N. Webber, L. Packman, D. J. Chapman, J. Barber, and J. C. Gray, *FEBS Lett.*, *242*, 259–262 (1989).

114. K.-D. Irrgang, L.-X. Shi, C. Funk, and W. P. Schröder, *J. Biol. Chem.*, *270*, 17588–17593 (1995).

115. M. Okamura, Ki. Satoh, R. A. Isaacson, and G. Feher, in *Progress in Photosynthesis Research*, Vol. 1 (J. Biggins, ed.), Martinus Nijhoff, Dordrecht, 1987, pp. 379–381.

116. H. P. Michel, D. F. Hunt, J. Shabanowitz, and J. Bennett, *J. Biol. Chem.*, *263*, 1123–1130 (1988).

117. J. Sharma, M. Panico, C. A. Shipton, F. Nilsson, H. R. Morris, and J. Barber, *J. Biol. Chem.*, *272*, 33158–33166 (1997).

118. M.-A. Takahashi, T. Shiraishi, and K. Asada, *FEBS Lett.*, *240*, 6–8 (1988).

119. Y. Takahashi, H. Nakane, H. Kojima, and Ki. Satoh, *Plant Cell Physiol.*, *31*, 273–280 (1990).

120. A. K. Mattoo, H. Hoffman-Falk, J. B. Marder, and M. Edelman, *Proc. Natl. Acad. Sci. USA*, *81*, 1380–1384 (1984).

121. E.-M. Aro, I. Virgin, and B. Andersson, *Biochim. Biophys. Acta*, *1143*, 113–134 (1993).

122. B. Andersson and J. Barber, in *Photosynthesis and the Environment* (N. R. Baker, ed.), Kluwer Academic, Dordrecht, 1996, pp. 101–121.

123. B. Andersson and E.-M. Aro, *Physiol. Plant.*, *100*, 780–793 (1997).

124. M. Kobayashi, H. Maeda, T. Watanabe, H. Nakane, and Ki. Satoh, *FEBS Lett.*, *260*, 138–140 (1990).

125. K. Gounaris, D. J. Chapman, P. Booth, B. Crystall, L. B. Giorgi, D. R. Klug, G. Porter, and J. Barber, *FEBS Lett.*, *265*, 88–92 (1990).

126. C. Eijckelhoff, H. Van Roon, M. L. Groot, R. van Grondelle, and J. P. Dekker, *Biochemistry*, *35*, 12864–12872 (1996).

127. A. Trebst, *Z. Naturforsch.*, *41c*, 240–245 (1986).

128. H. Michel and J. Deisenhofer, *Biochemistry*, *27*, 1–7 (1988).

129. R. Hienerwadel and C. Berthomieu, *Biochemistry*, *34*, 16288–16297 (1995).

130. J. P. M. Schelvis, P. I. van Noort, T. J. Aartsma, and H. J. van Gorkom, *Biochim. Biophys. Acta*, *1184*, 242–250 (1994).

131. D. Koulougliotis, J. B. Innes, and G. W. Brudvig, *Biochemistry*, *33*, 11814–11822 (1994).

132. D. H. Stewart, A. Cua, D. A. Chisholm, B. A. Diner, D. F. Bocian, and G. W. Brudvig, *Biochemistry*, *37*, 10040–10046 (1998).

133. R. J. Debus, B. A. Barry, G. T. Babcock, and L. McIntosh, *Proc. Natl. Acad. Sci. USA*, *85*, 427–430 (1988).

134. W. F. J. Vermaas, A. W. Rutherford, and Ö. Hansson, *Proc. Natl. Acad. Sci. USA*, *85*, 8477–8481 (1988).

135. R. J. Debus, B. A. Barry, I. Sithole, G. T. Babcock, and L. McIntosh, *Biochemistry*, *27*, 9071–9074 (1988).

136. J. G. Metz, P. J. Nixon, M. Rögner, G. W. Brudvig, and B. A. Diner, *Biochemistry*, *28*, 6960–6969 (1989).

137. B. Svensson, I. Vass, E. Cedergren, and S. Styring, *EMBO J.*, *9*, 2051–2059 (1990).

138. S. V. Ruffle, D. Donnelly, T. L. Blundell, and J. H. A. Nugent, *Photosynth. Res.*, *34*, 287–300 (1992).

139. B. Svensson, C. Etchebest, P. Tuffery, P. Van Kan, J. Smith, and S. Styring, *Biochemistry*, *35*, 14486–14502 (1996).

140. J. Xiong, S. Subramaniam, and Govindjee, *Photosynth. Res.*, *56*, 229–254 (1998).

141. H. B. Pakrasi and W. F. J. Vermaas, in *The Photosystems: Structure, Function and Molecular Biology* (J. Barber, ed.), Elsevier, Amsterdam, 1992, pp. 231–257.

142. W. F. J. Vermaas, *Annu. Rev. Plant Physiol. Plant Mol. Biol.*, *44*, 457–481 (1993).

143. B. A. Diner, X.-S. Tang, M. Zheng, G. C. Dismukes, D. A. Force, D. W. Randall, and R. D. Britt, in *Photosynthesis: From Light to Biosphere*, Vol. 2 (P. Mathis, ed.), Kluwer Academic, Dordrecht, 1995, pp. 229–234.

144. W. J. Coleman, P. J. Nixon, W. F. J. Vermaas, and B. A. Diner, in *Photosynthesis: From Light to Biosphere*, Vol. 1 (P. Mathis, ed.), Kluwer Academic, Dordrecht, 1995, pp. 779–782.

145. S. A. Merry, P. J. Nixon, L. M. Barter, M. Schilstra, G. Porter, J, Barber, J. R. Durrant, and D. R. Klug, *Biochemistry*, *37*, 17439–17447 (1998).

146. L. B. Giorgi, P. J. Nixon, S. A. Merry, M. Joseph, J. R. Durrant, J. De Las Rivas, J. Barber, G. Porter, and D. R. Klug, *J. Biol. Chem.*, *271*, 2093–2101 (1996).

147. M. T. Lince and W. F. J. Vermaas, *Eur. J. Biochem.*, *256*, 595–602 (1998).

148. J. M. Peloquin, X.-S. Tang, B. A. Diner, and R. D. Britt, *Biochemistry*, *38*, 2057–2067 (1999).

149. T. M. Bricker, *Photosynth. Res.*, *24*, 1–13 (1990).

150. J. B. Innes and G. W. Brudvig, *Biochemistry*, *28*, 1116–1125 (1989).

151. Y. Isogai, S. Itoh, and M. Nishimura, *Biochim. Biophys. Acta,* *1017,* 204–208 (1990).

152. Y. Kashino, I. Enami, S. Igarashi, and S. Katoh, *Plant Cell Physiol.,* *33,* 259–266 (1992).

153. A. A. Moskalenko, R. Barbato, and G. M. Giacometti, *FEBS Lett.,* *314,* 271–274 (1992).

154. N. Krauss, W.-D. Schubert, O. Klukas, P. Fromme, H. T. Witt, and W. Saenger, *Nature Struct. Biol.,* *3,* 965–973 (1996).

155. W. D. Schubert, O. Klukas, N. Krauss, W. Saenger, P. Fromme, and H. T. Witt, *J. Mol. Biol.,* *272,* 741–769 (1997).

156. O. Klukas, W. D. Schubert, P. Jordan, N. Krauss, P. Fromme, H. T. Witt, and W. Saenger, *J. Biol. Chem.,* *274,* 7351–7360 (1999).

157. O. Klukas, W. D. Schubert, P. Jordan, N. Krauss, P. Fromme, H. T. Witt, and W. Saenger, *J. Biol. Chem.,* *274,* 7361–7367 (1999).

158. W. F. J. Vermaas, *Photosynth. Res.,* *41,* 285–294 (1994).

159. P. Fromme, H. T. Witt, W.-D. Schubert, O. Klukas, W. Saenger, and N. Krauss, *Biochim. Biophys. Acta,* *1275,* 76–83 (1996).

160. W. D. Schubert, O. Klukas, W. Saenger, H. T. Witt, P. Fromme, and N. Krauss, *J. Mol. Biol.,* *280,* 297–314 (1998).

161. G. Shen, J. J. Eaton-Rye, and W. F. J. Vermaas, *Biochemistry,* *32,* 5109–5115 (1993).

162. G. Shen and W. F. J. Vermaas, *Biochemistry,* *33,* 7379–7388 (1994).

163. J. T. Wu, N. Masri, W. Lee, L. K. Frankel, and T. M. Bricker, *Plant Mol. Biol.,* *39,* 381–386 (1999).

164. P. Manna and W. F. J. Vermaas, *Eur. J. Biochem.,* *247,* 666–672 (1997).

165. W. F. J. Vermaas, M. Ikeuchi, and Y. Inoue, *Photosynth. Res.,* *17,* 97–113 (1988).

166. J. J. Eaton-Rye and W. F. J. Vermaas, *Plant Mol. Biol.,* *17,* 1165–1177 (1991).

167. R. Barbato, G. Friso, F. Rigoni, F. Dalla Vecchi, and G. M. Giacometti, *J. Cell Biol.,* *119,* 325–335 (1992).

168. W. R. Widger, W. A. Cramer, M. Hermodson, and R. G. Herrmann, *FEBS Lett.,* *191,* 186–190 (1985).

169. J. Sharma, M. Panico, J. Barber, and H. R. Morris, *J. Biol. Chem.,* *272,* 3935–3943 (1997).

170. G.-S. Tae, M. T. Black, W. A. Cramer, O. Vallon, and L. Bogorad, *Biochemistry,* *27* 9075–9080 (1988).

171. O. Vallon, G.-S. Tae, W. A. Cramer, D. Simpson, G. Hoyer-Hansen, and L. Bogorad, *Biochim. Biophys. Acta*, *975*, 132–141 (1989).

172. G.-S. Tae and W. A. Cramer, *Biochemistry*, *33*, 10060–10068 (1994).

173. G. T. Babcock, W. R. Widger, W. A. Cramer, W. A. Oertling, and J. G. Metz, *Biochemistry*, *24*, 3638–3645 (1985).

174. W. A. Cramer, G.-S. Tae, P. N. Furbacher, and M. Böttger, *Physiol. Plant.*, *88*, 705–711 (1993).

175. C. A. Buser, B. A. Diner, and G. W. Brudvig, *Biochemistry*, *31*, 11441–11448 (1992).

176. G. M. MacDonald, R. J. Boerner, R. M. Everly, W. A. Cramer, R. J. Debus, and B. A. Barry, *Biochemistry*, *33*, 4393–4400 (1994).

177. F. Morais, J. Barber, and P. J. Nixon, *J. Biol. Chem.*, *273*, 29315–29320 (1998).

178. V. P. McNamara, F. S. Sutterwala, H. B. Pakrasi, and J. Whitmarsh, *Proc. Natl. Acad. Sci. USA*, *94*, 14173–14178 (1997).

179. C. Francke, R. Loyal, I. Ohad, and W. Haehnel, *FEBS Lett.*, *442*, 75–78 (1999).

180. H. B. Pakrasi, K. J. Nyhus, and H. Granok, *Z. Naturforsch.*, *45c*, 423–429 (1990).

181. H. B. Pakrasi, P. De Ciechi, and J. Whitmarsh, *EMBO J.*, *10*, 1619–1627 (1991).

182. V. K. Shukla, G. E. Stanbekova, S. V. Shestakov, and H. B. Pakrasi, *Mol. Microbiol.*, *6*, 947–956 (1992).

183. N. Mizusawa, T. Yamashita, and M. Miyao, *Biochim. Biophys. Acta*, *1410*, 273–286 (1999).

184. J. Barber and J. De Las Rivas, *Proc. Natl. Acad. Sci. USA*, *90*, 10942–10946 (1993).

185. W. A. Cramer and J. Whitmarsh, *Annu. Rev. Plant Physiol.*, *28*, 133–172 (1977).

186. L. K. Thompson, A.-F. Miller, C. A. Buser, J. C. de Paula, and G. W. Brudvig, *Biochemistry*, *28*, 8048–8056 (1989).

187. I. Iwasaki, N. Tamura, and S. Okayama, *Plant Cell Physiol.*, *36*, 583–589 (1995).

188. I. Ahmad, L. B. Giorgi, J. Barber, G. Porter, and D. R. Klug, *Biochim. Biophys. Acta*, *1143*, 239–242 (1993).

189. J.-M. Briantais, C. Vernotte, M. Miyao, N. Murata, and M. Picaud, *Biochim. Biophys. Acta*, *808*, 348–351 (1985).

190. D. F. Ghanotakis, C. F. Yocum, and G. T. Babcock, *Photosynth. Res.*, *9*, 125–134 (1986).

191. J. C. de Paula, P. M. Li, A.-F. Miller, B. W. Wu, and G. W. Brudvig, *Biochemistry*, *25*, 6487–6494 (1986).

192. V. P. McNamara and K. Gounaris, *Biochim. Biophys. Acta*, 1231, 289–296 (1995).

193. N. Mizusawa, M. Miyao, and T. Yamashita, *Biochim. Biophys. Acta*, *1318*, 145–158 (1997).

194. G. N. Johnson, A. W. Rutherford, and A. Krieger, *Biochim. Biophys. Acta*, *1229*, 202–207 (1995).

195. M. Rova, F. Mamedov, A. Magnuson, P. O. Fredriksson, and S. Styring, *Biochemistry*, *37*, 11039–11045 (1998).

196. J. De Las Rivas, J. Klein, and J. Barber, *Photosynth. Res.*, *46*, 193–202 (1995).

197. L. Nedbal, G. Samson, and J. Whitmarsh, *Proc. Natl. Acad. Sci. USA*, *89*, 7929–7933 (1992).

198. M. Poulson, G. Samson, and J. Whitmarsh, *Biochemistry*, *34*, 10932–10938 (1995).

199. H. P. Michel and J. Bennett, *FEBS Lett.*, *212*, 103–108 (1987).

200. H. L. Race and K. Gounaris, *FEBS Lett.*, *323*, 35–39 (1993).

201. S. R. Mayes, J. M. Dubbs, I. Vass, É. Hideg, L. Nagy, and J. Barber, *Biochemistry*, *32*, 1454–1465 (1993).

202. T. Tomo, I. Enami, and Ki. Satoh, *FEBS Lett.*, *323*, 15–18 (1993).

203. M. Ikeuchi, V. K. Shukla, H. B. Pakrasi, and Y. Inoue, *Mol. Gen. Genet.*, *249*, 622–628 (1995).

204. L. K. Lind, V. K. Shukla, K. J. Nyhus, and H. B. Pakrasi, *J. Cell Biochem.*, *268*, 1575–1579 (1993).

205. M. Ikeuchi, B. Eggers, G. Shen, A. N. Webber, J. Yu, A. Hirano, Y. Inoue, and W. F. J. Vermaas, *J. Biol. Chem.*, *266*, 11111–11115 (1991).

206. Z.-H. Zhang, S. R. Mayes, I. Vass, L. Nagy, and J. Barber, *Photosynth. Res.*, *38*, 369–377 (1993).

207. P. R. Anbudurai and H. B. Pakrasi, *Z. Naturforsch.*, *48c*, 267–274 (1993).

208. H. Hoshida, R. Sugiyama, Y. Nakano, T. Shiina, and Y. Toyoshima, *Biochemistry*, *36*, 12053–12061 (1997).

209. K. Kitamura, S. Ozawa, T. Shiina, and Y. Toyoshima, *FEBS Lett.*, *354*, 113–116 (1994).

210. M. Ikeuchi, H. Koike, and Y. Onoue, *FEBS Lett.*, *253*, 178–182 (1989).

211. A. Lautner, R. Klein, U. Ljungberg, H. Reiländer, D. Bartling, B. Andersson, H. Reinke, K. Beyreuther, and R. G. Herrmann, *J. Biol. Chem.*, 263, 110077–10081 (1988).

212. C. Funk, W. P. Schröder, B. R. Green, G. Renger, and B. Andersson, *FEBS Lett.*, *342*, 261–266 (1994).

213. C. Funk, W. P. Schröder, A. Napiwotzki, S. E. Tjus, G. Renger, and B. Andersson, *Biochemistry*, *34*, 11133–11141 (1995).

214. C. Funk, I. Adamska, B. R. Green, B. Andersson, and G. Renger, *J. Biol. Chem.*, *270*, 30141–30147 (1995).

215. I. Adamska, C. Funk, G. Renger, and B. Andersson, *Plant Mol. Biol.*, *31* 793–802 (1996).

216. I. Adamska, *Physiol. Plant.*, *100*, 794–805 (1997).

217. C. Monod, Y. Takahashi, M. Goldschmidt-Clermont, and J.-D. Rochaix, *EMBO J.*, *13*, 2747–2754 (1994).

218. A. Kapazoglou, F. Sagliocco, and L. Dure, III, *J. Biol. Chem.*, *270*, 12197–12202 (1995).

219. Z. J. Lorkovic, W. P. Schröder, H. B. Pakrasi, K.-D. Irrgang, R. G. Herrmann, and R. Oelmüller, *Proc. Natl. Acad. Sci. USA*, *92*, 8930–8934 (1995).

220. L. X. Shi and W. P. Schröder, *Photosynth. Res.*, *53*, 45–53 (1997).

221. S. K. Kim, D. Robinson, and C. Robinson, *FEBS Lett.*, *390*, 175–178 (1996).

222. K. V. Kowallik, B. Stoebe, I. Schaffran, P. Kroth-Pancic, and U. Freier, *Plant Mol. Biol. Rep.*, *13*, 336–342 (1995).

223. I. Z. Zubrzycki, L. K. Frankel, P. S. Russo, and T. M. Bricker, *Biochemistry*, *37*, 13553–13558 (1998).

224. N. Lydakis-Simantiris, R. S. Hutchison, S. D. Betts, B. A. Barry, and C. F. Yocum, *Biochemistry*, *38*, 404–414 (1999).

225. R. S. Hutchison, S. D. Betts, C. F. Yocum, and B. A. Barry, *Biochemistry*, *37*, 5643–5653 (1998).

226. I. Enami, M. Kamo, H. Ohta, S. Takahashi, T. Miura, M. Kusayanagi, S. Tanabe, A. Kamei, A. Motoki, M. Hirano, T. Tomo, and Ki. Satoh, *J. Biol. Chem.*, 273, 4629–4634 (1998).

227. M. Miyao and N. Murata, *Biochim. Biophys. Acta*, *977*, 315–321 (1989).

228. K. Kavelaki and D. F. Ghanotakis, *Photosynth. Res.*, *29*, 149–155 (1991).

229. C. Leuschner and T. M. Bricker, *Biochemistry*, *35*, 4551–4557 (1996).

230. I. Enami, M. Kaneko, N. Kitamura, H. Koike, K. Sonoike, Y. Inoue, and S. Katoh, *Biochim. Biophys. Acta*, *1060*, 224–232 (1991).

231. Q. Xu and T. M. Bricker, *J. Biol. Chem.*, *267*, 25816–25821 (1992).

232. S. D. Betts, J. R. Ross, E. Pichersky, and C. F. Yocum, *Biochemistry*, *36*, 4047–4053 (1997).

233. A. Seidler, *Biochim. Biophys. Acta*, *1277*, 35–60 (1996).

234. T. M. Bricker and L. K. Frankel, *Photosynth. Res.*, *56*, 157–173 (1998).

235. T. M. Bricker, W. R. Odom, and C. B. Queirolo, *FEBS Lett.*, *231*, 111–117 (1988).

236. W. R. Odom and T. M. Bricker, *Biochemistry*, *31*, 5616–5620 (1992).

237. H. Ohta, N. Yoshida, M. Sano, M. Hirano, K. Nakazato, and I. Enami, in *Photosynthesis: From Light to Biosphere*, Vol. 2 (P. Mathis, ed.), Kluwer Academic, Dordrecht, 1995, pp. 361–364.

238. I. Enami, A. Tohri, M. Kamo, H. Ohta, and J. R. Shen, *Biochim. Biophys. Acta*, *1320*, 17–26 (1997).

239. I. Enami, S. Ohta, S. Mitsuhashi, S. Takahashi, M. Ikeuchi, and S. Katoh, *Plant Cell Physiol.*, *33*, 291–297 (1992).

240. T. M. Bricker, *Biochemistry*, *31*, 4623–4628 (1992).

241. R. L. Burnap and L. A. Sherman, *Biochemistry*, *30*, 440–446 (1991).

242. J. B. Philbrick, B. A. Diner, and B. A. Zilinskas, *J. Biol. Chem.*, *266*, 13370–13376 (1991).

243. S. R. Mayes, K. M. Cook, S. J. Self, Z. Zhang, and J. Barber, *Biochim. Biophys. Acta*, *1060*, 1–12 (1991).

244. R. Bockholt, B. Masepohl, and E. K. Pistorius, *FEBS Lett.*, *294*, 59–63 (1991).

245. M. Miyao, N. Murata, J. Lavorel, B. Maison-Peteri, A. Boussac, and A.-L. Étienne, *Biochim. Biophys. Acta*, *890*, 151–159 (1987).

246. R. L. Burnap, J.-R. Shen, P. A. Jursinic, Y. Inoue, and L. A. Sherman, *Biochemistry*, *31*, 7404–7410 (1992).

247. M. R. Razeghifard, T. Wydrzynski, R. J. Pace, and R. L. Burnap, *Biochemistry*, *36*, 14474–14478 (1997).

248. I. Vass, T.-A. Ono, and Y. Inoue, *FEBS Lett.*, *211*, 215–220 (1987).

249. H.-A. Chu, A. P. Nguyen, and R. J. Debus, *Biochemistry*, *33*, 6150–6157 (1994).

250. R. L. Burnap, M. Qian, and C. Pierce, *Biochemistry*, *35*, 874–882 (1996).

251. N. Murata, M. Miyao, T. Omata, H. Matsunami, and T. Kuwabara, *Biochim. Biophys. Acta*, *765*, 363–369 (1984).

252. B. Andersson, C. Larsson, C. Jansson, U. Ljungberg, and H.-E. Åkerlund, *Biochim. Biophys. Acta*, *766*, 21–28 (1984).

253. H. Wincencjusz, C. F. Yocum, and H. J. van Gorkom, *Biochemistry*, *37*, 8595–8604 (1998).

254. K. A. Campbell, W. Gregor, D. P. Pham, J. M. Peloquin, R. J. Debus, and R. D. Britt, *Biochemistry*, *37*, 5039–5045 (1998).

255. A. Boussac, J.-L. Zimmermann, and A. W. Rutherford, *FEBS Lett.*, *277*, 69–74 (1990).

256. J. R. Shen, M. Ikeuchi, and Y. Inoue, *J. Biol. Chem.*, *272*, 17821–17826 (1997).

257. J.-R. Shen, W. F. J. Vermaas, and Y. Inoue, *J. Biol. Chem.*, *270*, 6901–6907 (1995).

258. J.-R. Shen and Y. Inoue, *Biochemistry*, *32*, 1825–1832 (1993).

259. I. Enami, S. Kikuchi, T. Fukuda, H. Ohta, and J. R. Shen, *Biochemistry*, *37*, 2787–2793 (1998).

260. J. R. Shen, M. Qian, Y. Inoue, and R. L. Burnap, *Biochemistry*, *37*, 1551–1558 (1998).

261. J.-R. Shen, R. L. Burnap, and Y. Inoue, *Biochemistry*, *34*, 12661–12668 (1995).

262. D. Koulougliotis, X.-S. Tang, B. A. Diner, and G. W. Brudvig, *Biochemistry*, *34*, 2850–2856 (1995).

263. X.-S. Tang, D. A. Chisholm, G. C. Dismukes, G. W. Brudvig, and B. A. Diner, *Biochemistry*, *32*, 13742–13748 (1993).

264. B. A. Diner, D. A. Force, D. W. Randall, and R. D. Britt, *Biochemistry*, *37*, 17931–17943 (1998).

265. D. F. Ghanotakis, C. T. Yerkes, and G. T. Babcock, *Biochim. Biophys. Acta*, *682*, 21–31 (1982).

266. G. T. Babcock, D. F. Ghanotakis, B. Ke, and B. A. Diner, *Biochim. Biophys. Acta*, *723*, 276–286 (1983).

267. S. Un, X.-S. Tang, and B. A. Diner, *Biochemistry*, *35*, 679–684 (1996).

268. K. A. Campbell, J. M. Peloquin, B. A. Diner, X. S. Tang, D. A. Chisholm, and R. D. Britt, *J. Am. Chem. Soc.*, *119*, 4787–4788 (1997).

269. C. Tommos, L. Davidsson, B. Svensson, C. Madsen, W. F. J. Vermaas, and S. Styring, *Biochemistry*, *32*, 5436–5441 (1993).

270. C. W. Hoganson, M. Sahlin, B.-M. Sjöberg, and G. T. Babcock, *J. Am. Chem. Soc.*, *118*, 4672–4679 (1996).

271. F. Dole, B. A. Diner, C. W. Hoganson, G. T. Babcock, and R. D. Britt, *J. Am. Chem. Soc.*, *119*, 11540–11541 (1997).

272. C. Tommos, C. Madsen, S. Styring, and W. F. J. Vermaas, *Biochemistry*, *33*, 11805–11813 (1994).

273. P. Manna, R. LoBrutto, C. Eijckelhoff, J. P. Dekker, and W. F. J. Vermaas, *Eur. J. Biochem.*, *251*, 142–154 (1998).

274. R. Ahlbrink, M. Haumann, D. Cherepanov, O. Bögershausen, A. Mulkidjanian, and W. Junge, *Biochemistry*, *37*, 1131–1142 (1998).

275. H. Kless and W. F. J. Vermaas, *Biochemistry*, *35*, 16458–16464 (1996).

276. D. A. Force, D. W. Randall, R. D. Britt, X.-S. Tang, and B. A. Diner, *J. Am. Chem. Soc.*, *117*, 12643–12644 (1995).

277. X.-S. Tang, M. Zheng, D. A. Chisholm, G. C. Dismukes, and B. A. Diner, *Biochemistry*, *35*, 1475–1484 (1996).

278. C. Berthomieu, R. Hienerwadel, A. Boussac, J. Breton, and B. A. Diner, *Biochemistry*, *37*, 10547–10554 (1998).

279. A.-M. A. Hays, I. R. Vassiliev, J. H. Golbeck, and R. J. Debus, *Biochemistry*, submitted.

280. R. A. Roffey, D. M. Kramer, Govindjee, and R. T. Sayre, *Biochim. Biophys. Acta*, *1185*, 257–270 (1994).

281. R. A. Roffey, K. J. van Wijk, R. T. Sayre, and S. Styring, *J. Biol. Chem.*, *269*, 5115–5121 (1994).

282. H.-A. Chu, A. P. Nguyen, and R. J. Debus, *Biochemistry*, *34*, 5839–5858 (1995).

283. F. Mamedov, R. T. Sayre, and S. Styring, *Biochemistry*, *37*, 14245–14256 (1998).

284. A.-M. A. Hays, I. R. Vassiliev, J. H. Golbeck, and R. J. Debus, *Biochemistry*, *37*, 11352–11365 (1998).

285. B. A. Diner and P. J. Nixon, in *Photosynthesis: Mechanisms and Effects*, Vol. 2 (G. Garab, ed.), Kluwer Academic, Dordrecht, 1999, pp. 1177–1180.

286. A. Kanazawa, A. Roberts, and D. M. Kramer, Seventh Western Regional Photosynthesis Conference, Pacific Grove, CA, January 8–11, 1998, Abstract 4-7 (1998).

287. M. Haumann, A. Mulkidjanian, and W. Junge, *Biochemistry*, *38*, 1258–1267 (1999).

288. R. J. Debus, K. A. Campbell, D. P. Pham, A.-M. A. Hays, J. M. Peloquin, and R. D. Britt, in *Photosynthesis: Mechanisms and Effects,* Vol. 2 (G. Garab, ed.), Kluwer Academic, Dordrecht, 1999, pp. 1375–1378.

289. B. Svensson, J. Minagawa, and A. R. Crofts, in *Photosynthesis: Mechanisms and Effects,* Vol. 2 (G. Garab, ed.), Kluwer Academic, Dordrecht, 1999, pp. 1451–1454.

290. H.-A. Chu, A. P. Nguyen, and R. J. Debus, *Biochemistry*, *33*, 6137–6149 (1994).

291. X.-S. Tang, B. A. Diner, B. S. Larsen, M. L. Gilchrist, Jr., G. A. Lorigan, and R. D. Britt, *Proc. Natl. Acad. Sci. USA*, *91*, 704–708 (1994).

292. T. Noguchi, T.-A. Ono, and Y. Inoue, *Biochim. Biophys. Acta*, *1228*, 189–200 (1995).

293. N. Tamura, K. Noda, K. Wakamatsu, H. Kamachi, H. Inoue, and K. Wada, *Plant Cell Physiol.*, *38*, 578–585 (1997).

294. A. Magnuson and L.-E. Andréasson, *Biochemistry*, *36*, 3254–3261 (1997).

295. M. L. Ghirardi, T. W. Lutton, and M. Seibert, *Biochemistry*, *37*, 13559–13566 (1998).

296. M. L. Ghirardi, C. Preston, and M. Seibert, *Biochemistry*, *37*, 13567–13574 (1998).

297. G.-S. Tae and W. A. Cramer, *Biochemistry*, *31*, 4066–4074 (1992).

298. H.-A. Chu, A. P. Nguyen, and R. J. Debus, *Biochemistry*, *34*, 5859–5882 (1995).

299. P. J. Nixon and B. A. Diner, *Biochemistry*, *31*, 942–948 (1992).

300. R. J. Boerner, A. P. Nguyen, B. A. Barry, and R. J. Debus, *Biochemistry*, *31*, 6660–6672 (1992).

301. J. P. Whitelegge, D. Koo, B. A. Diner, I. Domian, and J. M. Erickson, *J. Biol. Chem.*, *270*, 225–235 (1995).

302. B. A. Diner and P. J. Nixon, *Biochim. Biophys. Acta*, *1101*, 134–138 (1992).

303. A. E. Martin, B. K. Burgess, C. D. Stout, V. L. Cash, D. R. Dean, G. M. Jensen, and P. M. Stephens, *Proc. Natl. Acad. Sci. USA*, *87*, 598–602 (1990).

304. Y. Kim, D. Misna, A. F. Monzingo, M. P. Ready, A. Frankel, and J. D. Robertus, *Biochemistry*, *31*, 3294–3296 (1992).

305. C. L. Stone, T. D. Hurley, L. M. Amzel, M. F. Dunn, and W. F. Bosron, in *Enzymology and Molecular Biology of Carbonyl Metabolism*, Vol. 4 (H. Weiner, ed.), Plenum Press, New York, 1993, pp. 429–437.

306. P. J. Nixon and B. A. Diner, *Biochem. Soc. Trans.*, *22*, 338–343 (1994).

307. T. N. Sorrell, P. K. Martin, and E. F. Bowden, *J. Am. Chem. Soc.*, *111*, 766–767 (1989).

308. J. C. Ferrer, J. G. Guillemette, R. Bogumil, S. C. Inglis, M. Smith, and A. G. Mauk, *J. Am. Chem. Soc.*, *115*, 7507–7508 (1993).

309. M. Ubbink, A. P. Campos, M. Teixeira, N. I. Hunt, H. A. O. Hill, and G. W. Canters, *Biochemistry*, *33*, 10051–10059 (1994).

310. K. Choudhury, M. Sundaramoorthy, A. Hickman, T. Yonetani, E. Woehl, M. F. Dunn, and T. L. Poulos, *J. Biol. Chem.*, *269*, 20239–20249 (1994).

311. C. Preston and M. Seibert, *Biochemistry*, *30*, 9625–9633 (1991).

312. M. W. Calhoun, L. J. Lemieux, J. W. Thomas, J. J. Hill, V. Chepuri Goswitz, J. O. Alben, and R. B. Gennis, *Biochemistry*, *32*, 13254–13261 (1993).

313. P. J. Nixon, J. T. Trost, and B. A. Diner, *Biochemistry*, *31*, 10859–10871 (1992).

314. M. Hundelt, A.-M. A. Hays, R. J. Debus, and W. Junge, *Biochemistry*, *37*, 14450–14456 (1998).

315. M. Qian, L. Dao, R. J. Debus, and R. L. Burnap, *Biochemistry*, *38*, 6070–6081 (1999).

316. C. Chen, J. Kazimir, and G. M. Cheniae, *Biochemistry*, *34*, 13511–13526 (1995).

317. W. F. J. Vermaas, J. Charité, and G. Shen, *Biochemistry*, *29*, 5325–5332 (1990).

318. S. Ermakova-Gerdes, S. Shestakov, and W. F. J. Vermaas, *Plant Mol. Biol.*, *30*, 243–254 (1996).

319. B. Eggers and W. F. J. Vermaas, *Biochemistry*, *32*, 11419–11427 (1993).

320. E. Haag, J. J. Eaton-Rye, G. Renger, and W. F. J. Vermaas, *Biochemistry*, *32*, 4444–4454 (1993).

321. H. M. Gleiter, E. Haag, J.-R. Shen, J. J. Eaton-Rye, Y. Inoue, W. F. J. Vermaas, and G. Renger, *Biochemistry*, *33*, 12063–12071 (1994).

322. H. M. Gleiter, E. Haag, J.-R. Shen, J. J. Eaton-Rye, A. G. Seeliger, Y. Inoue, W. F. J. Vermaas, and G. Renger, *Biochemistry*, *34*, 6847–6856 (1995).

323. T. R. Morgan, J. A. Shand, S. M. Clarke, and J. J. Eaton-Rye, *Biochemistry*, *37*, 14437–14449 (1998).

324. C. Putnam-Evans and T. M. Bricker, *Biochemistry*, *31*, 11482–11488 (1992).

325. C. Putnam-Evans and T. M. Bricker, *Biochemistry*, *33*, 10770–10776 (1994).

326. C. Putnam-Evans, R. L. Burnap, J. Wu, J. Whitmarsh, and T. M. Bricker, *Biochemistry*, *35*, 4046–4053 (1996).

327. J. Wu, C. Putnam-Evans, and T. M. Bricker, *Plant Mol. Biol.*, *32*, 537–542 (1996).

328. C. Putnam-Evans and T. M. Bricker, *Plant Mol. Biol.*, *34*, 455–463 (1997).

329. S. M. Clarke and J. J. Eaton-Rye, *Biochemistry*, *38*, 2707–2715 (1999).

330. M. Tichy and W. F. J. Vermaas, *Biochemistry*, *37*, 1523–1531 (1998).

331. M. Qian, S. F. Al-Khaldi, C. Putnam-Evans, T. M. Bricker, and R. L. Burnap, *Biochemistry*, *36*, 15244–15252 (1997).

332. M. G. Kuhn and W. F. J. Vermaas, *Plant Mol. Biol.*, *23*, 123–133 (1993).

333. N. Knoepfle, T. M. Bricker, and C. Putnam-Evans, *Biochemistry*, *38*, 1582–1588 (1999).

334. J. Hanley, Y. Deligiannakis, A. Pascal, P. Faller, and A. W. Rutherford, *Biochemistry*, *38*, 8189–8195 (1999).

335. C. Büchel, J. Barber, G. Ananyev, S. Eshaghi, R. Watt, and G. C. Dismukes, *Proc. Natl. Acad. Sci. USA*, (in press).

Subject Index

A

A.

actinomycetemcomitans, see
    Actinobacillus
eutrophus, see Alcaligenes
globiformis, see Arthrobacter
missouriensis, see Actinoplanes
niger, see Aspergillus
oryzae, see Aspergillus
proteolytica, see Aeromonas
putrefaciens, see Alteromonas
vinelandii, see Azotobacter
Ab initio calculations, 646
Absorption (*see also* Metabolism)
    of manganese, 92–95, 112
Absorption bands and spectra (*see
    also* Infrared spectroscopy,
    Spectrophotometry, *and* UV

[Absorption bands and spectra]
    absorption), 379, 395, 432, 455,
    563, 564, 599–601, 628, 667
    visible, 379, 508, 628
Accumulation in plants of
    cadmium, 38, 43, 44
    cobalt, 44
    copper, 43, 44
    manganese, 36, 38–52
Acetate (or acetic acid), 21, 238,
    482, 474, 534
    as inhibitor, 448, 454
    kinase, *see* Kinases
    manganese complexes, 432, 435–
    439
    phenyl-, *see* Phenylacetate
    oxalo-, *see* Oxaloacetate
Acetone, 20, 488
    vanillyl, 561

K

K. aerogenes, see Klebsiella
Kainate, 144
α-Ketoglutarate, 227
Keto group, *see* Carbonyl group
Ketones (*see also* individual
  names), 489
Kidneys (containing), 408
  aluminum, 127, 129, 130, 132–
    134
  copper, 128, 129, 131–135
  iron, 127–130, 135
  manganese, 92, 95, 105, 110, 111,
    128, 129, 131–134
  pig, *see* Pig
  rat, 127–135
  selenium, 128, 129, 131–133, 135
  zinc, 127, 129, 131–135
Kinases, 96, 228–231, 663
  acetate, 229
  adenylate, 229
  -associated protein phosphatase,
    311
  cAMP-dependent protein, 229
  carboxy-, *see* Carboxykinase
  creatine, 199
  crystal structures, *see* X-ray
    crystal structures
  glycerol, 229
  nucleoside diphosphate, 229
  phophoenolpyruvate, 229
  phosphatidylinositol, 229
  phosphoglycerate, 199, 229
  phosphorylase, 229, 230
  protein, 312
  pyruvate, 199, 229–231, 385,
    519
Kinetic studies (*see also* Rates of
  reactions *and* Stopped flow
  studies)
  Michaelis-Menten, *see* Michaelis-
    Menten kinetics
  transient-state, 577
Klebsiella aerogenes, 319
Kramer doublets, 188, 381, 515

L

L.
  edodes, see Lentinus
  lactis, see Lactococcus
  odoratus, see Lathyrus
  plantarum, see Lactobacillus
  sake, see Lactobacillus
  sativus, see Lathyrus
Lactate (or lactic acid), 39, 561
  L-phospho-, 231
Lactobacillus sp., 216, 376, 588
  plantarum, 39, 213, 431, 434,
    438, 528–532, 534–536, 539–
    541, 543–549
  sake, 237
Lactococcus lactis, 223
Lactuca sativa, 87
Lakes (*see also* Water)
  anoxic, 26
  Bret, 26, 27
  eutrophic, 26
  manganese in, 9, 14, 26, 27
  Oneida, 21
  oxic, 26
  Sempach, 26, 27
Lanthanides (*see also* individual
  elements), 477, 566, 574
Lanthanum(III), 477
Lathyrus
  odoratus, 226
  sativus, 226
Lead (different oxidation states), 43
  in brain, *see* Brain
  in cerebrospinal fluid, *see*
    Cerebrospinal fluid
  in xylose isomerase, 380
Leaves, 71–73, 77
Lectins, 253, 279–299
  animal, 298
  bacterial, 298
  legume, 295–298
  plant, 280, 298
  viral, 298
Legumes (*see also* individual
  names), 224